The World Of

CHILD DEVELOPMENT

The World Of

CHILD DEVELOPMENT

Conception
To
Adolescence

 DELMAR PUBLISHERS INC.

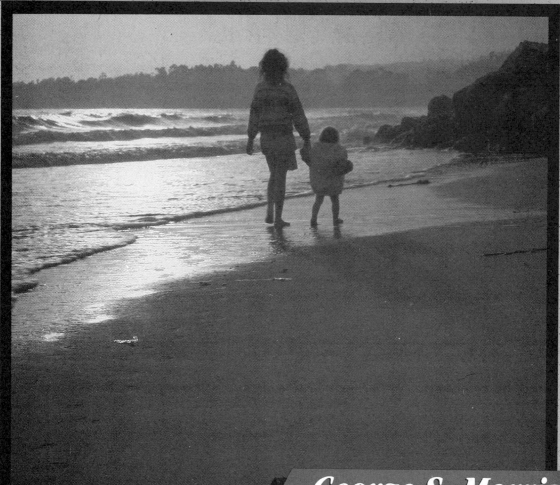

George S. Morrison

NOTICE TO THE READER

Publisher and author do not warrant or guarantee any of the products described herein or perform any independent analysis in connection with any of the product information contained herein. Publisher and author do not assume, and expressly disclaim, any obligation to obtain and include information other than that provided to them by the manufacturer.

The reader is expressly warned to consider and adopt all safety precautions that might be indicated by the activities described herein and to avoid all potential hazards. By following the instructions contained herein, the reader willingly assumes all risks in connection with such instructions.

The publisher and author make no representations or warranties of any kind, including but not limited to, the warranties of fitness for particular purpose or merchantability, nor are any such representations implied with respect to the material set forth herein, and the publisher and author take no responsibility with respect to such material. The publisher and author shall not be liable for any special, consequential or exemplary damages resulting, in whole or in part, from the readers' use of, or reliance upon, this material.

Figure 6-7 from *Infant Development,* by Lisa Barclay, copyright © 1985 by Holt, Rinehart and Winston, Inc.; reprinted by permission of the publisher.

Dedication:
To Betty Jane;
For all she has done, for all she does, for all she is.

Cover photo by Mark Roberts

Delmar Staff
Associate Editor: Jay Whitney
Project Editor: Carol Micheli
Production Supervisors: Karen Seebald and Larry Main
Design Coordinator: Susan C. Mathews

Photos by Ruby Gold: 1-1, 3-1, 3, 16, 19, 4-13, 6-1, 3, 6, 10, 12, 13, 15, 7-7, 9, 10, 11, 12, 13, 14, 8-2, 3, 9, 10, 9-2, 4, 5, 6, 7, 11, 10-10, 11-1, 4, 5, 6, 12-17, 13-3, 4, 5. Also chapter openers 3, 4, 8, 9, 11. And vignettes in chapters 8, 9 and 11.

For information, address Delmar Publishers Inc.,
2 Computer Drive West, Box 15-015
Albany, New York 12212

COPYRIGHT © 1990
BY DELMAR PUBLISHERS INC.

Printed in the United States of America
Published simultaneously in Canada
By Nelson Canada
A Division of The Thomson Corporation

10 9 8 7 6 5 4 3 2

Library of Congress Cataloging-in-Publication Data

Morrison, George S.
    The world of child development : conception to adolescence / George S. Morrison.
        p.   cm.
    Includes bibliographical references.
    ISBN 0-8273-3116-9. — ISBN 0-8273-3117-7 (instructor's guide)
    1. Child development. 2. Fetus—Growth. 3. Prenatal diagnosis.
4. Pregnancy, Complications of.   I. Title.
RJ131.M664 1989
612.6′5—dc20   89-23284
                                                                                  CIP

CONTENTS

PREFACE xiii

CHAPTER 1   THE WORLD OF CHILD DEVELOPMENT:
AN OVERVIEW xviii

    Vignettes 2
    What is Child Development? 3
    Developmental Processes 4
    Why Study Child Development? 8
    Career Choices and Child Development 9
    Personal Story: Maureen Reilly 9
    Personal Story: Paul Grolitzer 11
    Personal Story: Anne DeHaan 12
    Ways to Study Children 12
    Research: Answering Questions 14
    Research Methods for Studying Children 16
    Gathering Research Data 18
    Research Design for Determining Development 20
    Research Dissemination 22
    Analyzing Research 22
    The Ethics of Child Development 22
    Current Influences in Child Development 25
    What Would You Do? 28
    Summary 29

CHAPTER 2   THEORIES OF DEVELOPMENT 36

    Vignettes 38
    Theories of Development 39
    Why Are Theories Important? 40
    Sigmund Freud and Psychoanalytic Theory 42
    In the Spotlight: Permissive Parenting 48
    Erik Erikson and Psychosocial Theory 49
    The Cognitive Development Theory of Jean Piaget 57
    Skinner and Behaviorism 65

v

Maslow and Humanistic Theory 72
What Would You Do? 76
Summary 76

CHAPTER 3   BECOMING A PARENT 86
Vignettes 88
Contemporary Parents and Families 90
How Families Have Changed 92
The Shrinking Family—One is Enough 93
There's More Than One Way to Have a Baby 97
Stork in a Test Tube 98
Ethical Issues of Reproductiveness 100
Fertilization 100
In the Spotlight: A New Look at Abortion 101
When Does Human Life Begin? 103
Heredity 104
Why Do I Act the Way I Do? 108
Genetic Screening 111
Boy or Girl? 113
Twins—Triplets and More .114
Chromosome Abnormalities 115
Sex Chromosome Abnormality (SCA) 116
Genetic Diseases 117
What Would You Do? 119
Summary 120

CHAPTER 4   THE BEGINNING: PRENATAL DEVELOPMENT
AND BIRTH 130
Vignettes 132
Prenatal Stages of Development 134
In the Spotlight: How Do I Know I'm Pregnant? 137
A Primer of Prenatal Development 146
Fetal Circulatory System 148
Prenatal Personality Development 150
Prenatal Sensory Development 150
In the Spotlight: How Do We Know What Babies Know? . . .152
Fetal Biology 152
Fetal Medicine 156
Fetal Therapy—Accelerating Development 156
Medical Use of Fetal Tissues 157
Fetuses' vs Woman's Rights 157

What Would You Do? 158
Is There a Best Time to Be Born? 158
Pregnancy as a Developmental Process 158
Labor 159
Birthing Practices 160
Personal Story: Pattricia Lanius .165
Influences on Pregnancy 166
Summary 172

CHAPTER 5   THE NEONATE: LIFE'S FIRST MONTH 182
Vignettes 184
First Appearances: What Does the Neonate Look Like? 185
What's in a Name? 189
In the Spotlight: High-Risk Pregnancies—AIDS at Birth 189
Adjustments to the New World .190
Neonatal Assessments 193
In the Spotlight: Circumcision 195
Reflexes 195
Neonatal States 198
What Is the Neonate Able to Do? 199
Cognitive Development 204
Neonatal Learning 206
χ Neonates at Risk 208
Personal Story: Meredith Nelson—Neonatal Nurse 212
In the Spotlight: Is Life at Any Cost Worth It? 217
In the Spotlight: Preventing Prematurity 217
In the Spotlight: Getting in Touch With Your Baby 219
What Would You Do? 221
Social Development 221
The Individuality of Newborns .223
Psychosocial Development 224
Language Development 224
Caring for the Neonate 224
In the Spotlight: Naming Baby .225
Summary 231

CHAPTER 6   INFANCY: LIFE'S FIRST YEAR 240
Vignettes 242
Changing Views of Infancy 243
In the Spotlight: Brian's Weekly Schedule 245
The Importance of Infancy 246

Models of Development 246
Physical Development. 246
In the Spotlight: Is Beauty in the Eye of the Beholder? 252
Intellectual Development 254
Language Development 257
In the Spotlight: Motherese 260
Attachment. 262
Nutrition. 266
Parenting the Infant 269
In The Spotlight: Dr. Spock—Common Sense and
Parenting 269
In the Spotlight: Where Should Baby Sleep? 270
Caring for the Infant 271
Stranger Anxiety 272
What Would You Do? 273
Child Care for Infants 273
In the Spotlight: Is Child Care Good for Infants? 275
Summary 276

CHAPTER 7   THE TODDLER: EXPLORATION AND
INDEPENDENCE 284
Vignette 286
Physical Development. 287
Motor Development 289
Perceptual Development 291
Independence. 292
Safety 292
Nutrition. 293
Toilet Training 294
Intellectual Development 295
Language Development 298
Psychosocial Development 304
Developmental Milestones 304
Parenting the Toddler. 305
In the Spotlight: Superbaby. 307
In the Spotlight: Playtime With a Purpose 308
What Would You Do? 309
Toddler Child Care. 309
Summary 312

CHAPTER 8 THE PRESCHOOL YEARS 320
    Vignette 322
    Physical Development.........................324
    Motor Development 325
    Intellectual Development 328
    Language Development 330
    What Would You Do? 332
    Psychosocial Development 332
    Gender Development 334
    Development of Aggression 335
    Why Do Children Play?.......................336
    Classifications of Play.....................337
    The Competencies of Play 338
    Preschool Play Environments 339
    In the Spotlight: Preschool Fitness 340
    Accidents: Causes and Prevention 340
    Tantrums 340
    What Kind of Parent Should I Be?...........341
    In the Spotlight: Homeless Children 346
    Children With AIDS 347
    Summary 350
CHAPTER 9 LEARNING AND EDUCATION IN THE
PRESCHOOL YEARS 358
    Vignettes...................................360
    Preschool Enrollment 362
    Reasons for the Popularity of Preschools ...362
    Visions of Young Children 363
    Preschool Programs..........................365
    Nursery Schools 366
    Head Start 368
    The Montessori Program 370
    Bank Street Program: A Developmental-Interactionist
        Approach 372
    The High/Scope Curriculum 375
    Transitions 377
    Predicting Preschool Success 377
    Do Preschool Programs Make a Difference? ...379
    Facilitating Preschoolers' Language Development 380

Facilitating Preschoolers' Literacy Development 381
Communication in the Preschool Years 383
In the Spotlight: Preschool Peer Interaction 385
Special Needs Preschoolers 387
Preschool Issues 392
What Would You Do? 394
In the Spotlight: Crisis and Stress in Children's Lives 394
Summary 396

CHAPTER 10 MIDDLE CHILDHOOD: DEVELOPMENT DURING
THE ELEMENTARY SCHOOL YEARS 404
Vignettes 406
Physical Development 408
Nutrition During the Middle Years 411
Motor Development 415
In the Spotlight: Little League Baseball 416
Cognitive Development 417
Language Development 421
Psychosocial Development 422
Aggression 423
What Would You Do? 424
Peer Relationships 424
Psychosexual Development 425
In the Spotlight: Why Do Boys Do Better in Math Than
    Girls? Could Mind Sex Be the Answer? 426
In the Spotlight: Is Biology Destiny or Can We Have
    Androgyny, Too? 427
Moral Development 428
Gifted Children 431
In the Spotlight: Understanding Measurement Terms 432
Summary 434

CHAPTER 11 LEARNING AND EDUCATION DURING THE
MIDDLE YEARS 442
Vignettes 444
In the Spotlight: Just Say "No" to Guns 445
Cooperative Learning 446
Teaching Thinking 448
Thinking: What Is It? 448
Information Processing and Cognitive Development 451
Information Processing at Work 451

The Two Brains. 455
In the Spotlight: The Right Brain in Action 456
Kindergarten Education 457
In the Spotlight: School Readiness—Who Gets Ready for
Whom? 459
Emerging Literacy 461
Bilingualism—Making Children Literate in Two Languages . .463
In the Spotlight: A Just Community. 465
What Would You Do? 466
Child Care for School-Age Children 467
Transitions 470
In the Spotlight: The Dieting Craze 472
Summary 473

CHAPTER 12   DEVELOPMENT DURING THE ADOLESCENT
YEARS. 480
Vignettes. 482
Why an Adolescent Period of Development? 483
Physical Development. 484
In the Spotlight: Preventing Bone Loss 490
In the Spotlight: Cracking Voices 491
In the Spotlight: Winning and Losing an Olympic
Gold Medal 493
Puberty and Self Image 493
Adolescents and Suicide. 494
Personal Story: Carmen Espinosa and Project TRUST 495
In the Spotlight: Mirror, Mirror, On the Wall. 498
Madonna Wannabees 499
Parenting and Adolescent Conflicts 499
Recklessness and Foolish Risks 499
Anorexia Nervosa 500
In the Spotlight: Understanding Anorexia Nervosa 501
Bulimia 502
Peer Groups. 502
The World of Work 503
Adolescent Runaways 504
Juvenile Delinquency 506
Teenage Alcoholism 507
Why Do Adolescents Engage in Substance Abuse? 507
Teenage Sex. 509

Teenage Pregnancy—Premature Parenthood 509
In the Spotlight: A Freudian View of Teenage Pregnancy . . .511
In the Spotlight: A Dollar a Day Keeps the Stork Away 514
What Would You Do? 515
In the Spotlight: TAPP (Teenage Parenting Program) 518
Homosexuality 520
Summary 522

CHAPTER 13   LEARNING AND EDUCATION IN THE
ADOLESCENT YEARS 530
Vignettes 531
Schooling and Transitions 533
Educational and Social Policy Implications 534
Essential Features of Middle Schools 534
In the Spotlight: Loggers' Run Middle School 536
High Schools 538
In the Spotlight: Students Helping Students 540
Dropping Out 541
Remembering You 543
In the Spotlight: Reconsidering Adolescent Development 544
What Would You Do? 546
Character Education in the High Schools 546
Parenting the Teenager 546
In the Spotlight: The Shopping Mall as Surrogate Family . . .547
Prevention Programs 548
Summary 549

APPENDIX 556
BIBLIOGRAPHY 560
INDEX 581

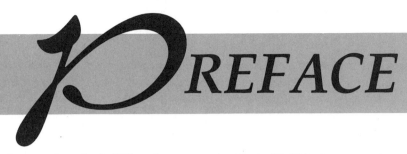

PREFACE

I'm frequently asked "Why do you write books?" This is a question most authors are asked, usually when a book is finished. A variation on this basic question is "Why are you writing the book?" This is a question most authors ask themselves, especially when it is very late at night or during a holiday or when many other "urgent" matters—like writing one's annual report—are also clamoring for attention. A trite answer to the first question is "Because I always wanted to," and a trite, but sometimes honest answer to the second question is "I need to get promoted." For me, neither of these answers is appropriate or sufficient. I have written a number of other books, so it wasn't as though I had to do something I had never done before. Likewise, I don't need to write in order to get promoted. I'm a full professor and have been for a number of years. So, I'll confess to the truth. I like to write. I enjoy the creative process, especially during those times when I have the time to write for extended periods of time—such as a whole day or for several days in a row. During these times I have visions in which I see myself as a full time writer. But, then reality intrudes and I realize that the ebb and flow of preparing for classes, teaching and researching—and other professorial functions and obligations—contribute to the writing process and are probably essential for a research-based developmental book.

A second answer to the "why do you write" question is that I feel fulfilled as a professor and a person. For me, writing is what being a professor is all about. While writing, I'm fulfilling what I envision as *my* professorial and creative role. Certainly, other professors have a vision of what being a professor is supposed to be. But *writing*, the creative act, is what the fulfilling part of the professorship is for me. I don't need to write a book to be promoted, but I do need to write a book in order to be a "good" professor.

A third answer is that I believe I am positively contributing to the relationships and interactions between children, parents, teachers, health workers and other child care professionals by presenting child development information in a readable and understandable manner. I'm affecting and influencing the lives of the nation's youth and the careers and parenting patterns of adults who work with and rear children and youth. This may sound maudlin or sentimental but, for me, positively influencing others is a worthy and noble calling. In this regard, I consider myself to be operating in Maslow's stage of Self Actualization and Erikson's stage of Generativity.

The World of Child Development: Conception to Adolescence is an accurate and up-to-date source of research, theory and information that instructors can use to provide an interesting, informative and meaningful course for students desiring a solid background in child development. A number of qualities make *The World of Child Development: Conception to Adolescence* appealing to professors and students. Taken as a whole they provide a rationale for adoption and the opportunity for interesting reading and learning.

Relevant and Up-to-Date

The contents of *The World of Child Development: Conception to Adolescence* are relevant, current and up-to-date. Where appropriate, classic research is cited to illustrate important concepts and theories. As an author, I used thoughtful and informed deliberation and decision making to assure that information is accurate, relevant, meaningful and understandable.

Vignettes

Program and biographical *Vignettes* show how child development information is applied to real life situations. Both the Vignettes and sections on *Implications for Parents and Professionals* provide a unifying theme of practicality and application to child rearing and care. They also provide a context within which students can understand how parents and professionals use child development information to guide daily decisions.

Comprehensive

The contents and sequence of *The World of Child Development: Conception to Adolescence* provide a comprehensive, research-based survey of child development. All major developmental topics from conception to adolescence are presented in a relevant, interesting manner. In addition, chapters are included on: An Overview to Child Development, Theories of Child Development and Becoming a Parent.

Chronological and Topical Approach

The World of Child Development: Conception to Adolescence provides both a chronological and topical coverage for each stage of development. Each stage of chronological development—prenatal, the neonate, infancy, toddler, preschool, middle childhood, and adolescence—has a unifying core of domains: physical, motor, perceptual, cognitive, language, personality, social and emotional, and applied sections on how to care for children in each stage of development.

Readability

The textural material is readable and interesting. The writing style is clear, smooth and easy to comprehend. As a result, the reader is able to understand concepts and ideas essential to the field of child development.

Pedagogical Aids

The liberal, yet selective use of graphs, tables, figures, charts, and photos promotes comprehension and encourages the retention of textual material. Whenever possible, data are presented graphically in order to stress the importance of written material and call visual attention to conclusions and important points. Visual materials also assist students with study and retention by providing a quick and easy reference to salient points. In addition, the many pedagogical aids address the multiple learning styles students bring to the written page and the field of child development.

The chapter format of *The World of Child Development: Conception to Adolescence* facilitates student learning. Each chapter has the following elements specifically designed to maintain student interest and involvement.

Outline of Chapter Headings.   An outline of headings and main topics visually and cognitively orients the reader and creates a positive learning set for important concepts and ideas.

Implications for Parents and Professionals.   Many topics in all the chapters contain sections devoted to how developmental information and concepts apply to the real world of parenting, caring for, working with and understanding child behavior. These discussions bridge the gaps that frequently exist between developmental theory and the real world in which people must apply theory as they function in their many roles.

In the Spotlight.   In all chapters, certain topics of a controversial, urgent or particularly interesting nature are placed *In the Spotlight*. This emphasis shows students how child development information and concepts are topics of discussion, affect people's lives and are used as a basis for public policy recommendations and decision making. These *In the Spotlight* accounts are set off from the rest of the textual material as a means of focusing attention and not interfering with the logical presentation of textual material.

Summary.   All chapters have a summary which asssists with the recall of major concepts. The summary also directs the reader's attention to important topics and assists with comprehension and retention.

Questions to Guide Your Review.   Questions at the end of each chapter bring textual material into sharper focus, reinforce major points and challenge readers to test their knowledge and comprehension.

Key Terms and Concepts With Definitions.   Key terms and concepts are defined at the end of each chapter. They assist with comprehension and serve as an additional review. These concise, end-of-chapter definitions also provide a convenient reference resource for future study.

Enrichment Through Further Reading.   At the end of each chapter a select list of annotated readings is provided as a means of encouraging students to enrich, extend and supplement knowledge acquired through textual material. All recommended readings contribute to the reader's further understanding of child development.

As always when I write I have the help, support and goodwill of many people without whom it would be difficult, if not impossible, to undertake and complete a book such as this.

The first person who deserves thanks is my wife Betty Jane, who by her love and unselfishness keeps our life free from turmoil and uncertainties. Second are those who help me with the word processing. While I wrote the text on a computer, using Wordperfect 4.2, Nancy Lodeiro competently and ably inserted many handwritten additions, spell-checked and ran off numerous verisons of each chapter. Jose Gonzalez was a whiz at finding references and all the right articles when I needed them. And, when he returned for the summer to his native El Salvador, Cristina Larrea and Jilma Lasso ably continued the research process. Other persons who provided wise counsel, advise and information are: Frank Pedersen, Maureen Riley, Marcia Orieveto, Chris Hollicek, and Ann Dehaan. Sue Stuka, from Front Range Community College, read an early draft of several chapters and provided valuable advise. Jacqueline Hartley, Florida International University, reviewed Chapters 4, 5, and 6 for accuracy and content. Special thanks also to other reviewers.

Ken Campbell
Auburn University

Kay Weese
West Liberty State College

Laurence Simon
Kingsboro Community College

E. Dean Schroeder
Laramie County Community
   College

Sally A. Jennings
St. Louis Community College
   Forest Park

Joanna Jones
Chaffey College

Margaret Budz
Triton College

Carol Gestwicki
Central Piedmont Community
   College

Drennan Nichols
Gulf Coast Junior College

Vernon Estes Jr.
San Antonio Community
   College

Ilene Hunter
Julie Brennan
Solano College

Joan Cook
County College of Morris

Mary Beth Mann
Northwestern State University
   of Louisiana

I would like to thank the people at Delmar Publishers for their constant support and encouragement. Karen Lavroff convinced me that I could do the project. Cynthia Haller provided many good suggestions. Jay Whitney was always calm, rational, helpful and professional. Suellen Wenz was an ideal copy editor—accurate, knowledgeable, concerned, helpful and pleasant. Project editor Carol Micheli handled all the details necessary to assure that the book was published on time.

George S. Morrison

July 4, 1989

$\mathcal{P}$ROLOGUE

I was very obsessed with the idea of growth, and I used to think that if I grew too much I would overshadow my younger brothers or even my father, which was a terrifying thought. Now I don't know where I got the idea that I was growing into a giant redwood tree, or I could possibly take the sunlight from other trees, but I really did. That was a tremendously erroneous concept, for I discovered that when a human being grows, this growth positively affects her environment, it affects the people around her and actually urges them to their own growth rather than the other way around. Our growth doesn't wither other people around us, it incites others to do the same. It inspires. I found that the more I expanded, the more I grew, the better it was for my environment. The effect of this would always be positive and would always be setting others on fire. (From *A Woman Speaks—Nintz, the Lectures, Seminars and Interviews* (p. 37) by Evelyn J. Nintz (Ed.), 1975, Chicago: The Swallow Press.)

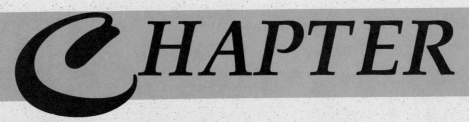

CHAPTER ONE

The world of child development: an overview

◆

VIGNETTES
INTRODUCTION
WHAT IS CHILD
   DEVELOPMENT?
DEVELOPMENTAL PROCESSES
Biological Processes
Environmental Processes
Critical Periods
Nature or Nurture?
Learning Processes
Interaction of Developmental
   Processes
WHY STUDY CHILD
   DEVELOPMENT?
CAREER CHOICES AND CHILD
   DEVELOPMENT
Personal Story: Maureen Reilley
Personal Story: Paul Grolitzer

Personal Story: Anne DeHaan
WAYS TO STUDY CHILDREN
Age–Stage Approach
Topical Approach
Life-span Approach
Multidisciplinary Approach
Ecological Approach
RESEARCH: ANSWERING
   QUESTIONS
Interest in Child Development
   Research
A Definition of Research
The Scientific Method
Stating a Hypothesis
Applying the Scientific Method
RESEARCH METHODS FOR
   STUDYING CHILDREN
Descriptive Research

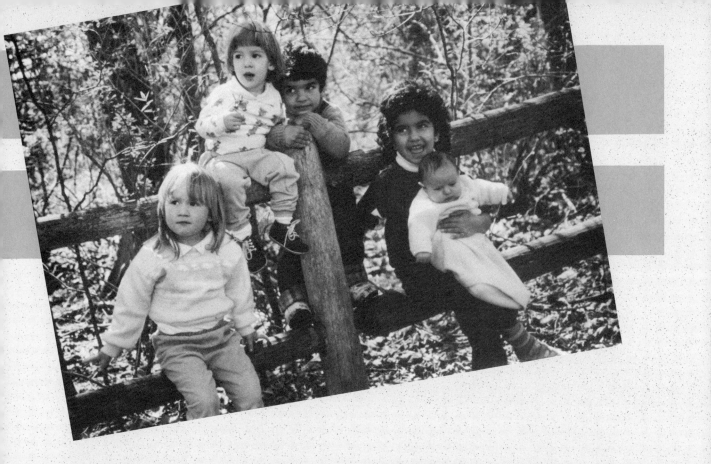

Correlational Research

The Experimental Method

GATHERING RESEARCH DATA

Questionnaires, Surveys, and
Interviews

Gathering Data through
Observation

Research Design for Determining
Development

Longitudinal Method

Cross-sectional Method

RESEARCH DISSEMINATION

ANALYZING RESEARCH

THE ETHICS OF CHILD
DEVELOPMENT

Ethical and Legal Issues

CURRENT INFLUENCES IN
CHILD DEVELOPMENT

Life-span Development

Renewed Areas of Interest

Early Learning

The "Plasticity" of Child
Development

Sociobiology

Ecological Considerations

Social Policy

What Would You Do?

SUMMARY

QUESTIONS TO GUIDE YOUR
REVIEW

ACTIVITIES FOR FURTHER
INVOLVEMENT

KEY TERMS

ANSWER TO "WHAT WOULD
YOU DO?"

BIBLIOGRAPHY

♡ VIGNETTES

Ramon was born at thirty-three weeks gestation via a cesarean section, weighed three pounds twelve ounces and was sixteen inches long. His head circumference was eleven and one half centimeters (four and one half inches). Ramon had a 40-percent oxygen deficiency, a rapid heart rate, and was in neonatal intensive care for twenty-three days. When discharged, he weighed four pounds, fourteen ounces. Today, Ramon is eighteen months old, weighs twenty-two pounds, and is twenty-nine and one quarter inches in height. He is developmentally delayed and his pediatrician is concerned about his overall growth pattern. Ramon's mother wanted to return to work, but the pediatrician has advised against placing him in child care at this time.

Latrenda is two years old and lives with her younger brother, seventeen-year-old mother, and grandmother in two rooms of a housing project in a major urban city. The neighborhood is still scarred by the riots of several years ago. Many social and educational agencies have opened storefront clinics in the area. The family's social worker is very concerned about Latrenda. She has referred her and her mother to a neighborhood child and family development clinic. In her referral report, the social worker noted that "Latrenda seems uninterested in events around her and is generally unresponsive to external stimuli."

Four-year-old Robyn lives with her parents, both attorneys, in a high-rise condominium. Robyn can't wait to go to her Montessori preschool in the morning, because, as she exuberantly exclaims, "I want to learn everything." Robyn enjoys reading books as she says, "All by myself." When adults ask her what she likes to do, she unhesitatingly responds, "I like learning." Robyn's parents believe she is gifted and have made arrangements to have her tested by a psychologist.

Seth and Lath live with their parents in a remote, rural township in the Midwest. The trailer in which they live is neat but sparsely furnished. Their mother prides herself on being a good housekeeper and makes a point of not letting the twins play with more than one toy at a time so they "won't make a mess." Seth and Lath will start first grade in the fall, but their mother is concerned about how they will get along. As she says, "They haven't played much with other kids, and Lath, he don't catch on as quick to things as his brother."

Tom, age eight, attends third grade in an eight-hundred-pupil elementary school. He recently moved with his parents from a "rust belt" city in the Northeast. He is a bright boy and has always made above-average grades. However, as the "new kid on the block," he is having trouble adjusting to school and is described by one of his teachers as "a blossoming discipline problem."

Sarah, a sixth-grade middle school student, lives in a rural area of the South with her mother, stepfather, and two older stepsisters. Her parents were divorced a year ago and her mother recently remarried. Sarah is a "B" student and babysits to earn extra money so she can buy the fashionable clothes she likes to wear. She is adjusting well to her role in the newly blended family, and looks forward to when she is old enough to get a better job.

Robert, sixteen, is a sophmore at a new high school in an affluent, fast-growing suburb of a Sun Belt city. He arrives at a corner not far from the school an hour before classes so he can sell "joints" to a group of eager peers. He clears about $200 per week. Robert's teachers describe him as bright, articulate, personable, and an underachiever. Robert's thoughts are not on school. In fact, he is thinking of quitting at the end of the year. He lists his priorities in life as, "My new red Camaro, girls, and how to keep from getting busted."

Myrna, age eighteen, has won just about all the awards her high school has to offer. In addition, she was recently nominated for a community leadership award for the many after-school hours she spends tutoring elementary school children in reading. Myrna is a member of the English honorary society and editor of its literary magazine, *The Mirror*. Although she originally selected journalism as a career, her tutoring experiences changed her mind. She now wants to be a teacher, "Because I want to bring happiness to others by helping them learn how to read and write."

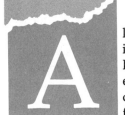

All these children are different, yet in many ways they are all alike. How are they alike and yet different? Why are they alike and yet different? How do genetics, family, friends, and environmental factors and forces influence them and cause them to be alike and yet different? What factors in their lives influence their growth—positively and negatively? What can parents, teachers, care-givers, and other professionals do to promote the positive development of these and other children? Through your study and involvement in child development you will learn much useful and interesting information that will enable you to answer these and other questions about the fascinating world of child development.

WHAT IS CHILD DEVELOPMENT?

Child development is the sum total of the physical, intellectual, social, emotional, and behavioral changes that occur in children from the moment of conception through the adolescent years. These changes make children the unique persons they are. Keep in mind that *human development* is a never-ending process through our life span from conception to death. Therefore, in our study of child development we must not forget that this time period from conception to adolescence is an integral part of and not separate from the rest of human development. The current interest in *life-span development* from conception to death reminds us of the importance of events throughout life, not just in certain time periods.

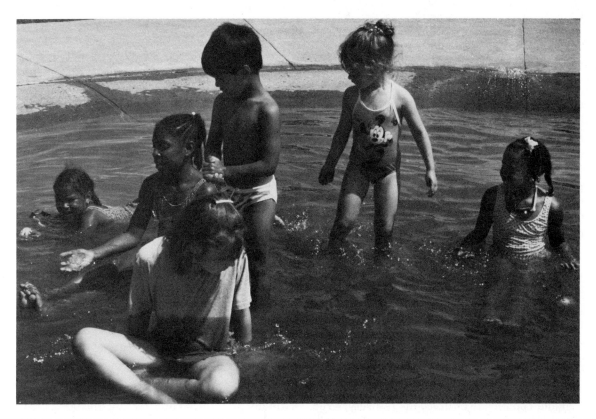

FIGURE 1-1 Children are alike in many ways, yet each child is a unique individual.

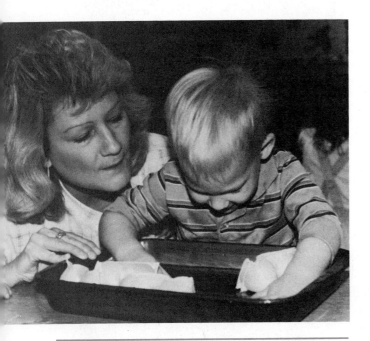

FIGURE 1-2   Care-givers contribute to children's development by nuturing and interacting with them.

The study of child development involves the exploration of how children change physically, intellectually, socially, and emotionally from conception to adolescence. This examination of maturation and change includes studying the impact of environment on development, and how people—teachers, parents, siblings, peers, care-givers, agencies, and children themselves—influence development.

The term *growth* is frequently identified with the term *development*, as in the phrase "child growth and development." These are not synonymous terms. Growth means the qualitative change in children that can be measured and described in inches, pounds, and numbers. For example, Andrea, one and one-half years old, weighs twenty-four pounds, is thirty-two inches tall, and has fourteen teeth.

Development on the other hand is an "increase in skill and complexity of function" (Lowery, 1986, p. 12). Child development theory describes child

behavior and development and helps explain why all children are the same and why individual children are different from each other. It predicts what children will be like and provides suggestions, ideas, and guidance to foster normal development. The study of child development provides direction for intervention strategies and therapy to people working with children with suspected or identified developmental problems.

DEVELOPMENTAL PROCESSES

Changes in children result from *developmental processes* that foster development. These processes are responsible for why you are who you are, and why others are the persons they are. Our understanding of developmental processes adds tremendously to our insights about children and helps explain behavior and development.

Biological Processes

Much of child development results from biological processes by which growth occurs and progresses in response to a genetic plan. This genetic plan, unique to each individual, determines the complexity, integration, organization, and function of individual parts of the organism as well as the whole of the individual. Genetic codes control many of the physical attributes of children, from physical stature to eye and hair color. Many child development experts believe that language acquisition and personality development are biologically based. We will discuss these and other biological influences in succeeding chapters. As you read, keep in mind that biological processes play a significant role in determining the "who," "what," and "why" of child development.

Environmental Processes

Biological processes are greatly influenced by environmental processes such as: nutrition; culturally prescribed child-rearing practices; the nature and quality of the home environment; parenting

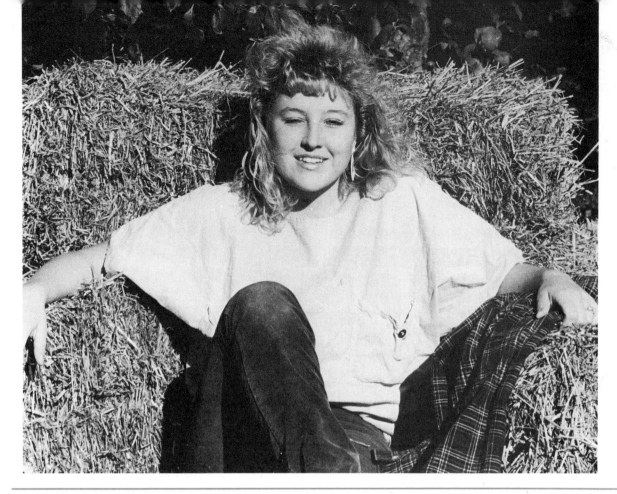

FIGURE 1-3 Development in the adolescent years can be and is for many bright and cheerful teenagers a positive, happy and rewarding experience.

styles; experiences with people, places, and objects; and social interactions with siblings and peers. We should expect environmental influences to cause differences in children. How dull and uninteresting life would be if everyone were alike!

Environmental processes can have long-lasting, negative effects on development. Lack of proper prenatal nutrition, for example, may result in premature birth and/or low birth weight. Other environmental influences that could have long-term negative consequences on children may have short-term or no developmental consequences depending on the nature of the intervention program designed to help them. For example, there is now ample evidence that the environments of poor, disadvantaged children can be counteracted by quality

early childhood education programs designed specifically for them (Sweinhart & Weikart, 1985).

There is a great deal of debate today in early childhood and child development circles about the nature and appropriateness of interventions for children. Child development professionals are very much involved in this discussion and are helping answer questions relating to the design and effectiveness of such programs.

The environmental influences just mentioned are the obvious ones that come to mind when talking about children. However, there are many environmental influences that affect children's behavior. Toys and other "hardware" of child rearing receive copious public attention regarding their ability to influence children's behavior. Currently many parent groups are opposed to the sale of "toys of violence" because of their negative behavioral influences on children. Television, a constant environmental influence (98 percent of all homes have at least one television), has the power to shape and influence children. The point is this: the environment is a very real, pervasive, and remarkably significant force in the process of child development.

Risk describes vulnerabilities that children face during the process of development. The domain of risk—what influences a child's development and to what extent—is highly dependent on the child's age and developmental stage as well as the nature and severity or mildness of risk. Genetic, biological, and environmental influences contain elements of risk for developing children.

Although lead poisoning may not receive daily attention, it nonetheless " . . . is probably the most serious underdiagnosed and undertreated childhood debilitating disease in the United States." (Chaiklin, Mosher & O'Hara, 1985, p. 63)

According to the Agency for Toxic Substances and Disease Registry (1988), the extent of lead poisoning in children is indeed extensive.

In short, about 2.4 million white and black metropolitan children [ages 6 months to 5 years] or about 17% of children in U.S. SMSAs [standard metropolitan statistical areas] are exposed to environmental sources of lead at concentrations that place them at risk for adverse health effects. This number approaches 3 million black and white children if extended to the entire U.S. child population (Agency for Toxic Subjects and Disease Registry, 1988, p. 4.)

An example helps place in perspective an environmental risk factor for children. The Center for Disease Control in Atlanta estimates that lead poisoning is causing neurological damage and behavioral difficulties in at least 700,000 children. The major source of poisoning is lead-based paint found in many older homes. Children eat the paint, which has a sweet taste, by chewing on windowsills and picking up flakes from the floor.

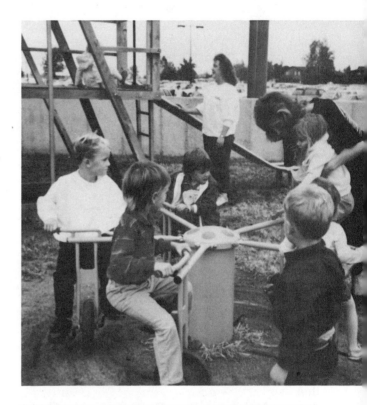

FIGURE 1-4   Teachers and other professionals who have a strong foundation of child development information are better able to work with and provide for the needs of children.

Though now banned for in-home use, lead-based paint was widely used in previous years and estimates of the number of homes and apartments that still have lead-painted surfaces range as high as twenty-seven million. Many of these are in poor, inner-city neighborhoods. Lead poisoning, then, is a major "risk" factor for many developing children.

Critical Periods

Colombo (1982) describes a *critical period* as one in which the developing organism is more sensitive to beneficial stimulation and more susceptible to detrimental influences. Children are more vulnerable to environmental risk factors, both internal and external, during these critical or sensitive periods. These periods occur during the time when a body system or organ part is growing most rapidly. If a child is subjected to risk during a critical period, then development can be permanently affected. On the other hand, a child can benefit from positive influences during a critical period. The majority of critical periods occur prenatally and in the early years. For example, there is a high incidence of hearing loss in children whose mothers contract rubella or German measles during the first trimester (the first three months of prenatal life), because this is the critical period for auditory development.

Nature or Nurture?

Which factor plays the dominate role in determining the course of development—heredity or environment? This question is the focus of a never-ending debate. At this time, there is no one, right, and true answer to this question, and it is unlikely that there ever will be. One reason is that answers depend on many things. For example, eye color is determined by heredity and can be changed by cosmetic lenses or surgery. In this regard, heredity is dominate. On the other hand, a child may encounter a risk in the environment, such as lead poisoning, that interferes with development. In this case, the environment is dominate. Political ideals also play a role in answering the question. Many socialist governments, for example, believe that heredity plays little, if any, role in development. They structure environments and child-rearing practices to accomplish their political goal of rearing children who will be good citizens. In such cases, hereditary influences are minimized. So, in an attempt to answer our original question, we have to consider how hereditary and environmental influences interact to make children the individual and unique persons they are.

Furthermore, and of equal importance, is the concept that being advantaged or disadvantaged by heredity or environment does not guarantee either a positive or negative outcome. As Sameroff and others (1989) point out:

> Where family and cultural variables have fostered development, children with severe perinatal [immediately after birth] complications have been indistinguishable from children without complications. Where these variables have hindered development, children from good preschool intervention programs like Head Start have developed later severe social and cognitive deficits.

Learning Processes

Learning processes also contribute to development. One of the primary ways children learn is through conditioning or reinforcement of behavior. The following interesting and very typical example helps emphasize the power of conditioning in learning. Many states have laws that require young children to be in car safety seats while traveling in a car. A young mother was stopped by a state trooper because her child was not restrained. She explained that it was impossible for her to get her child to stay in the car seat because every time she tried to put him in he would cry. The mother had reinforced the child's crying behavior by removing him from the car seat when he cried. The child learned how to stay out of the car seat. Needless to say, the mother received a citation.

Practice and repeated attempts in learning a particular behavior also play an important role in learning. All young toddlers, for example, spend vast amounts of time and energy practicing their emerging skill of walking.

Interaction of Developmental Processes

Developmental processes interact in the course of development. The average child will walk unassisted at one year of age. However, other factors, such as nutrition, opportunity or the lack of opportunity to practice, and the child's individual genetic code all interact with each other to deter-

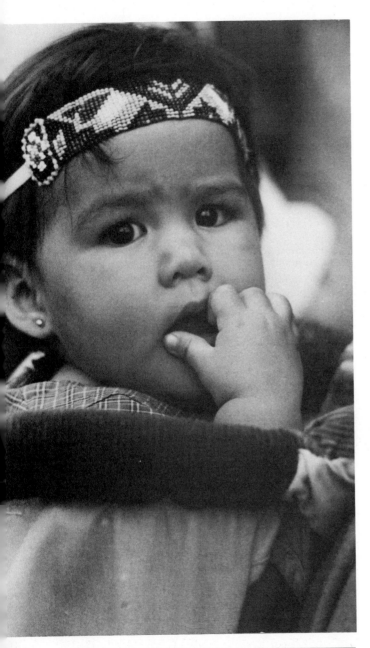

FIGURE 1-5 Environments and cultures in which children are reared help determine the nature and direction of developmental processes.

mine when a particular child begins unassisted walking. Heather used the kitchen table leg to pull herself to a standing position at six months and walked unassisted at nine months. Jason, on the other hand, didn't stand until twelve months and walked unassisted at fifteen months. Yet the average age of unassisted walking for these two children is twelve months, the average for all children.

WHY STUDY CHILD DEVELOPMENT?

Part of the American character includes the idea that everything must have a utilitarian purpose. In the context of child development, that utilitarianism is manifested in the question, Why should I study child development? There are a number of good answers to this question.

First, the study of child development provides self-insight and self-knowledge. Stop for a minute and ponder some intriguing questions. Who am I? How did I become the person I am? What makes me human? By studying children, we come to know ourselves. Children are the precursors of adults. What you are like today is in part because of what you were like as a child. Who you are today is partly a result of the experiences you had as a child. Without a knowledge of child development, answers to the above questions would not be complete, accurate, or satisfying.

Second, as we learn more about children and ourselves, we also learn more about others. As our knowledge of child and human development grows, we start to say such things as, "Now I know why my brother did that!" and "If only I had known that, I could have helped her more."

Third, the study of child development helps us understand how people are alike and yet different. Knowing the shared common elements of child development helps us understand the uniqueness of each child. Such knowledge helps all who work with children provide for their needs so they can achieve their full potential.

Knowledge of child development helps prepare people for parenthood and for careers involving children. All members of the "helping" professions who work with children and their families in any capacity—teachers, social workers, child care providers, nurses, home economists, counselors—must know about child development in order to do their jobs well.

Fourth, child development information and research play a significant role in the drafting of public policies relating to children. All who work with young children and their families should understand the effects such social forces as illiteracy, changes in the family structure, single parenting, lower school entrance ages, television programming, and child abuse have on young children. Public policy debate and implementation should be conducted within a context of what is best for children and their families. A discussion of legislation to provide federal support for establishing child care facilities for children of adolescent parents in public schools, for example, should involve knowledge about the impact of such services on adolescent parents and their children.

CAREER CHOICES AND CHILD DEVELOPMENT

Child development information is very useful, worthwhile and applicable to everyday, real-life events. The following vignettes relate how individuals in various fields and occupations use child development information to make day-to-day decisions about what is best for the children they work with, care for, and parent. The point is this: hundreds of thousands of decisions are made everyday by people in their relationships with children. These decisions affect children positively and negatively, and influence their growth and development. Better by far that these decisions are based on the best information we have at the time rather than on no information or the wrong information.

Personal Stories

MAUREEN REILLY, R.N., M.S.N.— PEDIATRIC NURSE PRACTITIONER

I am a pediatric nurse practitioner in the Child Development Center at Georgetown University Hospital. We have a government-funded project involving sixteen high-risk, chronically ill, medically fragile infants. I work with these infants and families while the infants are hospitalized and also assist in discharge planning. I accompany the doctors on their discharge rounds in the transitional nursery where the actual discharge plans for the babies are formed and reviewed. I then contact the family regarding the discharge plans and work with them to make the transition from the Child Development Center to the home as stress-free as possible.

When the infants are home, I do frequent medical/nursing evaluations and provide parents with psychological support. I actively listen to the parents' concerns and child care questions, and address these in positive ways. If parents are in need of specific medical information, for example, I provide it. I also support parents with infant education and development information by helping them select infant activities and toys that are appropriate for each child's developmental level. For example, I help parents decide which type of rattle is more appropriate (e.g., one with a very small circumference), what to look for in a crib mobile and how to hang it, and what toys will help them stimulate their babies. Some of the parents need basic teaching in child care, for example, bathing, how to care for diaper rash and the proper way to hold their babies.

My role recently expanded to include work with parents and infants at the craniofacial clinic. This clinic helps children who have craniofacial malformations, such as cleft lips and palates. I set up a schedule with the parents for clinic

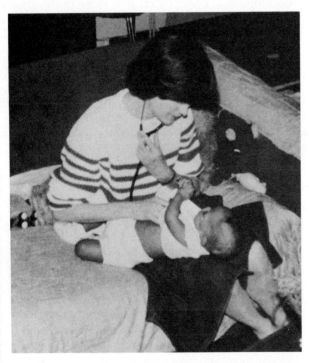

FIGURE 1-6 Maureen Riley, pediatric nurse practitioner, uses her knowledge of child development in her work with children and their families.

visitation and assist in pre- and postoperative teaching. When a baby is born with a craniofacial malformation, I visit the parents and teach them special child care techniques and introduce them to special equipment and materials for feeding. Babies with cleft palates, for example, need bottles and nipples designed especially for them. I also do home visitations when the babies are discharged.

Last June, a couple who were adopting a baby with a cleft palate came to the clinic. I counseled them and provided parenting and child care information. I told them to give me a call when the baby came. They called last week to let me know they had a lovely four-month-old girl! I went to their home and administered the Denver Developmental Screening Test. I also took along a lot of bottles and nipples and did an evaluation of what kind was best for the baby. The parents will be bringing her back in two weeks for a full evaluation.

Both in the craniofacial clinic and in homes, I administer the Denver Developmental Screening Test. Whenever I detect a developmental lag I refer the infant and parents for further testing to the Child Development Center. I also go over the results with a staff special educator and help her design a developmental educational stimulation program to use with each infant.

I also do home environment evaluations to determine if the environment supports children's learning. I use the Caldwell Home Assessment Scale. I observe the children's developmental behaviors in the home and make suggestions to parents for supporting and developing appropriate behavior.

I use child development knowledge and skills on a daily basis as an integral part of my job. I find myself constantly studying and looking for new information and ideas to help me help the families and children I serve.

Personal Stories

PAUL GROLITZER, B.S., M.A.— TEACHER, SEVERELY EMOTIONALLY DISTURBED ADOLESCENTS

I teach a group of 10 severely emotionally disturbed adolescents between the ages of thirteen and nineteen at the Family and Adolescent Development Center, Miami, Florida. Most of the youth have trouble behaving. They act out behaviorally and hit, curse, and yell, so I emphasize developing appropriate social behaviors. In addition to teaching basic academic skills, I also teach employability skills, such as how to arrive at work on time, how to work cooperatively with others, and how to dress for the job.

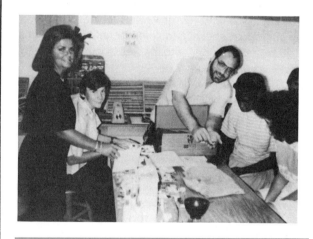

FIGURE 1-7 Paul Grolitzer, teacher of severely emotionally disturbed adolescents, finds many practical applications for his knowledge of child development.

I write an individual education plan for each youth in which I establish educational goals within a framework of their future goals. For example, I base my plan on what I and other staff members think their future holds, such as going on to a vocational training center or working in a sheltered workshop. I also make this plan as developmentally appropriate as I can for each youth. I take into consideration their learning styles and their developmental levels.

Last year, the other staff members and I felt we needed a different type of behavior management system for the center, so we designed a behavior modification point system. This is when my knowledge of child development was really put to good use. In our system, students earn points for appropriate behavior. Points are then spent for different rewards, such as videotapes and field trips. We have a canteen where they can use points to purchase special items such as cameras and radios.

We have weekly staff meetings in which teachers, two social workers, and a clinical psychologist come together to discuss the students. We use a lot of child development knowledge to determine ways to best meet the students' needs. We consider their academic/cognitive needs, social needs, and affective needs. For example, I needed some help with Susan, age fifteen. She was verbally aggressive, used a lot of profanity, was constantly out of her seat, and disturbed other children by hitting them. To meet her affective needs, we decided that when she started to get upset, I would involve her in relaxation techniques. So I have been teaching her and the rest of my class relaxation skills. To help Susan academically, the group suggested I try giving her smaller assignments, and now she seems to be able to accomplish more.

It is hard for me to imagine doing a good job without really knowing children and their development. The more I know about children in general and my group in particular, the better it is for them and me.

Personal Stories

ANNE DEHAAN, B.S., M.A.—CHILD CARE PROGRAM DIRECTOR

Coordinating all aspects of a child care program for 150 children requires the constant practice and application of child development theory. I use my theoretical and practical knowledge of child growth and development in decisions relating to center policies and procedures, curriculum planning, the assessment of children's progress and achievement, parent involvement, and staff development.

Every day I integrate knowledge of child development with program operations. When I assess lesson plans, for example, I assist the staff by suggesting ways in which an open-ended activity can challenge a five-year-old, yet not frustrate a two-and-a-half-year-old. I try to facilitate teachers' growth by giving suggestions about how to conduct a group time activity that is appropriate for the ages and abilities of the children. A new teacher is frequently uncertain in many situations, so I provide support, guidance, and explanations about why some activities are developmentally appropriate while others are not.

I also use a working knowledge of child development to formally and informally assess all children. When this assessment raises questions about a child's development, I help teachers and families seek the answers. We have a good network of referral agencies, and I find my background in child development helps me in my work with other professionals.

As early childhood programs continue their struggle for an enhanced professional image, it is imperative that they combine a strong theoretical base with nurturing and caring. A program founded on these principles benefits young children and families, and serves society as well.

WAYS TO STUDY CHILDREN

People who work in the field of child development use *theories* to help explain how children grow and develop. As such, a *theory*, according to Salkind, (1985) is "a group of logically related statements (for example, formulas, ideas, or rules) that explain events that have happened in the past as well as predict events that will occur in the future." Theories are very important to the study of children for they guide our thinking and research. Theories generally change and are revised over time as research confirms and/or rejects certain parts. A few of those theories are detailed next.

Age–Stage Approach

The field of child development is organized in several ways to facilitate study and understanding. The most common and popular organization is the *age–stage approach*, based on significant developmental processes that occur during distinct life periods. These age–stages are traditionally categorized as: prenatal (in utero—before birth), neonatal (the first month), infancy (the first year), toddlerhood (ages two and three), preschool and kindergarten (ages four through six), primary—grades one through three (ages six through eight), middle childhood—grades four through six (ages nine through twelve), and adolescence—grades seven through twelve (ages thirteen through eighteen). The primary developmental processes studied during each life stage are the physical, intellectual/cognitive, language, and social-emotional processes.

A major *advantage* of the age–stage approach is that it facilitates an understanding of the total range of development in each life period. As a result, the focus of attention is the developing child rather than the developmental processes themselves. This is as it should be, since it is children who give meaning to development.

A *disadvantage* to the age–stage approach is the danger of viewing child development as compartmentalized into ages and stages rather than as a continuous flow across the life span. This disadvantage is overcome, however, by integrating developmental processes in one life period to developmental processes in other life periods.

This textbook is based on the age–stage approach. The life periods are integrated so you have a sense of the continuity of development across the life span. Also, the textual material integrates developmental processes with life periods so you can understand how, for example, cognitive development progresses from conception to adolescence.

Topical Approach

The *topical approach* is another way of organizing the study of child development. The major topics of development are studied in their entirety across the life span from conception to adolescence. For example, language development is studied from the first cries of birth through and including the slang and special words of the adolescent years.

The *advantage* of the topical approach is that it provides a continuity in understanding a particular developmental process. On the other hand, one *disadvantage* is that there may be a tendency to not fully appreciate the interrelatedness between all the developmental processes. A second disadvantage may be that the focus of importance and study becomes the developmental process rather than the child.

Life-span Approach

During the last decade, life-span development has caught the attention of the public, and especially developmentalists. Developmental studies have broken out of the traditional conception-to-adolescence orientation. We now recognize the importance of studying the developing person across the life span from conception to death. Life after age twenty-one has been rediscovered! As a result of the graying of America due to the growing numbers of senior citizens, *life-span development* emphasizes that the human life cycle is a journey from conception to death, with many individual variations and possibilities. While we often don't have the time or inclination to study the entire life span, we should not forget that life is a continuous whole and that significant life events, such as marriage, divorce, remarriage, children leaving home, second careers, and retirement occur after adolescence. In addition, there has been in the past a tendency to stress how early events affect later life. While this is true, our view of the influence of these events is not as deterministic as it once was. Humans are capable of change, and change occurs across the entire life span.

Multidisciplinary Approach

No single discipline is capable of describing the incredible wonders, beauty, significance, and events of child development. The high drama about how children develop is described and written about utilizing all the disciplines relating to the field. Child development experts use a *multidisciplinary approach* and utilize theories, research, and ideas from disciplines such as early childhood, elementary, and special education, home economics, psychology, pediatrics, nursing, social work, anthropology, sociology, biology, medicine, and psychiatry. The interrelatedness of these disciplines, focused on learning more about how children develop, contribute to our understanding of children and provide a better life for them and their families.

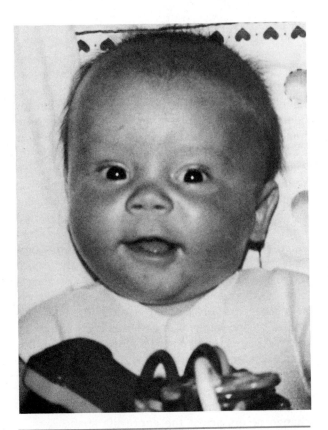

FIGURE 1-8   Today, infants are viewed as competent and skillful learners capable of interacting with and learning from their environment. (Photo courtesy of Teresa Hunt Gifford)

Ecological Approach

The *ecological approach* to child development emphasizes that the environment plays a tremendous role in the lives of children and influences their development. Many environmental influences are not always obvious to us because we do not always think of them as having a direct influence on children. We acknowledge the influence of a child's parents and home, but what influences do those who take care of her at the child care center have on her? Also, what are the influences of the center itself? Likewise, how does the state legislature, which we don't often think of as part of children's environment, but which is, influence

them? The researcher who got us thinking about the ecology of child development is Urie Bronfenbrenner, who argues for a new perspective in studying human development, namely one that focuses on the interactions between human development and environments. For Bronfenbrenner (1979), development is "a lasting change in the way in which a person perceives and deals with his environment" (p. 3). Bronfenbrenner sees development as influenced by three environmental influences.

The first consists of influences that immediately affect children. They take place in the home and classroom. The second sphere comprises the relationships *between* environments. As Bronfenbrenner (1979) points out, "A child's ability to learn to read in the primary grades may depend no less on how he is taught than on the existence and nature of ties between the school and home" (p. 3). The third sphere involves relationships and influences that occur in places and settings far removed from the child, yet which nonetheless influence development. These events usually result from public policy in the form of legislation, agency directives, and government regulations. For example, what effect does legislation increasing by three months the age for kindergarten enrollment have on children and their parents?

Undoubtedly, environmental influences on child development will continue to receive more attention from all who work with and study children.

RESEARCH: ANSWERING QUESTIONS

Interest in Child Development Research

"Christina is gifted." A young couple makes this proud pronouncement about their thirteen-month-old daughter to all who will listen. The headlines in the science section of a national newspaper declares: "Child Development: Language Takes on New Significance—Experts Believe That

Linguistic Markers Can Help Predict Problems" (*The New York Times*, 1987, p. 23). Signs in bars and other places where alcoholic beverages are served warn about the dangers of drinking during pregnancy. Parent groups advocate more federal funds to support preschool programs for children of low-income parents. Child advocates lobby against the violence contained in children's television programming.

In all sectors of society, from child care to public policy, people are talking about and are interested in information involving child development. With all this interest and talk targeted on child development, perhaps you have wondered, "How do we know if what we know and say about child development is true?"

There are many ways people come to "know" children's development. From ancient times to the present, philosophers, religious leaders, educators, and parents have offered explanations about children's growth and behavior. These beliefs are frequently based on feelings, emotions, single encounters with children, and the advice of others handed down from generation to generation. Until quite recently some parents believed, for example, that unless children with measles were kept in totally dark rooms, they would go blind; that babies could see little, if anything, at birth, and that they could not feel pain, taste or smell.

But, how do we know if such beliefs are true? Is our knowledge about children always based on the best information available? Pause for a moment to think about one of your beliefs about children. How do you know if your belief is true? Is it based on fact, on what you think is right, or on what others say is true? How can we determine if our "common-sense" solutions to questions of child rearing are indeed "right"? Are personal experiences people have while growing up and helping others grow up sufficient bases for determining how we will treat children? While common sense, personal experiences, and the advice of friends and relatives can be good sources of information, there is another, more significant way we can come to know what is or isn't "true."

A Definition of Research

Research helps find answers to questions so that we do not have to rely only on our experiences and the authority of others for child development knowledge. *Research* is the formal, systematic application of the scientific method to the study of problems or questions (Gay, 1987, p. 4)—in our case, questions about child development.

The Scientific Method

The *scientific method* is an objective and orderly process that consists of defining a problem, formulating a hypothesis or educated guess about the outcome of the research, collecting and analyzing data, and making conclusions about verifying or not verifying the hypothesis.

The following four steps result when the scientific method is applied to research. They constitute the research process: (1) selecting and defining a problem; (2) executing research procedures; (3) analyzing data; and (4) drawing and stating conclusions (Gay, 1987, p. 5).

Stating a Hypothesis

Researchers' problem statements and questions concerning child development are often stated in the form of *hypotheses*, which are reasonable, testable statements about what they believe their research will reveal. Notice in the following passage how the researchers state their three hypotheses (italics mine).

The purpose of the present study was to identify gender differences and similarities in the way preschool children interact in a same-sex group problem-solving situation requiring that the individual child engage in a range of behaviors in order to obtain a source. Given results from the earlier studies, *it was expected that there would be significant individual differences in resource acquisition. It was also hypothesized, in light of the general notions mentioned above [in the authors' introductory statement] concerning the universal necessity for and ability to acquire resources regardless of gender, that girl groups and boy groups would obtain the same amounts of resources, that is, movie viewing time. However, given what we know from the gender-differences literature, it was expected that girls and boys would go about doing so using different behavioral strategies* (Charlesworth and Dzur, 1987, p. 192).

Applying the Scientific Method

Researchers use the scientific method to learn many interesting things related to child growth and development. Today, with more women already in and entering the work force than ever before, many questions are raised about the effects of maternal employment on children. But does maternal employment have the same effect on boys *and* girls? Let's look at how researchers (Ansul, DiBase, & Weintraub, 1987) used the scientific method to answer these questions.

Research title: "The Effects of Maternal Employment and Child Sex" Selection and definition of a problem (research questions or hypotheses):

1. Do boys and girls differ in their responses to separation in the laboratory and at home?
2. Is the maternal employment history related to children's responses to separation?
3. Does maternal employment status differentially affect boys' and girls' responses to separation?

Execution of research procedures: The responses of eighteen-month-old boys (n = 13) and girls (n = 18) to maternal separation were observed in the laboratory and in the home. Measures of separation distress included the frequency of calling mothers, the amount of time the child spent crying, playing alone, playing with a stranger, and quietly interacting with a stranger. Children were also rated on how easy or difficult they were for a stranger to soothe.

Families in the study included mothers who returned to full-time work within the first four months after the child's birth and mothers who did not return to the labor force.

Data Analysis:
The researchers used statistical analysis to assess the effects of child sex and maternal employment on children's responses to separation.

Drawing and stating conclusions:
Based on the analysis of their data, the researchers concluded that:

> Our findings support previous research documenting sex differences in separation distress. Boys tend to be more distressed, play less, and soothe less easily than girls when separated from their mothers. However, when maternal employment status is taken into consideration, sex differences attenuated [reduced in amount]. Boys with employed mothers are *less distressed* during separation than boys with nonemployed mothers. Girls with both employed and nonemployed mothers were not different in their separation responses.

In discussing their conclusions, the researchers noted a number of possibilities raised by their data. First, maternal employment may serve to reduce boys' separation distress by providing more familiarity with the separation. Second, maternal employment may somehow affect mothers' interactions with their sons such that sons develop the ability to function adaptively in their mothers' absence.

RESEARCH METHODS FOR STUDYING CHILDREN

When researchers apply the scientific method to the solution of a problem, they have to decide what research method is most appropriate. The majority of child development research procedures fall into one of three broad categories: descriptive, correlational, and experimental.

Descriptive Research

Researchers utilize *descriptive research* to ascertain the characteristics, opinions, and attitudes of subjects; gather demographic information; and determine conditions and procedures. "A descriptive study determines and reports the way things are" (Gay 1987, p. 189). When child development researchers observe how parents soothe their stressed children or determine which toys children play with the most, they are conducting descriptive research based on their observation of the subjects. Researchers gather descriptive data primarily through questionnaires/surveys, interviews, and observation. These methods of gathering data will be discussed later in this chapter.

Developmental and Follow-up Studies Developmental and follow-up studies are included in descriptive research. Developmental studies examine the behavior, growth, and development variables that characterize children at different chronological ages and stages of development.

Researchers oftentimes want to follow up subjects who participated in research. They conduct a follow-up study when they examine the performance of second graders to determine if a particular preschool method had a lasting influence on their school achievement. Follow-up research is valuable and essential in determining the effects of practices and procedures.

Correlational Research

Correlational research describes in quantitative terms how variables are related. A correlation is the relationship between two or more variables, hence the name for this research method. For example, researcher Diane E. Field wanted to determine whether children's coviewing television— watching television with a parent—predicts children's performance on cognitive tasks. Field (1987) analyzed her data and concluded that "cognitive performance was not strongly predicted by coviewing. In fact, the small negative relationships suggest that coviewing at home may be distracting rather than facilitative."

As in Field's study, correlational research is used to predict the relationship between variables. If two variables are highly related, the researcher will obtain a *correlation coefficient* of near + 1.0 if the relationship is positive, and - 1.0 if the relationship is negative. If the variables are not related, the researcher obtains a relationship of .00. The more highly related the two variables are, that is, the nearer the relationship is to 1.0, the more accurate are predictions about relationships based on that relationship.

While correlational studies predict relationships and show how changes in one variable are *related* to changes in another variable, they do not show cause-and-effect relationships. Researchers who use correlational studies are not manipulating variables and therefore they cannot say that a change in one variable *causes* a change in another variable. Field's study examined the relationship between coviewing and cognitive performance by comparing coviewing time to indicators of cognitive performance. She is legitimately able to state the relationship between these two variables—a small negative relationship—but she cannot say that coviewing *causes* a change in cognitive performance.

The Experimental Method

When researchers conduct research studies, especially those with an experimental design, they often compare the performance of two (or more) groups of children. One group receives the treatment—the program or experience the researcher wants to study—and one group does not receive the treatment. The group that receives the treatment is the *experimental group,* the group that does not receive the treatment is the *control group.* Either nothing is done to the control group or they may receive another, entirely different treatment. The performance or behavior of the experimental group that received the treatment is compared to the performance or behavior of the control group that did not receive the treatment in order to determine the effect of the treatment. Without a control group, researchers would be unable to determine the true effect of the treatment.

The *experimental method* is the procedure of choice for researchers who want to test hypotheses involving cause-and-effect relationships. In an experimental study, the researcher carefully manipulates or controls an *independent variable* to determine the effect, change, or influence it has on the *dependent variable*. The independent variable, which is also referred to as the *experimental variable* or *treatment*, is the activity or process that the researcher believes will have a cause-and-effect influence on the dependent variable. The dependent variable is given that name because it is contingent on the independent variable, which the researcher controls. Let's look at an experimental study to see how it is used to test hypotheses.

You have probably heard the expression, "Actions speak louder than words." Common sense tells you it is so. But is it *really* true with very young children? This question intrigued Patricia Murray (1987) so she conducted an experimental study to see if infants responded better to actions-modeling or words-telling.

Murray randomly assigned seventy-two infants between the ages of fifteen and twenty-one months to either a modeling group or an instruction group. In the modeling group, Murray simply modeled a behavior—putting a hat on her head. In the instruction group, she instructed the infants to "see this, put this (hat) on your head." Murray found that asking infants to perform a *familiar* task was as effective as showing them what to do. However, when infants were taught an unfamiliar task, modeling was significantly more effective in teaching a new skill for boys and less effective in teaching a new skill for girls. So, in answer to her question, Murray emphasizes "the power of the spoken word, even to infants who are just beginning to speak. Simply asking an infant to do something is often as effective as showing them what to do."

In this study, the independent variables are the two teaching methods—modeling and verbal instructions. Murray's direct manipulation of the infants by these variables differentiates experimental research from all other methods of research. Put in another way, Murray decided who would get what. The behavior of the infants, that which Murray predicted would be affected by the independent variable, is the dependent variable.

Murray also used *random assignment* of the infants to the two groups. Each infant in her experiment had an equal chance of being assigned to one of the two groups. There are many ways to influence random selection, such as using a book of random numbers or drawing the names of the participants out of a hat. The important thing is that all have an equal opportunity to participate or not participate, or to be assigned to various groups.

Although, as indicated, experimental research is the preferred method of testing cause-and-effect predictions, a number of factors can still cause "problems." First, researchers have to make sure that the treatment is of sufficient duration for it to have an opportunity to "work." For example, researchers who want to determine the abilities of a new reading curriculum to increase achievement would not expect a student involvement of a week or two to be long enough to judge if the program is effective.

Second, keep in mind that although experimental research is the only type of research that can establish cause-and-effect relationships, there are many instances when it is inappropriate because there are many questions we may want to answer that cannot be answered by the experimental method. Researchers have to match the questions they want to answer with the method that will best answer their questions.

GATHERING RESEARCH DATA

Once researchers select their research method, they then must decide how to gather their data.

Questionnaires, Surveys, and Interviews

Popular and often-used methods for gathering research data, especially in descriptive research, are questionnaires, surveys and interviews. In fact, the questionnaire is the most widely used technique for obtaining information from subjects (McMillan & Schumacher, 1984, p. 140). *Questionnaires* can consist of statements or questions, but in all cases, subjects are responding to something written. *Interviews* are essentially vocal questionnaires. In a *survey*, the researcher selects a sample of respondents and administers a questionnaire or conducts an interview to collect data. Chances are fairly good that you have participated—or have been asked to participate—in a survey regarding topics ranging from dating habits to cereal preference.

A major problem with a questionnaire is it is difficult to get subjects (respondents) to return them. If a researcher sends a questionnaire to one hundred parents to determine their opinions about child care, and if only twenty parents, all of whom are dissatisfied with their child care arrangements, return it, conclusions drawn from such data will be very different from results obtained if we had data from *all* parents.

In addition, some researchers question the usefulness of data collected through questionnaires and other self-reporting methods. What parents report about how they discipline their children and how, in fact, they do discipline them may be two different things.

The problems encountered in gathering self-report data are exacerbated when working with children. Children may be less attentive than adults, and may have difficulty comprehending questions and expressing their feelings and opinions.

Because of shortcomings involved in interviews and questionnaires, many researchers prefer to gather their information directly through observation.

Gathering Data through Observation

Researchers use observational methods and procedures to directly observe—visually and auditorily—some phenomena and make a record of their observations. Observers avoid affecting the observed situation in any way. In this sense, they are literally "on the outside looking in."

In *naturalistic observation*, researchers observe behavior in a familiar setting because they believe it is more authentic than behavior observed in a laboratory setting. This method is frequently referred to as *ecological research*. Researchers believe that there is a greater likelihood the behavior they wish to observe will more likely occur in a natural setting. Thus, a researcher conducts naturalistic observation of parent-child interactions in the home rather than in a laboratory.

The ecological context of the family currently plays a pronounced role in research related to child development. The family represents the primary child development framework and more research efforts are now directed toward understanding the processes whereby it influences that development.

In the research of Ansul and others mentioned earlier, they were interested in observing the separation of young children from their mothers in the home *and* in the laboratory. Research with titles such as the following are becoming more commonplace in journals and magazines: "A Naturalistic Study of Humorous Activity in a Third, Seventh, and Eleventh Grade Classroom" (Fabrizi & Pollo, 1987).

In *simulated observation*, the researcher creates the observational setting and the activity for the subjects. For example, in the Charlesworth and Dzur study, the children were brought to the laboratory room and told about the movie viewer and how it worked. The researchers then turned the viewer over to the children and left to let them play. One of the problems with simulated observation is that it is not natural. On the other hand, such simulation allows researchers to use equipment and procedures that would be impractical to use in natural settings. Researchers can control variables they might not otherwise be able to control in natural settings, and create situations and events they might otherwise have to wait a long time to observe.

In *participant observation*, researchers use subjects who participate in an experiment as observers to help them gather data. The rationale for using participant observers is that they can provide useful information and insights that otherwise might not be available. Participant observers must receive special training so they know what to observe and how to record it.

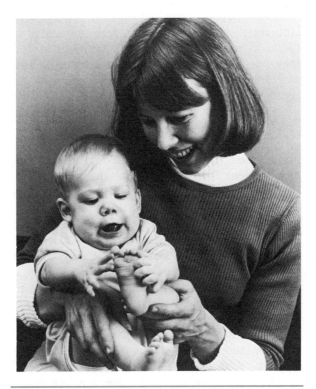

FIGURE 1-9 Adults have a strong and powerful influence on young children as they guide and direct their development. (Courtesy of Gerber Products Company)

The Technology of Observation More and more, researchers avail themselves of advances in technology to make their observations more effective. Charlesworth and Dzur used a video camera to record (observe) children's play interactions. Such technology has several advantages. First, it is unobtrusive, that is, it does not get in the way as humans tend to. Second, researchers have the recorded behavior available to them for review and continuing analysis.

RESEARCH DESIGN FOR DETERMINING DEVELOPMENT

Much of children's development is age related. Many developmental processes are tied to chronological age. Although age per se is no predictor of physical development or behavior, and although

variations from child to child in the emergence of physical and behavioral characteristics are normal, age-related descriptions are a valuable tool for all involved in child development. First, these descriptions help us know what to expect in terms of average, normal development. Second, discrepancies from the norm act as signals to alert caregivers to the need for close observation and the possibility of professional referral.

Children's development is frequently standardized according to age. There are growth and behavior charts (many of which appear in this text) depicting average ages for physical development and behavioral characteristics. For example, Table 1-1 shows the *average* ages for linguistic and auditory milestones in children during the first year (Capute, Shapiro, Wachtel, Gunther, & Palmer, 1986, p. 695).

TABLE 1–1

LINGUISTIC AND AUDITORY MILESTONES—THE FIRST YEAR	
Age in Months	Milestone
1	Is alert of bell, rattle, or voice
2	Produces social smiles
3	Coos
4	Orients to voice; Laughs aloud
5	Orients to bell (localizes laterally); Makes razzing sound; Says "Ah-goo"
6	Babbles
7	Orients to bell (localizes directly)
8	Uses "dada" indiscriminately
9	Understands "no"; Uses gesture language (waves "bye-bye" or plays "pat-a-cake")
10	Orients to bell (localizes directly; Uses "dada" and "mama" discriminately
11	Says one word other than "dada" and "mama"
12	Understands one-step command (with gesture); Has two-word vocabulary (other than "dada" and "mama")

Let's suppose we wanted to confirm in our own minds that linguistic and auditory development do indeed emerge in the order and at the chronological ages depicted in Table 1–1. There are several ways for us to gather such data—the longitudinal method and the cross-sectional method.

Longitudinal Method

In a *longitudinal study*, researchers gather data—in our case linguistic and auditory ability in the first year of life—on the *same* group of children over a period of a year. Many kinds of data are gathered using this method, from a single characteristic, such as weight, to the relationship between age and the emergence of cognitive behavior. While longitudinal studies allow researchers to observe and gather data about growth and development over time, there are nonetheless a number of disadvantages.

First, many longitudinal studies require a lot of time. In the case of linguistic milestones, it would take a year to gather data. Some researchers spend a lifetime gathering data on a particular group. This is precisely what Nancy Bayley did. She studied growth over long periods of the human life cycle. Her famous Berkley Growth Study (still in progress) gathered data relating to behavior, IQ, motor skills, physical development, influences of maternal behavior on offspring, rates of physical maturation, and body build (Corsini, 1984).

Subject attrition is a second disadvantage of longitudinal research. Let's suppose that in our study of linguistic and auditory abilities, some of the families moved away or, for some reason, did not want to participate anymore. The number of children in our study is reduced, affecting the amount and kind of data we are able to collect. Researchers who use the longitudinal method often make special efforts to retain as many of the original subjects in their study as possible. One researcher, William Baily, regularly contacts families participating in his studies. He sends the children birthday cards, sends all families cards during the holidays; writes letters to the families telling them about his research, and sends parents abstracts of his research reports. His efforts pay off. He reports no further attrition after starting his contact program (1987). Baily's efforts are an example of the dedication and extra efforts researchers make in their quest for knowledge.

Cross-sectional Method

A *cross-sectional* design is another method we can use to gather data. Using this method we simultaneously assess the linguistic abilities of groups of children of different ages, for example, one week, four weeks, six weeks and so forth, to determine their language competence. In the cross-sectional method, researchers gather data on groups of children of different ages. Put another way, a longitudinal study gathers data on the same children over time, whereas the cross-sectional study gathers data *at one time* on different children of different ages. (Researchers use the term *cohort* to describe people born in the same year or time period.)

An advantage of the cross-sectional design is that it enables researchers to gather data on a developmental process in a relatively short period of time. Instead of waiting a year to have data on linguistic development, it is possible to have it in a matter of weeks or months. However, this very advantage is also a disadvantage.

This disadvantage relates to gathering data on different cohort groups of children born at different times. Rather than following the linguistic and auditory development of a group of children over time, researchers gather data on children born in different time periods. The problem is they are not always sure what environmental, cultural, and social factors have influenced children's language and auditory development. These *generational influences* may influence the data collected. Consequently, it is different from data collected through the longitudinal design. Increased public awareness about early language development, for example, has encouraged many parents to increase language activities, such as talking with and reading to their children. These activities may enhance language development. In the cross-sectional design, researchers must assure themselves they are selecting children that are truly representative of each age level and who are comparable to each other in characteristics such as intelligence and cultural background.

While it is doubtful if there ever will be the perfect design for gathering data, this does not and should not prohibit researchers in their efforts to test hypotheses and open further the gates of knowledge. There are a number of safeguards built into the generic research process. First, most researchers are aware of the limitations of research designs. Second, readers of research are becoming more sophisticated in their knowledge of research processes and are quick to raise questions about research. Third, as previously noted, researchers replicate the research of others as a means of confirming and verifying research results.

RESEARCH DISSEMINATION

Researchers are obligated to disseminate research results. After all, of what use is knowledge and truth unless others know about it? Researchers use scholarly journals such as *Child Development* to publish their results. This is how Charlesworth and Dzur disseminated their research. Other journals that publish research and information about child development are listed in Appendix I. Also, the sources your author cites prove an appreciation for child development sources. Researchers also attend conventions, conferences, and seminars to disseminate information about their work and research, which is what Ansul, DiBase, and Weintraub did.

ANALYZING RESEARCH

Readers and users of research should ask the following questions:

1. *Is the research reported in a reputable journal or presented as a paper at a conference of a professional society?* Many professional journals have a policy of peer review and recommendation for publication. Practitioners review or *referee* submitted articles to uphold high standards of research and research reporting.

2. *Do I have all the information I need?* Many magazines and journals designed for public distribution frequently report only research conclusions without publishing supporting information. This is perfectly acceptable, but you should understand the necessity of knowing the purpose and nature of the study before basing judgments and decisions on those conclusions.

3. *Does the research clearly communicate what was done, how it was done, and the conclusions?* Generally, research reports contain the following: (1) an introduction, (2) a statement of the problem (also stated as a hypothesis or aim of the study), (3) the method, which states what was done and to whom and how it was done, (4) the results—what the researcher found—the data and how it was analyzed, (5) the conclusions—based on the data, and (6) a discussion in which the researcher explains the results and makes suggestions for further research.

4. *To what extent can the results of a study be generalized to other children?* For the most part, laboratory studies can be generalized only to laboratories. We can legitimately ask the question, will children play in their home environments the same way they do in a laboratory playroom setting? Increasingly researchers are finding that there is a difference. Therefore, answers to questions such as this one explain why there is so much interest in naturalistic research.

THE ETHICS OF CHILD DEVELOPMENT

All who conduct research with children should act with integrity and respect. Respect implies that all who work with children value children and in no way do anything to violate the essential nature of their physical, intellectual, or emotional growth.

Integrity implies that researchers will not compromise children's or parents' rights in efforts to conduct research, and that the intent, purpose, and procedures involved in the research will be honestly explained to all involved. Those who are the subjects of research and their guardians have a right to know in what they are participating and the intended purpose, results, and range of dissemination.

Ethical and Legal Issues

Researchers who involve human and or animal subjects in their research must be guided by proper ethics and legal responsibilities. The Society for Research in Child Development (Charlesworth, 1987) provides a set of ethical principles for research with children. As you read the principles in Table 1–2, think about their application and how they might influence researchers and subjects.

TABLE 1–2

ETHICAL STANDARDS FOR RESEARCH WITH CHILDREN		
Principle	Explanation	Example
Non-harmful procedures	The investigator should use no research operation that may harm the child either physically or psychologically	It would be unethical, for example to inflict pain on a newborn to determine newborns' sensitivity to pain. Likewise, if a researcher wanted to determine the nature of fearfulness in young children, she would have to take precautions that her procedures did not develop fear in her subjects.
Informed Consent	Before seeking consent or assent from the child, the investigator should inform the child of all features of the research that may affect his or her willingness to participate and should answer the child's questions in terms appropriate to the child's comprehension.	A researcher has the obligation to explain fully what he is going to do, how he is going to do it and to whom he is going to do it. In the case of young children, parents must be involved in this process. One 13 year old, after listening to a proposed study involving sexual behavior felt that participation would "be an invasion of my privacy", even though she was assured she would remain anonymous.
Parental Consent	The informed consent of parents, legal guardians or those who act in loco parentis (e.g., teachers, superintendents of institutions) similarly should be obtained, preferably in writing.	One parent, after listening to a researcher's plan for studying the growth of empathetic behavior in young children decided not to participate because she thought it would be too stressful for her child.
Additional Consent	The informed consent of any persons, such as school teachers for example, whose interactions with the child as the subject of the study should also be obtained.	In a study relating to the effectiveness of teacher praise on the vocabulary learning ability of young children, the teacher or teachers involved must also agree to participate. They should not be told by their principal or anyone else that they must participate. One researcher made some changes in her research design after discussing her project with a teacher.

TABLE 1-2 (Continued)

Incentives	Incentives to participate in a research project must be fair and must not unduly exceed the range of incentives that the child normally experiences.	Children are very susceptible to enticement and the prospect of getting things that they see advertised on television. If they are participating in a behavior reinforcement study involving earning tokens to "spend" on toys, then the toys should be of equal value and quality to what they as a group are normally used to.
Deception	Although full disclosure of information during the procedure of obtaining consent is the ethical ideal, a particular study may necessitate withholding certain information or deception.	A researcher for example, investigating the relationship of schizophrenia to heredity and environment may say that she is studying personality development in adopted children rather than tell the adopted couple to unduly infer their child is a schizophrenic.
Anonymity	To gain access to institutional records, the investigator should obtain permission from responsible authorities in charge of records. Anonymity of the information should be preserved and no information used other than that for which permission was obtained.	The assurance of anonymity is standard operating procedure for researchers. Most participants are assigned numbers or code names to assure and protect anonymity. One researcher was faced with this dilema. Two parents participating in her study on infant stimulation asked her for the names of participants so they could add them to mailing list of a new toy company they started. The researcher refused.
Mutual Responsibilities	From the beginning of each research investigation, there should be clear agreement between the investigator and the parents, guardians or those who act in loco parentis, and the child, when appropriate, that defines the responsiblities of each.	Everyone participating in a research project should fully understand their responsibilities. One researcher lost valuable time and good will with a group of parents because half way through his research study on parent-child interactions the parents suddenly "discovered" they had to implement a behavior reinforcement procedure they felt violated their parenting styles. They withdrew and the researcher was left without a project!
Jeopardy	When, in the course of research, information comes to the investigator's attention that may jeopardize the child's well being, the investigator has a responsiblity to discuss the information with the parents and with those expert in the field in order that they may arrange the necessary assistance for the child.	Following initial screening of children in a research project, data revealed a child who was suspected of being learning disabled. The researcher discussed the results with the parents and assisted them in a referral for further testing to a child development clinic.
Unforseen consequences	When research procedures result in undesirable consequences for the participant that were previously unforseen, the investigator should immediately employ ap-	One researcher began to interview parents and children for participation in a study of parents' methods of punishment. She quickly realized that what she was asking parents to do might result in an increase in punitive punishment.

TABLE 1-2 (Continued)

	propriate measures to correct these consequences, and should consider redesigning the procedures if they are to be included in subsequent studies.	She redesigned her study to eliminate this possibility.
Confidentiality	The investigator should keep in confidence all information obtained about research participants.	Researchers frequently learn information about others that individuals, parents and children would not want revealed. For example, in the study on parental punishment parents would not want the public or others to know the nature and frequency of their conflicts with their children.
Informing Participants	Immediately after the data are collected, the investigator should clarify for the research participants any misconceptions and inform them of general findings. Withholding information should have no damaging consequences for participants.	Many researchers provide parents and childrren written reports, in language they can understand, relating to their research reuslts.
Reporting Results	Because the investigator's words may carry unintended weight with parents and children, caution should be exercised in reporting results, making evaluative statements, or giving advice.	Many children and parents are in awe of the scientific and educational communities. When a teacher or researcher says something they believe it and may think they are a "bad" parent or child if they don't do what the researcher concluded. One researcher discovered that a parent was in danger of malnourishing her baby because of her interpretation of his discussion of the results of his study relating to overfeeding and obesity in young children.
Implications of Findings	Investigators should be mindful of the social, political and human implications of their research and should be especially careful in the presentation of findings from the research.	A number of examples relating to this ethical principle frequently appear in the popular press. Two currently receiving a great deal of attention are the effects of work-place radiation on the fetuses of pregnant women and the influences of child care on infants.

Ethical Dilemmas   Many ethical dilemmas arise in child research that are not neatly covered by ethical guidelines. Frequently researchers must make difficult decisions about their research. A researcher may choose not to conduct a particular research project, or will adopt another method, as a result of ethically based decisions.

CURRENT INFLUENCES IN CHILD DEVELOPMENT

In many ways, the field of child development is no different from other professions. Many issues influence the study of child development and certain topics attract special attention. Following is a discussion of some current influences in child development.

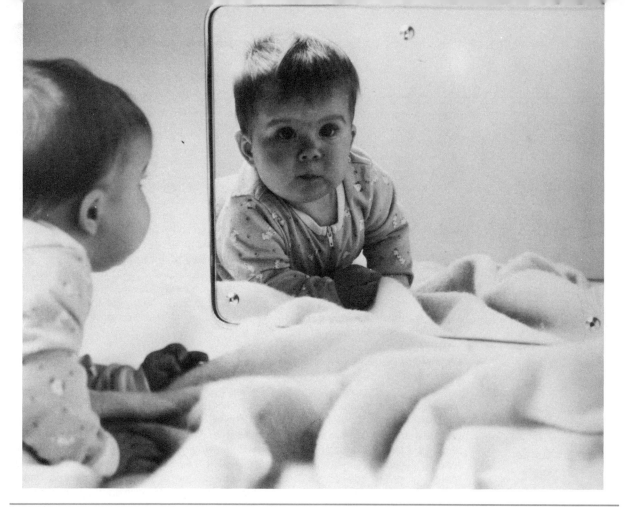

FIGURE 1-10 Researchers are constantly discovering how remarkably competent babies are and are dispelling many of the myths relating to their lack of capacities and abilities.

Life-span Development

Today, instead of viewing life as a series of distinct steps or stages (with some stages being more important and worthy of study than others), we now view as equally important the entire span of life from conception to death. The life span is a continuous flow from beginning to end. Just as the early years of development have been rediscovered, so, too, we realize that life does not end after adolescence or early adulthood.

Renewed Areas of Interest

There is always a tendency to focus on and give more attention to certain periods or stages of development than others. In the past, while particular areas were not completely ignored, they did, however, languish in the backwaters of inattention. Until recently, four of these areas were prenatal life, infancy, adolescence, and late adulthood. They now enjoy top billing as the stars of human development.

A prime candidate for center stage is the prenatal period. While two decades ago the fetal period was viewed as merely a preparation for the outside world, today there is a growing interest in the nature and influences of prenatal experiences and their role in development.

Babies are "in." Research is changing practitioners' and the public's estimation of an infant's abilities. For example, in research relating to habituation (becoming accustomed to a stimulus through frequent repetition), when a baby receives a sight or sound stimulus several times in a row, she usually pays less attention to it each time, indicating she has seen it several times and is less interested in it. When a new stimulus is presented, however, she pays attention, indicating she distinguishes between the two. Habituation studies provide evidence relating to brain and nervous system functioning.

Articles relating to adolescents are popular in newspapers and magazines. Stories about drugs, teenage pregnancies, and school dropouts are but a few topics that have grabbed the nation's attention. While many of these topics are negative in nature, they do call attention to this turbulent period in the life span. For example, peer pressure is considered a powerful influence in adolescent development and efforts are underway to examine how it can be employed in the fight against drug abuse.

America is graying. More people are living longer and are enjoying, rather than fearing, the "senior" years. Today there are twenty-eight million people older than sixty-five, up from eighteen million in 1965. Senior citizens, those sixty-five years old and above, are expected to comprise 20 percent of the population by the year 2000. There is more interest in the process aging and, as a result of research and increased public awareness, we now understand that the period of late adulthood does not automatically doom one to physical and intellectual failure.

Early Learning

There is much emphasis currently on early learning—in determining what infants know and how they come to learn it. At another level, there is much interest in the influences of early learning and the effects of practices that promote early learning. The term "superkid" is used to describe a child who is encouraged to do better earlier. Elkind's (1987) remark, "The pressure to make ordinary children exceptional has become almost

an epidemic in sports" (p. 60), applies equally well to most areas of young children's lives. There will continue to be heated debate in this area, and undoubtedly child development researchers will help provide additional information on which to base decisions about what is best for children.

The "Plasticity" of Child Development

How do early life events influence children's later development? Twenty years ago, it was commonly believed that there was a direct cause-and-effect relationship between children's early life events (including their socioeconomic conditions) and later accomplishments, such as school achievement. Now, rather than rigidly adhering to such a deterministic point of view, most child development practitioners believe children possess a remarkable resiliency that enables them to overcome early negative influences. While our awareness of this plasticity of human development should not be interpreted to mean that we should desire anything but the best for all children, it does nonetheless demonstrate that humans can, with the proper help and support, overcome less-than-ideal influences early in life.

Sociobiology

Why do humans behave as they do? Answers to this and other questions about human behavior are coming from the field of *sociobiology*, which is concerned with the biological and genetic bases of behavior. Sociobiologists hypothesize that human response strategies to certain social situations may have a genetic base, such as the tendency of parents to form attachment bonds with their children. This field is growing and provides much opportunity for exploring the antecedents of human behavior.

Ecological Considerations

Researchers are interested in examining the behavior of children in their natural environments—their home, school, family, and peer group. They are also interested in the influences of these environments on children's behavior. For example, because of current public awareness of child abuse, researchers want to know how families, which are young children's primary environments, contribute to, or insulate children from, abuse.

Social Policy

Many agencies, including local, state, and federal government agencies, develop policy when they react to new legislation, make regulations, and issue directives that influence children and their families. Such policies should be based on principles of child growth and development, the results of research, and the best interests of children and their families. Child advocates are insisting that public policy developers take into consideration evidence from child development research to determine how proposed policies will benefit or harm children and families. Sometimes social policy results when people, agencies, and government decide to do nothing. If an agency fails to make a statement about an issue, overcoming poor infant nutrition, for example, then the agency is expressing a "hands-off" policy.

There are many instances of social policy being implemented through specific legislation. For example, Project Head Start (see chapter nine) is a federally sponsored preschool program designed to assist disadvantaged children with schooling and to assist their families in achieving economic self-sufficiency (Slaughter, Oyemade, Washington, & Lindsey, 1988). Head Start began in the summer of 1965 and continues to serve the needs of about 20 percent of the children that need it.

In 1988 Congress passed Public Law 100-403, which funded the Comprehensive Early Childhood Development Program. This program was designed to establish demonstration projects providing a comprehensive set of supportive services to low-income children from birth to school age, and necessary services for parents and other family members. Also in 1988, Congress, through Public Law 100-435, improved nutritional benefits for

children in the School Breakfast and Child Care Food Program (CCFP). This legislation also authorized that children who are in child care for more than eight hours will be given an extra meal or snack through CCFP.

Two excellent sources for reports regarding social policy and national legislation are: the Children's Defense Fund, 122 C Street, N.W., Washington, D.C., 20004, and the Committee on Child Development and Social Policy of the Society for Research in Child Development, 100 North Carolina Avenue, S.E., Suite 1, Washington, D.C., 20003.

What Would You Do?

The following is an ethical dilemma faced by a researcher involving disclosure of intent. She wants to know how anxiety in pregnant women correlates to prenatal development and complications in childbirth. Several problems can arise if she tells an expectant mother she is studying the relationship of anxiety to pregnancy outcome. First, the discussion about the research topic could have a sensitizing effect on the participants. They could monitor their own emotional states and develop defense mechanisms, making it more difficult for the researcher to determine the influence of anxiety on prenatal development and childbirth. Second, stating the research question may make the participants more anxious. Whatever the participants were anxious about before, the researcher has now given them something else to be anxious about. Third, creating anxiety in the participants could trigger other responses, such as smoking and alcohol intake, which are detrimental to the fetus.

What should the researcher do? What should she disclose to the participants? Turn to the end of the chapter to find out what the researcher did *only* after you have decided what you would do.

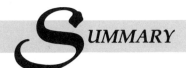

SUMMARY

- Children are alike and yet different in many ways. These similarities and differences make them the unique individuals they are. All who work with children in any capacity must recognize, appreciate, and provide for the individual needs of each child.

- Child development is the sum total of children's physical, cognitive, social, emotional, and behavioral changes. The study of child development involves how children change from conception to adolescence.

- Biological, environmental, and learning processes foster and direct development. These three processes interact to make children unique. Children's growth is influenced positively and negatively during critical periods.

- The study of child development provides for self-insight, learning about others, understanding how children are unique, and preparation for careers. People in many careers use child development information.

- The field of child development is organized in several ways to facilitate study and understanding. The age–stage approach is the most popular and is based on the study of developmental processes during distinct life stages. The topical approach examines developmental processes across the life span. Regardless of which of these two approaches is adopted, the study of child development is also a multidisciplinary effort, with many professions contributing to our knowledge of children. The ecological approach involves an examination of the influence of environments on child development.

- Research helps answer questions about children and is the formal, systematic application of the scientific method to problems or questions. Questions are often stated in the form of hypotheses, which are reasonable, testable statements.

- The research process consists of the following steps: selecting and defining a problem; executing research procedures; analyzing data; and drawing and stating conclusions.

- Researchers use a number of methods to gather age-related data. The longitudinal method gathers data on the same group of children over a period of time. With the cross-sectional method, data is gathered on different groups of children of different ages.

- There are three basic methods for conducting child development research: descriptive, correlational and experimental. Descriptive research gathers information to describe the way things are. Correlational research describes in quantitative terms how variables are related. Researchers use experimental research to explain cause-and-effect relationships. They manipulate an independent variable to test its effect on a dependent variable.

- Readers of research should consider three things in their evaluation of research findings: the method used to disseminate the research; how and what the researcher writes and communicates; and the applicability of the conclusions to other settings.

- All who work and research with children should be guided by the fourteen ethical principles of the Society for Research in Child Development.
- Child development is a dynamic field. Many influences help direct attention and research. Currently, attention is focused on prenatal life, babies, and adolescents. In addition, social policy issues, sociobiology, life-span development, and the influences of environments on behavior are topics of interest.

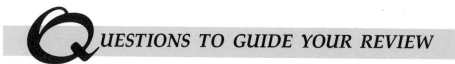

QUESTIONS TO GUIDE YOUR REVIEW

1. How are children alike?
2. How are children different?
3. What is child development?
4. What are the processes that cause likenesses and differences in children?
5. What are the differences between growth and development?
6. What are developmental processes? How do they influence development?
7. What role does risk play in development?
8. What are critical periods and what influences do they have on child development?
9. Why is the study of child development important?
10. What are the similarities and differences between the topical and age–stage approaches to studying child development?
11. What is research?
12. Why is research important?
13. What are the four major steps of the scientific method?
14. What are the differences between longitudinal and cross-sectional research?
15. What are the major purposes of descriptive, correlational, and experimental research?
16. What are important things to consider when analyzing research?
17. What method of research would you use if you wanted to show a cause-and-effect relationship?
18. What method of research would you use to determine parents' preferences for child care?
19. Why is it important to have ethical principles to govern child development research?
20. What are current influences in child development?

*A*CTIVITIES FOR FURTHER INVOLVEMENT

1. As discussed in this chapter, developmental processes are influenced in significant ways by environment factors. Based on interviews with professionals in the field and from your reading in journals and newspapers, list at least five examples of how environment influences development.
2. One purpose of the vignettes in this chapter is to help you see the relationship between child development and everyday life events and career occupations. Interview professionals in order to determine how child development information and knowledge contribute to understanding children in everyday settings and activities.
3. The ecological approach to studying children is gaining wider influence in child development circles. The word *ecology* is derived from the Greek for home or homeland. In this sense, we are interested in observing children's behavior in many different contexts in order to better understand the many influences on child development. Develop an observation form similar to the one shown to gather information about a child's social interactions. Observe one child in different contexts—at home, in school, at the shopping center, on the playground, and so forth.

SOCIAL INTERACTIONS

Child's Name:
Age:
Date:
Time:
Place:

1. Does the child get along with peers? Siblings? Adults?
2. Is the child confident in her/his relations with others?
3. Does the child express himself to others?
4. Does the child participate in activities?
5. What routines does the child follow?

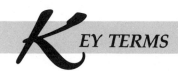

KEY TERMS

Age–stage approach The study of children based on significant developmental processes that occur during distinct life periods.

Child development The sum total of the physical, intellectual, social, emotional, and behavioral changes that occur in children from the moment of conception through the adolescent years.

Cohort group People born in the same year or time period.

Control group The group that does not receive the independent variable or treatment in a research study.

Correlation coefficient A numerical measure of relationship.

Correlational research Describes in quantitative terms how variables are related.

Critical periods Times during development when children are most vulnerable to risk factors.

Cross-sectional study Gathering data *at one time* on different children of different ages.

Dependent variable The variable in a research study that is contingent or dependent on the independent variable, which the researcher controls.

Descriptive research Research that determines and describes the way things are.

Development Increase in skill and complexity of function.

Developmental processes The genetic, biological, environmental, and learning processes that influence children's development.

Ecological approach The study of the effects and influences of environments on development and behavior.

Ethics The principles of conduct that guide the behavior of individuals and groups.

Ethological research The study of animal behavior in natural settings.

Ethology The study of animal behavior.

Experimental method The research method used to test cause-and-effect relationships.

Generational influences The environmental, cultural, and social influences on a generation of people.

Growth The qualitative change in children.

Human development The sum total of the physical, intellectual, social, emotional, and behavioral changes in people from conception to death.

Hypotheses Reasonable, testable statements about what researchers believe their research will reveal.

Independent variable The activity or process that the researcher believes will have a cause-and-effect influence on the dependent variable.

Life-span development Development from conception to death.

Longitudinal study Gathering data on the *same* group of children over a period of time.

Multi-disciplinary Researchers from specific disciplines and areas such as child development, nursing and early childhood are cooperatively researching and working on problems and issues relating to children, youth and families. Also, as professionals from different disciplines cooperate and work together, they share ideas and research methodologies.

Naturalistic observation Observation of behavior in familiar settings, such as in the family and home.

Participant observation Observation of behavior by subjects who are participants in an experiment as observers to help the researchers gather data.

Random assignment Assignment of children to groups so that they all have an equal chance of being assigned to a particular group.

Research The formal, systematic application of the scientific method to the study of problems or questions.

Risk Vulnerabilities children face during development.

Scientific method An objective and orderly process that consists of defining a problem, formulating a hypothesis or educated guess about the outcome of the research, collecting and analyzing data, and making conclusions about verifying or not verifying the hypothesis.

Simulated observation Observation of behavior in a setting and with an activity created by the researcher.

Sociobiology The study of the biological and genetic bases of behavior.

Subject attrition A situation in which subjects leave or drop out of a research project.

Theories Statements about how something happens.

Topical approach The study of topics or processes of development, for example, language development, as they occur from conception through adolescence.

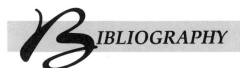

ANSWER TO "WHAT WOULD YOU DO?"

The researcher did not disclose the full intent of her study. She felt that the concerns cited in the dilemma justified her decision. She informed the participants that she was studying feelings and emotions during pregnancy and the role these play in the transition to parenthood.

BIBLIOGRAPHY

Agency for Toxic Substances and Disease Registry (July, 1988). *The nature and extent of lead poisoning in children in the United States: A report to congress July, 1988.* Atlanta, GA: Agency for Toxic Substances and Disease Registry. p. 4.

Ansul, S. E., DiBase, R., & Weintraub, M. (1987, April). *The effects of maternal employment and child sex.* Paper presented at the bienniel meeting of the Society for Research in Child Development, Baltimore, MD.

Baily, W. T. (1987, Spring). On avoiding subject attrition in longitudinal research. *SRCD Newsletter,* p. 2.

Bronfenbrenner, U. (1979). *The ecology of human development.* Cambridge, MA: Harvard University Press.

Capute, A. J., Shapiro, B. K., Wachtel, R. C., Gunther, V. A., & Palmer, F. B. (1986). The clinical linguistic and auditory milestone scale (CLAMS): identification of cognitive defects in motor delayed children. *American Journal of Diseases of Children, 140,* 694–698.

Chaiklin, H., Mosher, B. S. & O'Hara, D. M. (March, 1985). The social and the emotional etiology of childhood lead poisoning. *Journal of sociology and social welfare, XII,* 62–78.

Charlesworth, W. R., (1987, March). *Revision submitted to Council for the Committee for Ethical Conduct in Child Development Research.* Chicago: Society for Research in Child Development. Approved by the Governing Council of SRCD at the Biennial Meeting of the SRCD. Kansas City, April 1989.

Charlesworth, W. R., & Dzur, C. (1987). Gender comparisons of preschool behavior and resource utilization in group problem solving. *Child Development, 58,* 192.

Child development: Language takes on new significance, (1987, May 5). *The New York Times,* p. 23.

Colombo, J. (1982). The critical period concept: Research methodology and research issues. *Psychological Bulletin, 81,* 260–275.

Corsini, R. J. (Ed.). (1984). *Encyclopedia of Psychology* (Vol. 2). New York: John Wiley & Sons.

Elkind, D. (1987, May). Superkids and super problems. *Psychology Today,* p. 60.

Fabrizi, M. S., & Pollo, H. R. (1987). A naturalistic study of humorous activity in a third, seventh, and eleventh grade classroom. *Merrill-Palmer Quarterly, 33,* 107–128.

Field, D. E. (1987, April). *Television coviewing related to family characteristics and cognitive performance.* Paper presented at the bienniel meeting of the Society for Research in Child Development, Baltimore, MD.

Gay, L. R., (1987) *Educational research: Competencies for analysis and application,* Columbus, OH: Merrill.

Lowery, G. H., (1986). *Growth and development of children* (8th ed.) Chicago: Year Book Medical.

McMillan, J. H. & Schumacher, S. (1984). *Research in education: a conceptual approach.* Boston: Little, Brown & Co.

Murray, P. (1987, April). *Infants' responsiveness to modeling vs. instruction.* Paper presented at the biennial meeting of the Society for Research in Child Development, Baltimore, MD.

Salkind, N. J. (1985). *Theories of human development.* New York: John Wiley & Sons, p. 6.

Sameroff, A. J., Seifer, R., Baldwin, C., & Baldwin, A. (1989, April). *Continuity of risk from early childhood to adolescence.* Paper presented at the biennial meeting of the Society for Research in Child Development, Kansas City, MO.

Schweinhart, L. J., & Weikart, D. P. (1985). Evidence that good early childhood programs work. *Phi Delta Kappan, 66,* 545–548.

Slaughter, D., Oyemade, U. J., Washington, V. & Lindsey, R. W., (1988, Summer). Head Start: A backward and forward look. *Social Policy Report: Society for Research in Child Development,* 1–19.

CHAPTER TWO

Theories of development

◆

VIGNETTES

INTRODUCTION

THEORIES OF DEVELOPMENT

What are Theories of
  Development?

Why are Theories Important?

Stage and Nonstage Explanations
  of Development

SIGMUND FREUD AND
  PSYCHOANALYTIC THEORY

Basic Theory

Development of Personality Traits

Defense Mechanisms

Criticisms and Controversies
  Relating to Freudian Theory

Implications for Parents and
  Professionals: Meeting the Needs

of the Sensual Child

In the Spotlight: Permissive
  Parenting

Freud in the Depth of Childhood

ERIK ERIKSON AND
  PSYCHOSOCIAL THEORY

Psychosocial Theory

The Stages of Psychosocial
  Development

Implications for Parents and
  Professionals

Strengths and Weaknesses of
  Erikson's Psychosocial Theory

THE COGNITIVE
  DEVELOPMENT THEORY OF
  JEAN PIAGET

Piaget's Clinical Method

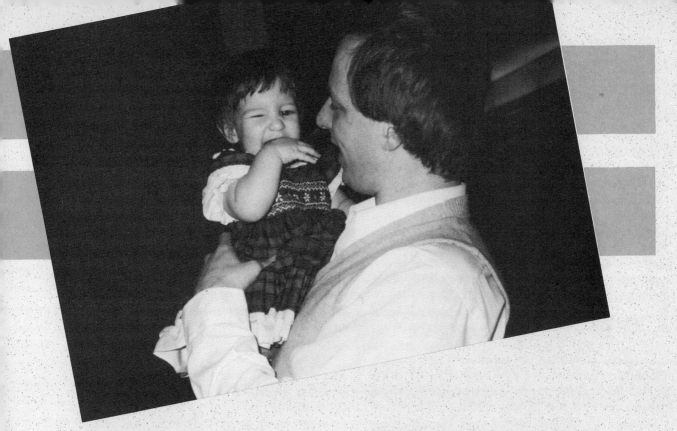

The Cognitive Development
  Theory
Equilibrium
Constructivism and Activity
Stages of Development
Strengths and Weaknesses of
  Piaget
SKINNER AND BEHAVIORISM
How to Keep a Room Clean
Skinner and Operant Conditioning
Skinner and "Teaching Machines"
The Baby-Tender
Basic Behaviorist Principles
A Glossary of Behaviorist Terms
Social Learning Theory
Advantages and Disadvantages of
  Behaviorism

MASLOW AND HUMANISTIC
  THEORY
The Hierarchy of Needs
Implications of Humanism
Strengths and Weaknesses of
  Humanism
What Would You Do?
SUMMARY
QUESTIONS TO GUIDE YOUR
  REVIEW
ACTIVITIES FOR FURTHER
  INVOLVEMENT
KEY TERMS
ENRICHMENT THROUGH
  FURTHER READING
ANSWER TO "WHAT WOULD
  YOU DO?"
BIBLIOGRAPHY

⏼IGNETTES

Two-year-old Heidi Kohl is standing in her front yard with her legs tightly crossed. Although it is difficult to stand this way, on the sides of her small feet, Heidi is determined that she is not going to let go of anything. Her face is contorted into a slit-eyed grimace and is red from the effort. A sheen of perspiration covers her forehead and cheeks. Heidi is showing remarkable determination. She has been standing this way for twenty minutes, emitting occasional grunts, whines, and groans.

While Heidi is engaged in her private battle with inner forces, her neighborhood playmates go about their games and activities as though nothing is wrong, seemingly unconcerned about her determined efforts to keep her feces to herself. When Heidi first started crossing her legs, her playmates found her behavior both puzzling and amusing. They would ask their mothers, "Why does Heidi cross her legs like that?," to which they would get an answer something like, "She's having trouble going to the bathroom." Some children still mimic Heidi's behaviors as a means of indicating that another child is stupid or clumsy.

Heidi's parents are very concerned about her behavior and have taken her to a series of pediatricians in order to find out what her problem is. Although they wish they didn't have to deal with what is frequently an embarrassing situation for the entire family, and feeling that they are a little old to have to go through the stresses and strains of child rearing again (Heidi was a "surprise baby") they nonetheless hope that they can find help and a solution to Heidi's problem. A new pediatrician, finding nothing physically wrong with Heidi, has advised the Kohls to make an appointment with Hans Duerf, a respected psychiatrist who specializes in children's psychological problems.

As an infant care-giver at Holy Cross Child Care Center, Silvia LaVilla knows there is more to taking care of infants than merely meeting their physical needs. Silvia believes that social development begins at birth and that she and the parents are the means by which infants will come to know about the world and themselves.

Silvia gives much of the credit for her success as a care-giver to Professor Amy Noskire at P. S. Segats Community College. In her child development classes, Professor Noskire emphasized the importance of providing for children's individual needs within a trusted framework of their cultural life-styles. Silvia tries to put into practice ways to make the infants feel good about her and themselves. She believes that care-givers like her are critical environmental influences in children's lives as they develop their unique personalities.

Also, Silvia knows that careful planning and adherence to daily routines makes the infants she cares for physically secure and, as a result, they will come to trust her and the world in which they are growing. Silvia believes that developing trust in "her babies" is an essential part of their development, and the means by which they will develop a positive and healthy self-esteem. Silvia makes a point of seeing to it that they can trust her for safe, sensitive, consistent, and loving care. She uses a pleasing, warm tone of voice with the infants, and she is often seen smiling and heard giggling, cooing, and talking with the children.

Ricky Gordon teaches children with special needs at Walden Elementary School. Three-year-old Reba has just been assigned to Ricky's classroom. Reba is mentally retarded and is lagging in her social development. After a few days of close observation, Ricky also believes that Reba is behind other children in her play behaviors. She interacts very little with the other children and does not seem to know how to play with toys. From her classes at the university and her past experience with other special-needs children, Ricky knows that one reason for the developmental delay in Reba's play skills is the close relationship between play and cognitive development.

In order to be sure about her initial observations, Ricky uses an observation form and, for several days, gathers data regarding Reba's play behavior. When Ricky gives Reba toys to play with, Reba seldom manipulates them, and when she does, she does so at a rudimentary level by putting them in her mouth. Reba believes that one way to begin to help Reba's cognitive and social development is to teach her how to play. Specifically, she decides to teach Reba how to play with toys.

However, in order to be certain about her observations and plans, Ricky has a meeting with Fred Renniks, the school psychologist. He concurs with Ricky's observations and agrees with her plan for teaching Reba how to play with toys. In her plan, Ricky will first try modeling child/toy interactions. She will first pick up a rattle toy, shake it and say "Oh, my goodness! It shakes and makes noise!" This may be enough stimulus to get Reba to begin playing. When she does play with the toy, Ricky will use positive reinforcement such as praise to promote the desired responses. If this method of teaching Reba how to play does not work, Ricky will next try a program of partial physical assist, using prompts. Regardless, Ricky knows that with time and the appropriate reinforcements, Reba will learn to play with toys and that, as a result, this will enhance Reba's social and cognitive skills.

When Debbie was perhaps nine months old, I was holding her in my lap. The room grew dark, and I turned on a table lamp beside the chair. She smiled brightly, and it occurred to me that I could use the light as a reinforcer. I turned it off and waited. When she lifted her left hand slightly, I quickly turned the light on and off. Almost immediately she lifted her hand again, and I turned the light on and off again. In a few moments she was lifting her arm in a wide arc "to turn on the light." She had behaved as our pigeon had behaved that day in the flour mill, and I was amazed. But, why should I have been? If I had put a rattle in her hand, and she had moved it slightly, and heard the noise, I should not have been at all surprised if she had then shaken it vigorously. But there was a difference. The contingencies which reinforced rattle-shaking were built into the rattle. I had contrived my contingencies, and their effect was therefore surprisingly conspicuous (Skinner, 1979, p.293).

THEORIES OF DEVELOPMENT
What Are Theories of Development?

People develop theories to explain and answer questions relating to what, how, when, where, and why of human existence. We can credit much of our understanding about our world and life around us to those who develop theories. There is a "black hole" theory to explain the beginnings of the universe; a theory of relativity to explain the enigmas of energy; and there are theories to explain how children grow and develop.

A *theory* is a systematic set of statements and assumptions about relationships, principles, and data designed to explain and predict behavior and events. Theories are the raw material, the essential building blocks necessary for understanding how children grow and develop, and for making decisions about how to support and enhance that development. Researchers use theories as a starting point to develop hypotheses (tentative explanations of behavior) and conduct research. Research data helps theorists and others support, revise, enrich, and expand theories. Theories are not, as they say in the popular vernacular, engraved in stone, and should not be viewed as permanent and unchanging. They are revised and changed over time as a result of new data, fresh insights, and research.

WHY ARE THEORIES IMPORTANT?

Theories serve several important functions. First, they explain past and present behavior and they predict future behavior. Second, they contribute direction and insight for making decisions about how to rear, educate, and care for children. Third, they serve as the theoretical framework for social policy, legislation, and agency decisions. Fourth, they act as a source of inspiration and a catalyst for other researchers who want to test concepts of the theory and explore its implications and applications. Piaget's theory, for example, spawned over 2,000 related studies between 1950 and 1980 (Cohen, 1983, p. 5).

Stage and Nonstage Explanations of Development

If a new parent asked you to explain her baby's growth and development, what would you say? You could frame your response in one of two ways. You could stress the *continuity* of her baby's development and explain it as a continual and gradual process. Language acquisition, as depicted in Table 1–1, could be explained as a gradual and cumulative process with few sudden changes. This *nonstage theory* depicts development as an additive and accumulative process. New development is merely an improved version of previous development. According to the nonstage view, development at any point of life is the sum of the development that preceded it. Most behaviorists ascribe to the nonstage theory and believe development is the sum total of learning experiences.

TABLE 2–1

MAJOR DEVELOPMENTAL THEORIES AND THE AREAS ADDRESSED		
Theorist	School	Theory Deals With
Sigmund Freud	Psychoanalytic	Psychoanalytic/ psychosexual development
Erik H. Erikson	Psychoanalytic	Psychoanalytic/ psychosocial development
Jean Piaget	Cognitive	Cognitive/ intellectual development
B. F. Skinner	Behavioral	General learning
Albert Bandura	Behavioral	Social learning
Abraham Maslow	Humanistic	Motivational/ psychosocial development

Stage theory is another, more popular way of explaining child growth and development. Stage theory is based on the premise that growth and development consist of discrete and recognizable stages, with development in one stage different and distinct from development in a previous stage. In this sense, stage theory emphasizes the discontinuity inherent in development. A four-year-old thinker, for example, is more than just an improved version of a two-year-old thinker. The four-year-old can and does think in ways that are not explained solely on the basis of simple improvements upon how she thought as a two-year-old. Her thinking is *qualitatively* different and results from new forms of development. Although Table 1–1 can be used to support the nonstage explanation of language development, you can also with more confidence use Table 1–1 to illustrate stages of language development. You can point out to the parent such milestones as the first use of "da-da"

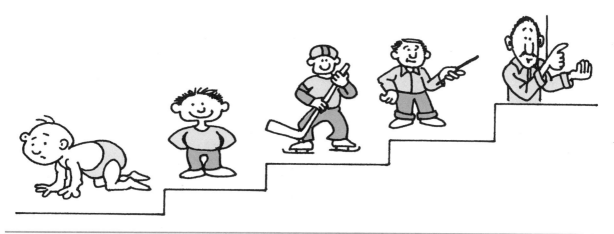

FIGURE 2-1 Stage theory holds that all children progress through the same stages of development in the same sequence.

and "ma-ma," the first word, and the first sentence.

Stage theory, like nonstage theory, depicts development as linear and logically progressive. However, later stages of development are more complex than earlier stages, as shown in Figure 2–1. Accomplishments of later stages, the ability to think logically, for example, depend on the nature of development in previous stages.

Stage theory portrays *all* children progressing through the same stages of development in the same, invariant sequence. Although the ages at which individual children exhibit the developmental characteristics of particular stages may vary, children do not skip stages. An infant does not skip a stage of cognitive development and suddenly start thinking like a preschooler, nor does a two-year-old get up one morning and ask, "What's for breakfast?"

The stage view is the most popular and generally accepted approach to child growth and development used today. This textbook reflects such an approach, and the majority of our discussions use stage theories to explain development. Not all developmentalists agree that such an approach is a good idea. They caution against compartmentalizing children into stages and ignoring or overlooking the continuity of development.

Common Features of Stage and Nonstage Theories All developmental theories, regardless of whether they are stage or nonstage, maintain that certain *functional invariants* operate at all ages. These invariants are like a recurring theme in a song, which continually restates a melody and gives form and substance to the composition. Sigmund Freud, for example, believed pleasure-seeking forms the basis for much of human behavior. Jean Piaget stresses activity as a functional invariant in developing intelligence. Behaviorists emphasize environmental stimuli as the sources of learning. We will examine more of these functional invariants as we discuss individual developmental theories.

It may be helpful to keep in mind that a specific theory generally addresses a specific area of development (see Table 2–1). Although you may hear someone refer to Piaget's theory of child development, such a statement is not accurate. Piaget's theory relates to cognitive development, although it has implications for all areas of development. We must avoid making a theory apply to a developmental area to which it is not applicable.

Also, keep in mind that children are integrated beings. They are not compartmentalized or made up of separate developing areas. The intellectual capacities of a child do not function separately from the social-emotional aspects. The sum total of children's development in all areas is greater than the mere additive sum of their development in each particular area.

SIGMUND FREUD AND PSYCHOANALYTIC THEORY

Sigmund Freud (1856–1939) lived in Vienna, Austria almost all his life. He was the eldest of seven children and the indisputable favorite of his mother (Jones, 1961, p. ix). It seems plausible that growing up the eldest and favored son in a large family made Freud especially aware of the intri-

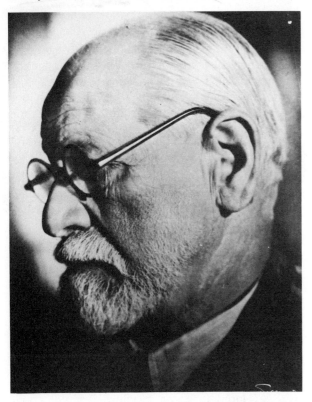

FIGURE 2-2   Sigmund Freud developed the psychoanalytic theory which has a powerful influence on our views of how children develop. (Photo courtesy of the Bettmann Archive)

cacies of family relationships and these impressions and insights influenced his theory. At age seventeen, Freud entered the University of Vienna to pursue a medical career.

Freud's theory of personality and psychosexual development is based on the ideas that humans are governed and, indeed, driven in their daily actions and behaviors by influential emotional and sexual impulses hidden in the subconscious. These impulses frequently trigger physical and emotional symptoms interpreted as hysteria and other mental disorders. Freud discovered that the way to help individuals was to have them lie on a couch and talk about whatever came to their mind. Such "free associations" relaxed their conscious censoring and revealed past memories, fears, desires, and hidden, unconscious sexual desires.

Freud also developed the idea of *infantile sexuality*, which maintains that beginning about age one, children have sexual desires and fantasies. This belief is attributed in part to Freud's own self-analysis, through which "he discovered in himself the passion for his mother and jealousy of his father; he felt sure this was a general human characteristic. . . ." (Jones, 1961, pp. 227–228).

Basic Theory

Freud believed that *libido* (general sexual or psychic energy) is the driving force in people's lives. The *id* of the human psyche (psychological structure), including the conscious and unconscious, controls this sexual energy and releases it through instinctual impulses, innate drives, reflexes, and impulses. The id's job is to bring immediate satisfaction, primarily through the *erogenous zones* of the mouth, anus, and genital organs. This constant drive for pleasure—known as the *pleasure principle*—is a basic operational characteristic and is a continuous theme throughout human development. Children derive much pleasure from oral gratification (sucking and eating), elimination of body wastes, and masturbation. Indeed, Freud called the mouth "the oral sexual organ." Likewise, adults also derive much erogenous plea-

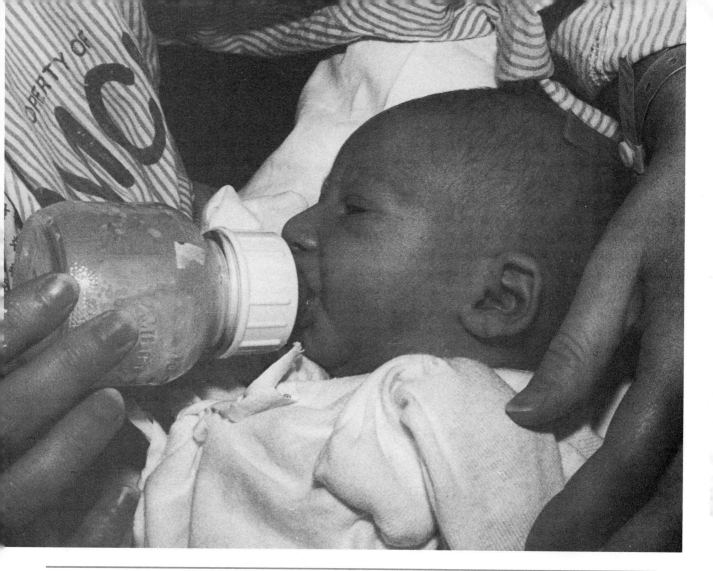

FIGURE 2-3 During the oral stage of psycho-sexual development and the sensorimotor stage of cognitive development the infant enjoys sucking on bottles, rattles, and other objects.

sure from eating, smoking, chewing gum, sucking on candy and pipes, sexual relations, and other sensual experiences. In fact, many popular self-help books, such as *The Joy of Sex* and *The Art of Sensual Massage*, are designed to help people maximize erotic, sensual, and psychic pleasure in socially acceptable and non-guilt-producing ways.

As you know, however, life is not one continuous journey devoted to bacchanalian delights. Constant pleasure-seeking is brought under control by the *ego* (Latin word for "I"). The ego brings as much pleasure as possible while controlling behavior within the boundaries of societal norms, the realities of everyday living, and the constraints of what is considered right and wrong. This restraining process is called the *reality principle*.

According to Freud, children are *amoral*, that is, they have no knowledge of right or wrong, good or evil. Parents have the responsibility for helping children learn right from wrong and de-

TABLE 2–2

	FREUD'S STAGES OF PERSONALITY DEVELOPMENT	
Stage	Age	Resolutions
Oral Much of the child's gratification comes orally.	Birth through one year	Gratification of oral pleasure; development of warm, loving relationships with care-givers. How parents satisfy their children's needs through feeding and weaning are important considerations.
Anal Attention on anal area.	Two to three	Toilet training; meeting with parents' demands for control of elimination and cleanliness. It is critical for parents to demonstrate love, support, and reassurance during this stage.
Phallic or Oedipal (Infantile– Genital) Attention on genital areas.	Three to four	Pleasure comes from playing with sex organs—penis, clitoris and vulva—and masturbation. Resolution of the Oedipal conflict, sex-role development and moral development usually occurs through repression of sexual desire for opposite-sex parent and identification with same-sex parent.
Latency Sexual and aggressive fantasies are now latent.	Five to thirteen (beginning of puberty)	Control of sexual thoughts and desires; continued solving of the Oedipus and Electra conflicts. Physical and psychic energies are directed to physical and intellectual achievements.
Mature Genital Freedom from parents; leaving home.	Twelve or thirteen to eighteen (adolescence)	Freedom from parents and leaving home. Continued resolution of Oedipus and Electra complexes; involvement in heterosexual activity within the limits of societal taboos and restrictions.

veloping a moral system that will assist them in governing their actions. Between the ages of four and five, the *superego* develops and becomes the child's conscience of what is right or wrong. Feelings of guilt, shame, and punishment originate from the operation of the superego. Daily living, then, is a constant tension between the id on the one hand, demanding pleasure and gratification, and the superego on the other hand, demanding rigid obedience to a moral standard of what is right or wrong. The ego mediates between these two. The result of this mediation enables children and adolescents to have pleasure in socially acceptable and approved ways. Yet, the pressure from society and peers may cause them to participate in activities their moral code says they shouldn't, such as shoplifting, premarital sex, and drug abuse. When this happens, depending on the strength of the superego and the moral system it enforces, feelings of guilt can manifest themselves in a number of ways. Transgressors may need to talk to a guidance counselor or other person, may have nightmares, and may live with a fear of being caught and punished.

According to Freudian theory, personality development progresses through a series of psychosocial stages. How children learn to expend libido during each stage determines their personality, including the nature and kind of adult *neuroses*, which are functional disorders of the mind and emotions, such as anxieties and phobias.

The five developmental stages as conceived by Freud are shown in Table 2–2. The ages at which children progress through these *qualitatively* different stages are not exactly fixed and vary from child to child. Also, a child is not entirely in one stage or another at any one time. It is likely that a child will be in several stages at one time with one stage predominating. Freud (1973) stated that "It would be a mistake to suppose that these three phases (oral, anal, and genital) succeeded each other in clear fashion. One may appear in addition to another; they may overlap one another, may be present alongside one another" (p. 12).

Oral Stage   During the *oral stage*, physical and psychic energy is directed toward gaining gratification through the mouth. Remember, Freud called the mouth "the oral sexual organ." The child achieves pleasure by sucking everything—breast, bottle, thumb, pacifier, blanket—and orally investigating anything put in or placed near her mouth. Oral and instant gratification of all physical needs plays a major role in the child's life. Loving, attentive, and consistent care-givers help children learn to delay gratification of their needs and communicate their needs in socially acceptable ways. Care-givers can help make weaning a pleasurable, nontraumatic experience. Freud believed weaning and feeding play critical roles in children's physical and psychic lives.

Anal Stage   The anal stage begins at age two and lasts until age three. Toilet training is a major developmental task of this period. A child, used to eliminating when and wherever he pleases, now finds that others participate in making these decisions. With assistance and guidance from parents or other care-givers, he must learn how to control bowels and bladder. Freud believed that personality characteristics are determined by how parents and others treat children during this process. Rigid demands for cleanliness, for example, may result in overattention to cleanliness as an adult.

Phallic Stage   The *phallic* or *infantile–genital* period occurs between ages three and four. Children's pleasure focuses on the genital areas of the penis, clitoris, and vulva. During this period, the male is sexually attracted to his mother. This sexual desire of a male child for his mother is termed the *Oedipus complex*. (In Greek legend, Oedipus, unaware of his relationship to his parents, killed his father and married his mother.) The father prevents the child from fulfilling his sexual desires and this is the psychosocial conflict that must be resolved.

A female likewise develops a sexual attraction for her father and competes with the mother for his affections. This is known as the *Electra complex*. (In Greek legend, Electra persuaded her brother to kill their mother and her lover, who had previously killed their father.)

This critical phallic stage involves the beginning of the development of appropriate sex-role identification and the emergence of the superego as a means of helping control sexual urges. Resolution occurs when children reject their sexual feelings for the opposite parent and identify with the parent of the same sex. Freud believed that resolution of the phallic stage is different for males and females. A male utilizes a process of identification, whereby he literally becomes like his father, adopting his mannerisms and ethical code of what is right and wrong.

Freud thought the first step in the resolution of the phallic phase for females occurs through *penis envy*, when they discover they do not have a penis. Normal female development occurs when a girl substitutes her desire for a penis with a desire for a child. Her father becomes the love object and the mother becomes the object of her jealousy. Freud believed that the ultimate satisfaction of a child's desire occurs much later with the birth of a son and the long-desired penis.

Latency Period   The *latency period* begins at about age five and lasts until about age twelve. During this period, children suppress their sexual urges and tend to act as though the opposite sex does not exist. Preference for playing almost exclusively with members of the same sex is a sign of children's efforts to control sexual thoughts.

Mature Genital Period   The *mature genital* period is the final stage of Freud's psychosexual stages of development and extends from puberty (beginning at about age twelve) and continues through adolescence (to about age eighteen). This period is characterized by the increased growth of sexual organs and related physical features that distinguish males and females. Pleasure gratification revolves around the mature sex organs. Adolescents are faced with the developmental dilemma of how to satisfy or control sexual urges in socially accepted and approved ways. This, as you know, is not an easy task and is fraught with uncertainty and guilt. Teenagers must resolve their sexual desires within the framework of what is parentally, religiously, socially, and, now with the AIDS epidemic, medically sanctioned.

Development of Personality Traits

Freudians believe that the ways in which children and adolescents resolve the crises of each developmental stage influence adult personality traits. Failure to resolve a particular developmental task can result in *fixation*, characterized by adults who satisfy needs in childish or inappropriate ways characteristic of a particular stage. An adult who seeks oral gratification through cigarette and pipe smoking, gum chewing, and nail biting, for example, may be fixated in the oral stage. Stinginess with emotional responses and physical possessions may indicate anal stage fixation. Some theorists believe that homosexuality has its beginnings in the phallic stage and that inappropriate patterns of interpersonal relationships, especially with members of the opposite sex, have their roots in the latency period.

Defense Mechanisms

The growth of the superego during the mature genital period determines the extent and nature of the *defense* or *adjustment mechanisms* individuals use throughout life. These defense mechanisms originate in the ego, whose job it is to manage the conflicts that arise between the id and the superego. Some of the more often used and recognized defense behaviors follow.

1. *Regression* is a return to childhood behaviors. A child who has a new sister may feel threatened by a perceived loss of his parents' love and regress to the anal stage and subsequent bedwetting. Regression to the oral stage is quite common on the part of children and adults, characterized by thumb sucking, placing objects in the mouth, and overeating.
2. *Repression* occurs when an experience is so painful or upsetting that the child forgets it ever happened. For example, a child who is sexually abused by a parent or relative may forget the incident or incidents and deny any molestation by others.
3. *Rationalization* is the overexplanation and justification of actions and decisions, so that the real motive is replaced by an alternative—usually a more pleasurable and less demanding motive. You have heard the com-

mercial, "You deserve a break today." This is an example of rationalization. A teen-ager, rather than staying home and finishing her final term report, rationalizes and says it is good enough as it is and gives in to the pleas of her friends to join them in partying. "After all," she says, "I've earned the right to have some fun."

4. *Sublimation* is the diverting of sexual energies to socially accepted activities, such as athletics. A teen-ager, for example, may channel his sexual energy and desires into developing his body through weight-lifting.

5. *Projection* is attributing to others the feelings a person denies exist in her. A sixth grader, who is stingy with her possessions, complains that her friend Nancy is selfish because she will not share her new cosmetics.

Freudians believe these and other defense mechanisms, designed to defend the personality from hurt and harm, are used by the majority of children and adults to resolve problems of adjustment that occur in the give and take of everyday living.

Criticisms and Controversies Relating to Freudian Theory

Although Freud's theory is not quite as popular now as it was several decades ago, there is nonetheless a noticeable renewal of interest in Freudian ideas. Critics find a number of faults with Freud's theory. First, it does not lend itself to scientific testing, which causes difficulty in replicating and confirming his conclusions through empirical research. Second, many case studies from which Freud formulated his theories were based on his clients' remembrances of their past experiences. This retrospection, or looking back, is not an ideal method for gathering data. People forget, exaggerate their experiences, and tend to recall only selected events. Third, people are reared in different societies and cultures, and these influence personality development and adjustment. Freudian

critics are quick to point out that life and experiences in nineteenth- and early twentieth-century Vienna were quite different from how life is now in the United States and other countries in the last decade of the twentieth century.

Many feminists find Freud's theory objectional because of his belief that female personality development centers around penis deprivation and envy. They contend that this view encourages inferior roles for women based on a male standard of masculinity, the penis. Many women believe they should not be reared under or judged by a theory that does not adequately account for their biological uniqueness. Consequently, Freud's theory is perceived as suppressive of female development and part of a male conspiracy to perpetuate the inferior status of women.

Implications for Parents and Professionals: Meeting the Needs of the Sensual Child

Freudian theory is deeply ingrained in the hearts and minds of many parents and professionals and exerts considerable influence in their daily interactions with children, often without their being fully aware of it.

1. Freud's views of children focus attention on the importance of the early years. Childhood experiences are seen as critical determinants in the process of human development. The interactions between parents and children are instrumental in forging and molding personality development. What children are like and what they will be like as teenagers and adults is based in large measure on how parents help them in their resolution of the conflicts associated with each psychosexual stage.

2. Many daily acts of child rearing have implications for parents from a Freudian perspective. The current interest in baby massage illustrates how parents believe that the sensual satisfaction of infants soothes the muscles as well as the psyche.

*I*N THE SPOTLIGHT

PERMISSIVE PARENTING

Freudian theory was and is widely applied to child-rearing practices. Freud taught that the essential foundations of personality are constructed by age three, and that later life events can modify, but not alter, the traits established (Jones, 1961, p. 13). This explains, in part, why Freudians ascribe critical importance to the nature and kind of encounters between parent and child. One of the basic and persistent practices resulting from this application is the advice to parents to refrain as much as possible from creating traumatic experiences in their children that might arrest or interfere with their developmental progression through the psychosexual stages. This belief maintains that when development is arrested or interfered with, the foundation is laid for later behavior and personality disorders. The result is *permissive parenting,* in which parents pursue a *laissez-faire* attitude toward their children and let them do pretty much as they want. Permissive parenting consists of a cluster of four parental behaviors:

1. The ideological belief that it is "right" for children to display their feelings and emotions. This belief, however, can lead to frustration with children's behavior and can result in harsh punishment.
2. Inattention.
3. Indifference.
4. Nonintervention in children's affairs because of tiredness, depression, or preoccupation (Maccoby & Martin, 1983, p. 39).

Parents further justify their noninvolvement on the basis that they don't want to traumatize their children.

The results of such parenting are several. Children of permissive parents are immature and their behavior is characterized by a lack of impulse control, self-reliance, independence, and social responsibility (Baumrind, 1971).

Permissive parents are likewise influenced by their adopted parenting style. First, permissive parents are always tentative and cautious in their relationships with their children and when discipline happens, the parents feel "guilty." They also worry about the past and future implications of their parenting behavior. They speculate how a child's present inappropriate behavior may be rooted in a particular past parent-child encounter that they mishandled in some unknown way. Or they second-guess themselves and say "Well, I suppose that I've done something I may be sorry for later on."

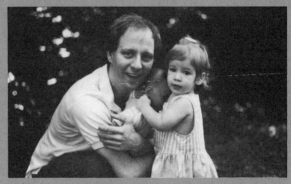

FIGURE 2-4 Parent-child interactions, although happy and placid to outward appearance, may be the root causes of future conflicts.

Second, children can add to their parents' guilt later in life by saying such things as, "I am like I am because of you." Parents are thus caught between their own acts and the recriminations of their children. Guilt plays a very large role in Freud's view of development.

Third, permissive parenting frequently results in unruly and ungovernable children. Most parents sooner or later discover, often to their chagrin, that children left to their own devices do not develop the strong superego they need to help govern their behavior.

The beginning of what is known as *teething* (the eruption of the deciduous or primary teeth) occurs in the oral stage. The first teeth, the lower central incisors, erupt at between six and eight months. This period begins a difficult time in the child's life as well as that of the parents. Oral gratification and comfort are a primary way parents can assist their children in resolving the trauma of the oral stage.

Freud in the Depth of Childhood

Life and contemporary culture abound with Freudian ideas, symbolism, and suggestions. The following passage from Kenneth Lynn's (1987) biography of Ernest Hemingway illustrates the influence Freudian themes play in the analysis of the life and contributions of great people, including this Nobel laureate.

At Walloon Lake in 1900, the summer of Ernest's first birthday, he and Marcelline [His sister, eighteen months older] had played naked on the beach in front of their parents' newly completed cottage. Dr. Hemingway's snapshots of them in the buff, duly pasted into scrapbooks by Grace, [Ernest's and Marcelline's mother] are charming. But while splashing his feet in the water and exploring the rowboat pulled up on the shore, it can be presumed that Ernest had ample opportunity to notice—if he had not done so already—that he and his sister were not built identically.

Did the infant boy take pride in the equipment that set him apart from Marcelline? Or did the sight of her smoothness make him think that she had suffered some sort of dreadful accident which might soon befall him as well? Or were pride and fear intermingled in his turbulent imagination? Familiar Freudian speculations these, which acquire extra force in this case because Ernest would soon become aware that he and Marcelline were being treated like twins of the same sex. And in years to come, the horrific image of phallic loss would be made light of by Hemingway in jokes about such matters as the hazards of skiing in subzero temperatures, dealt with seriously in two anguishing works of fiction, ''God Rest You Merry, Gentlemen'' and *The Sun Also Rises* (p. 53).

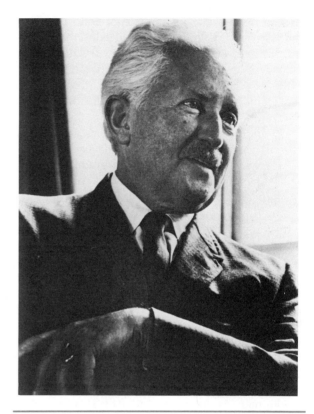

FIGURE 2-5 Erik Erickson used Freud's theory to develop his theory of psycho-social development. (Photo courtesy of the Bettmann Archive)

ERIK ERIKSON AND PSYCHOSOCIAL THEORY

When Erik Erikson (1902–   ) graduated from high school at eighteen, he wandered throughout Europe for a year before deciding to study art (Coles, 1970, p. 14). Erikson finally decided, however, that formal schooling was not for him, so he traveled to Florence, Italy to immerse himself in the rich Renaissance tradition. While there, he received a letter from his high school friend Peter Blos, who offered him a job teaching art at his school in Vienna. Erikson accepted the offer. The life of the free-spirited, wandering artist changed dramatically, and so began a significant turning point in his life and in the field of child development as well. Erikson was introduced to the Freuds and, in time, was invited to begin psychoanalytic training with Anna Freud as his analyst. A tenet of the psychoanalytic movement is that anyone who wants to be an analyst must be thoroughly analyzed.

In addition to undergoing analysis with Anna, Erikson began psychoanalytic study and Montessori teacher training. In 1931, he graduated from the Vienna Psychoanalytic Society and moved with his wife and two children to Boston where he became the city's only child analyst. In his practice he treated children from a wide spectrum of various backgrounds: well-to-do professional families, children of poverty, and young delinquents. At first, Erikson found it difficult to work with children who were not typically middle-class psychoanalytic fare. Over time, however, he discovered behind children's very different exteriors the hopes and fears common to all children. Building on his psychoanalytic foundation, Erikson added to his theory the contributions and influences of society in shaping human behavior. For Erikson, psychosocial development is largely a matter of identity—with parents, family, neighbors, and culture.

Psychosocial Theory

Psychosocial or personality development, according to Erikson, results from the interplay between maturational processes, biological needs, and the social forces of everyday life. Erikson theorizes eight qualitatively different stages in psychosocial development. (See Table 2–3.) These stages are governed by underlying maturational forces, and each stage confronts individuals with a conflict between their biological *needs* and social demands. Such conflict must be resolved before individuals can progress to the next stage of development.

Erikson believes the ego mediates and shapes development through the eight stages. In one sense, Erikson views the ego in much the same way as Freud, as the executor of realistic behavior and the intermediary between the primitive urges of the id and the societal mores of the superego. Additionally, however, Erikson believes the ego is present at birth and is the place where developmental crises are resolved. Favorable resolution of identity crises at each stage facilitates resolution and "normal development" at later stages across the life span. Erikson describes an *ego crisis* or basic conflict that individuals experience during each developmental stage. The conflict or crisis must be successfully resolved, enabling a positive quality, for example, trust rather than mistrust, to be incorporated into personality. Ideally each individual resolves conflicts with a minimum of crisis, resulting in a positive ego state.

The Stages of Psychosocial Development

Stage 1—Oral-sensory: Basic Trust vs. Mistrust (Birth to Eighteen Months) During this stage children learn to trust the world. This is possible when, according to Erikson (1963), "one has learned to rely on the sameness and continuity of the outer providers, but also that one may trust oneself and the capacity of one's own organs to cope with urges" (p. 248). A key to the development of trust in the wonderful process of growing in the first year-and-a-half of life depends on the "sensitive care of the baby's individual needs and a firm sense of personal trustworthiness within the trusted framework of their culture's lifestyle" (p. 248). While for Erikson the mouth is a primary "zone" charged with significance in meeting children's basic nutritional and psychological needs, the total process of development in a particular child-rearing context is also important. Care-givers and parents must provide an environment and relationships characterized by love, warmth, and support so that children can learn trust. An added advantage of such an environment of trusting and being trusted is that, "One may say (somewhat mystically, to be sure) that in thus *getting what is given*, and in learning to *get somebody to do* for him what he wishes to have done, the baby also

TABLE 2–3

ERIK ERIKSON'S EIGHT AGES OF MAN				
Stage	Approximate Ages	Developmental Task— Resolution of Psychological Conflict	Care-giver Tasks/Roles	Intended Outcome
1. Oral-Sensory (similar to Freud's oral stage)	Birth to eighteen months	Basic trust vs. mistrust	Children learn to trust when their basic needs are met with consistency, continuity, and sameness.	Children view the world as safe and dependable.
2. Muscular-Anal	Eighteen months to three years	Autonomy vs. shame and doubt	Encourage children to do what they are capable of doing. Avoid shaming for any behavior.	Children learn independence and competence; develop confidence to deal with the environment.
3. Locomotor-Genital (similar to Freud's phallic stage)	Three to Five years (to beginning of school)	Initiative vs. guilt	Encourage children to engage in many activities. Provide environment in which children can explore language development.	Children are able to undertake a task, be active and involved; are not hesitant, guilty or afraid to do things on their own.
4. Latency	Five to eleven years (elementary years)	Industry vs. inferiority	Help children to win recognition by producing things. Recognition results from achievement and success.	Feelings of self-worth and industry; the ability to accomplish.
5. Puberty and Adolescence	Twelve to eighteen years (adolescence)	Identity vs. role confusion	Help teenagers develop independence from parents. Resolve confusion about sex role and occupation.	Develop ego identity as a result of sameness and continuity from others about self.
6. Young Adulthood	End of adolescence to middle adulthood	Intimacy vs. isolation	Support efforts at establishing intimate relationships.	Intimate relationships.
7. Adulthood	Thirty-five to forty-five years	Generativity vs. stagnation	—	—
8. Maturity	Mid-life to death	Ego integrity vs. despair	—	—

develops the necessary ego groundwork to *get to be a giver*" (Erikson, 1963, p. 76). On the other hand, when infants are treated and cared for in ways that teach them to mistrust others, then the psychosocial outcome is mistrust.

Stage 2—Muscular-anal: Autonomy vs. Shame and Doubt (Eighteen Months to Three Years) The developmental task learned here is control of behavior and an understanding of the body's limits in relation to key developmental functions such as: the newly developed skill of walking to explore the environment, rapid language development, the beginning of cooperative play, and learning to control the bowels and bladder. During this time children become more independent. They want to do things for themselves and explore the environment. Care-givers should avoid being overprotective *and* overrestrictive while providing opportunities for children to do things for themselves and in facilitating opportunities for them to learn about their environment. Too often during this stage, care-givers want to control children and seek to unnecessarily restrict their movements so they "won't get into things and make a mess." Erikson views such restrictions as undermining children's resolution of the autonomy/shame conflict.

What is the toddler's favorite word? Anyone who has cared for and worked with young children can easily answer this question. Toddlers' frequent use of the word "No," combined with a desire to do things for themselves, can be frustrating and exasperating to parents who overreact to the growing autonomy of children. Picture a mother and her two-year-old waiting in a supermarket checkout line. The child eagerly and enthusiastically walks up to the candy display and grabs a handful of candy and gum. The mother tells the child to put the things back and the child in her most affirmative manner says "No." The mother then grabs the child, gives her a swift smack on the bottom while admonishing, "Don't say no to me! When I tell you to do something, you better do it." It is easy for the casual onlooker, who is emotionally detached from the parenting process,

to judge the mother as harsh and punitive. She may, indeed, appear to be so in this instance, but it is just such situations in daily parenting that shape children's behavior and personality. Parents are both juggler and judge. They must find a satisfactory balance between their wills and desires and those of their children. They must make the judicious decisions necessary to support a child's need for autonomy while, at the same time, helping the child grow and develop within the bounds of safety and socially acceptable norms.

Toilet training, or toilet learning as it is more frequently referred to, also places great demands on children and parents. Psychosocially, children are involved in learning to keep and let go. Toilet training at one level is largely a matter of recognizing that children need to be physically ready for learning and that training should be conducted in nonpunitive ways to help children understand that they have control over their behavior. Care-givers must avoid "shaming" children, for example, "Jason, why can't you learn to go to the bathroom like other kids do?" and "Jessica goes to the bathroom by herself and she's younger than you."

Stage 3—Locomotor-genital: Initiative vs. Guilt (Three to Five Years) The psychosocial task during this stage involves becoming independent from parents while continuing to explore the limits of one's potential. Initiative goes beyond autonomy in that the child is both independent *and* an active initiator of events. Erikson believes children need opportunities to respond with initiative to activities and tasks so that they will experience accomplishment *and* gratification. Many household and preschool activities offer opportunities for children to initiate and experience a sense of purposefulness and accomplishment. Care-givers and parents support children in these efforts when they provide a physical setting for initiative and greet children's accomplishments with enthusiasm, approval, and encouragement.

Erikson characterized the learning of children at this stage as *intrusive*, that is, leading away from her as a person to new knowledge and activities.

While initiating activities children often encounter conflicts as they intrude into the lives, space, and feelings of others. When children are treated punitively, are discouraged from initiating activities, and are restricted in doing things for themselves, uncomfortable feelings and guilt may ensue. Resolution of this psychosocial crisis depends very much on how care-givers and parents provide freedom within limits and help children feel proud rather than guilty about themselves and their accomplishments.

Stage 4—Latency: Industry vs. Inferiority (Five to Eleven Years—The Elementary Years) When children enter school they enter the world of adults as "grown-ups." They are full of confidence, enthusiasm, and energy, and are ready to engage the world and master it. The grown-up world is ready to teach a child new things and he is anxious and eager to learn. Children have literally put away—at least for now—what seem to them useless things, such as wishing for the opposite sex parent, and are ready to concentrate on the business of mastery and industriousness. Sexual desires, including those for the opposite sex parent, are latent. The child sublimates and energetically engages in play, the work of childhood. During this period children learn how to be productive and successful. They seek recognition for their industrious nature and attitudes. Adult responses to children's efforts and initiatives assist or hinder their development of a positive self-image. When children's growing abilities are routinely and harshly criticized and when they are unfairly compared to others, inferiority results. The psychosocial risk during this stage is that children will learn a sense of inadequacy and inferiority rather than industry and accomplishment.

Home and school, in particular, provide settings for children to learn much about the American society's emphasis on values associated with the work ethic, achievement orientation, and accomplishment. These two institutions must help children develop skills necessary for achieving important societal tasks. Feelings relating to industry and inferiority emanate from many school and school-related tasks. Reading and writing are critical schooling processes. Under the wise and patient tutelage of caring teachers, children lay the foundation for future success and an industrious outlook on life. Through success in literacy activities, children develop a feeling that they can "handle life." Failure to learn to read and write in the early elementary years makes future school success and, in many respects, future life success if not impossible, then unnecessarily difficult.

Stage 5—Puberty and Adolescence: Identity vs. Role Confusion (Twelve to Eighteen Years—Adolescence) This fifth stage involves children's search for identity as individuals and members of society. As Erikson explains it, children are "now primarily concerned with what they appear to be in the eyes of others as compared with what they feel they are" (Erikson, 1963, p. 261). In other words, children are searching for role identity, an individually appropriate sex role, and their place in society. During this time, belonging to a group is very important, and peer opinions and ideas exert powerful influences. Through group identity each child develops a sense of personal identity.

In addition to group identity, several other facets of adolescent life play important and powerful roles. Teenage romances assist with identity development since they provide the opportunity for individuals to clarify who they are. Career decisions literally force adolescents to answer questions such as, "Who am I?" and "What do I want to do with my life?" Positive psychosocial development outcomes of this stage depend, in part, on the individual's ability to develop an identity. If an individual is confused about the purpose of life or does not have clear-cut feedback from parents, family, and society, then an ill-defined sense of self results. This stage, perhaps more than any other, reflects the critical role of socialization on development. Think for a moment about contemporary times and local, state, national, and inter-

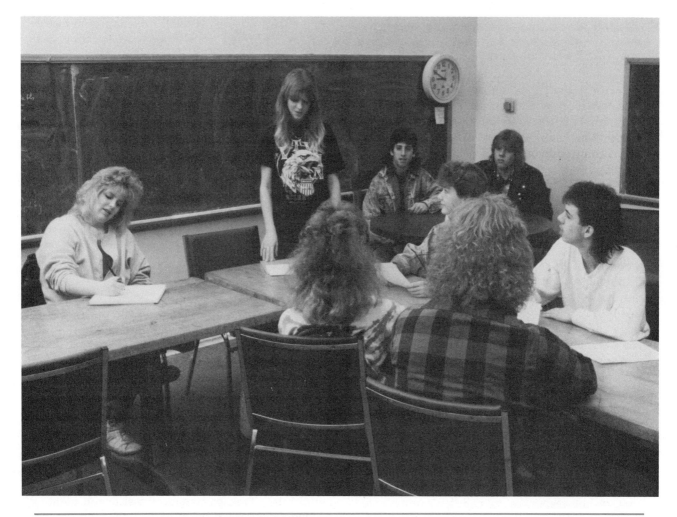

FIGURE 2-6 Teenagers share similar dress and hairstyles. Belonging to a group and fitting in is an important part of teenage development. (From Bailey *Working Skills for a New Age*, copyright 1990 by Delmar Publishers Inc.)

national issues relating to crime, discrimination, poverty, drugs, and abuse. In the context of these powerful negatives and in opposition to the many positive influences of society, is it any wonder that many children have trouble defining their roles in life and developing a set of standards to which they can adhere? Individuals who have difficulty dealing with the task of identity development may demonstrate "childish" behaviors and seem to take a long time to "grow up."

Stage 6—Young Adulthood: Intimacy vs. Isolation (End of Adolescence to Middle Adulthood). During this stage individuals develop intimate relationships with others and learn to give fully of themselves. The intimacy of this stage is both general and specific. It involves relating to others regardless of sex or closeness of personal ties. The development of intimate relations is important. If little or no intimacy is experienced, then the adult feels isolated and becomes preoccupied with his own affairs and manifests feelings of low self-esteem.

Stage 7—Adulthood: Generativity vs. Stagnation (Thirty-five to Forty-five Years) Generativity, according to Erikson (1963) is "primarily the concern in establishing and guiding the next generation" (p. 267). The psychosocial task is contribution to society. Productivity, rearing and teaching children, and other activities that support and develop the next generation are ways of avoiding the stagnation of self-centeredness.

Stage 8—Maturity: Ego Integrity vs. Despair (Mid-life to Death) As individuals mature and grow older, they look back over their lives and determine if they were worthwhile. This represents the ultimate developmental task. To the question that all persons eventually must ask about themselves—"Was my life meaningful?"—Erikson provides this answer, "Only in him who in some way has taken care of things and people and has adapted himself to the triumphs and disappointments adherent to being the originator of others or the generator of products and ideas—only in him may gradually ripen the fruit of these seven stages." This ripening of the fruit, and the realization that the fruit is sweet and good rather than shriveled and sour, Erikson identifies as *ego integrity.* Despair comes from realizing that life is too short to start again or to select alternative paths that could lead to integrity.

These, then, are the eight stages of life that all of us, according to Erikson, must encounter and master to the best of our abilities. As a participant yourself in this process and as one who is in a helping role for others, keep in mind several things. First, the behaviors or ego qualities Erikson describes typically occur at the end of a stage, and the "conclusion" of a stage is characterized by the mastery, in some form and to some degree, of the conflict. Second, the sequential order of Erikson's stages are invariant. Children and adults must progress from one stage to the other, with each stage related to the one previous to it. Third,

individuals wrestle with and confront their developmental conflicts in their own ways and in the context of their families, societies, and cultures. Consequently, the resolutions are unique for each individual in each time and place. Erikson continually stresses that the personality of an individual is the sum total of his or her ego's synthesizing resolutions of the developmental conflicts. One's life history is made throughout life, across the eight stages, not in just one particular stage.

Implications for Parents and Professionals

Erikson's theory offers parents and professionals many opportunities to apply his ideas to their daily interactions with children.

1. Caregivers and parents are very active participants with children in assisting in the resolution of ego conflicts. They provide guidance, support, and direction at each stage of development.
2. Although Erikson talked about the traits of each stage as absolutes, in reality they are not. Rather, they exist along a continuum from one extreme to the other, for example, absolute trust to absolute mistrust. As Murray Thomas (1979) points out:

Between these extremes are gradations that the individual may attain. In reality, no one reaches either extreme. Each personality represents some mixture of self-trust and mistrust, as well as some combination of trusting and mistrusting other people and the world in general. Consequently, one way of describing the configuration of a given child's or adolescent's personality within Erikson's system would be to identify where, along each of these scale lines, the individual stands at any particular time (p. 267).

The key, then, in child rearing and guidance is to help children develop attributes and behaviors that will enable them to have personalities identifiable with the positive end of each of the stages.

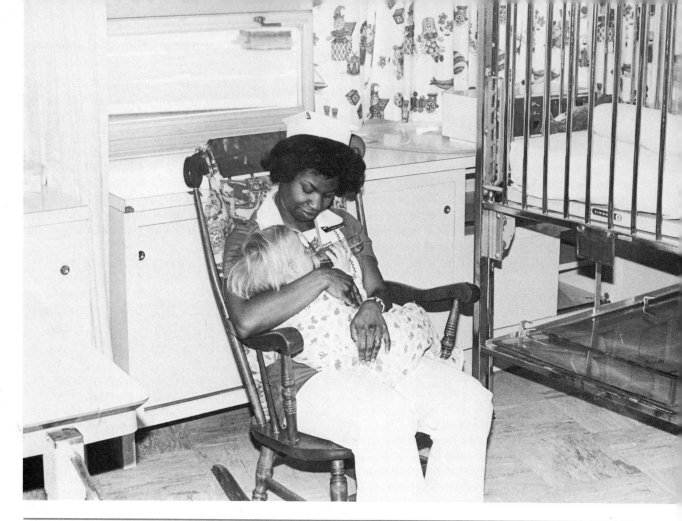

FIGURE 2-7 Erickson's theory has many practical applications to child rearing and care for nurses, teachers and parents. (From Lesner *Pediatric Nursing*, copyright 1983 by Delmar Publishers Inc.)

Strengths and Weaknesses of Erikson's Psychosocial Theory

Erikson's theory has a number of strengths.

1. Erikson's theory is neo-Freudian, meaning that he has taken Freud's ideas and added to them. This has the benefit of making some of Freud's ideas and psychoanalytic theory more understandable and acceptable to the general public.
2. Erikson's theory, unlike Freud's, which focused on the early years, extends across the human life span. Consequently it provides more interest in and adds more significance to the whole range of human development.
3. Erikson's theory allows for its practical application to child rearing, child care, teaching, and the professions involving children, youth, and adults. As part of the current interest in infant development and care, there is a marked emphasis on the application of Erikson's theory to care-giver training and everyday interactions with children.

On the other hand, there are several weaknesses to Erikson's theory.

1. The concepts embedded in Erikson's theory are not always easy to test and replicate because much of his data comes from personal observations and his synthesis of ideas.
2. Just as Freud's theory was developed from a limited population in Viennese society, critics claim that Erikson's theory relies too heavily on critical life events in European and North American societies.
3. Modern critics say that elements of American society, particularly the home and family, have changed considerably over the last several decades with the growing numbers of single parent and two-income families, and that Erikson's theory does not adequately account for these changes.

THE COGNITIVE DEVELOPMENT THEORY OF JEAN PIAGET

Jean Piaget (1896–1980) was born in Neuchatel, Switzerland. He was very close to his father, a university professor, and they spent many hours discussing academic topics. His mother was very religious and it can be argued that she instilled in her son a need for absolute truths in the best Calvinist tradition (Cohen, 1983, p. 8). His mother was also prone to emotional disturbances and Piaget coped with the family turmoil by identifying with his father and taking refuge in intellectual tasks (Fancher, 1979, p. 341). This immersion in things intellectual is reflected in Piaget's early precociousness. He wrote his first article about a partly albino robin at the age of ten. This paper was the beginning point for the 40 books and 500 articles he wrote throughout his life—a prodigious outpouring relating to cognitive development, knowledge, and knowing.

At the age of twenty-two, Piaget graduated with a Ph.D. in natural sciences after writing a dissertation on mollusks. He then journeyed to

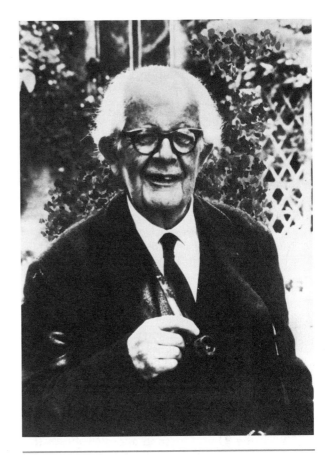

FIGURE 2-8 Jean Piaget developed a theory of cognitive development which provides teachers and child development professionals with insights into how to teach and care for children. (Photo courtesy of the Bettmann Archive)

Zurich and attended lectures given by Carl Jung, a former follower of Freud, who had established his own system of psychoanalysis. This involvement with psychiatry formed the basis of his now famous "clinical method," whereby he questioned or interviewed children as a means of determining how they think and view the world.

Piaget's Clinical Method

Piaget adapted the psychiatric interview to learn how children think. At the time Piaget adopted and adapted the psychiatric interview, it was based on the premise that people with mental disorders view reality differently from normal people. One "cure" consisted of attempting to get them to see how "wrong" their thinking was. Since Piaget said he was more interested in children's "wrong" answers than in their "right" answers, it is understandable that he would adopt the clinical interview as a method for understanding the reasons behind children's thinking. Piaget was intrigued by the idea that children's thinking was not "wrong," but qualitatively different from adult thought. As Piaget himself explains it:

> Thus I engaged my subjects in conversations patterned after psychiatric questioning, with the aim of discovering their right, but especially their wrong answers. I noticed with amazement that the simplest reasoning task involving the part in the whole [finding the part common to two wholes] . . . presented for normal children up to the age of eleven or twelve difficulties unsuspected by the adult (Evans, 1973, pp. 118–119).

This *clinical method* seeks to assess the *quality* of the child's thinking, regardless of the answer given. The following example illustrates the interactive nature of the clinical method and also shows that the child has an understanding of one-to-one correspondence but not of equivalence of corresponding sets.

> Hoc (Four years, three months). "Look, imagine that these are the bottles in a cafe. You are the waiter, and you have to take some glasses out of the cupboard. Each bottle must have a glass." He put one glass opposite each bottle and ignored the other glasses. "Is there the same number?" *Yes.* (The bottles were then grouped together). "Is there the same number of glasses and bottles?"— *No.* "Where are there more?" *There are more glasses.* The bottles were put back, one opposite each glass, and the glasses were then grouped together. "Is there the same number of glasses and bottles?"— *No.* "Where are there more?"—*More bottles.* "Why are there more bottles?"—*Just because* (Piaget, 1965, p. 44).

Piaget also worked with Theodore Simon, who had assisted Alfred Binet in the development of his intelligence test. Simon asked Piaget to standardize a series of reasoning tests for children. This experience further motivated Piaget to determine how children think. This work resulted in the publication of some of his first articles, such as "On Studying the Explanations of Children." In 1921, Piaget was invited to be the director of the Institute Jean-Jacques Rousseau in Geneva, Switzerland, a position he held all his life and where he was affectionately known as *le patron* or "the boss." It was at the kindergarten associated with the institute that Piaget observed children, questioned them on a wide variety of topics, and gathered much data that would form the basis for his many writings about his famous theory.

Piaget gathered and harvested abundant data from another, more personal source. For him, all babies but especially his own children, were exciting and anything but boring. The three Piaget children, Jacqueline, Lucienne, and Laurent, are famous for their roles in the explanation of their father's theory. The very first observation of Laurent is noteworthy for a number of reasons. First, it illustrates Piaget's ecological and naturalistic observation. Second, the sucking reflex, which plays a major role in the development of sensorimotor intelligence, is observed and recorded.

> Observation 1. From birth sucking-like movements may be observed: impulsive movement and the protrusion of the lips accompanied by displacements of the tongue, while the arms engage in unruly and more or less rhythmical gestures and the head moves laterally, etc. (Piaget, 1952, p. 25).

The Cognitive Development Theory

Piaget presents a very positive and optimistic picture of children. For him, there are no enduring conflicts, no suppressed sexual desires that act as hidden wells of aggressive energy, and no personality deficits or flaws traceable to the early years. Instead, he views children as wondrous beings, highly involved in the development of their own intelligence, and capable of remarkable thinking. Piaget invests children with a grandeur and majesty that is like a breath of fresh air wafting across the field of psychological developmental theories.

Piaget's *cognitive development* theory is about how children develop cognitively, that is, intellectually. And, it is important to keep in mind that biology plays a powerful role in his theory. Many of his concepts relate to biological processes. In biology, it is the structure that changes and adapts to biological and environmental processes and influences. For Piaget, *scheme* is the cognitive correlate for a biological structure. A scheme is a mental idea, design, or blueprint. For example, if you think about your high school, the mental picture that comes to mind is a scheme consisting of a building, trees, classmates, teachers, sport events, pep rallies, smells from the cafeteria, your first date, and so on.

According to Piaget, there are two types of schemes. The first schemes are not mental, but *overt* actions demonstrated through reflexive, sensorimotor activities such as sucking and grasping. These schemes change in response to the environment, experiences, and *active involvement of the child.* Sucking soon becomes differentiated between nutritive and nonnutritive and changes in form to accommodate the cup and spoon. Piaget believed that the child from birth to age two does not have internalized "thinking" processes or "thoughts of the mind." Rather, infants come to know their world through overt sensorimotor actions. Sensorimotor schemes help the young child know her world because they are used in new ways, thereby expanding her cognitive development. Another infant sensorimotor scheme, for example, is grasping. It consists of looking, opening the hand, closing the fingers, retracting the fingers, and finally, grasping. This scheme functions with toys, books, bottles, the breast, clothing, and noses! Sensorimotor schemes, then, exist only through the actions of the infant. Infants "know" their world by acting upon it with action-based schemes including sucking, grasping, pulling, shaking, and looking.

The second schemes, the *cognitive schemes,* develop from approximately two years of age and are the method by which children organize and classify their world. Cognitive schemes include our number system, concepts of space and time, and the laws of logic. Cognitive schemes enable children to know their world by helping them understand how objects, experiences, and events are related. These cognitive schemes form a child's *cognitive structure.* Just as the skeletal structure organizes our physical appearance, so, too, cognitive structures organize cognitive development.

Schemes develop primarily through the process of *adaptation,* which is the basis for any developmental change in intelligence. You are very much aware of the process of physical adaptation, whereby an individual, when stimulated by environmental factors, reacts and adjusts physically and behaviorally. Piaget applied this concept to cognitive development.

> *Adaptation* is for Piaget the essence of intellectual functioning, just as it is the essence of biological functioning. It is one of the two basic tendencies inherent in all species; the other is organization, the ability to integrate both physical and psychological structures into coherent systems. Adaptation takes place through organization; the organism discriminates among the myriad stimuli and sensations by which it is bombarded and organizes them into some kind of structure (Pulaski, 1980, p. 6).

Piaget believed adaptation is comprised of two interrelated and simultaneously operating processes, *assimilation* and *accommodation.* Assimilation is the process of taking in experiences, impressions, sensations—sounds, sights, smells—and incorporating them into existing schemes. As Richmond (1970) explains it:

> Every experience we have, whether as infant, child or adult, is taken into the mind and made to fit into the experiences which already exist there. The next experience will need to be changed in some

degree in order for it to fit in. Some experiences cannot be taken in because they do not fit. These are rejected. Thus the intellect assimilates new experiences into itself by transforming them to fit the structure which has been built up (p. 68).

Accommodation occurs when a child changes her present way of thinking, believing, and behaving to fit incoming information. Again, Richmond (1970) explains it this way:

Now with each new experience, the structures which have already been built up will need to modify themselves to accept that new experience, for, as each new experience is fitted in to the old, the structures will be slightly changed. This process by which the intellect continually adjusts its model of the world to fit in each new acquisition, Piaget calls accommodation (p. 68).

An example will help you understand how assimilation and accommodation work in real life. A young child in the preoperational stage has never experienced crayons before. His mother buys him a pack and places them in front of him. He reaches for the pack, picks it up, and the crayons tumble out. He picks up a crayon, adjusting his grip to the size and shape of the crayon. By accommodating his grip to the crayon, he is able to pick it up. At the same time, he assimilates the crayon into his other schemes of things to pick up, look at, and with which to scribble. Gradually, through these reciprocal procedures of assimilation and accommodation, he will develop a scheme for crayons as objects with which to scribble, color, and write.

Equilibrium

Just as Erikson, and Freud before him, perceived a need for emotional equilibrium, so Piaget saw a need for cognitive equilibrium. Cognitive equilibrium is maintained in the developing individual through a four-step process of *equilibration*. First, a child assimilates information in accordance with her cognitive structures at a particular stage of intellectual development. Second, the child

encounters information that does not fit her cognitive structures. Third, this encounter sets off a state of *disequilibrium* in her cognitive structures. Fourth, this disequilibrium causes the cognitive structures to change or *accommodate* the new information. For example, three-year-old Odalys goes to the park daily with her babysitter. Odalys likes to feed the ducks and from her experiences with ducks, she has developed a mental scheme for ducks as two-legged animals that have feathers and that waddle and quack. This scheme is based on the similarities of ducks.

Last week, Odalys' mother took her to a petting zoo, where she encountered chickens for the first time. She said to her mother, "Duck!" She asked for bread to feed the new "ducks." As she ran toward a chicken, it clucked and ran away from her. Odalys was quite surprised. Her mother said, "That's a chicken, Odalys." Odalys tried to assimilate the new experience with the chicken into her scheme of ducks. The experience didn't quite fit, and disequilibrium was introduced into Odalys' thinking. She was able to accommodate and develop a new scheme—chickens—based on her new experience. As a result, equilibrium—a balance between assimilation and accommodation—was restored to her thinking. As time goes by and as Odalys has additional experiences, she will refine her schemes for ducks and chickens, and will develop new ones as well.

Constructivism and Activity

Piaget placed heavy emphasis on the role of activity in cognitive development. Sensorimotor intelligence, for example, stems directly from the motor movements of the baby. He believed that children literally *construct* their knowledge of the world through the process of self-directed activity. Each child organizes, structures, and restructures experiences in accordance with his or her schemes of thought through the process of equilibration. Experiences provide the raw material for constructing schemes. Constance Kamii (1981) explains that "constructivism refers to the fact that knowledge is built by an active child from the inside

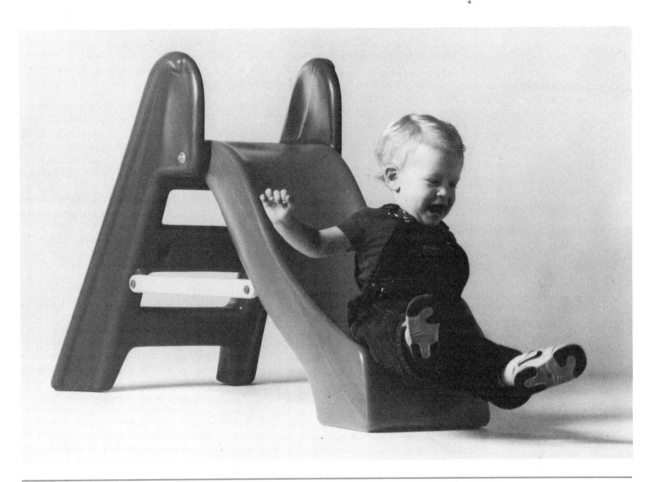

FIGURE 2-9 Activity plays an important role in the intellectual development of young children.

rather than being transmitted from the outside through the senses." Children literally create their intelligence by experimenting with the world.

Stages of Development

Piaget established four stages of cognitive development. These stages are the same for all children and children progress from one stage to another in the same sequence. The ages he assigned to each stage are approximate and vary for individual children. Stages are defined by the *qualitatively* different cognitive structures of each stage. To say that one child has "graduated" from one stage to another is to say that the child has a new and different set of cognitive structures. Piaget's stages of cognitive development are shown in Table 2-4. In addition to the information provided here, each stage is discussed in greater detail in succeeding chapters.

TABLE 2-4

PIAGET'S STAGES OF COGNITIVE DEVELOPMENT

Sensorimotor Stage (Birth to two years)	Uses behaviors such as sucking, grasping, and gross body activities to build schemes. Begins to develop the concept that things exist even when not visible. Dependent on real objects. The frame of reference is the world of here and now.
Preoperational Stage (Two to seven years)	Language development accelerates. Self-centered in thought and action. Thinks everything has a reason or purpose. Makes judgments primarily on basis of how things look.
Concrete Operations Stage (Seven to eleven years)	Capable of reversing thought processes. Ability to conserve or undo thought processes. Still dependent on how things look for decision making. Less self-centered. Is able to organize time and space. Begins understanding of numbers.
Formal Operations Stage (Eleven to fifteen years)	Capable of dealing with word and hypothetical problems. Ability to reason scientifically and in a logical manner. No longer bound to concrete objects in thinking. Can think using words or numbers.

Sensorimotor Stage (Birth to Two Years) The sensorimotor stage begins at birth and lasts until about age two (with the beginning of symbolic thought characterized by the use of language). Beginning with innate sensory and reflexive schemes or actions such as looking, sucking, and grasping, the child develops an increasingly complex, unique, and individualized hierarchy of sensorimotor schemes. The sucking scheme, for example, is adapted to include nipple, thumb, blanket, and toys. The child's cognitive development depends on such sensorimotor functions and interactions.

This stage has six independent but interrelated substages, each of which is described in detail in later chapters.

1. *Reflexive Action*—Infants are ruled by their reflexive actions yet through practice they assimilate, accommodate, and build schemes.
2. *Primary Circular Reaction*—Modification of reflexive actions in Stage 1 continues and infants begin to direct their behavior rather than being totally dependent on reflexive actions. Primary circular reactions begin, for example, infants use their bodies to initiate and repeat many pleasurable actions such as thumb-sucking.
3. *Secondary Circular Reaction*—This is the stage of "making interesting things happen." The infant reproduces events with the *intent* of sustaining or repeating acts. The infant attempts to elicit a response from a secondary source, such as a toy or care-giver.
4. *Coordination of Secondary Schemes*—During this stage, the infant uses means to achieve ends. She will move objects out of the way, for example, to get another object.
5. *Experimentation (Tertiary Circular Reactions)*—This stage marks the beginning of truly intelligent behavior. Novelty is interesting for its own sake and the toddler experiments in many ways with a given object. For example, he may use a small shovel to dig a hole, bang a bucket, pat down sand for a mud pie, and hit the child beside him.

6. *Representational Intelligence (Intention of Means)*—This is the stage of transition from sensorimotor thought to symbolic thought. Toddlers are liberated from sensorimotor actions as the *only* means of intellectual development.

During the sensorimotor period, children are *egocentric*. They see and judge everything from their own point of view. Children are the center of their own worlds and believe they are all that matters. This egocentrism should not be confused with selfishness, as experienced in adults. For the young child, there is literally no other point of view other than his own because of his developmental stage.

Children also begin to develop a knowledge of *object permanence* during the sensorimotor stage. Between birth and eight months, infants have no understanding that an object or person exists when not physically observable. They believe that "out of sight is out of mind." This explains why a mother can take a favorite teddy bear from a six-month-old child and the child immediately loses interest. However, when she attempts the same thing with her eighteen-month-old child, he cries because he knows it still exists and he wants it back! Now!

Preoperational Stage (Two to Seven Years)

The *preoperational stage* begins at age two and ends at age seven. The preoperational child possesses an increased ability to internalize events or to think by utilizing words and numbers in place of concrete objects. An understanding of the concept of operation will help us better understand the preoperational stage. When Piaget uses the word *operation*, he means "an action that can be internalized: that is, it can be carried out in thought as well as executed materially. Second, it is a reversible action; that is, it can take place in one direction or in the opposite direction" (Piaget, 1970, p. 21). Operations are reversible and they can be performed mentally in the child's mind.

To be preoperational means that the child cannot perform operations. An example will help illustrate this point. Place two identical glasses filled with equal amounts of milk in front of a four-year-old child. Then introduce two new glasses, one tall and thin, the other short and squat. Pour the milk from one glass into the tall glass and the milk from the other glass into the short glass. Ask the child which glass has more milk, and she will tell you the tall glass has more because it is "fuller." The child could not mentally reverse the event. Reality for her is what she sees, because she is perceptually bound as part of her egocentric condition.

Concerning egocentrism, the preoperational child believes everyone thinks as she thinks and that they act the way she does for the same reasons. She cannot, therefore, put herself "in someone else's shoes." To ask her to do so, either mentally or emotionally, is asking her to go beyond her cognitive ability.

Also, preoperational children act as though everything has a reason or purpose. This accounts for a child's constant and recurring questions about why things happen and how something works. This also explains the corresponding exasperation of parents and care-givers in having to answer questions, many of which don't have neat and readily available answers.

Concrete Operations Stage (Seven to Eleven Years)

The stage of *concrete operations* begins at age seven and ends at about age eleven. During this stage a child's thinking is more internalized, logical, and reversible, and he is more capable of engaging in problem-solving. But there is a catch. He can only figure things out if all the necessary information is presented *concretely*. Concrete does *not* mean, as is sometimes erroneously thought, that the child must physically touch, feel, and handle the objects. Rather as Thomas (1979) explains " 'Concrete' means that the problems involve identifiable objects that are either directly perceived or imagined. In the later formal operations period the child is able to move ahead to deal with problems that do not concern particular objects" (p. 313).

In this sense, then, concrete means that an addition word problem, for example, should be stated this way: If Jennifer has three oranges and Josh gives her two oranges, how many oranges will she have altogether? In this case, the child imagines "oranges" in her problem solving. In the beginning phases of concrete operations, however, children should be given objects to manipulate as they solve problems. This is also an example that "telling is not teaching." An obvious implication is to structure teaching so that children have many experiences with real objects and with people other than the teacher.

A child of seven in the beginning of concrete operations stage knows that when two equal pieces of clay are rolled out, there is not more clay in the "long one." Thus, while he understands conservation of size, he will not understand conservation of weight until age nine or ten and conservation of volume (displacement in water) until about age eleven or twelve.

Concerning egocentrism, the child becomes more of a social person during this stage. The increased use of language in particular enables her to interact with others and better understand the views of others. Piaget advocated the importance of involving children with other people as a context for helping them develop out of their egocentrism. Consequently, children need to have experiences where they can learn to take many aspects of a situation into account. Having the opportunity to hear other people express their feelings, opinions, and points of view help children to do this.

Formal Operations Stage (Eleven to Fifteen Years) *Formal operations*, the second part of operational intelligence, is the ultimate, the summit of intellectual development and occurs between the ages of eleven and fifteen. During this stage, adolescents are increasingly capable of understanding complex verbal and hypothetical problems such as, "What would happen if there were no more oil in the world?" They are literally released from the mental bondage of being dependent on the world of things and the here and now. Instead of being tied to concrete mental images of the world,

they can now engage in thinking *about* the world. Adolescents' thinking ranges over the wide time span of the past, present, and future. They can reason scientifically, logically, and abstractly. They can develop hypotheses and engage in their solutions.

The Pendulum Problem The pendulum problem is a classical experimental situation Piaget used to determine the nature and extent of adolescents' logical thinking. Subjects are shown a pendulum hanging from a string and are instructed how to vary the length of the string, change the weight of the pendulum, release the pendulum from various heights, and propel it with differing forces. This problem, often included in an introductory physics class, asks the experimenter to determine which of the four factors—length, weight, height, and force—affects the frequency of swing. The adolescent in formal operations is able to plan for how to solve the problem, observe the results of her experimentation, and draw logical conclusions based on the data, as illustrated in the following account:

> EME (Fifteen years, one month). After having selected 100 grams with a long string and medium length string, the 20 grams with a long and short string, and finally 200 grams with a long and short, concludes: "It's the length of the string that makes it go faster or slower; the weight doesn't play any role." She discounts likewise the height of the drop and the force of her push (Piaget & Inhelder, 1958, p. 75).

When the adolescent demonstrates logical thinking in this manner, she is, in Piagetian terms, an adult. This does not mean she is finished with her mental development. Quite the contrary, she will continue to add to her mental schemes and finish rounding out her knowledge of the world. In fact, the process of scheme and knowledge acquisition is a lifelong process.

However, unless we envision too perfect a picture of intellectual development, we must understand that not all adolescents or, for that matter, all adults reach and function at the formal operations level (Kuhn, 1984). Reasons for this failure to reach formal operations are educational attainment, experiential background, and general intellectual functioning.

Egocentrism in the formal operations stage takes on another wrinkle in relation to self-centeredness. Teenagers see themselves as others see them. Such egocentrism leads to group conformity and reinforces the adoption of faddish behavior that is so characteristic of teenagers, yet exasperating for parents.

The acquisition of logical thought also helps explain two other adolescent characteristics—argumentativeness and idealism. Teenagers' new-found ability to reason logically encourages them to engage in sometimes heated and argumentative debates involving the nuances of a topic, often to their parents' and teachers' exasperation. Elkind (1984) encourages adults to deal with the principles involved in such arguments and avoid becoming embroiled in personalities.

Emotionally, an adolescent can, as Ginsburg and Opper (1979) explain it, not only "love his mother or hate a peer, now he can love freedom and or hate exploitation. The adolescent has developed a new mode of life: the possible and the ideal captivate both mind and feeling" (p. 201).

Strengths and Weaknesses of Piaget

As we have previously indicated, Piaget has undoubtedly had a tremendous influence on the fields of psychology, education, and child development. In many ways, Piaget's theory is very practical and applicable. His theory and ideas have challenged researchers to test his hypotheses, develop and test their own hypotheses, explain his theory to others, and change and revise it as necessary.

Educators are consistently seeking ways to apply Piaget's ideas to classroom and educational practice. For example, *Young Children in Action: A Manual for Preschool Educators* by Hohmann, Banet, and Weikart (Ypsilanti, MI: High/Scope Press, 1979)

and *Young Children Reinvent Arithmetic: Implications of Piaget's Theory* by Kamii (New York: Teachers College Press, 1985) are two books designed to help educators bridge the gap between Piaget's theory and classroom practice.

Most practitioners in child development (including your author) rely heavily on Piaget's theory to explain children's intellectual development. They also make applications of Piagetian theory to child rearing, agency programs, and public policy pronouncements. The primary reason for this is simple—there is no other theory of choice. Piaget's theory is the only theory that explains fully and in detail human intellectual development.

On the other hand, Piaget has been criticized for many things, including the informal nature of his experiments, his intolerance for the ideas of others with regard to intellectual development, the use of his children in his studies, and the difficulty of interpreting many of his writings.

Also, the ages for the stages of development specified by Piaget don't seem to hold for today's children. Many children engage in cognitive behaviors earlier than they are expected to do so. However, Piaget was concerned more with characteristics of cognitive behavior at a particular stage rather than with rigid age/time frames. We will discuss such discrepancies in forthcoming chapters.

Behaviorists in particular believe that Piaget underestimated the importance experience plays in cognitive development. Training, education, and feedback may play greater roles in intellectual development than Piaget theorized.

SKINNER AND BEHAVIORISM

Burrhus Frederick Skinner (1904–), better known as B. F. Skinner, was born in Susquehanna, Pennsylvania. His father was a self-taught lawyer and Skinner described his mother as "bright and beautiful" (Fancher, 1979, p. 355). Skinner showed an early talent for writing and, like Piaget before him, published his first work at ten, a poem entitled "The Pessimistic Fellow." Skinner entered Hamilton College where his writing for the college

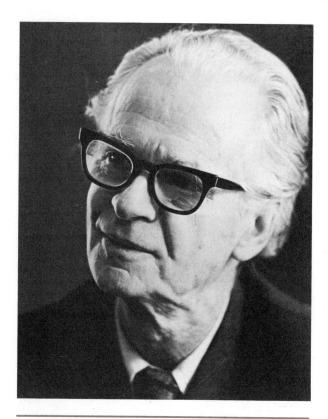

FIGURE 2-10 B.F. Skinner is famous for his many applications of behaviorism to child rearing and teaching. (Photo courtesy of the Bettmann Archive)

newspaper and literary magazine intensified his ambition to be an author. Following graduation, he returned to his parents' home, built a study in the attic and settled down to the life of a writer. But the literary life, at least as Skinner had envisioned it, was not meant to be, for the rewards were quite the opposite of what he expected. Frustrated and dejected with writing, Skinner turned to psychology as an alternative method for studying human behavior. The ideas Skinner embraced and the movement he would head for many decades are popularly known as *behaviorism*. In a strict sense, behaviorism is not a theory of development, but a theory of learning.

Behaviorism plays down the roles of biology, maturation, and time in learning, and instead stresses the role of the environment. For behaviorists, critical factors in development are not biology and time, but the environment and the opportunity to learn. Behaviorists see development as a continuous set of changing behaviors governed by the principles of learning, rather than as a series of age-bound behaviors. Age and stage descriptions of development are irrelevant because development results from children's interactions with the environment and the reward system inherent in the environment. Change in behavior is a function of learning, not age or changes in cognitive schemes or hidden psychic forces. Change is a function of learning.

Behaviorism's beginnings and foundation involve primarily three people—a biologist, Ivan Pavlov, and two psychologists, J.B. Watson and Edward Thorndike. Ivan Pavlov (1849–1936) won a 1904 Novel Prize for his work on animal digestive systems. He was interested in how biological events such as digestion systematically relate to changes in the environment. The application of this interest to learning was truly revolutionary. Pavlov knew that a hungry dog salivates when presented with meat. The meat is the *unconditioned stimulus* and the salivation is the *unconditioned response*. Pavlov *conditioned* or trained a dog's salivary response by providing meat simultaneously with the ringing of a bell. After several repetitions, Pavlov could merely ring a bell and the dog would salivate. The bell became a *conditioned* stimulus because it took the place of food, an *unconditioned* stimulus. Salivating became a *conditioned response*, because when the dog heard the bell ring—the conditioned stimulus—it salivated. This process of conditioning a response is called *classical conditioning*. The process sounds familiar, doesn't it? How is your life influenced by conditioned responses? Do you salivate or "get hungry" at the sight of a picture of your favorite food?

J. B. Watson (1878–1958) is considered the founder of behaviorism. He expressed this view rather well when he said, "Psychology as the behaviorist views it is a purely objective natural science. Its theoretical goal is the prediction and control of behavior" (Watson, 1913, p. 158). The three key terms of this definition are *objective*, *prediction*, and *control*, for they emphasize the behaviorists' focus on observable, external behavior not emotions, the prediction or specification of intended behavioral outcomes, and the management or control of the environment to assure the intended outcomes.

Important concepts for Watson were: (1) *stimulus*, which is any form of energy that stimulates a *sensory receptor* or a nerve ending specialized to receive stimuli, and (2) *response*, which is an observable reaction of the body, typically motor reactions. These stimulus-response pairs or connections are at the heart of Watson's theory of behavior. He examined behavior and saw it to be a system of stimulus-response associations. Behaviorism views development as the culmination of an individual's learning experiences. Without learning experiences, there is no development, only physical growth.

Watson applied many of his ideas to child rearing and wrote a very popular child-rearing guide. He gave parents the advice that rearing children is not some mystical or mysterious process based on inner unfoldings or unconscious tendencies. Rather, Watson believed that child rearing is greatly enhanced by parents who exert purposeful and effective control over children's experiences. Watson emphasized purpose and intent and the careful control of the environment as the means for promoting desired behavior.

In fact, Watson (1924) maintained that he could take any normal child and raise him to be just about any person he chose.

> Give me a dozen healthy infants, well-formed, and my own specified world to bring them up in and I'll guarantee to take any one at random and train him to become any type of specialist I might select—doctor, lawyer, artist, merchant-chief and, yes, even beggar-man and thief, regardless of his talents, penchants, tendencies, abilities, vocations, and race of his ancestors (p. 104).

Edward Thorndike (1874–1949) popularized the *reinforcement theory* so often associated with behaviorism. Thorndike believed that behavior is strengthened by the effects it has on the doer. He believed people do things that bring them pleasure and avoid doing things that bring them pain. This is not a new idea for us since it is reminiscent of

Freud's pleasure-seeking principle. Thorndike, however, stated it behaviorally and said what today seems fairly obvious, namely that the consequences of a particular response determine whether or not the response will be continued and therefore learned. What happens to an individual following a behavior helps determine whether or not she will continue to act in the same manner. A child who cries and is given a cookie by her mother will likely learn to use crying as a means of getting cookies. Pleasurable responses increase tendencies to act; unpleasant consequences decrease a tendency to act. As you know from your own experiences, people don't usually do something in order to see how painful it is. As a matter of fact, they do quite the opposite. People generally do all they can to avoid pain, which is precisely the behavior many makers of pain relievers and similar products take advantage of in their advertising.

While others laid the groundwork for behaviorism, B. F. Skinner is the modern day popularizer. He has done more than any other individual to spread the behaviorist theory through words and accomplishments.

HOW TO KEEP A ROOM CLEAN

Although he may not have known it at the time, one of young Skinner's efforts to respond to his mother's constant admonitions to keep his room clean was behaviorist in nature. It also reflects the mechanical aptitude that would serve him well in the psychology laboratory. As Skinner (1967 describes it,

> A special hook in the closet of my room was connected by a string-and-pulley system to a sign hanging above the door to the room. When my pajamas were in place on the hook, the sign was held high above the door and out of the way. When the pajamas were off the hook, the sign hung squarely in the middle of the door frame. It read "Hang up your pajamas!" (p. 396)

Skinner and Operant Conditioning

One of Skinner's major contributions is a detailed explanation of the process of *operant conditioning*, which describes the process of learning that occurs when responses are followed by reinforcers. The term *operant* means that children (individuals) operate or act in and on the environment. As a result of this operation or interaction, certain behaviors are reinforced and learning results. Whereas Pavlov *created* a new stimulus response relation, in operant conditioning, an *already existing* response is strengthened or weakened. A child must emit a response *before* the response is conditioned.

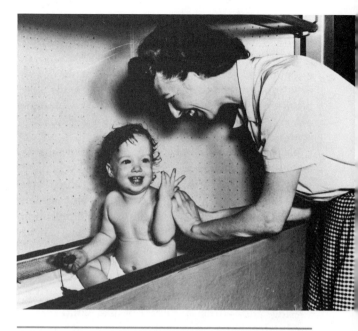

FIGURE 2-11 The baby tender is one of the research tools developed by Skinner to test his many ideas relating to behaviorism. (Photo courtesy of the Bettmann Archive)

THE BABY TENDER

Another of Skinner's inventions was his BABY-TENDER or Aircrib, as it was commercially known. To assist his wife in the care of their second child, Debbie, Skinner mechanized baby tending.

> I built a crib-sized living space that we began to call the "baby-tender." It had sound absorbing walls and a large picture window. Air entered through filters at the bottom and, after being warmed and moistened, moved upward through and around the edges of a tightly stretched canvas, which served as a mattress. A strip of sheeting ten yards long passed over the canvas, a clean section of which could be cranked into place in a few seconds (Skinner, 1979, p. 275).

So baby Skinner was comfortable, able to move about and, in theory at least, free from negative reinforcements. In addition, Mom had fewer clothes to wash! Skinner is still "pained" by rumors that Debbie grew up to be psychotic. On the contrary, she is a healthy, happy, productive woman (Goleman, 1987, p. 17).

For example, Melody Jacobs is desirous of having her eighteen-month-old son, J. P., learn names for things. She shows him many toys while saying their names. One day, much to Melody's delight, J. P. says "ball." She profusely praises J. P.: "Great, fantastic, good for you, J.P.! You know the name for 'ball.'" Consequently, when J.P. plays with his toys and touches, picks up, or otherwise interacts with a ball and says "ball," Melody praises him. Through such operant conditioning (the operant response, "ball," is followed by a reinforcer, praise) J.P. learns the name for "ball." It is in precisely this manner that behaviorists believe J. P. will not only learn language, but other behaviors as well. Life is full of other such examples.

One day thirteen-year-old Mandy wore a new hair style. All her friends complimented her on her "new look." Several days later when she wore her "old" hair style, no one complimented her, so the next day she wore her new look to renewed compliments. Now her new hair style is part of her daily attire.

A major contribution by Skinner to experimental psychology and our understanding of reinforcement and behavior was an ingenious piece of laboratory equipment called, appropriately enough, "The Skinner Box." It was designed to hold one rat and had a press bar and pellet cup mounted on one side. When a rat presses the lever, a food pellet is released as a reward and a cumulative record is kept of the frequency of lever pushing. The box is a convenient way to arrange *contingencies*, or situations, and record the *contingencies of reinforcement*, that is the relationship between a response and the presence or absence of a *reinforcer*.

Skinner and "Teaching Machines"

Skinner introduced to education and teaching the concept of programmed learning, whereby what students are to learn is programmed or arranged in a progressive series of small steps from simple or basic to complex. Students are rewarded or

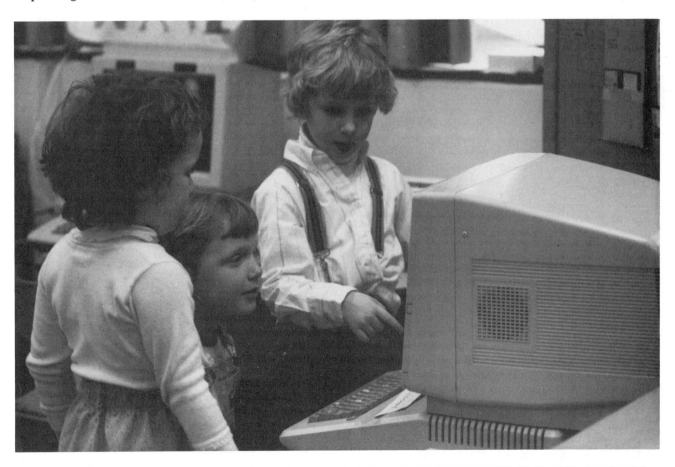

FIGURE 2-12 Computers and software programs use many stimulus-response interactions which promote interactive learning. (Photo courtesy of Jane Davidson, from Davidson, *Children and Computers in the Early Childhood Classroom*, copyright 1989 by Delmar Publishers Inc.)

reinforced with the right answer after each small step, a concept in keeping with Skinner's belief that knowing that one has answered a question correctly (in other words, positive feedback) is a powerful motivating force for children. Many of these programs were incorporated into "machines" whereby students opened a slot or window to reveal the correct answer. Several advantages of programmed learning are: learning is broken down into small, manageable units; students use the program themselves; and individuals progress at their own rate. Today, computer programs designed to teach colors, numbers, and other concepts are based on Skinnerian and behaviorist principles.

The following dialogue between Skinner and interviewer Richard Evans (1968) provides insight into Skinner's view of teaching:

> *Evans:* Dr. Skinner, to turn now to the field of education, I know this to be an area which is of profound interest to you. You were the significant developer of programmed learning. In describing this method of teaching, do you not use the term "teaching machines"?
>
> *Skinner:* Yes, I'm afraid I'm responsible for it. People advised me not to use the term, but a sewing machine sews, a washing machine washes and a teaching machine teaches. The original teaching machines were the equipment in operant laboratories which arranged contingencies of reinforcement. That's all teaching is, arranging contingencies which bring about changes in behavior. Machines bring them about more rapidly than the natural contingencies in daily life. The teacher expedites learning by arranging effective contingencies, at least in theory. The contingencies arranged without instrumental aid are often quite defective. You can teach more effectively with devices of one kind or another. In the future, they will be commonplace in all institutional situations (pp. 59–60).

Basic Behaviorist Principles

1. The environment is everything. Experiences come from environmental stimuli. In the nature/nurture–heredity/environment contro-versy, behaviorists are environmentally oriented and emphasize the role of the environment in controlling and determining behavior.
2. Observable behaviors are what is important, not what a person thinks. Actions speak louder than words.
3. The principles of learning hold true for people of all ages, across the life span from birth to death.
4. Learning, that is, development, is gradual and continuous, not stage-related. Behaviorists see development as an incremental sequence of specific conditioned behaviors.

A Glossary of Behaviorist Terms

1. *Classical conditioning*—The process of pairing a stimulus with a response resulting in a new form of learning. A new stimulus response connection is created.
2. *Operant conditioning*—The process whereby an already existing response is strengthened or weakened by reinforcement.
3. *Behavior modification*—The conscious use of reinforcers and contingency management to change behavior.
4. *Stimulus*—Any event that produces a physical or mental response.
5. *Response*—The reaction to a stimulus.
6. *Reinforcement*—Providing reinforcers to increase the frequency of response.
7. *Reinforcer*—Any stimulus that increases the likelihood that a response will be increased or strengthened.
8. *Positive reinforcer*—A stimulus, often referred to as a reward, that increases a behavior.
9. *Negative reinforcer*—A stimulus, such as the threat of punishment, that increases behavior necessary to avoid an unpleasant situation or punishment.
10. *Punishment*—A stimulus that suppresses or decreases a response.
11. *Development* (from the behaviorist perspective)—Learned responses.

12. *Contingency management*—The management of the behavior development and reinforcement processes. This usually involves the selection of desired behavior (the behavior that will be strengthened or weakened), the reinforcers, and the reinforcement schedule (the frequency and conditions under which reinforcers will be given).

13. *Extinction*—The disappearance of a response as a result of the removal of a reinforcer.

14. *Habituation*—A decrease in responsiveness or sensitivity as the result of the repetition of a stimulus. Satiation in relation to a stimulus.

Social Learning Theory

Not all behaviorists believe behavior can be explained solely on the basis of classical or operant conditioning. Albert Bandura (1925–) described *social learning theory* as "the explanation of human behavior in terms of a continuous reciprocal interaction between cognitive, behavioral, and environmental determinants" (Bandura, 1977, p. vii). Bandura believes that such a conception of behavior "neither casts people into the role of powerless objects by environmental forces nor free agents who can become whatever they choose. Both people and their environments are reciprocal determinants of each other" (p. vii). Thus people play a greater role in the development of their behaviors than traditional behaviorists ascribe to them. Bandura and other learning theorists believe learning occurs primarily through modeling, observation, vicarious experiences, and self-regulation.

There are basically four processes involved in modeling: attention to people, selecting behaviors to reproduce, remembering the observed behavior, and reproducing what was observed. Attention to people is based on their engaging qualities, their particular behaviors, and a child's frame of reference. Selecting what behaviors to reproduce is largely a matter of what the child values or what he sees others whom he admires valuing. Those behaviors that bring pleasure will more likely be modeled, while if a child sees a peer being punished for a particular behavior, she is less likely to model that behavior. Retention occurs through recalling the observed, because obviously if a child does not remember a behavior, she cannot be much influenced by it. Reproduction is more than a process of "monkey see, monkey do." Replication occurs best when a child has the requisite skills to perform the behavior and an opportunity to practice.

Social learning theorists believe that a child does not have to directly observe a behavior to model it, but that vicarious experiences serve as a model for behavior. Self-regulation, or the ability to use cognitive functions such as the manipulation of words and numbers, helps children verify experiences before they model a behavior and thus they are able to anticipate future benefits and difficulties.

Advantages and Disadvantages of Behaviorism

There are a number of advantages derived from the behaviorist view of development.

1. It is a neat, concise, economical and relatively uncomplicated way to describe human behavior.

2. It has been widely accepted and adopted in the classroom and by parents. Many teachers have been trained in its use, and school programs and curricula utilize its concepts and ideas. The field of special education in particular uses behavior modification techniques with significant success. Consequently, a practitioner finds wide and popular support for adopting a behaviorist approach to working with and rearing children.

3. The stimulus-response approach as a means of explaining behavior is relatively easy to understand. In addition, for a wide range of behaviors it is a plausible and reasonable explanation.

4. Many of the tenants of behaviorism are easy to apply in classroom, clinic, and home set-

tings. Furthermore, the application of behaviorist principles works. And since most people have a tendency to be result-oriented, a program that gets results is popular.

5. Social learning theory, with its emphasis on the role of the person as an intermediating force, changes the equation from S (Stimulus) → R (Response) to S (Stimulus) → person → R (Response). This is a much more enlightened view of human nature and casts children as less passive and more active in their development.

On the other hand, there are a number of weaknesses with the behaviorist view of learning. For example, the simplicity and economy of the S → R approach strikes many as too simplistic and oversimplified to explain human behavior. They believe that human learning is more complex and involves more than stimuli and responses. Take the example of J.P. and language learning. Is the S → R approach really adequate to fully explain how he will learn language?

Also, since behaviorists place great emphasis on observable behavior, critics contend that children's unobservable thoughts and feelings are overlooked in considering their behavior. In fact, some contend that a deemphasis on how children feel about something has two consequences. First, it leads to an uncaring attitude on those who are doing the reinforcing. Second, it fails to take into consideration the child's point of view—her feelings and emotions about a topic or behavior. This second point also touches on the issue of power. He who has the rewards has the power.

Many people are fearful of the methods and consequences of behavior modification. They claim that use of behavior modification is little more than manipulation of children. Certainly, we are all susceptible to manipulation, however, manipulation implies intent that is not in the best interest of others. This is where ethical principles and moral behavior are necessary to guide all we do.

Early childhood educators in particular object to the nature of the reinforcers sometimes used with young children. They contend that foods in particular are inappropriate for reinforcing behavior.

MASLOW AND HUMANISTIC THEORY

Abraham Maslow (1908–1970) was born and reared in Brooklyn, New York. Following graduation from high school, he entered the City College of New York and a year later transferred to the University of Wisconsin. It was here that he developed an enthusiasm for psychology and behaviorism. While his enthusiasm for psychology remained all his life, Maslow became disaffected with behaviorism. He believed that,

its fatal flaw is that it's good for the lab and in the lab, but you put it on and take it off like a lab coat. It's useless at home with your kids and wife and friends. It does not generate an [adequate] image of man, a philosophy of life, a conception of human nature (Lowery, 1973, p. 5).

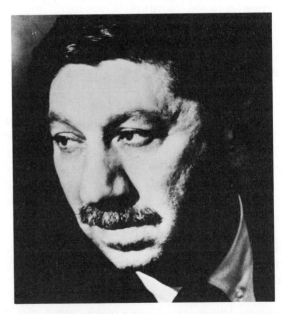

FIGURE 2-13 Abraham Maslow developed a theory based on human needs. (Photo courtesy of the Bettmann Archive)

This dissatisfaction with behaviorism as an adequate explanation for human behavior motivated Maslow to search for an alternative explanation. His starting point was the premise that humans, by nature, are good. Given this basic belief, it makes sense that Maslow would begin with humans in his search for human motivation. This is a key factor. Humanists look to humans for reasons, answers, and explanations. A major premise of *humanism*—as the term implies—is that humans, not a higher authority, provide the key to understanding human success and values. In other words, in searching for guidance and direction and the reasons for their behaviors and actions, humans must look to themselves, not to someone else or someplace else.

Maslow believed that in the search for guiding principles of good, bad, right and wrong, by which to live, people have tended to look outside themselves, to a God and to sacred sources. However, Maslow thought that this was unnecessary. He

dedicated himself to the theory that it was possible to discover the values to guide daily living by examining the lives and behaviors of "good" people. He felt that by observing the best of humankind, he could discover those values by which we all should govern our actions and lives.

In his search for the good in human behavior, Maslow also sought to explain why it is that people always don't demonstrate their basically good natures. He thought that nasty behavior was exhibited by basically good people and set out to determine why.

The "why" of his answer resulted in the development of his now-famous explanation of human needs toward the ultimate goal of *self-actualization*. Maslow believed, however, that this goal of self-actualization is not realized unless certain other basic human needs are met first. Humans have a hierarchy of needs that must be met or satisfied before self-actualization occurs. This hierarchy is depicted in Figure 2–14.

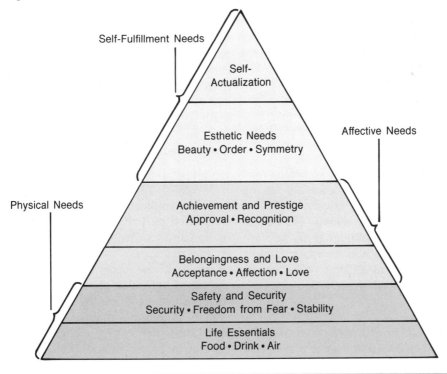

FIGURE 2-14 Maslow's "Hierarchy of Needs." (Reprinted with permission of Harper & Row Publishers, Inc. from Abraham H. Maslow (1970). *Motivation and Personality*.)

The Hierarchy of Needs

Level 1. Life Essentials   The first level involves those essential things that are necessary for maintaining life. These needs include food and air. These needs are necessary for survival and until they are satisfied, according to Maslow, nothing else matters. But merely getting or having food may not be enough. A child, for example, may eat too much junk food and not have his basic nutritional needs met. The point is that basic needs cover a wide range of continued applications in the daily lives of children and adolescents.

Level 2. Safety and Security   Once basic life essentials are satisfied, then the next level of needs emerge, the needs associated with safety, security, and protection. Safety exists at several levels—physical, emotional, and cognitive. Parents and care-givers provide for infants' physical protection and adults pay taxes for police protection and buy dead bolt locks for their doors in order to satisfy their safety needs. Parents provide for their children's emotional security by helping them to become confident and competent individuals. A solid and stable marriage provides emotional security for each partner. Knowledge frees people from fear and makes them feel secure. The knowledge that a parent is close by is comforting and reassuring to a child.

Level 3. Belongingness and Love   According to Maslow, belongingness, love, and affection are basic human needs. Belonging and love involve the reciprocal process of giving and taking. Humans want to love and be loved. Belongingness needs explain why people establish and maintain families, join organizations, become members of groups, and go to shopping malls when they don't need to buy anything.

Level 4. Achievement and Prestige (Self-esteem)   Achievement and prestige enable people to feel confident and worthy. Everyone needs to feel that what they do is significant and contrib-

utory. Children want to be involved in and do things so they may develop feelings of confidence and competence. Adults also want to feel that what they are doing is worthwhile. These are the basis for self-esteem.

Level 5. Aesthetic Needs   Everyone likes things that are aesthetically pleasing and beautiful. Appreciation of beauty is a basic human characteristic according to Maslow. A child comments on the beauty of her teacher's dress. Adults buy an otherwise useless object because it is pretty. Communities adopt "art in public places" policies in order to surround their citizens with beauty. In addition to beauty, other basic needs of this level of Maslow's hierarchy are goodness, justice, and truth.

Level 6. Self-actualization   At the apex of Maslow's hierarchy is self-actualization. The self-actualized person is a full human being, desirous of becoming all that she is capable of becoming. The self-actualized person possesses a joyous, contented feeling. She is an "actualized" person.

Much of the inspiration for self-actualization and qualities ascribed to the self-actualized person come from a journal Maslow kept. He referred to it as the "Good Human Being" notebook or the "GHB." In this notebook, Maslow kept notes regarding people—friends, acquaintances, and college students—and his efforts to identify good human beings and their characteristics.

Implications of Humanism

The application of humanistic ideas to education and parenting results in a number of child-rearing and curriculum practices. Current programs in and practices of "values clarification" are one example. These programs and curricula are designed to help children and adolescents "clarify" their values as a means of developing a value system. Humanists maintain that by helping children know what they believe, the children can develop a set of beliefs that will assist them in their journey toward self-actualization. On the other hand, conservative critics point out the "ungodly"

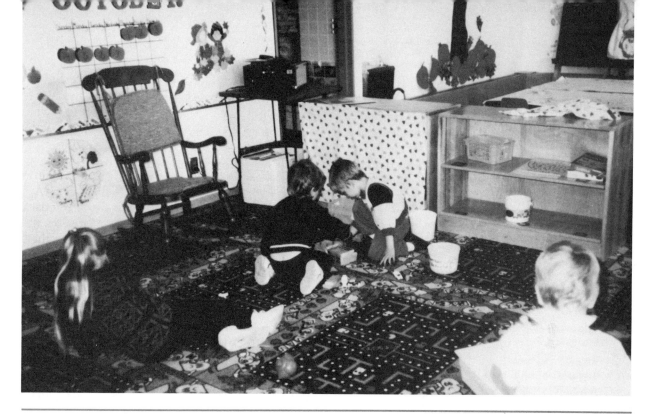

FIGURE 2-15 An important function of early childhood educators is to develop humane environments in which children are taught and cared for with respect and dignity.

nature of such an approach and assail humanistic attempts to substitute children's values for universal and "God-given" values.

In regard to child rearing, humanistic ideas lend themselves well to a child-centered and permissive approach. Humanists have a strong kinship to all—past and present—who advocate rearing children in an environment of freedom in which children follow their own timetables and guide and direct their own behavior. Children are loved, respected, and supported so that they have the opportunity to become whatever they want to be. But how do children and adolescents know what they want to become? The humanistic answer is deceptively simple, yet fraught with critical implications. According to Maslow (1968), "In the normal development of the healthy child, it is now believed that, much of the time, if he is given a really free choice he will choose what is good for his growth." Not everyone agrees this is the best way to rear children.

Humanistic educators tend to stress instructional practices that encourage children to accomplish learning tasks for "the joy of learning" rather than for a physical reward or grade. Teaching, therefore, is a process of helping children develop a desire to learn. This occurs best when teachers use interesting activities, follow the interests of children, and provide a classroom atmosphere that promotes autonomy. This contrasts sharply with the behaviorist conception of learning motivated by candy, stars, privileges, and grades.

Strengths and Weaknesses of Humanism

In the truest sense of the word, humanistic theory is not a theory of child development. Rather, it is a theory of development that focuses on self-actualization or fulfilling inner talents to their fullest extent. However, Maslow's ideas exert considerable influence on education and child-rearing practices as discussed, in part because it lends itself well to application in these areas.

A basic weakness of humanism, according to its critics, is that it looks to human beings rather than to external forces or a higher being for the explanation of human behavior. Maslow's basic assumption that the answers to behavior reside in humans immediately gets him into trouble with conservatives and religious fundamentalists. Much of the criticism relating to "secular humanism" involves this very issue.

Some critics also maintain that self-actualization is nothing more than giving people a license to "do their own thing," often at the expense of others and society.

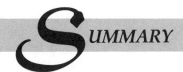

What Would You Do?

Nancy Rennik prides herself on being an organized and "with it" mother and wife. She combines rearing three children with a well-paying career as an interior designer. Nancy attributes part of her ability to manage all she does to some well-defined and reinforced rules, such as: the children can use the computer before school (something they love to do) only if they are dressed, and everyone must come to breakfast when called.

But there is trouble in the household and things are not going well. Lately, Nathan, age six, is so captivated with computer games he wants to do little else. He gets up before everyone else, goes to the computer room clad in his pajamas, "logs on," and becomes immersed and entranced by the latest game his dad, Charlie, has bought for him.

When Nancy calls Nathan for breakfast, he usually responds, "Mom, I can't now. I'm just about to solve this game!" When Nancy becomes insistent, "But you must come now! The rule is that when breakfast is ready, you have to come." Nathan responds, "No—and you can't make me! Besides, Daddy wants to see how well I'm doing on this game!"

Charlie seems to be taking Nathan's side in his increasing infatuation with computer games. For the past several mornings, he has joined Nathan in his before-school computer games. As Nancy and the two other children eat, you can hear Nathan and Charlie happily congratulating each other on their progress. When Nancy says anything to Charlie, he protests, "Come on, Nancy, you're taking all the fun out the things. Besides, you have no right to keep me from playing with Nathan."

Nancy has confided to her close friend, Joanne, that she is getting sick and tired of Charlie's behavior. "He's acting like a child! I know he's been having trouble at the office, but honestly, you'd think he'd grow up!"

Based on the theories you read in this chapter, how would you interpret the behaviors in the Rennik household? Write down your ideas before turning to the end of the chapter for ideas and suggestions.

Summary

- Theories help answer the what, how, why, and when of human development. A theory is a systematic set of assumptions about relationships, principles, and data designed to predict and explain human behavior and events. Theories serve many useful functions. They explain behavior, provide researchers with ideas, provide guidance for the education and care of children, and contribute to decisions regarding public policy.

■ Stage and nonstage theories help explain development. A stage theory views development as occurring in discrete and recognizable stages with development in one stage qualitatively different from development in a previous or future stages. A nonstage theory views development as acumulative with few, if any, discontinuities.

■ The following questions help assess a theory of development. Does it:
  ■ accurately reflect the world of children?
  ■ seem understandable?
  ■ explain the past and predict the future?
  ■ provide practical guidance for child rearing?
  ■ seem consistent?
  ■ stimulate new research?
  ■ explain development in a way that makes sense?

■ Sigmund Freud developed a theory of personality development based on ideas of infant sexuality and hidden sexual impulses. The libido is the sexual energy that drives people's lives. The ego acts as a mediating influence between the id and the superego or conscience.

■ Stages of Freudian personality development are: (1) Oral—birth to one year; (2) Anal—two to three years; (3) Phallic or Oedipal—three to four years; (4) Latency— five to thirteen years; and (5) Mature Genital—thirteen to eighteen years.

■ Freud believed how children and adolescents resolve the crises of each developmental stage determines the nature and kind of personality characteristics they develop.

■ Defense mechanisms that develop during the mature genital stage help people deal with stressful life experiences. Defense mechanisms include: repression, regression, rationalism, sublimation, and projection.

■ Criticisms of Freud's theory relate to the impossibility of testing his conclusions, the inapplicability of his stages to children of all cultures, the fact that his conclusions are based on remembrances, and its inadequacies in accurately explaining female social, sexual and moral development.

■ Erik Erikson developed a theory of psychosocial development based in part on Freudian ideas. Personality development is a product of the interplay between maturational processes, biological needs, and the social forces of everyday life.

■ Erikson's theory postulates eight qualitatively different stages of development. These stages are:
  ■ Stage 1—oral-sensory: basic trust vs. mistrust (birth to eighteen months)
  ■ Stage 2—muscular-anal: autonomy vs. shame and doubt (eighteen months to three years)
  ■ Stage 3—locomotor-genital: initiative vs. guilt (three to five years)
  ■ Stage 4—latency: industry vs. inferiority (five to eleven years—the elementary years)
  ■ Stage 5—puberty and adolescence: identity vs. role confusion (twelve to eighteen years: adolescence)

■ Stage 6—young adulthood: intimacy vs. isolation (end of adolescence to middle adulthood)

■ Stage 7—adulthood: generativity vs. stagnation (thirty-five to forty-five years)

■ Stage 8—maturity: ego integrity vs. despair (mid-life to death)

■ Basic strengths of Erikson's theory are that it makes basic Freudian ideas more useful and practical, provides for developmental stages across the life span, and provides information and ideas that are practical and applicable to child rearing and other child-related fields. On the other hand, critics maintain that his theory is difficult to verify with experimental methods, that it was formulated on too few cultural populations, and that it fails to adequately account for changes in contemporary families and life-styles.

■ Jean Piaget developed one of the most influential theories about children's cognitive development. Part of his procedure for gathering information about how children think is the "clinical method," based on psychiatric methods of interviewing.

■ Children develop mental schemes through the reciprocal processes of assimilation and accommodation. Children literally construct intelligence through physical and mental activity.

■ Piaget identified four stages of intellectual development. Stage 1—sensorimotor (birth to two years) has six independent substages: reflexive actions, primary circular reactions, secondary circular reactions, coordination of secondary schemes, experimentation, and representational intelligence. The other stages are: Stage 2—preoperational (two to seven years), Stage 3—concrete operations (seven to eleven years), and Stage 4—formal operations (eleven to fifteen years).

■ Many educators and child developmentalists use Piagetian theory as their "theory of choice." Piaget stimulated many others to study intellectual development and test his ideas. Critics fault Piaget's experimental methods, complain about the frequent obtuseness of his writings, and question the ages he specified for the stages of development.

■ Behaviorists emphasize the role of the environment in learning, and view development as a continuous set of changing behaviors governed by the principles of learning. Development results from children's interactions with reward systems in the environment.

■ Ivan Pavlov demonstrated the process of classical conditioning; J.B. Watson, the founder of behaviorism, introduced ideas relating to stimulus-response connections and contingency management; Edward Thorndike maintained people do those things that bring them pleasure and avoid those things that bring them pain.

■ B. F. Skinner popularized behaviorism and introduced the process of operant conditioning. His "Skinner box" enabled detailed and elaborate experiments involving conditioning. Many of Skinner's ideas are applied to education and child-rearing processes.

■ Social learning theorists led by Albert Bandura believe individuals act as mediators in stimulus-response situations. In addition, Bandura believes that modeling is a major factor in learning.

■ Abraham Maslow developed a theory of personality development based on a hierarchy of needs that consists of six stages: life essentials; safety and security; belongingness and love; achievement and prestige; aesthetic needs; and self-actualization.

QUESTIONS TO GUIDE YOUR REVIEW

1. What are theories of development?
2. What functions do theories serve?
3. Why are theories important?
4. What are the similarities of and differences between stage and nonstage theories of development?
5. What are the major purposes of the id, ego, and superego?
6. What are the stages of psychosexual development and the resolutions in each stage?
7. What are the major criticisms of Freudian theory?
8. What are the differences between psychoanalytic and psychosocial theory?
9. What are the stages of psychosocial development and what are the conflicts of each?
10. What are the differences between Freud's, Erikson's, and Piaget's theories?
11. What is Piaget's clinical method?
12. What is a scheme?
13. What is the relationship between assimilation and accommodation?
14. According to Piaget, what are the four stages of cognitive development?
15. What is behaviorism?
16. What are the major differences between operant conditioning and social learning theory?
17. What are the major advantages and disadvantages of behaviorism?
18. What is humanism?
19. What are the levels of Maslow's hierarchy of needs?
20. What are the major differences between psychoanalytic, psychosocial, cognitive, learning, and humanistic theories?

ACTIVITIES FOR FURTHER INVOLVEMENT

1. Behavior modification and reinforcement techniques are very popular with teachers, care-givers, special educators, and others. Visit schools, programs, and agencies to determine how practitioners use behavior modification techniques in their everyday work with young children.
2. Over a period of several weeks or a month, collect articles from newspapers and popular magazines relating to infants, toddlers, and preschoolers, and then:
   a. Categorize these articles by topics, for example, child abuse. What topics were given the most coverage? Why?
   b. What are the emerging topics or trends in early education according to newspaper and magazine coverage?
   c. Do you agree with everything you read? Can you find instances in which information or advice may be inaccurate, inappropriate, or contradictory?
3. The media is paying special attention to programs that involve infant stimulation and baby massage. Visit programs that are involved in such activities. How is what they are doing supported by the theories discussed in this chapter? Are any of the activities you observed contrary to the basic principles of the theories?
4. Interview professors and students from various disciplines to determine how the theories discussed in this chapter are incorporated into their disciplines and courses of study. For example, the other day, during a lecture on pediatric nursing, the professor said, "Of course, the nurse-practitioner will have to meet all of the infant's needs, both physical and psychosocial." What did she mean?
5. According to Maslow's theory, life essential needs, safety and security needs, and belongingness and love needs must be met in order for children to develop or advance to higher levels of development. Give examples of how society is and is not meeting these basic needs of the nation's children.

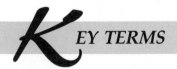

KEY TERMS

Accommodation The process of changing an existing scheme to include new information.

Adaptation The reciprocal process of assimilation and accommodation whereby a person adjusts to new ideas and experiences.

Adulthood The seventh stage of psychosocial development.

Anal stage The second stage of Freudian personality development. Pleasure focuses on the anal area.

Assimilation Taking in and incorporating new information into already existing mental schemes.

Behavior modification The conscious and planned use of reinforcers to change behavior.

Behaviorism The sch[ool of psychology that] ...view. Children believe
believes that human [...] ...d act as they do.
primarily through st [...] ...xual desire of a female

ronment.

Classical conditi[on] [...] ...**libration)** The mental
whereby a condition [...] ...ssimilation and accom-
a conditioned respo[nse] [...] ...lve cognitive conflict

Clinical method A [...] ...g experiences and per-
and interview pop[...]
which the interview[...] ...Areas of the body sen-
upon an individua[l...] ...mulation and arousal.
haviors. [...] ...isappearance of a re-

Cognitive develop[ment...] ...t of the removal of a
tal processes and ab[...]
edge and awarenes[...] ...in which an adult uses

Concrete operation[...] ...ate to a less mature stage
for the third stage of intellectual develop- ...especially the oral, anal,
ment. A child is able to use logical thinking and phallic stages.
but still must use real or "concrete" things
and symbols to assist with the thinking
process.

[Handwritten note overlaid:]
Teach the Erogenous zone
area of the body sensative
to sexual stimulation
and arousal
He responded well
to stimulation.
The habituation continue
until about February
I start see changes
Sex has something to do
with the Brain)

Formal operations stage The final stage
in Piaget's theory of cognitive development. The adolescent is able to think logically and develop and test hypotheses.

Conditioned response The result of conditioning whereby a conditioned stimulus
elicits a response.

Functional invariants Processes that are
critical to and influence behavior.

Conditioned stimulus A stimulus that is
conditioned by, or takes the place of another stimulus. In Pavlov's experiment, the
bell became the conditioned stimulus for
the meat.

Habituation A decrease in responsiveness
or sensitivity as the result of the repetition
of a stimulus. Satiation in relation to a
stimulus.

Constructivism The concept that knowledge is built by an active child from the
inside rather than being transmitted from
the outside through the senses.

Humanism A theory popularized by Abraham Maslow that humans, not a higher
authority, provide the key to understanding human success and values.

Id Source and controller of libido.

Contingency management The process of
managing or manipulating the reward system in order to promote a desired behavior.

Latency The fourth stage of Eriksonian
psychosocial development.

Defense mechanism Behavior or thought
patterns that originate in the ego. Defense
mechanisms are psychological processes
that operate unconsciously to help protect
the ego against reality.

Latency period The third stage of Freudian
personality development. The child has no
particular interest in erogenous zones or
sexual desire.

Libido General sexual or psychic energy.

Ego Latin word for "I." The reality force
of the human psyche; mediates between
the id and the superego.

Locomotor-genital The third stage of psychosocial development.

Mature genital period The fourth and last
stage of Freudian personality development.
The stage of mature sexuality.

Egocentric (egocentrism) Children's cognitive processes are governed by their own

Maturity The eighth stage of psychosocial
development.

Muscular-anal The second stage of psychosocial development.

Negative reinforcer A stimuli, such as the threat of punishment, that increases behavior necessary to avoid an unpleasant situation or punishment.

Neuroses Functional disorders of the mind and emotions, such as anxieties and phobias.

Nonstage theory Depicts development as an additive and cumulative process. New development is merely an improved version of previous development.

Object permanence The understanding that when things are not present or seen, they still exist.

Oedipus complex Sexual desire of a male child for his mother.

Operant The process of operating on one's environment.

Operant conditioning (instrumental conditioning) The procedure popularized by B. F. Skinner for promoting learning by reinforcing a particular behavior.

Oral-sensory The first stage of psychosocial development.

Oral stage The first stage of Freudian personality development. During the oral stage, physical and psychic energy is directed toward gaining gratification through the mouth.

Penis envy Freudian (psychoanalytic) belief that at about age four, girls become jealous when they realize boys have a penis and they do not.

Phallic stage Third stage of Freudian personality development. Pleasure focuses on the genital areas of the penis, clitoris, and vulva.

Positive reinforcer A stimulus, often referred to as a reward, that increases a behavior.

Preoperational stage Piaget's term for the second stage of intellectual development. Children at this stage do not have operational intelligence and cannot mentally conserve or reverse thought processes.

Primary circular reaction Piaget's term for the process whereby infants use their bodies to initiate and repeat many pleasurable actions such as thumb-sucking.

Projection Attributing to others the feelings persons deny exist in them.

Puberty and adolescence The fifth stage of psychosocial development.

Punishment A stimulus that suppresses or decreases a response.

Rationalization Overexplanation and justification of actions and decisions.

Regression Return to childhood behaviors.

Reinforcement The process of rewarding a behavior to increase or strengthen the likelihood of its occurrence.

Reinforcement theory The idea that behavior is strengthened by the nature and kind of reward or reinforcer that follows it.

Reinforcer Anything that increases the rate or nature of a response.

Representational intelligence (intention of means) The sixth and final stage of sensorimotor intelligence. The stage of transition from sensorimotor thought to symbolic thought.

Repression Unconsciously forgetting a painful or upsetting experience.

Response For behaviorists, any observable reaction.

Scheme (schema) A mental representation, idea, design, or blueprint used to organize events.

Secondary circular reaction Piaget's term for the process whereby infants reproduce events with the *intent* of sustaining or repeating acts. The infant attempts to elicit a response from a secondary source, such as a toy or care-giver.

Self-actualization The apex or final stage in Maslow's hierarchy of needs. The self-actualized person develops or is developing to his fullest potential.

Sensorimotor stage Piaget's first stage of

intellectual development during which the child acquires knowledge through sensory experiences and motor activities.

Sensory receptor A nerve ending specialized to receive stimuli.

Social learning theory That field of behaviorist psychology that believes that children play a mediating role in stimulus-response learning. Emphasis is placed on learning through modeling and observation.

Stage theory Based on the premise that growth and development consist of discrete and recognizable stages, with development in one stage qualitatively different and distinct from development in a previous stage.

Stimulus Any event that produces a physical or mental response.

Sublimation Diverting sexual energies to socially accepted activities.

Superego The conscious or moral code of an individual.

Tertiary circular reactions Piaget's term for sensorimotor actions in which the toddler does an interesting action for its own sake. The toddler experiments in many ways with a given object.

Theory A systematic set of statements and assumptions about relationships, principles, and data designed to explain and predict behavior and events.

Unconditioned response A response caused by an unconditioned stimulus.

Unconditioned stimulus A stimulus that causes a response without any prior learning.

Young adulthood The sixth stage of psychosocial development.

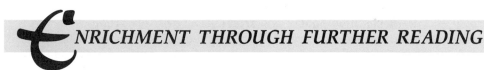

ENRICHMENT THROUGH FURTHER READING

Crain, W. C. (1980). *Theories of development: concepts and applications.* Englewood Cliffs, NJ: Prentice-Hall.

> From Locke to Maslow, this book discusses learning theories of the behaviorists, but most fully examines developmental theories. Easy-to-read and understand with many practical recommendations.

Dokecki, P. R., & Zaner, R. M. (Eds.). (1987). *Ethics of dealing with persons with severe handicaps: Toward a research agenda.* Baltimore: Paul H. Brooks.

> Deals with the issues and concerns in the many ethical dimensions and dilemmas involved in mental retardation. Helps all involved in the education and care of the handicapped make informed judgments about crucial ethical issues.

Gazda, G. M., Corsini, R. J., et al. (1980). *Theories of learning.* Itasca, IL: F. E. Peacock.

> This book concentrates on twelve major learning theories, because as the authors state: "Practically all human misery or happiness depends on a better understanding of the issue of learning. Such eminently practical problems as how to bring up children, how to have happy marriages, how to prevent wars, and how to make a living are essentially issues of learning."

Hergenhahn, B. R. (1982). *An introduction to theories of learning* (2nd ed.). Englewood Cliffs, NJ: Prentice-Hall.

> An easy-to-read discussion of the major learning theories. A concluding chapter provides applications to educational settings.

Thomas, M. R. (1979). *Comparing theories of child development*. Belmont, CA: Wadsworth. This is an interesting and informative explanation of how children learn, grow, and develop. Provides many practical insights and applications.

ANSWER TO "WHAT WOULD YOU DO?"

Behaviorists would maintain that Nancy needs to rearrange the contingencies and rewards associated with using the computer. Nancy could keep the computer games and give them to Nathan only after he was dressed or only after breakfast. After all, behavior is caused by rewards and punishments.

Since modeling plays a major role in social learning theory, an interpretation based on this point of view would examine ways to provide Charlie a role model for being a better husband and father.

Humanists would advocate the inherent ability of children and adults to make good and enlightened decisions. Consequently, Nancy should "back off" and give things an opportunity to work themselves out. Perhaps Nancy is causing part of the "problem" because she is too "controlling."

From a Piagetian perspective, Nathan is actively involved in "learning" that has the potential to contribute to cognitive growth. Some Piagetians would advocate that Nancy be more proactive in sharing her views with Nathan, enabling him to appreciate others' points of view and develop self-autonomy and responsibility for his actions.

Using Erikson's psychoanalytic theory, Nathan is in the industry vs. inferiority stage. It is important for him to develop feelings of self-worth and industry. Consequently, Nancy should seek ways for him to meet his "member-of-the-family" responsibilities without stunting his efforts of achievement.

Freudians would surely see Charlie's problem at work as a cause for regression to childish behaviors in order to cope with the realities of the work world. Also, he may unconsciously view Nancy as a mother figure. A recommendation would be counseling, perhaps involving Nancy.

The theory you choose by which to look at an incident—even a fairly uncomplicated, day-by-day family one involving Nancy and Charlie—makes a difference as to how you view the incident, what you will "read" into it, and the *limits* of what you can say about it. For example, a Piagetian perception limits what we can say about it because Piaget was interested in cognitive development and didn't emphasize behavioral problems or Charlie's adult/child behavior.

BIBLIOGRAPHY

Bandura, A. (1977). *Social learning theory*. Englewood Cliffs, NJ: Prentice-Hall.
Baumrind, D. (1971). Current patterns of parental authority. *Developmental Psychology Monograph* (4, Pt. 2).

Cohen, D. (1983). *Piaget: Critique and assessment.* New York: St. Martin's Press.

Coles, R. (1970). *Erik H. Erikson: The growth of his work.* Boston: Little, Brown.

Elkind, D. (1984). *All grown up and no place to go.* Reading, MA: Addison-Wesley.

Erikson, E. H. (1963). *Childhood and society* (2nd ed.) New York: W. W. Norton.

Evans, R. I. (1968). *B. F. Skinner: The man and his ideas.* New York: E. P. Dutton.

Evans, R. I. (1973). *Jean Piaget: The man and his ideas.* New York: Dutton.

Fancher, R. E. (1979). *Pioneers of psychology.* New York: W. W. Norton.

Freud, S. (1973). *An outline of psychoanalysis.* London: Hogarth.

Ginsburg, H. & Opper, S. (1979). *Piaget's theory of intellectual development.* Englewood Cliffs, NJ: Prentice-Hall.

Goleman, D. (1987, August 25). Embattled giant of psychology speaks his mind. *New York Times,* p. 17.

Jones, E. (1961). *The life and work of Sigmund Freud* (J. Trilling & S. Marcus, eds.). New York: Basic Books.

Kamii, C. (1981). Application of Piaget's theory to education: The preoperational level. In I. E. Sigel, D. M. Brodzinsky, R. M. Golinkoff (eds.), *New directions in Piagetian Theory and Practice.* Hillsdale, NJ: Lawrence Erlbaum Associates.

Kuhn, D. (1984). Cognitive development. In M. H. Bernstein & M. E. Lamb (Eds.), *Developmental psychology: an advanced textbook.* pp. 133–180. Hillsdale, NJ: Erlbaum.

Lowery, R. J. (1973). *A. H. Maslow: An intellectual portrait.* Belmont, CA: Wadsworth.

Lynn, K. S. (1987). *Hemingway.* New York: Simon and Schuster.

Maccoby, E. E., & Martin, J. A., (1983). Socialization in the context of the family: Parent-child interaction. In *Socialization, personality of social development:* E. M. Hetherington (Ed.), Vol. 4 of Paul H. Mussen (Ed.), *Handbook of child psychology* (4th ed.). New York: John Wiley.

Maslow, A. (1968). *Toward a psychology of being.* Princeton, NJ: Van Nostrand.

Maslow, A. H. (1970). *Motivation and personality.* New York: Harper & Row.

Piaget, J. (1952). *The origins of intelligence in children* (M. Cook, Trans.). New York: International Universities Press.

Piaget, J. (1965). *The child's conception of number.* New York: W. W. Norton.

Piaget, J. (1970). *Genetic epistemology* (E. Duckworth, Trans). New York: Columbia University Press.

Piaget, J., & Inhelder, B. (1958). *The growth of logical thinking from childhood to adolescence* (A. Parsons & S. Seagrin, Trans.). New York: Basic Books.

Pulaski, M. A. S. (1980). *Understanding Piaget* (rev. ed.). New York: Harper & Row.

Richmond, P. (1970). *An introduction to Piaget.* New York: Basic Books.

Skinner, B. F. (1967). Autobiography. In E. G. Boring & Gardner Lindzey (eds.), *A history of psychology in autobiography: Vol. 5* New York: Appleton-Century-Crofts.

Skinner, B. F. (1979). *The shaping of a behaviorist.* New York: Alfred A. Knopf.

Thomas, R. M. (1979). *Comparing theories of child development.* Belmont, CA: Wadsworth.

Watson, J. B. (1913). Psychology as the behaviorist views it. *The Psychological Review, 20,* 158.

Watson, J. B. (1930). *Behaviorism* (rev. ed.). Chicago: University of Chicago Press.

CHAPTER THREE

Becoming a parent

◆

VIGNETTES
INTRODUCTION
CONTEMPORARY PARENTS
  AND FAMILIES
HOW FAMILIES HAVE
  CHANGED
THE SHRINKING FAMILY—ONE
  IS ENOUGH
To Be—or Not to Be—a Parent
Implications for Parents and
  Professionals
Surrogate Parenting and
  Reproductive Technology
How Do You Define "Mother" and
  "Father"?
THERE'S MORE THAN ONE
  WAY TO HAVE A BABY
Adoption
STORK IN A TEST TUBE

In Vitro Fertilization (IVF) and
  Embryo Implantation
Catheter Fertilization
Gamete Intra-fallopian Transfer
  (GIFT)
Sperm Banks
ETHICAL ISSUES OF
  REPRODUCTIVENESS
In the Spotlight: A New Look at
  Abortion
FERTILIZATION
WHEN DOES HUMAN LIFE
  BEGIN?
HEREDITY
Laws of Inheritance
Sex-linked Inheritance
WHY DO I ACT THE WAY I DO?
Personality
Temperament

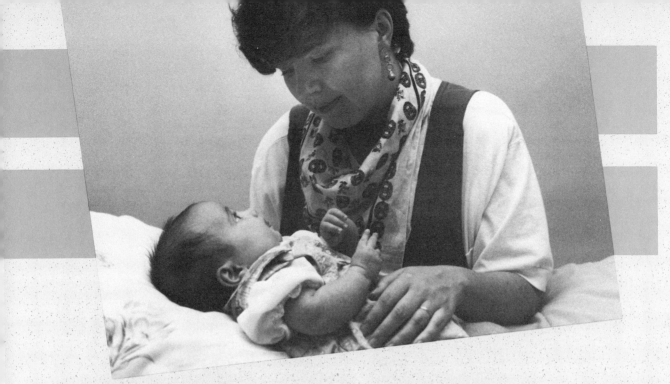

Intelligence
GENETIC SCREENING
Mapping Human Genes
Prenatal Fetal Genetic Screening
Gene Therapy
BOY OR GIRL?
Choosing Baby's Sex—With 80%
   Accuracy
TWINS, TRIPLETS, AND MORE
CHROMOSOME
   ABNORMALITIES
Down Syndrome (Trisomy 21)
SEX CHROMOSOME
   ABNORMALITY (SCA)
Turner Syndrome (TS)
Triple-X Syndrome (XXX)
Klinefelter's Syndrome (XXY)
XXY Syndrome

Fragile-X Syndrome
GENETIC DISEASES
Sickle-cell Anemia
Phenylketonuria (PKU)
Tay-Sachs Disease
Cystic Fibrosis (CF)
What Would You Do?
SUMMARY
QUESTIONS TO GUIDE YOUR
   REVIEW
ACTIVITIES FOR FURTHER
   INVOLVEMENT
KEY TERMS
ENRICHMENT THROUGH
   FURTHER READING
ANSWER TO "WHAT WOULD
   YOU DO?"
BIBLIOGRAPHY

⟲IGNETTES

On July 25, 1978, in Kershaw's Cottage Hospital in Oldham, Lancashire, Louise Brown was born. With her was born a new era in making babies. Until then, every human being had begun her or his existence deep inside a female body. There, unseen by human eyes and protected from any kind of outside interference, egg and sperm had fused and the fertilized egg had begun the process of dividing and growing that leads, if all goes well, to the birth of a baby nine months later.

Lesley and John Brown had been wanting children for several years, but Lesley Brown was infertile. Her ovaries produced eggs, but the eggs could not pass down the fallopian tubes to be fertilized. Surgery to remove the blockage proved unsuccessful. Then she was referred to Dr. Patrick Steptoe, an Oldham gynecologist, who, together with the Cambridge biologist Dr. Robert Edwards, was working on a novel method of overcoming infertility.

What Edwards and Steptoe did was to remove an egg from one of Lesley Brown's ovaries, place it in a glass dish, and then fertilize it with her husband's sperm. For the Browns, the significance of the technique was that it enabled them to have a longed-for child; but Edwards and Steptoe accomplished something much more momentous than that. For the first time, a human being had developed from an egg that was fertilized outside the female body. Thus Edwards and Steptoe opened a door to a host of new possibilities in the field of human reproduction (Singer & Wells, 1985, pp. vii–viii).

At thirty-five, Bonnie Benson was unmarried and childless. As she tells her friends, "I felt my biological time clock was ticking away and I wanted a baby before it was too late. So, I followed my heart and made a gut-level decision to have a baby. I knew there would be a lot of talk and gossip, especially at the high school where I teach, but this is not like thirty years ago when I would

have been a social outcast." Bonnie visited a local sperm bank and from a catalogue of donors selected the father-to-be of her child. Nine months after artificial insemination, Bonnie gave birth to Jennifer, now two-and-a-half. Bonnie doesn't regret her decision at all. "I couldn't have experienced the loving mother/child bond without Jennifer. Motherhood is very rewarding."

Artificial insemination didn't appeal to Alexis Masterson. "I wouldn't have felt right about carrying the baby of someone with whom I had no connection." Instead, she visited an attorney who specializes in helping clients adopt unwanted babies. Alexis paid all expenses—over $10,000—for the prenatal care of the natural mother during pregnancy and for the delivery of Josh, who is now two years old. Last week the attorney called Alexis to inquire if she wanted to adopt another child by the same mother. "I jumped at the chance," exclaims Alexis. "I just couldn't let the opportunity pass for Josh to have a brother or sister."

Patty and Pat lived together for five years before they decided on marriage and a family. "We felt comfortable with each other, but just didn't take the plunge into marriage," explains Pat. "I think it was our desire for children that helped us decide to get married." They now are the parents of two children, three-year-old Andrew and two-month-old Shelly. Patty thinks that postponing parenthood was good. "A period of time without children enabled us both to establish our careers and get ahead financially. I'm sure it has made supporting a family a lot easier."

When Paul Bradley learned he was going to be a father, he was ecstatic. "Linda and I had been trying to have a baby for years and we had just about given up hope. When we got the official confirmation from the doctor, it was as though all our dreams had come true. I attended Lamaze classes with Linda and did everything I could to help her have a healthy, normal pregnancy. When Adam was born, I was right there. I had heard so much about bonding at birth, there was no way I was going to miss anything!" Paul considers himself a truly equal parent. "Anything that needs to be done, I help Linda do it. I'm willing to share both the blame and the credit."

Gail Jordan was five months pregnant when she and her husband Tobias discovered she was going to have twins. Gail explains, "I went for a regular checkup and had a sonogram. When the doctor showed me two babies on the screen, I freaked out and started to cry. I had all these weird thoughts, like how was I going to take care of them and how could I get into a car with two babies! I knew from parenting seminars that the twinning rate for blacks is above average—about one in seventy-seven—but I never thought I would be the one!" Identical twins Yolanda and Tanya are two months old, healthy and normal. "Having twins really got me organized," says Gail. "I've learned how to do things quicker."

According to seventeen-year-old Rachel, "Being a pregnant teenager is *frustrating*. When you ride a bus, first people look at your belly and then at your finger. When they look at you like that, they just suck out all your self-confidence. For a while, I had no hope of succeeding." Thanks to her high school counselor, Rachel enrolled in a teenage parenting program where she received prenatal care and completed her high school degree. Today, one-year-old Brian receives child care while Rachel works as a checkout clerk in a grocery store. "Brian's father offered to marry me—after the fact—but I decided I didn't want a marriage because someone felt obligated to do it. Brian and me—we get along fine."

When Lourdes Menendez took her two youngest children, Carolina, age two, and Maria, age four, to a friend's birthday party recently, she felt more like an observer than a participant. "The other mothers were the same age as my older daughter. I was sitting there listening to how strict they were with their children and I thought, 'I must be doing something wrong or I must be a grandmother.'" Lourdes, forty-one, is a grandmother and, as a result of a divorce and remarriage, a "second-time-around mother" and an "encore parent". Lourdes believes she is much better equipped to handle the demands of parenting since she went through it once before. "I know these two children are my last ones, so I appreciate them more. I am less anxious about being a parent and know I can handle things as they come up. I don't make a lot of the mistakes I made the first time around. It's as though your parenting slate has been wiped clean and you can start again. Also, financially, it isn't a struggle to do nice things for the girls like it was for my other children when they were growing up."

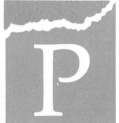arents, homes, and families play important roles in children's lives. Throughout this text you will read about how the interactions and attitudes of parents and the events of family life influence children and their development. Likewise, children have profound influences on parents, families, and the nature of family life. More and more, professionals who work with young children and their families realize that attitudes and perceptions brought to the marriage and parenting processes affect how parents interact with each other and their children. For example, in a study of the process of transition to parenthood, Marsha Kline (1989) found that when partners are dissatisfied in pregnancy, then this dissatisfaction is translated into parents' stress across the transition. Kline explains further:

> Two types of stress emerged as particularly salient for general well-being. Partners with lower well-being in pregnancy had higher parental stress (that is, they reported having a more difficult child and more difficult interactions with the child), and they had more family role strain (difficulty juggling houseperson, partner, and parent demands) when their child was eighteen months old (p. 4).

Consequently, the events surrounding and the process of becoming a parent should be of interest to all who parent or work with children. What persons will be like as parents and partners once children join the family, and what their children will be like, are the results of a process that begins long before conception and continues through all the stages of parenthood.

Also, throughout this book much emphasis is placed on *transitions*, and how these transitions affect children, youth, and adults as they grow, develop, and assume new roles throughout life; for example developmental changes from infancy to toddlerhood and social changes from nonparenthood to parenthood. In child development and early childhood circles, there is a tremendous amount of interest about the nature of life's many transitions and their influences on the people involved in them and how professionals and agencies can assist in these transitions.

CONTEMPORARY PARENTS AND FAMILIES

What would happen if society decided there would be no more children? There would be no child development, no schools, no future generations, and after several generations, no society. In fact, this is exactly what is happening to the Shakers, a religious community that does not believe in cohabitation. Before too long, their way of life will be extinct, because there are no children and, therefore, no future generation. The Shakers, known officially as the United States Society of Believers in Christ's Second Appearing, were introduced into the United States in 1774 by Englishwoman Anne Lee. The Shakers practice communal living and celibacy. At one time numbering 6000 in 19 villages in nine states, today only eight sisters remain in the two surviving villages, Sabbathday Lake, Maine and Canterbury, New Hampshire (Lindsley, 1987).

Government agencies and public institutions are interested in people's procreational attitudes and practices. Such interest is demonstrated through laws, policies, and economic support—or the lack of it—that influence people's reproductive decisions. When people have too few children to replace those who die, then society faces a shrinking work force and the threat of economic recession. On the other hand, too many children place a strain on economic resources. Such a situation currently exists in China, which has one of the toughest birth control programs in the world. Stringent provisions of China's population policy, including mandatory abortion, limits childbearing to one child per family.

In the Soviet Union, the government has a very strong "profamily" policy and offers mothers financial incentives to have babies. Certain inducements have been in effect since 1981, for example, mothers are provided a leave for one

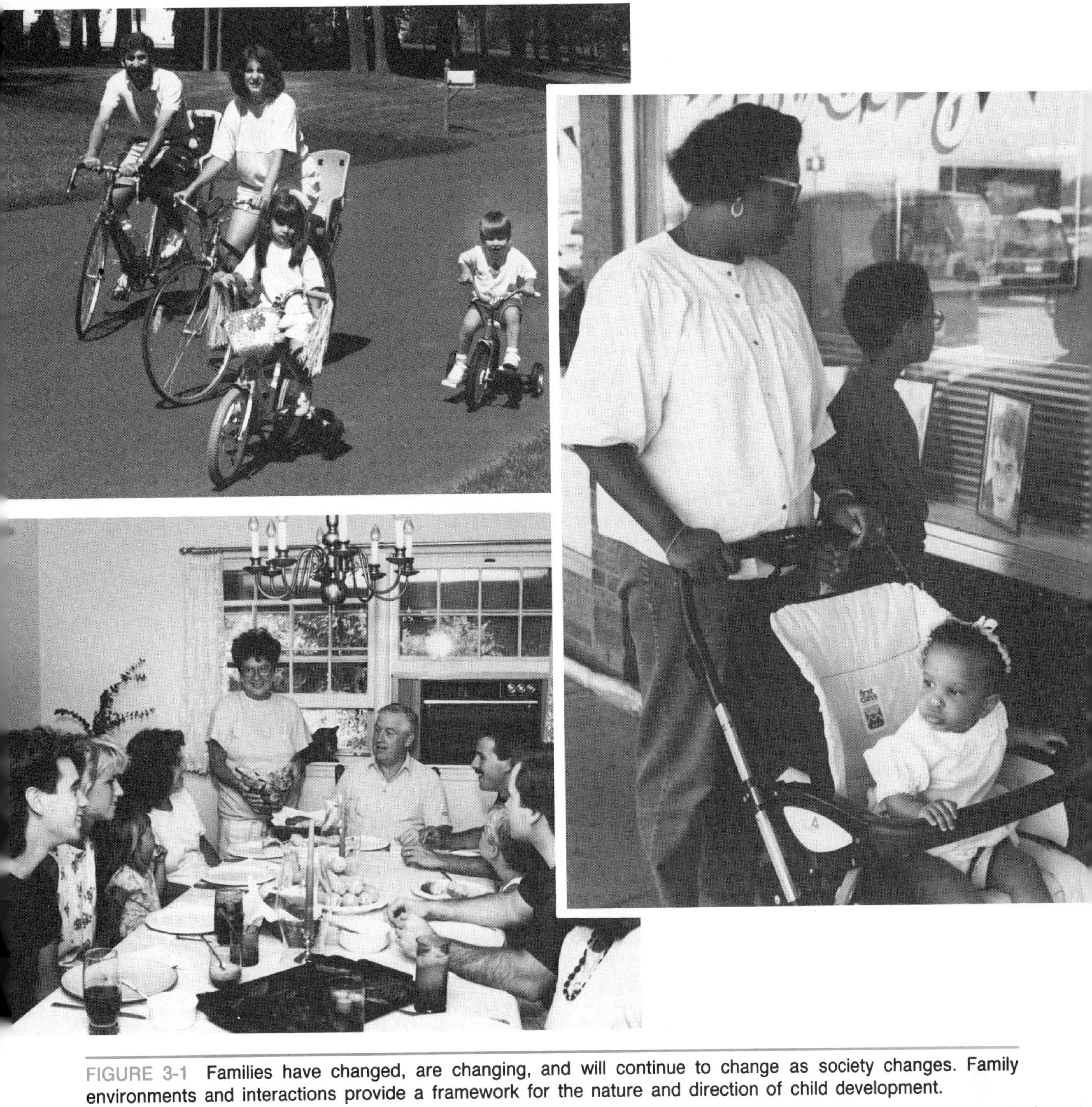

FIGURE 3-1 Families have changed, are changing, and will continue to change as society changes. Family environments and interactions provide a framework for the nature and direction of child development.

year with a monthly stipend; are paid bonuses for childbearing—about $80 for the first child and $100 for the second child—; and are given improved maternity care. These inducements are necessary in order to have a birthrate large enough to assure a population growth that will provide enough workers and military personnel (Keller, 1987).

Political leaders in Quebec, Canada, determined to protect and promote French culture, provide cash bonuses to encourage larger families (Jones, 1988). Paying bucks for babies is one way Quebec politicians see as reversing a demographic trend of declining birthrates. Politicians believe that by increasing the population they will be able to preserve the French culture. The profamily inducement amounts to $410 for each of the first two children and $2,460 for each child thereafter. Opponents of such pregnancy payoffs maintain that bribery is no way to build families and that bonuses may result in unwanted children.

In the United States, politicians draft profamily legislation to counteract antifamily cuts in support for child care and social services. In particular, increases in single parenting have generated tremendous interest in and demand for care for infants as young as six weeks of age. Some legislators would like to pass a law requiring companies with more than fifteen employees to provide unpaid maternity and paternity leave to mothers and fathers so they could spend time with their newborn children.

HOW FAMILIES HAVE CHANGED

Society has changed dramatically over the last decade and so have families. Much publicity and attention is given to the breakup and the breakdown of the American family. The demise of the family is blamed for and used to explain everything from the crime rate to AIDS.

The *nuclear* family, consisting of a married couple with children under eighteen living at home, is no longer the average family. In fact, it is a

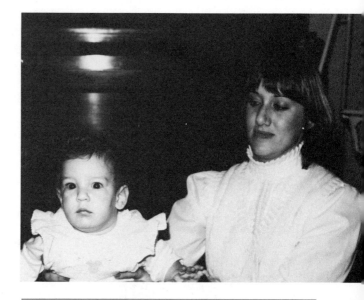

FIGURE 3-2 Single parenting and single parent families are more common today than they were in the past. Increasingly, people who work with children and families are being challenged to use their knowledge of child development to help single parents meet the challenges of single parenting.

minority family unit, with only 48 percent of families and 18 percent of households living in this arrangement (U.S. Bureau of the Census, 1987a, p. 1). As the traditional nuclear family undergoes transformation and possible dissolution, other kinds of families emerge to take its place and provide the traditional family functions of child rearing, economic and emotional support, socialization, education, protection, and satisfaction of basic human needs.

Other types of family units are: *extended* families, consisting of parents, children, and relatives, such as grandparents, aunts, and uncles; *single-parent* families (those headed by men are increasing in numbers), and, as a result of divorced people remarrying, *blended* or *stepfamilies*.

On the block where I live, there are twelve families. They include: a blended family of "his," "her," and "their" children; one family of two unmarried adults with children; two married couples with no children; an extended family of parents, children, and a grandmother; a single mother with two children; five married couples with children (comprising traditional nuclear families); and a homosexual couple with custody of a child from a previous marriage.

As families undergo changes and new families emerge, the rights of both children and parents are extended and modified. Stepparents in particular are enjoying rights they once did not have. Many states have laws that provide stepparents with the right to seek visitation and custody rights after a divorce. As one stepparent put it, "My wife's children by her former marriage spent more time living with me than with their biological father. We are very close and I didn't want to become a stranger to them after their mother and I divorced." Table 3–1 shows how families have changed over a fifteen-year period. A family household consists of two persons: the householder (the person, or one of the persons, who owns or rents the living quarters) and one or more additional persons who are relatives of the householder through birth, marriage, or adoption (U.S. Bureau of the Census, 1986, p. 1).

TABLE 3–1

HOW FAMILIES HAVE CHANGED—1970–1985 (NUMBERS IN THOUSANDS)			
	1970	1980	1985
Family Households	51,456	59,550	62,706
Married Couple Family	44,728	49,112	50,350
Male Householder	1,228	1,733	2,228
Female Householder	5,550	8,705	10,129
Non-Family Householder	11,945	15,557	24,082

Note. From "Household and Family Characteristics: March 1985" (Current Population Reports, Series P-20, No. 441), U.S. Bureau of the Census, 1986, p. 2.

THE SHRINKING FAMILY— ONE IS ENOUGH

Families have not only changed in composition. They are also changing—becoming smaller.

The number of children per family has dipped below two for the first time in decades, as shown in Table 3–2. One reason for the shrinking family is the drop in the *fertility rate*—the number of live births per 1,000 women. This rate has steadily dropped since 1957, the peak of the "baby boom" years of 1947 to 1964. Table 3–3 shows the extent of this decline.

TABLE 3–2

THE SHRINKING AMERICAN FAMILY		
Years	Average Family Size Including Children (All Children—All Ages)	Average Number of Children Per Family (Children Under 18)
1970	3.58	1.34
1971	3.57	1.32
1972	3.53	1.29
1973	3.48	1.25
1974	3.44	1.21
1975	3.42	1.18
1976	3.39	1.15
1977	3.37	1.13
1978	3.33	1.10
1979	3.31	1.08
1980	3.29	1.05
1981	3.27	1.03
1982	3.25	1.01
1983	3.26	1.00
1984	3.24	0.99
1985	3.23	0.98
1986	3.21	0.98
1987	3.19	0.96
1988	3.17	0.96
Projection 2000 (2)	3.07	0.92

Reasons for the shrinking family include: an increase in the number of women pursuing education and careers; postponement of marriage (in 1986, the median marriage age for men was 25.7 years and 23.1 years for women [Norton, 1987]); couples choosing between the quality of their lives and having children; and, as more families find they need the income of both parents to make

TABLE 3–3

FERTILITY RATE—1957 TO 1986	
Calendar Year	Fertility Rate (Live births per 1,000)
1957	122.7
1960	118.0
1965	96.6
1970	87.9
1975	66.0
1980	68.4
1986	64.9

Note. From "United States Population Estimates and Components" (Current Population Reports, Series P-25, No. 1006), U.S. Bureau of the Census, 1987, p. 4.

TABLE 3–4

THE COST OF RAISING AN URBAN CHILD—BIRTH TO AGE EIGHTEEN	
Geographic Region	Cost
Midwest	$ 90,100
Northeast	$ 94,976
South	$ 98,047
West	$100,151

Note. From "Updated Estimates of the Costs of Raising a Child," April 1986, Family Economics Review, 2, p. 34.

ends meet, the decision to be satisfied with one child.

Some couples who postpone childbearing find that time has passed them by and, as a result, may have only one child. They decide it is too late to have a larger family or they are divorced in the meantime (more than 35 percent of only children come from families where the parents are divorced).

Only children, or "onlies" as they are often called, are frequently stereotyped as "selfish," "lonely," or "maladjusted". While these stereotypes may motivate some parents to have a second child, it does not hold up under scrutiny. As Falbo (1984) points out, "Only children perform well on intelligence tests and achievement tests and do not differ consistently from other children in self-esteem or mental health" (p. ix). One reason only children tend to be brighter is the extended attention of their parents and the advantage of being reared in an environment undiluted by the presence of other children (Zajonc, 1987).

Increasingly, in the choice between upscale lifestyles and children, couples decide to remain childless. Such couples are referred to as "Dinks"—double income, no kids. Indeed, a child's economic demands on a family are considerable. The cost of raising a child from birth to age eighteen is shown in Table 3–4.

And, for those couples who want the feeling of having a baby but who don't want the diapers, midnight feedings, and other responsibilities, there is always Video Baby. Billed as "enjoyment without the commitment," Video Baby retails for about $19.95, and vicariously provides viewers with many of the pleasures associated with child rearing (Ricklefs, 1987).

To Be—or Not to Be—a Parent

Today, decisions about parenthood are more deliberate and planned. With advances in contraceptive methods, especially the pill, intercourse no longer necessarily results in parenthood. The widespread availability of contraceptive methods has had a pronounced impact on reproductive behavior. Indeed, the use of a contraceptive method is the rule rather than the exception. Of all women between the ages of fifteen and forty-four, 81.2 percent have used some contraceptive method, as have 94.6% of all sexually active women in the same age category. Contraceptive methods available to people and the extent of their use are shown in Table 3–5.

Sterilization as a contraceptive choice is growing in popularity. In 1984, 1,150,000 people had sterilizations—419,00 vasectomies and 731,000 tubal ligations ("An Increasing Proportion," 1987).

With the means and knowledge to prevent pregnancy and therefore parenthood, what motivates people to have children? Conception by choice

TABLE 3-5

AMONG ALL U.S. WOMEN AGED 15–44, AND AMONG THOSE AGED 15–44 WHO HAVE EVER HAD SEXUAL INTERCOURSE, PERCENTAGE WHO HAVE EVER USED VARIOUS CONTRACEPTIVE METHODS, 1982 NATIONAL SURVEY OF FAMILY GROWTH

Method	All Women (N = 54,099)	Sexually Active Women (N = 46,419)
Any method	81.2	94.6
Pill	65.9	76.8
Condom	44.7	52.1
Spermicides	28.8	33.5
Other*	25.6	29.9
Sterilization	17.8	20.8
IUD	15.9	18.5
Periodic absti-nence	15.8	18.4
Diaphragm	14.8	17.2

* Withdrawal, douche or other. Note: Ns in 000s.
Note. From "Has She or Hasn't She? U.S. Women's Experience with Contraception" by J. D. Forrest, May–June 1987, *Family Planning Perspectives,* 19, p. 113.

has a significant influence on reproductive behavior. For many couples, planning for parenthood is a reality. Indeed, most pregnancies within a marriage are reported to be planned and intended (Miller, 1983).

Frequently reported reasons for having children include: (1) to carry on one's name or physical characteristics; (2) to achieve adult status and social identity, and (3) to establish a family (Gromley, Gromley, & Weiss, 1987). Potts (1980) reports that decisions about having children revolve around the effect of the child on career, couple relationship, finances, and overall satisfaction and happiness (p. 631). Traditional sex roles also are part of decisions regarding childbearing. As Span, contributing editor of *Our Bodies, Ourselves,* suggests, "The mother role is probably the most satisfying part of the traditional complex of female roles" (Boston Woman's Health Book Collective, 1976, p.

103). Teenagers view childbearing as a way of recovering from an emotional loss, capturing a particular male, competing with the mother, escaping from an unhappy family life, and resolving a sense of deprivation and dependency (Phipps-Yonas, 1980).

Implications for Parents and Professionals

The reality of changing families has a number of implications for parents and those who work with and care for children and youth.

1. Older and more affluent parents are highly goal directed in matters relating to their children's education. They are willing to spend time and money on those programs and activities that promise to develop the intellectual abilities of their children. Consequently, there are more children attending academic preschools and infant stimulation programs than ever before.

2. Because of intentional parenthood, delayed parenthood, and planned parenthood, there is a decrease in the number of years people devote to childbearing. In developed countries, the duration of childbearing years ranges from a low of four in Japan and the Netherlands, to six in France, seven in Australia, to a high of ten in the United States ("Childbearing Occupies," 1987). This shortening of the childbearing years means that the number of children per family is likely to continue to decline. Also, parents will continue to invest more of themselves—monetarily and emotionally—in their few, and increasingly their only, children.

3. The labor force participation of women with young children has increased dramatically over the last decade. At the present time, over half of the mothers with children under three are employed outside the home. Also, women heading single-parent families are more likely to be employed than women from two-parent

homes and, as children grow older, the likelihood of the mother joining the labor force increases. Clearly, these kinds of demographic realities increase the demands for child care and have implications for parents, child care providers, and early childhood educators.

4. Parents will increasingly look to child development workers and researchers to help them and their children adjust to changing family conditions. Because of the trauma and stress involved in family breakups, there is a critical need for therapeutic and preventative child and family services. Researchers will be challenged to investigate the benefits, risks, and consequences of changes in family patterns that have occurred in the last decade and that are likely to continue into the twenty-first century.

5. Profamily legislation and family support services will increase. These efforts will include additional advocacy for unpaid and paid paternity leaves, extended counseling services, more extensive child care programs, and an expanded network of parenting support groups.

Surrogate Parenting and Reproductive Technology

Twenty years ago, most couples or individuals who were unable to achieve natural parenthood had two choices—childlessness or adoption. Today, they have available to them not only these choices but also a wide array of new biological and social techniques for achieving parenthood.

The vignettes at the beginning of this chapter depict some of the options individuals have in matters relating to parenthood. Probably one of the most celebrated and publicized cases involved the custody case of "Baby M." Mary Beth Whitehead, the surrogate mother, violated the terms of the surrogate contract and decided to keep Baby M rather than give her to William Stern, the biological father (through artificial insemination) and his wife, Elizabeth. After a lengthy court battle,

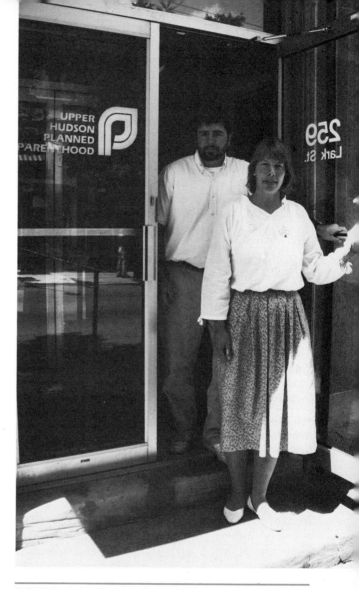

FIGURE 3-3 Today, there are many opportunities available to single persons and couples to become parents. Artificial insemination is one of these alternatives.

the Sterns were awarded custody of Baby M and Mary Beth Whitehead was awarded visitation privileges. She has also written an account of her experiences entitled *A Mother's Story*.

In another case of surrogate parenting, Pat Anthony of Johannesburg, South Africa gave birth to her daughter's triplets (as a result of embryo implants) and became the surrogate mother of her own grandchildren ("Surrogate Grandma," 1987).

Women give a number of reasons for their decisions to act as a surrogate. These include: enjoyment of pregnancy, a desire to help a childless couple, and a desire for money (Hanafin, 1987).

Typically, a surrogate mother receives $10,000–$15,000 (Mary Beth Whitehead received $10,000) for bearing a child. The total bill to the adoptive couple or parent can run from $25,000 to $45,000, including legal fees, insurance, and hospitalization. However, some states are attempting to make surrogate parenting illegal.

Surrogate parenting raises many knotty legal and ethical questions including: (1) the validity of the surrogate contract; (2) infants' rights; (3) the responsibilities of the surrogate mother and adoptive parents, especially in cases where the fetus is physically or mentally defective; and (4) the appropriateness of bearing a child for money, what some call reproductive prostitution and commercial procreation. Although some state legislators are considering bans on surrogate parenting for money, the demand for children is high, with more infertile couples seeking children than there are children to go around. Consequently, it may well be that efforts to regulate the practice of surrogate parenting could encourage a black market in bearing children for others.

Parents magazine conducted a national survey regarding surrogate parenting. The results indicated that "we as a society are not ready to embrace—unconditionally—the practice of surrogate motherhood. For example, 15 percent of the respondents approve of surrogate parenting under any circumstances; 43 percent approve only in certain circumstances; 32 percent oppose regardless of the circumstances, and 9 percent are not sure (Groller, 1987). Some states, such as Florida, have passed laws that prohibit childbearing for others for money.

How Do You Define "Mother" and "Father"?

Although many people would have little difficulty defining who is a "mother" or "father," it is not always as easy as you might think in this fast-paced world of reproductive technology and advanced medical practices. Indeed, the legal profession is having to redefine who is a "mother" and, as many people are learning, what they mean when they use the word is not what others have in mind. A mother can be the "genetic" mother, the person who gave the ovum. She can be the "carrying" mother, also known as the "birthing" mother, the one who carries and gives birth to the baby. Likewise, "father" may be the person who donates sperm—the biological father—or the person who resides with the mother and child.

THERE'S MORE THAN ONE WAY TO HAVE A BABY

Adoption

There are basically three ways to enter a family—birth, marriage, and adoption. Some persons see adoption as a highly desirable way to have the children they are not able to have through birth or marriage. Adoptions are usually arranged in one of three ways: through private agencies, through public agencies, or independently, usually with the assistance of an attorney. Some couples who want to adopt a baby are often frustrated by the likelihood of a long wait—perhaps five years or more—due to the increase in abortions and the growing tendency of many unwed mothers to keep their babies. Some childless couples consider adopting "hard-to-place" children, who have physical or intellectual handicaps, or older children. Others turn to agencies who specialize in transracial and international adoptions. The cost of an adoption ranges anywhere from $5,000 to $12,000. In an independent adoption, for example, these costs are typical: attorney's fees—$450–$3,000; medical and hospital costs for the birth mother—$5,000; housing and food costs for the birth mother during the last trimester—$4,000; and a home study and postplacement supervision—$1,700 (Schneider, 1987).

Adoption workers emphasis that everyone involved in the adoption process must keep the needs and rights of children in the forefront of their deliberations. In addition, such agencies as the American Adoption Congress advocate as standard practice "open adoptions," in which children have a right to be told of their adoption and information about their natural parents.

The National Committee for Adoption (P.O. Box 33366, Washington, DC 20033) publishes an in-depth *Adoption Factbook* that lists adoption agencies and much useful information about adoption.

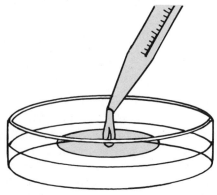

FIGURE 3-4

STORK IN A TEST TUBE
In Vitro Fertilization (IVF) and Embryo Implantation

The process of *in vitro fertilization* (IVF) begins when a laparoscope—a long tube with a light and magnification—is inserted through a small incision in the abdominal wall and ripe ova are removed from an ovary by aspiration. This procedure takes only a few minutes. (See Figures 3–4 and 3–5.) The ovum is placed in a petri dish and mixed with the husband's or donor's sperm. The fertilized egg or *zygote* develops for a few days in a laboratory incubator. There it grows to an eight- or sixteen-cell embryo and is then injected into the mother's womb.

Frequently, more than one embryo (usually three) are injected to assure implantation success. Ethical considerations of this and other procedures include: (1) decisions regarding whether to abort or not to abort any of the embryos after it is determined they have survived implantation; (2) the appropriateness of subjecting the mother to unwanted multiple births in order for her to be-

(1)

When it is seen under a microscope, the human egg looks just like a hen's egg.

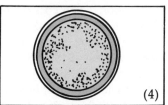

(2)

Following removal from body, the egg matures for three hours in an incubator.

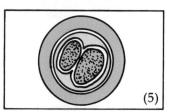

(3)

A few drops of sperm are combined with the egg in a solution in the petri dish.

(4)

The sperm (again, as seen in microscopic view) penetrates the membrane of the egg.

(5)

The single-cell, fertilized egg begins to divide. This represents the two-cell stage.

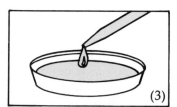

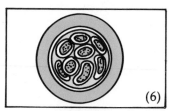

(6)

At the eight-cell stage, the embryo is ready to implant in the mother's uterus.

FIGURE 3-5

come a natural parent; (3) the risks to the mother in carrying a single child as compared to carrying two or three; and (4) the risks of survival and development for three babies in utero compared to the risks involved for only one.

In some instances, extra embryos are frozen for future use in the event that a woman does not become pregnant. The *cyropreservation* of embryos also allows for future implantation in women not genetically related to the donor. Interesting ethical questions are raised about the sharing or selling of genetic material. Also involved are issues relating to how many embryos should be frozen for future use; how long they should be stored; whether or not they should be used in research; and, who the embryos belong to when a couple divorces.

Catheter Fertilization

A new method of fertilization (Kolata, 1988) uses a very fine catheter to implant fertilized eggs directly into a fallopian tube. Fertilization normally occurs in the fallopian tube rather than in the uterus. Thus a fertilized egg inserted directly into the tube would have a better chance of surviving.

Gamete Intra-fallopian Transfer (GIFT)

Gamete intra-fallopian transfer (GIFT) uses much of the same technology as IVF. The eggs and sperm are mixed together and loaded into a catheter, which is then inserted through the laparoscope and the gametes discharged into the fallopian tube. Ideally, fertilization occurs in about thirty minutes. The fertilized egg then travels down the fallopian tube to the uterus where implantation occurs and pregnancy begins.

Sperm Banks

Many health and medical clinics around the United States have resources for the dissemination of fresh or frozen sperm. Proponents of *cyro-banking*, the storage of frozen sperm, contend that frozen sperm is safer than fresh sperm to use because a three-month waiting period permits testing for diseases prior to use. This testing is, for many hopeful parents, an essential process, especially because of the current AIDS epidemic. On the other hand, others may prefer fresh sperm because it can achieve pregnancy months sooner and it may have a higher motility rate, increasing the chances of pregnancy. Many sperm banks have a voluntary limit of ten to fifteen on the number of children a donor can sire. This reduces the possibility of half-sibling matings. Half-sibling matings, like full-sibling matings, increase the possibility for genetic diseases since the gene pool is so restricted.

Charges of *eugenics*, or the effort to improve the human gene pool by encouraging only the best and brightest to reproduce, are frequently leveled at sperm banks such as the Repository for Germinal Choice in Escondido, California. It was founded in 1980 by Robert Graham, a wealthy optometrist who envisions such centers creating a better world through brighter people. Originally this center was known as the Nobel Laureate Sperm Bank because it recruited semen donations from Nobel laureates. Today, it recruits persons who are renowned and leaders in their field. Clients are limited to married couples and women must be thirty-eight years of age or younger and of high intelligence. Semen is screened for all genetic diseases and motility—the ability to move spontaneously. Through 1987, the program was responsible for fifty-five births. Sperm is shipped to a couple's physician or directly to them if they choose to inseminate in the privacy of their own home. A donor's semen is not used a second time in the same geographic area to avoid the possibility of half-sibling marriages and individual donors are limited to eight pregnancies. Donors are not paid for their semen. Semen is provided without charge and the clients pay only a $50 application fee and the cost of the semen storage (Vaux, 1987).

The Cleveland Clinic recruits women to donate eggs for couples unable to have children. Donors and recipients are matched according to physical characteristics, but remain anonymous to each other ("Woman Pregnant," 1987).

ETHICAL ISSUES OF REPRODUCTIVENESS

As you undoubtedly suspect from our discussion of reproductive procedures, there are many troubling and critical ethical, legal, and social questions relating to artificial insemination, abortion, sterilization, surrogate parenting, and in vitro fertilization. These include:

1. Who should and should not be a recipient of sperm?
2. What are and what are not appropriate screening procedures for donors and recipients?
3. Should there be a mandatory limit on the number of children a donor can sire?
4. What legal and moral responsibilities do donors have to children if and when the children learn who donated egg or sperm?
5. Is it appropriate to try and "select" through sperm and egg donations only those who would make the "best" parents?
6. Should doctors experiment with embryos not used in transplants?
7. What should be done with unused embryos?

One of the problems facing all those involved in the area of reproductive technology is the absence of a federal code of ethics governing the field. The American Fertility Society, a nonprofit organization representing professionals in the field, has a nonbinding set of ethical considerations. For example, in the matter relating to embryo experimentation, the Society recommends that "it seems prudent at this time not to maintain human pre-embryos for research beyond the 14th day of post-fertilization development" (Ethics Committee of the American Fertility Society, 1986, p. 57S).

Advances in biology and medicine focus public and private attention on the many decisions and responsibilities involved in parenting. Rapid changes and discoveries in reproductive technology have a way of changing people's perspectives on life. Each new advance thrusts new choices and responsibilities upon parents and prospective parents, causing them to think differently about life. The ability to have children when the door to natural parenthood seemed closed; the ability to have someone else's child, and the ability to be the anonymous cause of enabling others to have children collectively raise awesome questions about parenting and human life, as well as issues relating to religious beliefs and practices.

Programs and clinics that provide hope and promise for solving infertility problems appeal to many prospective parents. About one million couples a year turn to in vitro fertilization (IVF) clinics, of which there are about 169 in the United States, and spend about $1 billion a year in attempts to cure their infertility and have children (Otten, 1988). However, a congressional research agency, the Office of Technology Assessment, warns couples that many of the clinics have low success rates.

FERTILIZATION

People's motivations and decisions relating to sexual intercourse and parenthood set off one of the most interesting and intriguing processes of child development.

Being in the right place at the right time is an important factor in numerous life events. Timing is critical for many developmental events as you will learn throughout this text. Timing also plays an important part in fertilization. *Ovulation*—the discharge of a female egg cell or *ovum*—occurs once every twenty-eight days, about midway through the menstrual cycle. During ovulation, a fluid-filled sac or *follicle* containing the ovum is released from the outer surface of one of the two *ovaries* into the abdominal cavity. From there, it is swept into one of the two fallopian tubes. Unlike the sperm, the ovum is not equipped for mobility, so its journey down the funnel-shaped fallopian tube is accomplished by contractions of the walls and the sweeping actions of hair-like *cilia*. The ovum (see Figure 3–6) is the largest cell in the human body and is 0.2 millimeter in size or about this (.) big.

*I*N THE SPOTLIGHT

A NEW LOOK AT ABORTION

On July 3, 1989, the Supreme Court gave individual states the right to set their own restrictions on abortion. While the Court did not overturn the landmark *Roe* vs. *Wade* decision that established women's constitutional right to abortions, giving states the freedom to set restrictions indicates the Court no longer believes abortion to be a constitutional right. (Greenhouse, 1989). The decision of the court up-held three provisions of a 1986 Missouri law. The decision:

1. Bars public employees from performing or assisting in abortions not necessary to save a pregnant woman's life. The Opinion said: ". . . .the due process clauses generally confer no affirmative right to governmental aid, even where such aid may be necessary to secure life, liberty, or property interests of which the government itself may not deprive the individual." (The New York Times, 1989).

2. Bars the use of public buildings for performing abortion, even if no public funds are involved.

3. Requires that doctors perform tests to determine whether the fetus can live outside the womb if they believe a woman requesting an abortion may be at least 20 weeks pregnant. The Opinion said: "After viability, when the State's interest in potential human life was held to become compelling, the State, may, if it chooses, regulate, and even proscribe abortion except where it is necessary, in appropriate medical judgment, for the preservation of the life or health of the mother. . . . The State here has chosen viability as the point at which its interest in potential human life must be safeguarded. (The New York Times, 1989).

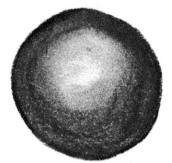

FERTILIZED OVUM

FIGURE 3-6 The female egg or ovum is the largest cell in the human body, and in the world of human cells is considered a giant. (From Anderson *Basic Maternal-Newborn Nursing*, copyright 1989 by Delmar Publishers Inc.)

At birth, a female's ovaries contain approximately 400,000 immature ova. Beginning at sexual maturity, she will ovulate one ovum a month and during her sexually mature years ovulates about 400 times. According to our understanding of time, the life of an ovum is not long, and can only be fertilized during an interval of ten to twenty-four hours (Nilsson, 1977, p. 22).

During the orgasm phase of intercourse, the male ejaculates *semen*, a liquid consisting of glandular secretions and *spermatozoa*, mature male germ cells. Each ejaculation contains about 300–500 million *sperm* (from the Greek word for seed), which are about 1/600 of an inch long, tadpole-like in

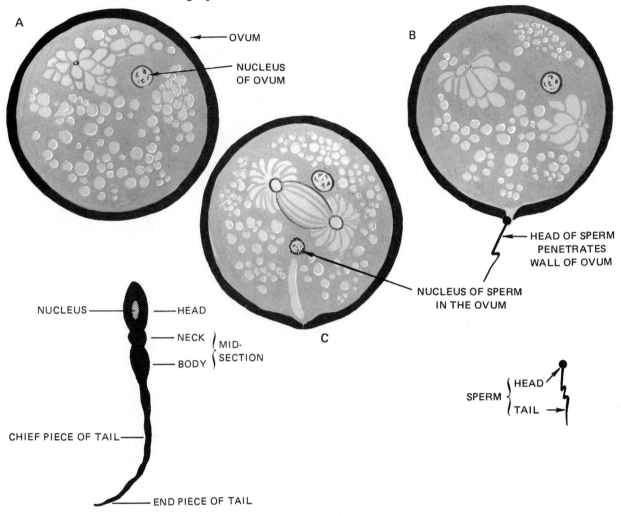

A

OVUM

NUCLEUS
OF OVUM

B

C

HEAD OF SPERM
PENETRATES
WALL OF OVUM

NUCLEUS OF SPERM
IN THE OVUM

NUCLEUS ——————— HEAD

NECK }
BODY } MID-SECTION

SPERM { HEAD
TAIL

CHIEF PIECE OF TAIL —

END PIECE OF TAIL

FIGURE 3-7 Male sperm, tadpole-like in appearance, are small in comparison to the ovum, and have a life span of 24–48 hours. (From Anderson, *Basic Maternal-Newborn Nursing*, copyright 1989 by Delmar Publishers Inc.)

appearance (see Figure 3–7), and have a lifespan of between twenty-four and forty-eight hours.

Why are 300–500 million sperm necessary to fertilize one ovum? First, sperm have a long way to travel. Through the whipping actions of their tails, they swim from the vagina, through the cervix into the uterus, and then up the fallopian tube where fertilization occurs (see Figure 3–8) (Craig, 1986, p. 60). Second, sperm enter either one of the two fallopian tubes. Only one tube has an egg

for fertilization, so half the sperm never reach the right place! Third, not all sperm are of equal vigor or *motility*. Some are deformed, others immature. The more sperm there are, the greater the chances that some will survive, thus increasing the likelihood of fertilization. Approximately an hour after ejaculation, about a hundred sperm reach the egg. However, only one fertilizes it. The reason only one sperm fertilizes an egg is that when the sperm makes contact with the egg membrane, a chemical

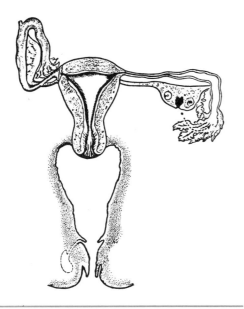

FIGURE 3-8 Fertilization—the uniting of sperm and egg, occurs in the fallopian tube and the resulting zygote implants into the wall of the uterus. (Reprinted with permission of Tambrands Inc. © 1989.)

reaction occurs, preventing entry of more sperm. If an ovum is not fertilized, it continues down the fallopian tube, into the uterus, and is discharged.

At fertilization, egg and sperm, each containing half of the heredity potential of the future individual, unite into a single cell called a *zygote* (from the Greek word *zygotos*, meaning "yoked" or "bound together") and the wonderful and remarkable process of child development begins.

Considering all the factors involved in fertilization, and taking into consideration that the "window of fertility" is at most forty-eight hours, timing does indeed play a major role in the beginning of human development.

WHEN DOES HUMAN LIFE BEGIN?

For our discussion, human development begins at the moment of conception with the union of sperm and ovum into a one-celled zygote. Al-

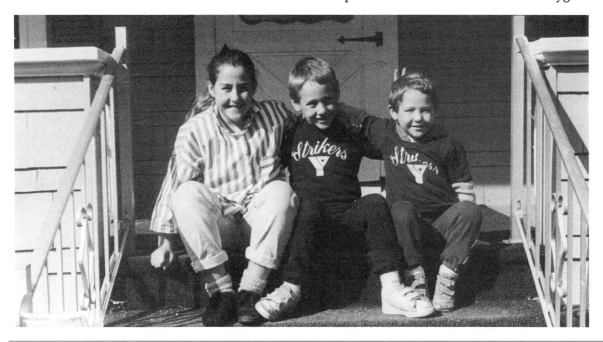

FIGURE 3-9 The interactions of environmental influences and heredity helps explain why all individuals are different from each other. Yet, it is apparent from strong family resemblances, that heredity does exert a powerful influence in child development.

though biological life begins at conception, when does human life begin? This is a much-debated question and one that does not have an easy or widely agreed-upon answer. The following constitute beliefs regarding the beginnings of human life:

- A fertilized egg is a distinct genetic entity and thus is the beginning of humanity.
- Many theologians believe that conception by humans constitutes humanity.
- Human life begins when the embryo implants into the uterus, about a week after conception.
- Human life begins when the heart of the embryo begins beating, about the fourth week of development.
- Human life begins when the embryo's central nervous system has developed to the point where simple reflexes are evident.
- Human life begins at the eighth week, when the embryo undergoes the transition to a fetus and is recognizable as a human.
- Human life begins when the fetus is "viable" and is sufficiently developed to survive outside the uterus. In 1973, the Supreme Court gave women the legal right to have abortions up to the moment of viability, which was placed at twenty-four to twenty-eight weeks.

HEREDITY

Look in the mirror. How many times have you asked yourself such questions as, "Why do I look the way I do?" or, "Why don't I have naturally curly hair like my father?" Equally interesting questions are, "Why doesn't everyone look alike?" and "Could my genetic material have been altered to make me look different from the way I do look?"

To answer the question about why you don't have naturally curly hair, we must discuss your *genotype*, or your genetic makeup. To respond to questions about why you look and behave the way you do, we must discuss your *phenotype*, or the outward manifestation of your genetic endowment. We can safely say that genotype influences phen-

otype, but there is more to inheritance of human characteristics than that. Heredity is not completely deterministic. Genotype does not completely determine phenotype. Who you are, including your appearance and behavior, is determined by your genotype *and* your environment. Even though a child's genetic code may indicate a particular trait—height, for example—poor nutrition may prevent her from growing to her full height.

All humans are the same in many general and specific ways. An observer from another planet would have no trouble determining that you and your best friend are both members of the species *Homo sapiens*. On the other hand, each and every human carries genetic instructions that makes him or her *unique* and different from everyone else.

All cells in the human body have forty-six chromosomes—with two exceptions. Sperm and ova, also called *gametes* or *germ cells*, each have twenty-three chromosomes. Developing children are constantly creating new cells as they grow. New cell growth occurs through *mitosis*, in which a new cell is a duplicate of the cell from which it divided. Gametes, on the other hand, divide through *meiosis*, or reduction division, whereby each new cell has half the chromosomes of the cell from which it divided. Meiosis is necessary in sex cell division because each gamete supplies twenty-three *single* chromosomes to form the twenty-three pairs of chromosomes in the zygote. If meiosis did not occur, at fertilization there would be forty-six *pairs* of chromosomes instead of twenty-three. In each chromosome there are thousands of genes composed of deoxyribonucleic acid or *DNA*. Another acid, ribonucleic acid or *RNA*, acts as a messenger, carrying directions from the DNA to the rest of the cell. These messages determine such things as what cells will be like—skin, nerve, muscle and their characteristics, as well the directional codes for structural and developmental process.

In 1962, James Watson, an American, and Francis Crick, an Englishman, won the Nobel Prize for their discovery of the double-helix structure of DNA. Their efforts unlocked the mystery of how

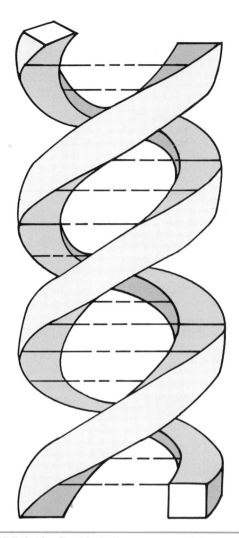

FIGURE 3-10 Double helix structure of DNA

Nucleotides

1. Nucleotides, four different kinds represented by the letters A, C. G, and T, are the smallest genetic unit and are paired in various combinations within the double helix of DNA.

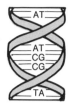

Genes

2. A gene contains thousands of the nucleotide pairs and has enough information in it to specify a particular protein.

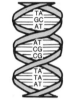

Chromosomes

3. A chromosome is a strand of DNA coiled and packed with proteins. A full set of 46 chromosomes contains about 100,000 genes.

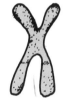

Cells

4. A cell contains the chromosomes in its nucleus and uses the information in the chromosomes to manufacture proteins.

The Human Body

5. The human body has about 10 trillion cells. Proteins determine the structure and function of each cell. Scientists are considering mounting a crash effort to determine the order of the three billion pairs of nucleotides that make up genes and chromosomes.

FIGURE 3-11 **The genetic primer.** (Adapted from and used with permission by *Chronicle of Higher Education* from a drawing by David Wheeler, September 3, 1986.)

genes and genetic inheritance work. Their model of DNA is a spiral-staircase-like "double helix," as shown in Figure 3–10. The two long strands are phosphate and sugar with the "rungs" or "steps" consisting of chemical bases connected by hydrogen, as shown in Figure 3–11. (Wheeler, 1986, p. 33).

When the two genetic codes—one half from the mother and one half from the father—unite, each pair is either homozygous or heterozygous. A gene pair is *homozygous* when the uniting genes

PARENT COMBINATION 1

Parent BB
Brown-eyed with both genes dominant
Homozygous

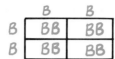

Parent BB
Brown-eyed with both genes dominant
Homozygous

The only possible combination in any offspring will be brown-eyed children.

PARENT COMBINATION 2

Parent BB
Brown-eyed with brown gene dominant
Homozygous

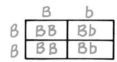

Parent Bb
Brown-eyed with brown gene dominant
Heterozygous

Again, only brown-eyed children will result, although 50 percent of the children have the chance to be heterozygous.

PARENT COMBINATION 3

Parent Bb
Brown-eyed with brown gene dominant
Heterozygous

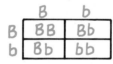

Parent Bb
Brown-eyed with brown gene dominant
Heterozygous

In this combination, there is a 25 percent chance of having a blue-eyed child.

PARENT COIMBINATION 4

Parent Bb
Brown-eyed with brown gene dominant
Heterozygous

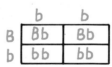

Parent bb
Blue-eyed with blue recessive genes
Homozygous

Again, the chance of this blue-eyed father and brown-eyed mother having a blue-eyed child are one in two.

PARENT COMBINATION 5

Parent bb
Blue-eyed with recessive genes
Homozygous

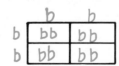

Parent bb
Blue-eyed with recessive genes
Homozygous

The only combination available is for all children to be blue-eyed. None will have brown eyes.

FIGURE 3-12 The five different possible combinations of parents with recessive and dominant genes.

carry the same instruction for a particular trait or characteristic. The pair is *heterozygous* when the genes carry two *different* instructions for a particular trait. When a gene pair carries two different instructions for a trait—such as height, which one controls development? Let's suppose, for example, stature is determined by either a gene *S*, for tall or *s* for short. If the father contributes an *S* and the mother contributes an *S*, then the child will be tall. If the father contributes an *s* and the mother contributes an *s*, the child will be short. However, what happens if the father contributes an *S* and the mother contributes an *s*? In this case, development is controlled by laws of inheritance.

Laws of Inheritance

Inheritance of a particular characteristic is determined by dominance relationships. Simply stated, the *dominant gene* determines the characteristic. In human development, the gene for brown eyes is dominant over the gene for blue eyes. If one parent contributes a gene *B* for brown eyes and the other parent contributes a gene *b* for blue eyes, then the child will have brown eyes. Since brown eyes are dominant over blue, you are probably wondering how you got your blue eyes. You inherited your blue eyes because two *recessive* genes—genes that are not dominant—combined into a homozygous pair. Parents who are blue-eyed will always have the *bb* genetic combination, which means they will have blue-eyed, not brown-eyed children. Brown-eyed parents can have blue-eyed children, but blue eyed parents will never have brown-eyed children. Figure 3–12 will help you understand why. Once you understand how the process works, draw diagrams for the following parent combinations showing what eye colors are possible in their children: *BB/bb, BB/Bb, BB/bb* and *Bb/bb.*

In humans there is seldom a one-to-one correspondence of genotype to phenotype. Literally thousands of combinations are possible in the very random process of mate selection and gene pairing. Also, gene combinations exert various influences, resulting in *codominance*, where the phenotype is a compromise between the two genes; and *incomplete dominance*, where the dominant gene, while still exercising its dominance, does not do so to its fullest extent. In reality, the inheritance of characteristics is a *polygenic* process whereby many genes acting together determine phenotype. The resemblance of some children to their parents makes it obvious to others that a particular child belongs to his parents while in other children it may be difficult to understand how the child "got into the family."

Some of the more common dominant and recessive human characteristics are shown in Table 3–6. Notice that most of the serious genetic dis-

TABLE 3–6

COMMON DOMINANT AND RECESSIVE CHARACTERISTICS	
Dominant Traits	Recessive Traits
Brown eyes	Gray, green, blue, hazel eyes
Curly hair	Straight hair
Dark hair	Baldness
Nonred hair (blond, brunette)	
Normal coloring	Red hair
	Albinism (lack of pigment)
Thick lips	Thin lips
Roman nose	Straight nose
Cheek dimples	No dimples
Extra, fused, or short digits	Normal digits
Double-jointedness	Normal joints
Normal color vision	Color blindness, red-green (sex-linked)
Normal vision	Myopia, nearsightedness
Farsightedness	Normal vision
Immunity to poison ivy	Susceptibility to poison ivy
Normal hearing	Congenital deafness
Normal blood clotting	Hemophilia (sex-linked)
Normal metabolism	Phenylketonuria
Normal blood cells	Sickle-cell anemia (related to race)

Note. From *Child Psychology: A Contemporary Viewpoint* (p. 57) by E. M. Hetherington and R. D. Parke, 1986, New York: McGraw-Hill.

eases, for example, *hemophilia* or bleeder's disease, are carried on recessive genes. This is fortunate for us, otherwise there would be many more people with these characteristics. (Hemophilia is a group of bleeding disorders resulting from a deficiency in one of the factors necessary for blood coagulation.)

Sex-linked Inheritance

Do you know anyone who is color-blind? If you do, you know they can't see red and green. How did they become color-blind? Color blindness is the result of the sex-linked inheritance of recessive traits. In sex-linked inheritance, a recessive trait—color blindness for example—is present only on the X chromosome. Remember that females have two chromosomes (XX) and that males have an X and a Y chromosome (XY). (See "Boy or Girl?" later in this chapter.) When a female carries the recessive trait for color blindness on one X chromosome, she usually also has a dominant gene for color vision on the other X chromosome. Consequently, she is seldom color-blind, but she is a *carrier*, or a person who does not have the trait, but who passes it on. So, when a female who has the recessive trait passes it on to her son (remember that males have only one X chromosome), then the male will have a 50 percent chance of being color-blind. Color blindness and hemophilia are examples of sex-linked traits that appear on the X chromosome.

Consanguineous relationships are those that exist between people who are related by blood. Have you ever wondered why there are taboos and laws prohibiting consanguineous or blood marriages? The laws of inheritance provide the answer. Recessive traits and diseases are passed on to children when both parents are recessive for a particular trait. The chances of marrying someone with a recessive gene is greater through "inbreeding" than when mate selection occurs from outside an inner circle of relatives.

More is inherited than physical features, in other words, more than just good looks. There is now evidence for the genetic basis for the mental

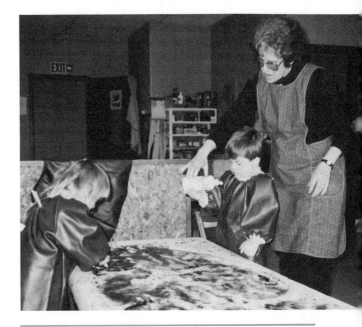

FIGURE 3-13 **One of the different ways children with Down syndrome can interact in their environment.**

disorder known as manic depression, in which a person alternates between periods of excitement and depression. Through research involving Old Order Amish in Lancaster County, Pennsylvania, researchers were able to identify a discrepancy in a region of chromosome 11 that led them to conclude that a gene or a group of genes confers a predisposition to manic depression. While there is presently no proof of a genetic basis for manic depression in non-Amish families, what is important is the discovery of such a link at all (Egeland et al., 1987).

WHY DO I ACT THE WAY I DO?

An age-old question that philosophers and scientists have been trying to answer for centuries is, "Why do people act the way they do?" As you might expect, the answers are varied, conflicting, and often controversial. More often than not, ex-

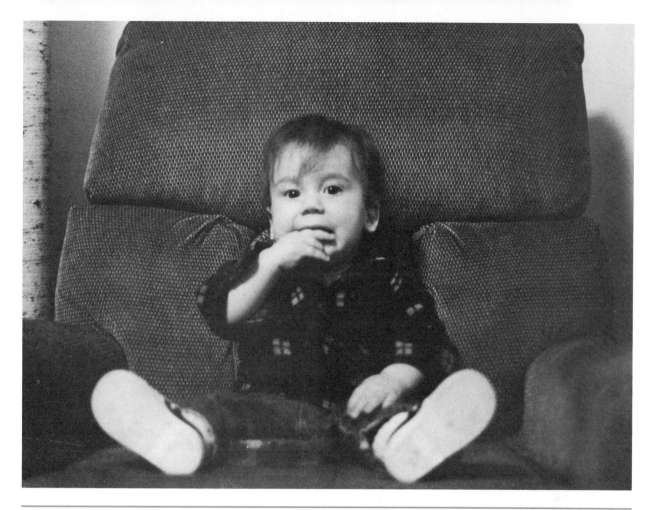

FIGURE 3-14 Infants are born with different temperaments which determine how they respond to the world around them. Children's individual temperament also determines how their parents will react to them.

perts have ascribed differences in human behavior to differences in both heredity and environment, with environment frequently getting most of the credit. Now, however, psychologists Sandra Scarr and Kathleen McCartney propose that only after a child is genetically receptive is the environment able to have any real effect on his or her behavioral development (Guillen, 1984). Children's environments are tailored in passive ways by parents who are their genetic "look-alikes." If a child is predisposed to read, for example, then she likely has parents who are also so predisposed. They provide an environment conducive to reading. Children influence their environment *evocatively* by encouraging some responses and discouraging others.

As Scarr and McCartney explain it: "Cooperative, attentive preschoolers receive more pleasant and instructional interactions from adults around them than the uncooperative, destructible children" (Guillen, 1984, p. 72). As children grow, they actively influence their environments "by literally seeking and settling into conditions that satisfy their native biases" (Guillen, 1984, p. 73).

Personality

Have you sometimes wished that you were more socially adept, mixed more easily with others and were more often the center of attention? Perhaps you put the blame for your social timidity

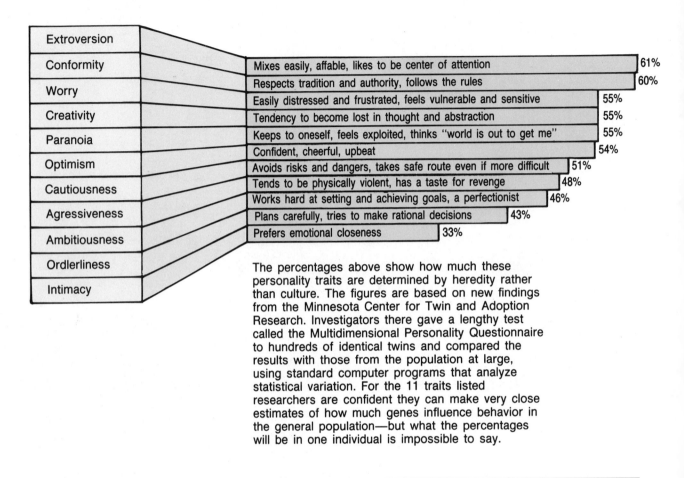

The percentages above show how much these personality traits are determined by heredity rather than culture. The figures are based on new findings from the Minnesota Center for Twin and Adoption Research. Investigators there gave a lengthy test called the Multidimensional Personality Questionnaire to hundreds of identical twins and compared the results with those from the population at large, using standard computer programs that analyze statistical variation. For the 11 traits listed researchers are confident they can make very close estimates of how much genes influence behavior in the general population—but what the percentages will be in one individual is impossible to say.

FIGURE 3-15   It is surprising how much of one's personality are attributable to heredity. The above figure shows the extent of heredity influence. (Adapted from and used with permission by *U.S. News and World Report* from an article by Stanley Wollborn, April 13, 1987).

on a traumatizing early experience or may have blamed your parents. Well, the case may be with your genes instead. Figure 3–15 shows the percentages of personality traits that are determined by heredity (Wellborn, 1987).

Studies of twins, especially identical twins reared apart, reveals the strong influence of heredity on personality development. Thanks to the University of Minnesota longitudinal study of twins, more information than ever before is revealed about the inheritability of personality characteristics. Some traits that have more than a 50 percent chance of being determined by heredity include: leadership, obedience to authority, vulnerability or resistance to stress, and fearfulness or risk-seeking (Tellegen, 1987). Rather than there being one gene for a particular personality trait, such as obedience, there are a host of genetic influences that contribute to development. Results of studies of identical twins reared apart by the Minnesota Center for Twin and Adoption Research reveal that these siblings as adults are similar in posture and expressive style. Twins tend to have similar mannerisms, gestures, speed and tempo of talking, habits, and jokes. (Holden, 1987).

Temperament

Infants have individual, biologically determined behavioral characteristics or ways of responding to the world. These characteristics taken as a group constitute *temperament* and include: motor activity rhythm and regularity of functions, acceptance or rejection of a new person or experience, adaptability, sensitivity to stimuli, intensity of energy level, general mood, distractibility, attention span, and persistence (Thomas, Chess, & Birch, 1970). Depending on the presence or absence of temperament characteristics, some babies are considered temperamentally "difficult." They have biological irregularities in sleep, feeding, and elimination; are slow to adapt to new situations; and are generally fussy. Difficult children are irregular in body functions, tense in their reactions, tend to withdraw from new stimuli, are slow to adapt to changes in the environment, and are generally negative in mood. "Easy" babies, on the other hand, are friendly, happy, adaptable, and smile a lot. They are positive in mood, regular in body functions, have a low or moderate intensity of reaction, and show adaptability and a positive approach to new situations. "Slow-to-warm-up" children have a low activity level, are slow to adapt, withdraw from a first exposure to new stimuli, are somewhat negative in mood, and respond with a low intensity.

Intelligence

Perhaps you have also speculated about the inheritability (the capability of being inherited) of intelligence, especially as it relates to you and your family. I'm sure you have heard someone remark, "Where did they get all their brains?" The answer lies in the genes. The heritability of IQ in adults is about .55 (DeFries, Plomin, & LaBuda, 1987), which means that over half of that which is measured as IQ can be accounted for by genetic influences. So while as far as IQ is concerned, biology may not necessarily be destiny, it certainly does play a large role.

A caveat is in order, however. We should not and must not allow such data to lead to deterministic conclusions about children. Many environmental factors in childhood and adulthood diminish or amplify genetic influences during the course of human development. For example, Scarr (1984) believes there is a *reaction range* within which the environment can influence intelligence. Everyone has a reaction range for potential. For example, a child with genes for average height may not reach the average because of a poor nutritional environment. On the other hand, another child with genes for average height may exceed the average because of a superior nutritional environment. Likewise, a child's intelligence may be enhanced by being reared in an environment in which parents provide many enriching opportunities and experiences. One of the challenges for all who participate in the process of child development is to determine the factors and processes that can enhance intellectual development *in all children*.

GENETIC SCREENING

Genetic screening is the process of examining a person's genetic make-up or *gnome*. Genetic screening helps identify genetic diseases and variations in the genes that might make a person more susceptible to diseases, e.g., lung cancer. The results of genetic screening are used in *genetic counseling*. Currently, we are aware of many genes that cause diseases and are beginning to uncover many that increase a person's susceptibility to others, such as heart disease, certain cancers, and insulin-dependent diabetes. The purposes of genetic testing are two-fold. First, such testing pro-

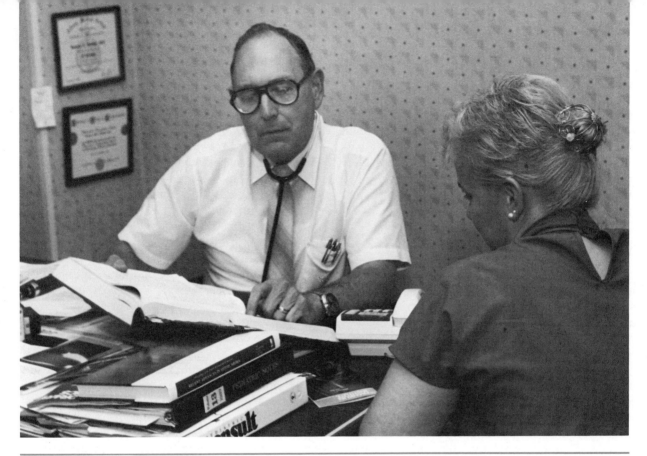

FIGURE 3-16 More couples are using genetic counseling to help them make decisions related to child bearing.

vides people with information to help them make decisions regarding marriage and child rearing. For example, a person may not know prior to screening that she carries the gene for cystic fibrosis. Upon learning she does, this information may cause her to readjust plans for child bearing. Second, such information enables people who carry genes that would predispose them to certain diseases to use preventative measures that might reduce their risk. This information is often provided in the form of a "risk profile" outlining a person's susceptibilities. This information enables that person: to take preventative measures, such as dieting and physical exercise, to reduce the chances of heart disease; and to avoid or eliminate the influences of environmental factors, such as an overexposure to sunlight that might facilitate skin cancer.

Some view genetic screening as a boon to humankind in terms of disease prevention and guidance for persons making decisions regarding marriage and children. Others view genetic screening differently because it conflicts with their notions of equality and fairness. Genetic screening is often viewed by union groups, women's organizations, and civil libertarians as antiegalitarian, racist, invasive of privacy, and a grave threat to democratic ideals.

The National Genetics Foundation (555 W. 57th St., New York, NY 10019) offers a form to establish an in-depth family health history. The information is fed into a computer, which produces a report on potential genetic risks. The charge is about $15 for an individual and $25 for a couple.

Mapping Human Genes

Currently, there is underway an ambitious project to locate and define all of the

50,000–100,000 genes which comprise the human *genome,* or entire set of genes. In the United States, this effort is headed by Dr. James D. Watson, co-discoverer of the DNA structure. Watson is the associate director at the National Institutes of Health for the Human Genome Studies (Schmeck, 1989). The mapping of the human genome will provide a number of useful purposes—the artificial duplication of genes, and the identification and detection of genetic diseases. Mapping of all the genes in the human genome involves finding the location of the genes of the 46 chromosomes. It is estimated that this project will take 15 years and cost billions of dollars (Schmeck, 1989).

Prenatal Fetal Genetic Screening

Prenatal fetal testing is an increasingly used method for the early identification of genetic diseases. This new method, developed by Scott Kogan (1987), a researcher at the University of California at San Francisco, allows medical workers to test small samples of fetal blood and tissue by looking directly at stained fragments of the DNA. This procedure promises to automate genetic testing and reduce or eliminate the need for radioactive "probes" and X-ray films, a lengthy and time-consuming procedure. Now, physicians and parents can have vital information within days.

Gene Therapy

Gene therapy involves splicing a gene into the genetic material of an individual's bone marrow cells. Performed successfully with monkeys and still in the experimental stage, the first human trials with gene therapy will likely involve the genetic disorder known as ADA deficiency, which destroys the immune systems of infants. This disease is fatal and involves a single gene that is easily cloned in the laboratory. Splicing this gene into an infant's genetic material enables the body to produce the ADA enzyme.

BOY OR GIRL?

Despite the popular sentiment that girls are made of "sugar and spice and everything nice," and boys are made of "snips and snails and puppy dog's tails," in the world of sex selection, they are made of X's and Y's.

A person's sex is determined at the moment of fertilization when the twenty-three single chromosomes from the sperm and the egg unite to form the normal forty-six-chromosome cell. The twenty-third chromosome of each sex cell determines the sex of the fertilized zygote. The female egg *always* carries the X or female-determining chromosome. The male sperm carries *either* an X, female-determining chromosome. *or* a Y, male-determining chromosome. At fertilization, when a sperm carrying an X chromosome unites with the egg, the result is XX—female. When a sperm carrying a Y chromosome unites with the egg, the result is XY—male. Sperm determine the sex of a child. However, throughout history women have been wrongly blamed for not giving birth to a male. One of history's most notorious "blamers" was Henry VIII of England, who resorted to marrying six times in order to have a male heir.

Although Aristotle believed that a father's degree of excitement at conception determined his offspring's sex (more excitement determined a boy), researchers now believe a single gene located on the Y chromosome is responsible for sex determination. Whenever that gene, known as the testes determining factor (TDF), is present in the chromosomes of the fertilized egg, the fetus develops testes and becomes a male. On an X chromosome where the gene is absent, the fetus develops ovaries and becomes female. Thus, the gene acts as a biological switch for sex development, turning other genes on or off (Schmeck, 1987).

Choosing Baby's Sex—With 80 Percent Accuracy

In this age of smaller families, many couples want to select the sex of their children. As Mary and Robert Quintano explain it, "We have two girls and we wanted a boy. Our decision was one of not having another child or trying to see if we couldn't increase our chances of having a boy." Couples use many methods to try to increase their chances of having a child of a particular sex. Harlap (1979) reports an incidence of male births ". . . significantly higher in the offspring of women who resumed intercourse two days after ovulation" (p. 1447).

Ronald Ericsson, a reproductive physiologist has developed and patented a method for separating sperm for the Y chromosome, a method that he maintains is 80 percent effective (Maranto, 1984). The process consists of having sperm swim through several albumin solutions. About 80 percent of the sperm that finish the journey carry the Y chromosome. The procedure costs about $500–$600.

Similar efforts to filter sperm that carry the X chromosome are underway but have not been as successful. Researchers are hopeful that the same 80 percent success rate for X-carrying sperm will be possible in the near future (Maranto, 1984).

The only relatively sure method of sex preselection is through *amniocentesis*—the examination of the amniotic fluid—and then abortion if the fetus is not of the parents' choice.

The ethical concerns of sex selection are basically the same as those associated with artificial insemination, embryo transplants, and surrogate parenting. Namely, it reduces babies to little more than commodities, and debases the value of marital relations and life in general. In addition, there is an even more important ethical question associated with sex selection. Given the universal preference for sons, selecting sons over daughters may skew the population ratio and relegate females to a subservient position for generations to come. On the other hand, advocates of sex selection say it enables couples who have children of one sex to have children of the other sex. Also, families with a genetic tendency toward hemophilia may, in the absence of sex selection, decide not to have children. However, the opportunity to select a female child would make parenthood acceptable for such couples.

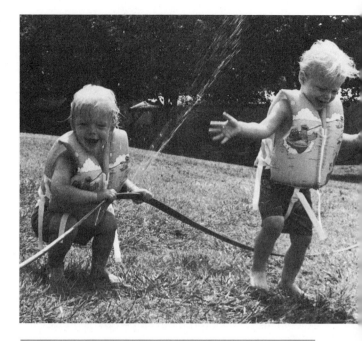

FIGURE 3-17 When two ova are fertilized, the twins are fraternal. When a fertilized egg separates, two individual persons, called identical twins, develop.

TWINS, TRIPLETS, AND MORE

Multiple births occur in several ways. During ovulation, one or more egg may be released and, if fertilized, twins, triplets, quadruplets, or quintuplets may result. When two ova are fertilized, the twins are *fraternal* or *dizygotic*. Each has its own unique genetic makeup, placental and umbilical cord. Brother and sister twins are always fraternal. If, however, a fertilized egg separates, two individual persons develop. Since they originated from the same zygote, they are called *identical* or *monozygotic twins*. The chances of bearing fraternal twins are about one in eighty, while the chances of having identical twins are about one in two hundred. Occasionally, the splitting of monozygotic twins is incomplete, resulting in conjoined or Siamese twins. This occurs about once in a possible 50,000 pregnancies (Neeson & May, 1986,

p. 495). Unlike other animal species in which multiple births are common, this is not so with humans. There may be a number of reasons for this. First, the human infant needs a long period of development after birth. Caring for multiple children of the same age taxes the abilities of parents. Second, a singleton has a greater chance of survival than do children of multiple births.

Daily media reports of women giving birth to three, four, and more children are almost commonplace with the increased use of fertility drugs. These drugs promote superovulation, or the release of many ova, which can result in multiple births.

There are many groups and organizations, such as the Mothers of Twins Clubs, Inc. (5402 Amberwood Lane, Rockville, MD 20853), that provide information and support to parents who have or are expecting twins, triplets, or more.

CHROMOSOME ABNORMALITIES

Sometimes children are born with *congenital birth defects*, which are not hereditary. They are caused by the improper union of genes or an error

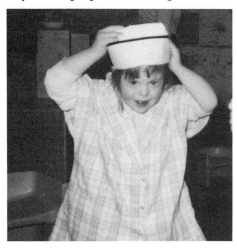

FIGURE 3-18 Today, because of earlier intervention, therapy and better care, many children with Down syndrome are not as limited by this genetic error as they once were.

in development. On the other hand, when defects are passed through the genes, they are called *hereditary* or *genetic disorders* or *diseases*, and will be discussed later in the chapter.

Down Syndrome (Trisomy 21)

One of the most common and widespread consequences of genetic error is *Down syndrome*, with a frequency of one in 700 live births. First described in 1866 by John Down, an English physician, it is the commonest cause of mental retardation in the United States (Patterson, 1987). Down syndrome children have a wide variety of anatomical and biochemical abnormalities, such as folds of skin on the sides of the nose and eyelids, a broad face, flattened nose, and protruding tongue. Forty percent of Down syndrome children have congenital heart defects, most have small brains, and many are at increased risk for developing cataracts (Patterson, 1987). (See Figure 3–18.)

The primary cause of Down syndrome is *nondisjunction*, the failure of chromosomes to separate properly while undergoing meiosis (cell division) during the production of the egg and sperm cells. Down syndrome children have three chromosome 21s in their cells rather than two. Therefore they have a total of forty-seven chromosomes rather than the normal forty-six. Because of the presence of the additional chromosome (2 plus 1) on chromosome 21—the smallest human chromosome—Down syndrome is frequently referred to as *trisomy 21*. Parents do not pass Down syndrome on to their children as an inherited characteristic. The disease results from an error in cell division.

Down syndrome is also an age-related chromosome disorder, because the possibility of women over age thirty-five bearing a Down syndrome child increases dramatically, with 50 percent of all such children born to this age group. (See Table 3–7.) One of the reasons for increased birth defects, such as Down syndrome, in children of older women may be that their eggs are exposed longer to environmental hazards, such as chemicals and radiation.

TABLE 3-7

RELATIONSHIP OF DOWN SYNDROME TO AGE OF MOTHER		
Woman's Age	Rate	Births
Under 30	1	3,000
30–34	1	600
35–39	1	280
40–44	1	80
40+	1	40

Note. From "Genetic Counseling: Learning What to Expect" by J. Willis, September, 1980, *FDA Consumer, 14,* pp. 11–13.

However, males also play a role in Down syndrome, with an estimated one-third of the cases caused by sperm deficiencies.

SEX CHROMOSOME ABNORMALITY (SCA)

Approximately one in 400 children are born with a sex chromosome abnormality. These occur at the time of conception and, as of now, are of unknown origin (Berch and Bender, 1987).

Turner's Syndrome (TS)

In Turner's syndrome, females are born with an *XO* combination instead of the typical *XX* combination. These single-X girls lack the second sex-determining chromosome and therefore have only forty-five chromosomes. These individuals are not likely to be mentally retarded or severely mentally ill, but they usually have specific cognitive deficiencies, are short in stature, and have short fingers and webbed necks. Most TS girls have normal verbal abilities, but their spatial skills are below normal, which may account for why they also have difficulties with mathematics, handwriting, copying, and drawing design (Berch & Bender, 1987). They tend to be very hyperactive in middle childhood and have trouble paying attention. Es-

trogen therapy—the administration of female hormones—at puberty enables Turner's syndrome females to develop sexually in a normal way, although they remain sterile.

Triple-X Syndrome (XXX)

In contrast to Turner's syndrome, some females have one more chromosome than they should (forty-seven), an abnormality called *triple-X syndrome.* These triple-X females are usually normal physically, but their overall level of mental functioning is lower than girls with Turner syndrome, and they manifest problems with a variety of verbal skills, including delayed speech development and defective speech articulation. Also, they have problems involved with balance, equilibrium, sensory integration, and short-term memory. Many also have difficulties forming relationships (Berch & Bender, 1987).

Klinefelter's Syndrome (XXY)

Males with *Klinefelter's syndrome* carry an extra X chromosome, resulting in an *XXY* combination rather than the normal *XY* male chromosome pattern. These males have problems with language skills as well as reading disabilities and neuromotor problems, such as primitive reflexes, poor sensorimotor integration, and trouble with fine and gross motor control. Their parents also report that they tend to be unreactive and withdrawn (Berch & Bender, 1987).

XYY Syndrome

Males born with the *XYY syndrome* carry an extra Y chromosome. Less is known about the mental abilities of these children, but data to date suggest that about half have problems with language, motor, and reading skills. Although it was once thought that extra Y males are prone to criminality, this belief no longer has the support it once did (Berch & Bender, 1987).

Fragile-X Syndrome

Some males carry a *fragile-X* [fra(X)] chromosome that is pinched or narrowed and subject to breaking. These males usually are mentally retarded (from severe to mild), have delayed speech, and demonstrate hyperactivity, self-mutilation, violent outbursts, autistic behavior, and psychosis. Physical characteristics include enlarged testes, a greater than normal ear length, short stature, a high, prominent forehead, a long rectangular face, and square hands with stubby fingers (Ho, Glahn, & Ho, 1988). Fifty percent of the women who carry the fragile gene pass it on to their sons. Although it was previously thought that women who were carriers of fra(X) did not demonstrate the symptoms, recent studies have found that some do (Ho, Glahn, & Ho, 1988).

Fragile-X syndrome is believed to be the second most common form of mental retardation after Down syndrome (Ho, Glahn, & Ho, 1988).

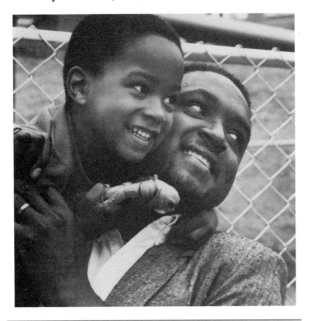

FIGURE 3-19 Sickle cell anemia affects about one in 400 black Americans. In this genetic disease, the red blood cells are affected, making it difficult for them to transport oxygen.

As more research is conducted regarding SCA children, several things are becoming clear. First, not *all* children involved have the serious behavioral problems, are as unlikely to be mentally retarded, and are not as prone to criminality as was once believed. Second, as a group, they are varied in their behavior and abilities. While some have serious learning disabilities, others do well in school and go on to college. Third, the environment is a critical factor in their development. Two leading researchers in the field succinctly summarize the outlook for SCA children this way: "It is likely that these children will lead normal, productive lives if they are reared by sensitive, realistic parents in supportive environments" (Berch & Bender, 1987, p. 57).

GENETIC DISEASES

Genetic diseases are passed from parents to children by the operation of normal genetic principles. Many of these have names you have probably heard—hemophilia, sickle-cell anemia, phenylketonuria, Tay-Sachs disease, and cystic fibrosis. All these diseases are single-gene defects because a single gene is the cause of the disease. Some of these diseases are sex-linked, meaning they are passed on by one parent to the opposite sex child. For example, hemophilia, or bleeder's disease, is passed on from mothers to sons. Mothers carry; sons inherit. The mother is a carrier because she transmits the disease.

Sickle-cell Anemia

Sickle-cell anemia affects the red blood cells. Normal red blood cells are circular, whereas in sickle-cell anemia, they are shaped like a sickle (or one of a pair of parentheses), hence the name. The shape of the cell makes it difficult to transport oxygen. In addition, sickle cells are brittle and break easily. As a result, the body cannot manufacture new ones fast enough and anemia results. About one in 400 black Americans inherit sickle-cell anemia.

Some individuals carry the trait for sickle-cell anemia, but do not have any of the symptoms. When both parents have the trait, there is a 25 percent chance that one of their children will have sickle-cell anemia.

Phenylketonuria (PKU)

Phenylketonuria or *PKU* is a genetic disorder that interferes with a child's ability to utilize an amino acid, phenylalanine, found in milk and milk products. Left untreated, it results in brain damage and mental retardation. PKU is an *inborn error of metabolism*, in which a substance (in this case, phenylalanine) necessary for a normal metabolic process is absent. It affects about one in 15,000 children. Most hospitals routinely test for PKU, and when present, it can be managed through diet. In infancy, a special milk substitute, *Leofenalac* (Mead-Johnson) is used. A special diet low in phenylalanine is usually continued until the child is about eight years old, when the majority of brain development has occurred.

Tay-Sachs Disease

Tay-Sachs disease is a metabolic disorder of the nervous system in which an enzyme necessary for metabolizing a particular fat is absent. When not metabolized, fat accumulates in the brain, interfering with neurological processes. There is no known cure and most children die by the age of four. Genetic counseling prior to pregnancy can help couples make important decisions. Also, amniocentesis can detect the presence of Tay-Sachs disease during pregnancy so that parents can make decisions regarding abortion.

Cystic Fibrosis (CF)

Cystic fibrosis is an inherited metabolic disorder that causes an overproduction of thick mucus throughout the body. This increase in mucus causes obstructions in the organs, especially the lungs. With improved diagnosis and medical care, such

as pulmonary therapy, many children who might have died in their teens are now able to live into early adulthood.

Types of genetic diseases that are hereditarily transmitted are found in Table 3–8. The number of people in the United States affected by various genetic diseases is shown in Table 3–9.

TABLE 3–8

TYPES OF GENETIC DISEASES		
Genetic Disease	Symptoms	Population
Phenylketonuria (PKU)	Short; light-skinned; mentally retarded; emotionally disturbed	all
Tay-Sachs disease (autosomal recessive*)	Affects brain; usually results in death by age four	Ashkenazic Jews of Eastern European origin
Hemophilia	Inability of blood to clot; affected male literally bleeds to death	all
Sickle-cell anemia (autosomal recessive*)	Anemia; severe pain in arms, legs, back, and stomach; leg ulcers	Blacks; in U.S., blacks of African origin
Cystic fibrosis	Lungs lose elasticity making oxygen exchange difficult. Child may die prior to adolescence, but enhanced health care and personal regimes may increase life expectancy.	Caucasians

* All chromosomes except the sex chromosomes are called *autosomes.*

TABLE 3–9

GENETIC DISEASES AND NUMBERS OF PEOPLE AFFECTED	
Adult polycystic kidney disease	500,000
AAT deficiency (emphysema)	120,000
Fragile-*X* syndrome	100,000
Sickle-cell anemia	65,000
Duchenne muscular dystrophy	32,000
Cystic fibrosis	30,000
Huntington's disease	25,000
Hemophilia	20,000
Phenylketonuria	16,000
Retinoblastoma (childhood eye cancer)	10,000

Note. From "Predicting Diseases," *U.S. News and World Report,* May 25, 1987, p. 65.

What Would You Do?

Linda and Harry James wanted a child for a long time before they learned that Harry was infertile. Harry's sperm do not have the motility necessary to reach Linda's ovum or the fertility to fertilize it. Linda and Harry decided to have a baby through artificial insemination by donor (AID). Together, they visited the medical center of a local university specializing in artificial insemination. And as a result of the artificial insemination, Linda became pregnant and later gave birth to a daughter, Cynthia.

Now, Linda and Harry have been talking about what they will tell their Cynthia about her parentage. They have discussed the possibility of telling her nothing and letting her go through life believing she is their natural child. Harry especially likes this idea. He sees no reason to tell Cynthia otherwise. As he puts it, "I want her to think I'm her father. There is no need to let her go through life wondering if the elderly gentleman sitting beside her on the subway is her father."

Linda, on the other hand, favors telling Cynthia all of the circumstances of her conception. She has kept a detailed record of events and data in case they decide to tell Cynthia everything. Linda believes Cynthia has a right to know and says, "Even though Harry is not her genetic father, he is the best father Cynthia could ever have."

What would you do? Would you tell Cynthia about her parentage and disclose the events and nature of her conception or would you let her think that Harry is her natural father?

SUMMARY

- Federal and state governments use social policy, legislation, and economic incentives to influence people's decisions regarding marriage, family living, childbearing and child rearing.
- The traditional nuclear family is no longer the "majority" family unit. It has been replaced by single-parent, extended, blended, and stepfamilies, which now provide traditional family functions.
- Women are having fewer children. The decline in the fertility rate is also accompanied by a decline in the numbers of children in a family.
- More families have only one child, and use of contraception is more widespread. Contrary to popular myth, only children, or "onlies" are not necessarily maladjusted, but are bright and similar to other children in health and adjustment.
- Child rearing in the 1990s is expensive. The cost for rearing a child to age eighteen is approximately $100,000.
- As more parents work, they need child care and family services as a means of supporting them in their tasks of child rearing.
- Reproductive technology is changing the way parents have children and enables more people to have children of their own. Surrogate parenting is growing in popularity, although many legal questions and social controversies are involved.
- Today, there are many ways to have babies. Adoption is one alternative for persons who want children. In vitro fertilization and embryo transplants are two methods frequently used to help parents have natural children.
- Sperm banks provide the opportunity for women and couples to have access to sperm and the possibility of parenthood. Some critics label sperm banks whose donors are limited to "the best and the brightest" as elitist.
- Many ethical and legal issues involving parents, unborn children, and the health professions are inherent in the use of reproductive technology.
- During ovulation, an ovum or egg is discharged into the fallopian tube where it has a life of ten to twenty-four hours. The male ejaculates semen that contains 300–500 million sperm having a life span of eighteen to twenty-four hours. Only one sperm fertilizes an egg.
- At fertilization, egg and sperm, each containing one-half of the future child's hereditary potential, unite into a zygote.
- Genotype constitutes genetic makeup, while phenotype is the outward manifestation of genetic heredity and environmental influences.
- All cells in the human body have forty-six chromosomes, with two exceptions, sperm and ova, also called gametes or germ cells, which have twenty-three. New cell growth occurs through mitosis, but gametes divide through meiosis, or reduction division. Each gamete supplies twenty-three single chromosomes to form the twenty-three pairs of forty-six chromosomes in the zygote.
- When the two genetic codes—one-half from the mother and one-half from the father—unite, each pair is either homozygous or heterozygous. A gene pair is homozygous when the uniting genes carry the same instruction for a particular trait, and heter-

ozygous when the genes carry two different instructions for a particular trait.

■ Inheritance of a particular characteristic is determined by dominance relationships. There is seldom a one-to-one correspondence of genotype to phenotype. Literally thousands of combinations are possible. Gene combinations exert various influences, resulting in codominance or incomplete dominance.

■ Many physical characteristics are inherited, from thickness of lips to dimples. Growing evidence supports the inheritance of manic depression. Some researchers believe the environment influences children's development most when they are "genetically ready."

■ Each infant has an individual temperament, a biologically determined set of behavioral characteristics or ways of responding to the world. Based on their temperaments, babies may be characterized as "easy" or "difficult," or "slow-to-warm-up."

■ Heredity plays a role in intellectual development. A little over half of what we measure as intelligence is attributable to heredity.

■ Genetic screening, or the process of examining a person's genome, is used as a counseling tool. However, many ethical and legal issues are involved.

■ Prenatal fetal testing is a growing and increasingly used method for the early identification of genetic diseases.

■ The female egg carries the X, or female-determining chromosome and the male sperm carries *either* an X, female-determining chromosome, or a Y, male-determining chromosome. When a sperm, carrying an X chromosome, unites with the egg, the result is XX—female. When a sperm carrying a Y chromosome unites with the egg, the result is XY—male.

■ Choosing a baby's sex is the object of much research and controversy. As researchers seek ways to refine the processes of sex selections, critics and proponents debate the many ethical and social issues involved.

■ Down syndrome is one of the most common and widespread consequences of genetic error, with a frequency of one in 700 live births. Commonly referred to as trisomy 21, it is caused by an error in cell division.

■ About one in 400 children are born with a sex chromosome abnormality. These include: Turner's syndrome, triple-X syndrome, Klinefelter's syndrome, XXY syndrome, and fragile-X syndrome.

■ Genetic diseases are passed from parents to children. Many have names you probably heard—hemophilia, sickle-cell anemia, Tay-Sachs disease, and cystic fibrosis. All are single-gene defects.

QUESTIONS TO GUIDE YOUR REVIEW

1. Why is the nuclear family no longer the predominant family in American society?
2. What are the reasons the fertility rate in the United States is declining?
3. What implications do changes in family patterns have for parents, children, and society?

4. In what ways has reproductive technology such as in vitro fertilization and embryo transplants changed the ways people are having babies?
5. Describe four examples of advances in reproductive technology.
6. What are sperm banks, how do they operate, and what are the controversies surrounding them?
7. What are the legal and ethical issues involved in reproductive technology and surrogate parenting?
8. How does fertilization occur in humans?
9. Describe genotype and phenotype and the relationship between them.
10. Do the gametes have forty-six chromosomes? Why?
11. Why was the discovery of DNA important?
12. Explain the difference between homozygous and heterozygous gene pairs.
13. List five human traits that are dominant and five that are recessive.
14. What characteristics (other than physical) and abilities are inherited?
15. What is genetic screening and why is it so useful and controversial?
16. How is sex determined? What procedures are being used to make it easier for parents to select the sex of their child? What are the issues involved in letting parents decide what sex child they want?
17. What is Down syndrome? What is the cause? What are the characteristics of children with Down syndrome? Is Down syndrome an age-related disorder? Why?
18. Describe four sex chromosome abnormalities and tell how they affect children.
19. Describe four genetic diseases.

CTIVITIES FOR FURTHER INVOLVEMENT

1. Contact different governmental agencies to gather information about single parenting, teenage parenting, legal separations, and the rights and custody of young children. How are these social forces affecting early childhood education programs and child development in your state and local community?
2. Visit a clinic or medical center that provides human artificial insemination services.
   a. What are the procedures and guidelines for using the program's services?
   b. What are the pros and cons of bearing children through artificial insemination?
   c. Would you use artificial insemination to bear a child? Would you approve of your spouse doing so? Why or why not?
   d. Identify and define the legal issues and concerns involved in the many technologies and procedures for promoting fertility, conception and childbearing.
3. Given the many different and unique types of families in American society, it is natural that the parents of such families would have unique needs.
   a. What are the unique needs of parents and children in the following families:
      1) Single-parent female   4) Extended
      2) Single-parent male   5) Foster
      3) Blended (mixed)
   b. How and in what way does child development information help these parents/families meet the needs you identified?

4. Visit a genetic counseling clinic/program.
   a. What are the pros and cons of such services?
   b. Would you consider using such services? Why? Why not?
   c. Have a genetic counselor share with you (anonymously) the results of a genetic screening and the recommendations based on it.
5. Interview these sets of parents:
   a. Teenage parents
   b. Single female divorced parents
   c. Parents who have delayed childbearing and rearing into their late thirties and early forties
   What similarities/differences do you find in their
   a. Attitudes toward their children
   b. Interactions with their children
   c. Need for parenting and child development information.

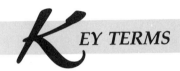 EY TERMS

Amniocentesis The process of removing amniotic fluid and examining it for the child's gender or the presence of chromosomal abnormalities.

Codominance Characteristic of two genes for a different trait being fully expressed without either being influenced by the other.

Congenital birth defects Birth defects that are not hereditary.

Cystic fibrosis An inherited metabolic disorder that causes an overproduction of thick mucus throughout the body. This increase in mucus causes obstructions in the organs, especially the lungs.

DNA Deoxyribonucleic acid.

Dizygotic twins See *Fraternal twins*.

Dominant genes Genes that exercise dominance over other genes.

Down syndrome A congenital birth defect in which children have a wide variety of anatomical and biochemical abnormalities, such as folds of skin on the sides of the nose and eyelids, a broad face, flattened nose, and protruding tongue.

Eugenics The science of, or efforts involved in, improving the gene pool.

Fertility rate The number of live births per 1,000 women.

Follicle A fluid-filled sac on the ovary containing the ovum.

Fragile-X syndrome An abnormality in which males carry a chromosome that is pinched or narrowed and subject to breaking. These males are mentally retarded, have severe behavioral problems, and have distinguishing physical characteristics.

Fraternal or dizygotic twins Result of two ova being fertilized. Each has its own unique genetic makeup, placenta and umbilical cord. Brother and sister twins are always fraternal.

Gamete intra-fallopian transfer (GIFT) Essentially the same process as IVF except that the gametes are injected into a fallopian tube.

Gametes Germ or sex cells.

Gene therapy The process of splicing a gene into the genetic material of an individual's bone marrow cells.

Genetic screening The process of examining a person's *genome*—their complete set of hereditary factors—for genes that cause or influence abnormalities and diseases.

Genome A person's complete set of hereditary factors.

Genotype Genetic makeup. *Genotype* refers to all the characteristics an individual has inherited, regardless of whether or not they are observable. The expression of the genotype in terms of appearance and behavior is known as the *phenotype* of an individual.

Hereditary (or genetic) disorders and diseases Defects passed from parents to children through the genes.

Heterozygous Characteristic of a gene pair carrying two *different* instructions for a particular trait.

Homozygous Characteristic of a gene pair carrying the *same* instruction for a particular trait or characteristic.

Identical or monozygotic twins Result of a fertilized zygote dividing into two, producing two identical individuals. See *Identical twins.*

In vitro fertilization The process of taking a ripe ova from a woman, mixing sperm with it, incubating the zygote, and injecting it into the uterus.

Incomplete dominance Characteristic of two genes being equally expressed; neither gene is recessive to the other.

Klinefelter's syndrome Abnormality in which males carry an extra *X* chromosome, resulting in an *XXY* combination rather than the normal *XY* male chromosome pattern.

Meiosis Reduction cell division whereby each new cell has half the chromosomes of the cell from which it divided.

Mitosis Cell division in which a new cell is a duplicate of the cell from which it divided.

Monozygotic twins See *Identical twins.*

Nondisjunction The failure of chromosomes to separate properly while undergoing *meiosis* (cell division) during the production of the egg and sperm cells.

Ovaries The female gonads or gamete-producing sex glands in which ova are formed.

Ovulation The discharge of a female egg cell or *ovum.*

Ovum Female egg.

Phenylketonuria (PKU) A genetic disorder that interferes with a child's ability to utilize the amino acid, phenylalanine, found in milk and milk products. Left untreated, it results in brain damage and mental retardation.

RNA Ribonucleic acid. Acts as a messenger, carrying directions from the DNA to the rest of the cell.

Recessive genes Genes that are not dominant.

Semen A liquid consisting of glandular secretions and *spermatozoa,* mature male germ cells.

Sickle-cell anemia A single-gene defect in which the red blood cells are impaired from transporting oxygen.

Sperm From the Greek word for seed; a mature germ cell. A sperm is about 1/600 of an inch long and tadpole-like in appearance. (Singular of *spermatozoa.*)

Tay-Sachs disease A metabolic disorder of the nervous system in which an enzyme necessary for metabolizing a particular fat is absent. When not metabolized, the fat accumulates in the brain, interfering with neurological processes. There is no known cure.

Temperament A child's characteristic way of responding to others and the world.

Triple-X syndrome Abnormality in which females have one more *X* chromosome than they should have.

Trisomy 21 Down syndrome.

Turner's syndrome A chromosome abnormality in which females have an *XO* instead of the typical *XX* chromosomal makeup and therefore have only forty-five chromosomes.

XYY syndrome Abnormality in which males carry an extra Y chromosome.

Zygote A fertilized egg formed by the union of the egg and sperm.

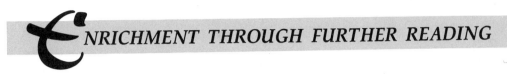

ENRICHMENT THROUGH FURTHER READING

Andrews, L. B. (1984). *New conceptions: A consumer's guide to the newest infertility treatments, including in vitro fertilization, artificial insemination, and surrogate motherhood.* New York: St. Martin's Press.

This is especially good reading for those faced with infertility problems. Contains much useful and practical advice for all who may use or are interested in the new reproductive technologies.

Arendell, T. (1986). *Mothers and divorce.* Berkeley, CA: University of California Press.

Reveals the harsh world of single parenthood for which some divorced women may not be emotionally or professionally prepared. Explores the realities of the economic and class effects divorce has on women.

Arnold, E. L. (Ed.). (1985). *Parents, children and change.* Lexington, MA: Lexington Books.

A very interesting and informative collection of chapters dealing with many important topics, such as: "Our Changing Society and Changing Families," "Nurturing the Parent-Child Relationship," "Food in the Future Family," and "When the Parent/ Child Relationship Goes Public."

Barrett, M. & McIntosh, M. (1982). *The anti-social family.* London: Verso Editions/NLB.

Clearly argued and well-written accounts of the socialist and feminist debates on the family.

Bayles, M. D. (1984). *Reproductive ethics.* Englewood Cliffs, NJ: Prentice-Hall.

This is an interesting and informative analysis of all you ever wanted to know about reproductive ethics. The reader will be well informed and thus able to discuss and appreciate the many issues involved in this important area.

Bettelheim, B. (1987). *A good enough parent.* New York: Alfred A. Knopf.

The major thesis of the book, as the title suggests is as Bettelheim himself says: ". . . .it is quite possible to be a good enough parent—that is, a parent who raises his child well. To achieve this, the mistakes we make in rearing our child—errors often made just because of the intensity of our emotional involvement in and with our child—must be more than compensated for by the many instances in which we do right by our child." The purpose of this book is to facilitate being such a good enough parent.

Fischhoff, A. (1987). *Birth to three: A self-help program for new parents.* Eugene, OR: Castalia.

Emphasizes the challenges parents face while acknowledging their competence. Tells how to organize a support group for parents.

Frank, D., & Vogel, M. (1988). *The baby makers*. New York: Carroll & Graf.
A compelling account of in vitro fertilization, artificial insemination, and surrogacy. Presents a balanced account of the many moral and ethical issues involved when infertile couples want to become parents.

Greenberg, M. (1985). *The birth of a father*. New York: Continuum.
A fascinating, first-person account of a psychiatrist's experiences of becoming a father. Full of practical advice that will help fathers become *engrossed* with their children.

Greenburg, D. (1986). *Confessions of a pregnant father*. New York: Macmillan.
A frank and often funny look at fatherhood by a person who never thought he would become a father.

Hochschild, Arli and Machung, Anne. (1989). *The second shift: Working parents and the revolution at home*. New York: Viking.
This is an insightful report on two career family life, and one that may surprise those who think that the majority of working women are liberated from the major responsibilities of domestic work, including child-rearing.

Merritt, S., & Steiner, L. (1984). *And baby makes two: Motherhood without marriage*. New York: Franklin Watts.
The results of a nationwide survey of single, adult women who became mothers, the authors provide a balanced view of single-by-choice parenting.

Singer, P. & Wells, D. (1985). *Making babies: The new science and ethics of conception*. New York: Charles Scribner's Sons.
An in-depth discussion of the scientific and sociological ramifications of alternative forms of conception. Examines the technology of fertilization as well as the many ethical, moral, and legal issues.

Walker, G. (1986). *Solomon's children*. New York: Arbor House.
An interesting account of the impact of divorce on children ages eleven to sixteen. Provides useful insights into families and stepfamilies.

Wallerstein, J. S. and Blakeslee, S. (1989). *Second chances*. New York: Ticknor & Fields.
What really happens to children after their parents divorce? As portrayed by the authors, the picture of life after divorce for both children and parents is grim. In only 10 percent of the families studied did the spouses build a happier life ten years after divorce. Provides good insights into the effects of divorce.

Whitehead, M. B. with Schwartz-Nobel, L. (1989). *A mother's story*. New York: St. Martin's Press.
"My name is Mary Beth Whitehead. I am the mother of Baby M." Thus begins the story of a surrogate mother who responded to a newspaper ad for women to bear children for other couples for a fee of $10,000. A moving and absorbing account of a mother who changed her mind and wanted her daughter back.

Yglesias, R. (1988). *Only children*. New York: William Morrow.
Depicts the joys and challenges of two couples as they rear their children in the 80s. Of special interest is the involvement of fathers in child rearing.

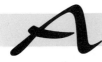# ANSWER TO "WHAT WOULD YOU DO?"

A committee appointed by the British government recommends that the husband of a woman receiving donated sperm be regarded as the father of the resulting child. The committee recommends that, at the age of eighteen, the child is entitled to learn about the sperm donor's ethnic origin and genetic health.

Another point of view is expressed by Michael Bayles (1984): Like many other people, AID children may desire to know their biological parents. Such a desire is emphasized in adoption situations. But is the desire a rational one? Finding out who one's genetic father is means learning his personal identity. Why would that be important? The mere knowledge does not entitle one to inheritance, other financial support, or love. What one's genetic father is or was—criminal, actor, politician, industrial worker— does not, except for certain genetic traits, determine or indicate what type of person one is or is going to become. Thus, although this desire is not necessarily irrational, if one fully understands what is involved in such information and its implications for one's own life, it probably would not be a strong desire. Much of the current interest is probably culturally conditioned (and exaggerated by the media). In addition, AID children may be significantly concerned about the possibility of inheriting a genetic disease. Such a concern certainly is rational, but fulfilling it does not require learning the donor's personal identity (p. 20).

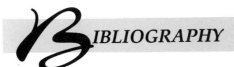# BIBLIOGRAPHY

"An increasing proportion of tubal ligations take place in outpatient units. (1987). *Family Planning Perspectives*, p. 276.

Bayles, M. D. (1984). *Reproductive Ethics*. Englewood Cliffs, NJ: Prentice-Hall.

Berch, D. B. & Bender, B. G. (1987, December). Margins of sexuality. *Psychology Today*, pp. 54–57.

Boston Woman's Health Book Collective, (1976). From infancy to old age: Development across the lifespan. *Our Bodies, Ourselves*. New York: Simon and Schuster.

Childbearing occupies short period of woman's life in developed world. (1987, March–April). *Family Planning Perspectives*, 19, 85.

DeFries, J. C., Plomin, R., & LaBuda, M. C. (1987, January). Genetic stability of cognitive development from childhood to adulthood. *Developmental Psychology*, 23, (1), 4–12.

Egeland, J. A., et al. (1987). Bipolar affective disorders linked to DNA markers on chromosome 11. *Nature*, 325, 783–787.

Ethics Committee of the American Fertility Society. (1986). Ethical considerations of the new reproductive technologies. *Fertility and Sterility Supplement 1, 46*, 57S.

Falbo, T. (ed.), (1984). *The single-child family*. New York: The Guilford Press.

Forrester, J. D. (1987, May–June). Has she or hasn't she? U.S. women's experiences with contraception. *Family Planning Perspectives*, 19, 113.

Greenhouse, L. (1989, July 4). A right is challenged—Justices accept more cases on the issue. *The New York Times*, p.1.

Groller, I. (1987, October). Is surrogate motherhood okay? *Parents,* p. 28.

Gromley, A. V., Gromley, J. B., & Weiss, H. (1987). Motivations for parenthood among young adult college students. *Sex Roles, 16,* 34–36.

Guillen, M. A. (1984, December). The first cause. *Psychology Today,* pp. 72–73.

Hanafin, H. (1987, August 28). *Surrogate parenting: Reassessing human bonding.* Paper presented at the convention of the American Psychological Association, New York.

Harlap, S. (1979, June 28). Gender of infants conceived on different days of the menstrual cycle. *New England Journal of Medicine, 300,* 1447.

Hetherington, E. M., & Parke, R. D. (1986). *Child psychology: A contemporary viewpoint.* New York: McGraw-Hill.

Holden, C. (1987, September). Genes and behavior: a twin legacy. *Psychology Today,* p. 18.

Ho, Hsiu-Zu, Glahn, T. J., & Ho, Ju-Chang. (1988). The fragile-x syndrome. *Developmental Medicine and Child Neurology, 30,* 252–265.

Jones, T. (1988, June 1). Quebec tries to buck trend, kindle baby boom with cash. *The Miami Herald,* p. 2A.

Keller, B. (1987, December 26). Mother Russia makes a comeback on births. *The New York Times,* pp. 1, 4.

Kline, M. (1989, April). *Work and family life during the transition to parenthood.* Paper presented at the "Becoming a Family" Project Symposium at the biennial meeting of the Society for Research in Child Development, Kansas City, MO.

Kogan, S. C., Doherty, M., & Gitschier, J. (1987, October 15). An improved method for prenatal diagnosis of genetic diseases by analysis of amplified DNA sequences. *New England Journal of Medicine, 317,* 985–990.

Kolata, G. (1988, October 4). New egg-implanting technique avoids surgery. *The New York Times,* p. 27.

Lindsay, B. as told to Cable Neuhaus. (1987). The shakers face their last amen. *People Weekly, 27,* 78–82.

Maranto, G. (1984, October). Choosing your baby's sex. *Discover,* pp. 25–27.

Miller, W. (1983). Chance, choice and the future of reproduction. *American Psychologist, 38,* 1198–1205.

Neeson, J. D., & May, K. A. (1986). *Comprehensive maternity nursing.* Philadelphia: J.B. Lippincott.

The New York Times, (1989, July 4). Excerpts from the court decision on the regulation of abortion, p. 10.

Nilsson, L. (1977). *A child is born.* New York: Delacorte Press/Seymour Lawrence, p. 22.

Otten, A. L. (1988, May 18). Study cites lack of success with in vitro fertilization. *The Wall Street Journal,* p. 33.

Norton, A. J. (1987, July–August). Families and children in the year 2000. *Children Today, 16,* p. 6.

Patterson, D. (1987, August). The causes of Down syndrome. *Scientific American, 257,* 52.

Phipps-Yonas, S. (1980, October). Teenage pregnancy and parenthood: A review of the literature. *American Journal of Orthopsychiatry, 50,* 403–431.

Potts, L. (1980, October). "Considering parenthood: group support for a critical life decision." *American Journal of Orthopsychiatry, 50,* 629–638.

Predicting diseases. (1987, May 25). *U.S. News and World Report*, p. 65.

Ricklefs, R. (1987, November 24). What a darling baby! Let's push rewind and see her again. *The Wall Street Journal*, pp. 1, 22.

Scarr, S. (1984, May). Interview. *Psychology Today*, pp. 59–63.

Schmeck, H. M., Jr. (1987, December 12). Single gene may determine the sex of a fetus. *The New York Times*, p. 1.

Schmeck, H. M. J. New methods fuel efforts to decode human genes. *The New York Times*. (1989, May 9) p. 23.

Schneider, P. (1987, November). What it's like to adopt. *Parents*, p. 178.

Singer, P., & Wells, D. (1985). *Making babies: the new science and ethics of conception.* New York: Charles Scribner's Sons.

Surrogate grandma has triplets. (1987, October 1). *Miami Herald*, p. 23A.

Tellegan, A. (1987, July). Recruitment bias in twin research: The rule of two-thirds reconsidered. *Behavior Genetics, 17*(4), 343–362.

Thomas, A., Chess, S., & Birch, H. (1970, August). The origin of personality. *Scientific American, 223,* 102–109.

Updated estimates of the costs of raising a child. (1986, April). *Family Economics Review, 2,* p. 34.

U.S. Bureau of the Census. (1986). (Current Population Reports, Series P-20, No. 441). *Household and Family Characteristics: March 1985.* Washington, DC: U.S. Government Printing Office.

U.S. Bureau of the Census. (1987a). (Current Population Reports, Series P-23, No. 150). *Population profile of the United States: 1984–85,* Washington, DC: U.S. Government Printing Office.

U.S. Bureau of the Census. (1987b). (Current Population Reports, Series P-25, No. 1006). *United States population estimates and components of change: 1970 to 1986.* Washington DC: U.S. Government Printing Office.

U.S. Bureau of the Census.

Vaux, D., Manager of the Repository for Germinal Choice. (1987, October 8). Information provided in a telephone conversation with the author.

Wellborn, S. N. (1987, April 13). Extroverts are born, not made. *U.S. news & world report. 102,* 62.

Wheeler, D. (1986, September 3). Researchers weigh a stepped-up effort to map the terrain of the human gene. *Chronicle of Higher Education.*

Willis, J. (1980, September). Genetic counseling: Learning what to expect. *FDA Consumer, 14,* 11–13.

Woman pregnant with twins frozen from embryos. (1987, July 15). *The Tampa Tribune,* p. 4A.

Zajonc, R. B. (1986). Decline and rise of scholastic aptitude scores. *American psychologist, 41,* 862–867.

CHAPTER FOUR

The beginning: prenatal development and birth

◆

VIGNETTES
INTRODUCTION
Prenatal Development Test
PRENATAL STAGES OF
    DEVELOPMENT
Gestation Period
Zygote Stage—Conception to Two
    Weeks
In the Spotlight: How Do I Know
    I'm Pregnant?
Embryo Stage—Three to Eight
    Weeks
Fetal Stage—Nine Weeks to Birth
A PRIMER OF PRENATAL
    DEVELOPMENT (FETAL AGE)
Month One—Zygote Stage and
    First Two Weeks of Embryo
    Stage
Month Two—Embryonic Stage
Month Three—End of First
    Trimester

Month Four
Month Five
Month Six—End of Second
    Trimester
Month Seven
Month Eight
Month Nine to Delivery—Third
    Trimester
FETAL CIRCULATORY SYSTEM
PRENATAL PERSONALITY
    DEVELOPMENT
PRENATAL SENSORY
    DEVELOPMENT
The Womb As a Classroom
In the Spotlight: How Do We
    Know What Babies Know?
FETAL BIOLOGY
Amniocentesis
Ultrasound
Fetoscopy
Chorionic Villus Sampling (CVS)

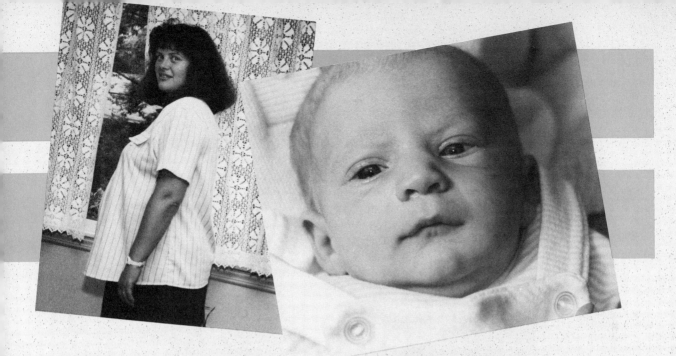

Alpha-Fetoprotein Test (AFP)
Percutaneous Umbilical Blood
  Sampling (PUBS)
FETAL MEDICINE
FETAL THERAPY—
  ACCELERATING
  DEVELOPMENT
MEDICAL USE OF FETAL
  TISSUES
FETAL RIGHTS—WOMEN'S
  RIGHTS
What Would You Do?
IS THERE A BEST TIME TO BE
  BORN?
PREGNANCY AS A
  DEVELOPMENTAL PROCESS
LABOR
Stages of Labor
BIRTHING PRACTICES
Natural Childbirth
Water Babies
Cesarean Births
Personal Story: Patricia Lanius—
  Becoming a Mother
INFLUENCES ON PREGNANCY

Teratogenic Substances
Chemicals
Drugs and Pregnancy
Radiation
Tobacco
RH Blood Factor
Rubella
Fetal Alcohol Syndrome (FAS)
Heroin
Caffeine
Maternal Nutrition
SUMMARY
QUESTIONS TO GUIDE YOUR
  REVIEW
ACTIVITIES FOR FURTHER
  INVOLVEMENT
KEY TERMS
ENRICHMENT THROUGH
  FURTHER READING
ANSWERS TO THE PRENATAL
  DEVELOPMENTAL TEST
ANSWER TO "WHAT WOULD
  YOU DO?"
BIBLIOGRAPHY

⟲IGNETTES

Seven months after Jean and Joe Canicatti were married, she became pregnant. However, the pregnancy ended in a miscarriage. For the next 2½ years, Jean and Joe tried to have a baby, but without success. "We really wanted a child, but doing what comes naturally wasn't working, so we decided I should see a doctor who specializes in fertility problems," says Jean. "I went to her, had a complete checkup, including Xrays to see if my tubes were blocked. I was fine, so for about a year I took Clomiphene, a fertility drug. Nothing happened. So the doctor put me on a stronger dose of Clomiphene. It was terrible. I gained a lot of weight and generally wasn't a very nice person to live with. In the meantime, Joe and I were doing all kinds of things to help me get pregnant, like taking my temperature every day to determine the days on which I was fertile. Finally, I said, 'This is crazy—we've got to do something else.'"

Jean went to another fertility expert for help. A complete physical examination revealed that both Jean's tubes were blocked. The doctor gave Jean and Joe three choices: surgery to unblock the tubes, in vitro fertilization, or adoption. "It was a hard decision for us," says Jean, "because I had just turned forty, and I felt time was running out. Also, I have two children by a previous marriage, a girl, age nineteen and a boy, age seventeen, who live with their father. But Joe never had children before, and he wanted a child of his own in the worst way."

Jean and Joe opted for surgery to unblock her tubes. "It was like a miracle!" Jean says. I had surgery on the first of October and a little over a month later, in November, I was pregnant!"

However, as Jean is quick to point out, "It has not been your 'normal' pregnancy. I haven't been able to enjoy the pregnancy as much as I would like to because I have been scared that something would go wrong. I've been doing all I have to do to carry the baby to term."

"At sixteen weeks I had amniocentesis. We were sitting on pins and needles all the time until we found out the results. I'm considered high risk because of my age, plus I'm Rh negative. But things are normal and the baby and I are both okay. In the beginning I wasn't getting too close to the baby, because I didn't want to feel too torn up in case I had to abort. It was like I was afraid of getting too attached.

"Now that everything is going well and as the time gets closer, both Joe and I are more involved with getting ready for our baby boy. We still haven't picked out a name for him yet. Maybe he'll be Joe, Jr.,—I don't know. We got new carpet for the house—we want it to look nice for him. We bought a baby crib with a waterbed mattress—we've heard that's supposed to be good for babies. We are going to put new wallpaper up in his room. Every weekend we do something to get ready for the baby. This coming week we are starting to attend childbirth classes. It includes breathing, exercising, films on normal birth, uses of different kinds of anesthesia, and so forth.

"Every time the baby moves, and he moves a lot, it brings a smile to my face. I say to Joe, 'Honey, come here! Feel it! Feel it! Feel your boy move!' Joe's already planning for the baby's future. He wants him to be a golfer and make lots of money! I just hope he gets here healthy and in good shape!"

Mario and Mayra Diaz became parents of a baby boy at 1:26 AM on May 13, 1989. Little Oscar weighed seven pounds, two ounces, and was born at Perdue Maternity Center. It was a normal delivery all the way. Mayra's contractions were about four and one-half minutes apart when she and Mario went to the maternity center. Mayra was in labor about four hours. Oscar was delivered by Elaine Spencer, one of two midwives at the Center. Mayra met Elaine at the Community Health Clinic of South Dade for the first time only three days before her delivery. "I was so surprised that I liked Elaine so much. I was concerned at first. They do a lot of births at Perdue, but with no doctor in attendance, I didn't know what to expect. On the day I gave birth, there were seven other births as well, so it is a busy place.

"I selected Perdue because I couldn't afford my own doctor. My husband has been unemployed for the last year, so we don't have any money. I presented my Medicaid card to Purdue, so they didn't charge me anything.

"When I got pregnant, it was a complete surprise to us—we didn't plan to have any other children. Yvette is eight years old and Mario Jr. is six, and we thought that would be it. But when I got pregnant, I said, 'Well, okay, I'll have it.' "

At the beginning of her pregnancy, Mayra went once a month to the Community Health Clinic for an examination. At the clinic, they examined Mayra, weighed her, and took her temperature and blood pressure. At every visit, the doctor measured Mayra around the stomach and checked her legs and ankles for swelling. At six months Mayra went to the clinic every three weeks, and at eight months she went every two weeks. During the last month she went every week.

"I did everything I was supposed to do during my pregnancy," explains Mayra, "and I didn't do anything I wasn't supposed to do. I don't drink or smoke and I wasn't sick a day. It was a good pregnancy. Thank God everything turned out alright."

As for Oscar, he is getting along well too. "He is a good boy," says Mayra. "He's not a baby that is crying all the time. The only time he cries is when he is hungry or if he is constipated a little bit—I can tell the difference and take care of him. Other than that, he sleeps most of the time. Plus, the other kids help me a lot with him. Mario Jr. helps watch him when I leave the room. Yvette is like a little mother herself. She loves to dress Oscar and she brings me the bottle and diapers and all the other things like that."

Mayra and Oscar will go to the community clinic to see the doctor for their first checkup in five weeks. "I'm glad we had the clinic and maternity center available to us," explains Mayra, "Otherwise, I don't know what we would have done."

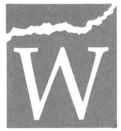

We all try to be sophisticated and up-to-date regarding our beliefs about pregnancy, birth, and parenting. However, we may not always know what we need to know. See how you do on the following prenatal development test. Answers are found at the end of the chapter.

Prenatal Development Test

1. A pregnant woman should avoid exercise and physical activity during pregnancy because this may cause the umbilical cord to wrap around her baby's neck. T __ F __
2. A missed menstrual period is one of the best ways to determine if a woman is pregnant. T __ F __

3. If an expectant woman in the last month of pregnancy is frightened by a vicious dog, her child will be born afraid of dogs. T __ F __

4. Nancy Hillard smokes a pack of cigarettes a day and enjoys a glass or two of wine with her evening meal. Nancy just learned she is pregnant. As Nancy's friend, the best advice you can give her is to cut back to half a pack of cigarettes and one glass of wine a day. T __ F __

5. The pregnant woman's blood and her baby's blood are separated by the placenta, which acts as a barrier to harmful drugs and toxic substances. T __ F __

6. The most critical period of prenatal development is during the last three months of pregnancy. T __ F __

7. The main purpose of fetal diagnostic procedures such as ultrasound imaging is to satisfy parents' desires to know the sex of their child and to view the fetus. T __ F __

8. Maria Figueroa is three months pregnant with her first baby and has Rh negative blood. Her husband is Rh positive. Their baby will be born anemic because of the incompatibility of the parents' blood. T __ F __

9. Rachel Stein has just learned she is pregnant. She hopes to resume her modeling career after the birth of her child and is concerned about putting on too much weight. She decides to limit her weight gain during pregnancy to under twenty pounds. Rachel has made the right decision for herself and her child. T __ F __

10. Labor is completed when the fetus is born. T __ F __

PRENATAL STAGES OF DEVELOPMENT

The wonderful and dynamic process of human development whereby a child grows from a microscopic being to a seven-pound "bundle of joy" begins at *conception*, with the fusion of the male and female *gametes,* or sex cells. Conception also marks the beginning of the *zygote stage* (also called the *germinal* and *ovum* stage), which includes the first two weeks of prenatal development. The *embryo stage* begins at three weeks and lasts through the eighth week. The developing child is in the *fetal stage* from the ninth week until birth.

Gestation Period

The chronology of pregnancy is referred to as *gestation* (from the Latin *gestare,* to carry), the period of time the child is in the uterus. This time period is divided in several ways, ten lunar months of four weeks each, or nine calendar months comprising three *trimesters.*

The first trimester is the first three months, the second trimester is from the fourth through sixth months, and the third trimester is from the seventh month to birth. Gestational time varies depending on the *beginning* reference point chosen to date the pregnancy, as shown in Table 4–1. From the moment of conception to birth, the fetus will be in the mother's womb about 266 days or 8¾ months. However, most physicians date the pregnancy from the first day of the mother's last menstrual period (LMP), giving a gestational age of 280 days. The LMP method for dating the pregnancy is most often used for the practical reason that most women can easily remember their last menstrual period.

TABLE 4–1

GESTATIONAL TIME BASED ON FERTILIZATION AND LAST MENSTRUAL PERIOD (LMP)		
	Fertilization (Fetal Age)	Last Menstrual Period (LMP) (Gestational Age)
Days	266	280
Weeks	38	40
Calendar months	8 ¾	9
Lunar months (28 days)	9 ½	10

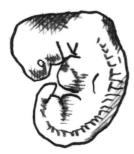

4 WEEKS — FIRST LUNAR MONTH

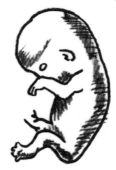

8 WEEKS — SECOND LUNAR MONTH

12 WEEKS — THIRD LUNAR MONTH

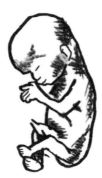

16 WEEKS — FOURTH LUNAR MONTH

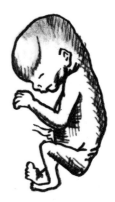

20 WEEKS — FIFTH LUNAR MONTH

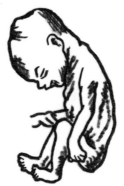

28 WEEKS — SEVENTH LUNAR MONTH

32 WEEKS — EIGHTH LUNAR MONTH

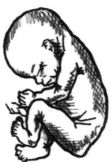

38 WEEKS — TENTH LUNAR MONTH

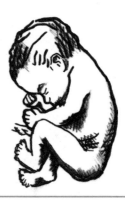

FIGURE 4-1 With the uniting of the ovum and sperm, the wondrous process of prenatal development begins. It ends nine months later with the emergence of the unique individual from her mother's womb. (Adapted from Lesner/PEDIATRIC NURSING, copyright 1983 by Delmar Publishers Inc.)

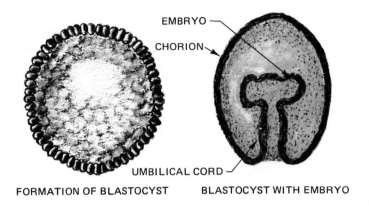

EMBRYO

CHORION

UMBILICAL CORD

FORMATION OF BLASTOCYST   BLASTOCYST WITH EMBRYO

FIGURE 4-2 The blastocyst, here shown in the early and late stages, is a hollow ball of cells that will implant in the wall of the uterus 7-10 days after fertilization. (From Anderson/BASIC MATERNAL-NEWBORN NURSING, 5th edition, copyright 1989 by Delmar Publishers Inc.)

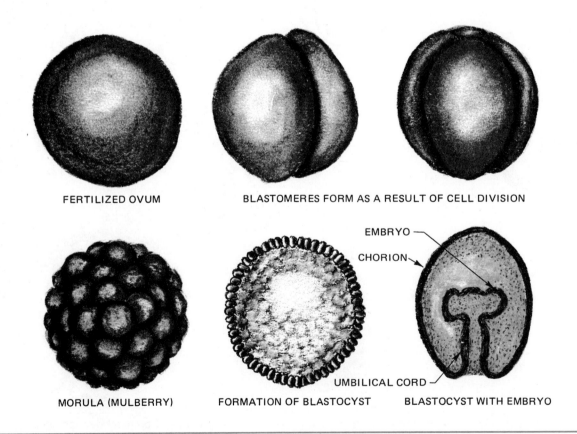

FERTILIZED OVUM   BLASTOMERES FORM AS A RESULT OF CELL DIVISION

EMBRYO

CHORION

UMBILICAL CORD

MORULA (MULBERRY)   FORMATION OF BLASTOCYST   BLASTOCYST WITH EMBRYO

FIGURE 4-3 The process of development from fertilization, cleavage, blastycyst formation and implantation. (From Anderson/BASIC MATERNAL-NEWBORN NURSING, 5th edition, copyright 1989 by Delmar Publishers Inc.)

Zygote Stage—Conception to Two Weeks

Prenatal development, like all human development, is predictable and orderly. At conception, the *zygote*, the cell formed when egg and sperm unite, is floating free in the fallopian tube and, through ciliary action and muscle contractions, moves down the fallopian tube. A period of rapid cell division called *cleavage* begins, and by the fourth day, the cells form a *blastocyst*, a hollow ball of cells. (See Figure 4–2.) Similar in appearance to a volleyball, the blastocyst consists of two layers of cells. The outer layer, the *trophoblast*, will become the *placenta*, the organ that connects the developing child to the mother and provides a system for prenatal nourishment, oxygen, and disposal of carbon dioxide and waste products. The inner layer is the developing child. The blastocyst is filled with fluid from the uterus and is still free floating in the fallopian tube.

By the sixth day the blastocyst completes its journey to the uterus where it begins *implantation*, the process of attaching to the nutrient-rich uterine wall. Implantation occurs when the trophoblast forms finger-like projections called *villi*, which attach to the uterus. Implantation is usually completed from seven to ten days after fertilization (Bobak & Jensen, 1987, p. 188). (See Figure 4–3.)

Implantation marks the beginning of pregnancy and is a *critical period* in development. Sometimes, implantation does not occur, in which case the blastocyst is discharged through the vagina. The usual site of implantation is the upper, posterior part of the uterus, but implantation may occur in any part of the uterus. Occasionally, implantation occurs outside the uterus or even in the fallopian tube. These *ectopic* pregnancies occur outside the uterus, in the fallopian tubes, ovaries, or the abdominal cavity. If the pregnancy occurs in the fallopian tube, the tube spontaneously bursts after about three months.

Ectopic pregnancies occur in about one in every 200 pregnancies and maternal death occurs in about one in 800 cases (Bobak & Jensen, 1987, pp. 818, 822).

*I*N THE SPOTLIGHT

HOW DO I KNOW I'M PREGNANT?

Presumptive Signs of Pregnancy The first group of pregnancy signs are called *presumptive* signs, and are symptoms of pregnancy. They are the least reliable signs of pregnancy and are not considered positive proof of pregnancy. Several signs or physical indicators of pregnancy are:

- A missed menstrual period, especially in women with regular cycles, is often used as a sign of pregnancy. However, unless a woman is anticipating pregnancy, she may not think she is pregnant because a missed period could be attributable to other factors, such as illness and stress.
- Nausea and vomiting are symptoms associated with pregnancy. These indications, present during the first trimester, usually occur early in the day and are popularly known as *morning sickness*. Long considered the bane of pregnant women, there is, however, a beneficial outcome to all the nausea and queasiness. In one study by researchers at the National Institutes of Health (Klebanoff, Koslowe, Kaslow, & Rhoades, 1985) "over half of all women vomited on at least one occasion during the first sixteen weeks. Vomiting began early, peaked in the second and third months, and was uncommon after twenty weeks" (p. 612). They also report that women who vomit early in pregnancy are less likely to experience miscarriages and deliver before thirty-seven weeks' gestation. As often happens

with good news, there is some bad news to accompany it. Researchers further report that women who vomit in one pregnancy are more likely to vomit in subsequent pregnancies.

■ Other presumptive signs of pregnancy include: excessive fatigue; frequent urination; changes in the breasts, including tenderness and increased pigmentation of the nipple and areola (the area around the nipple); *quickening* (the first fetal movement recognized by the mother); softening of the cervix; discoloration (bluish-red) of the mucos membrane of the cervix; and abdominal enlargement.

Probable Signs of Pregnancy There are objective changes in the woman's body that help indicate pregnancy. They are nonetheless considered probable signs because they are not definitive of pregnancy. These signs include: uterine enlargement, *ballottement* (from the French "to toss about") during a vaginal examination in which the fetus will rise in the amniotic fluid; uterine contractions known as Braxton-Hicks contractions or false labor; and pregnancy tests.

Pregnancy Tests Commercial, over-the-counter pregnancy test kits enable women to determine the possibility of pregnancy. These kits can be used as early as nine days after a missed period and manufacturers claim 99 percent accuracy. The tests work by mixing the first morning urine with the supplied chemical to determine the presence of *human chorionic gonadotrophin* (HCG), a hormone which is present following implantation. HCG is secreted through the kidneys and this is why urine is used in the test. Because these tests cannot conclusively prove pregnancy, they are categorized as probable indicators of pregnancy. The most accurate laboratory test, and the one used by most physicians, utilizes maternal blood serum to detect the presence of HCG.

Positive Signs of Pregnancy Four positive signs of pregnancy are: the fetal heartbeat, fetal movement felt by the physician, visualization of the fetus by ultrasound, and fetal EKG. A fifth way to positively determine pregnancy is through X-ray of the fetal skeleton. However, this may have a harmful effect on the developing fetus and therefore is seldom used.

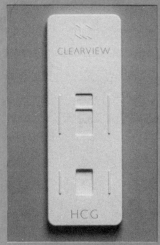
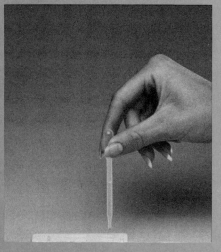

FIGURE 4-4A The accuracy rate of the modern pregnancy test is 99.1%, far more reliable than could have been expected even just a few years ago. (Photo courtesy of Sequoia-Turner Corporation)

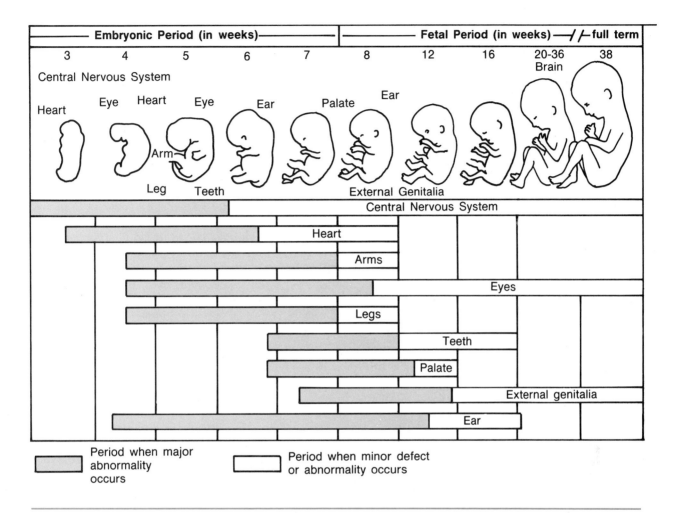

Embryonic Period (in weeks)					Fetal Period (in weeks) —//— full term				

FIGURE 4-4B The critical periods in prenatal development are shown and are the times when the embryo and fetus are most affected by negative influences. (Used with permission from White, *Before we are born*, p. 96, copyright W.B. Saunders, Co.)

As we discussed in Chapter One, a *critical period* is a period when pre- and postnatal development is most vulnerable to risk factors. The embryonic period of prenatal development is often viewed as the most critical period of development since this is when developing organs, systems and body parts are most influenced. Figure 4–4B shows the critical periods for the developing embryo and fetus and the area of development most seriously affected.

Embryo Stage—Three to Eight Weeks

The embryo period begins with the third week of pregnancy and concludes at the end of the eighth week (fifty-six days) when the embryo measures about three centimeters or 1.18 inch (Rosenblith & Sims-Knight, 1985, p. 24). (See Figure 4–5.) The embryonic period is one of rapid growth and tremendous developmental significance. It is

DEVELOPMENTAL MILESTONES OF THE EMBRYO (ROSENBLITH AND SIMS-KNIGHT, 1985)

3 weeks (15–20 days)	Development of three-layered (trilaminar) disc. Neural tube begins to form. Disc becomes attached to wall by short, thick umbilical cord. Placenta develops rapidly.
4 weeks (21–28 days)	Eyes begin to form. Heart starts beating. Crown-rump length 5 mm (less than ¼ in.); growth rate about 1 mm per day. Neural tube closes (otherwise spina bifida). Vascular system develops (blood vessels). Placenta maternal-infant circulation begins to function.
5 weeks	Arm and leg buds form.
7 weeks	Facial structures fuse (otherwise facial defects).
8 weeks	Crown-rump length 3 cm (slightly more than 1 in.); weight 1 g (about 1/30 oz). Major development of organs completed. Most external features recognizable at birth are present.

FIGURE 4-5 Developmental milestones of the embryo from weeks three through eight are shown above.

the most critical time in the development of an individual because all the main organ systems are established and the embryo develops uniquely human characteristics. The developing organ systems are most affected by and vulnerable to such damaging influences as drugs, viruses, radiation, infection, and poor nutrition. These negative influences can result in developmental *anomalies* (deviations from the normal) of various kinds, such as neural tube defects. Unfortunately for many children and parents, during this critical period of development some women may not realize they are pregnant and may expose the developing embryo to hazards that have serious short- and long-term consequences.

During the third week, the inner cells of the blastocyst *differentiate* into three germ layers: *ectoderm* (outside), *mesoderm* (middle), and *endoderm* (inner). Three major body systems develop from these specialized groups of cells. The ectoderm develops skin, nails, hair, eyes, mouth, and tooth enamel; the mesoderm produces the circulatory system, muscles, bones, kidneys, and the inner layer of skin and teeth (except enamel); and from the endoderm develops the internal organs, glands, lungs, digestive system, tongue, and auditory canal. (See Figure 4–6.)

The cardiovascular system is the first system to function in the developing human and at the end of the third week, a rudimentary heart is formed and is pumping blood (Bobak & Jensen, 1987, p. 197). Thus the mother's menstrual period—if she were to have one—would be only about a week late by the time her child's heart is beating! *Folding*, the process whereby the embryo transforms from a flat surface to a "C"-shaped cylinder with a distinguishable head and tail, also begins in the third week.

Arm and leg buds and rudimentary eyes are formed by the fourth week. In the fifth week, rapid brain development occurs and during this week, limb differentiation is apparent, with identifiable wrist and elbow regions and finger rays, denoting future fingers. (See Figure 4–7).

Neural Tube Defects During prenatal development, the neurological system may not develop properly, resulting in midline abnormalities of the spine or brain caused by a failure of the neural tube to properly close. These are referred to as

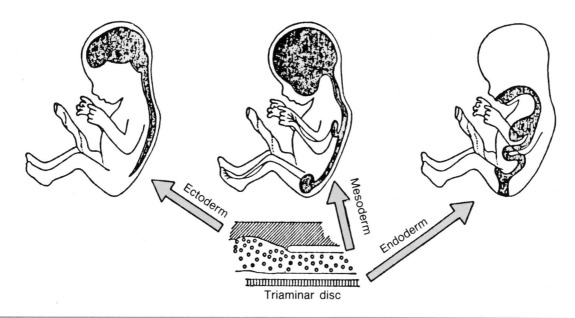

Triaminar disc

FIGURE 4-6   This figure depicts the development of the three different types of germ layers and the major body systems which develops from each. (Used with permission from Neeson & May, *Comprehensive maternity nursing: nursing process and the childbearing family,* copyright 1986 by J.B. Lippincott Co.)

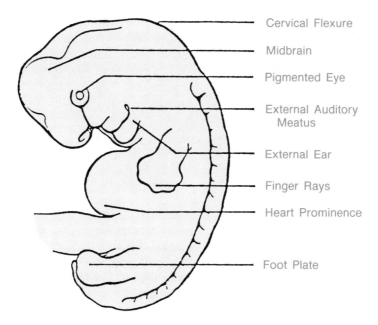

Cervical Flexure

Midbrain

Pigmented Eye

External Auditory Meatus

External Ear

Finger Rays

Heart Prominence

Foot Plate

FIGURE 4-7   The rapid development of the embryo period is shown above. Notice the development of various body features, especially eye, ear, finger and heart area.

neural tube defects and occur in the fourth week of development. When the neural tube is open at the top, the baby is born with a rudimentary brain or no brain at all, a condition known as *anencephaly*. These babies die at birth or within a day or two after. In other cases, the opening is along the spine and a portion of the spinal nerve column is exposed. This defect is known as *spina bifida*, or *cleft spine*. These babies are often paralyzed below the portion of the open spine. Children with spina bifida may be mentally retarded and frequently have no bowel or bladder control. Some babies also have *hydrocephaly*, whereby fluid accumulates in the head and can result in brain damage. Neural tube defects occur in about one in 700 pregnancies (Neesen & May, 1986, p. 237).

Most parents-to-be want to do all they can to assure that they will have a healthy and developmentally normal baby. Some mothers may be overwhelmed by what they must do, e.g., stop smoking and drinking, that they wish there were something relatively easy they could do to help prevent prenatal developmental problems such as neural tube defects (see chapter 5). Well, there may be. Researchers (Mulinare et al, 1988) have found that there is ". . . an overall protective effect of periconceptional (from three months before conception through the third month of pregnancy) multivitamin use on the occurence of neural tube defects. . . ." A number of cautionary notes are in order however. The study was a retrospective one (meaning that the researchers asked women after the fact if they took vitamins before and after pregnancy) and, women who use multivitamins are different from those who do not. So, there may be other factors involved such as the overall quality and nature of prenatal care. Nonetheless, for women of child bearing age, adding a multivitamin to their diets may be worth it not only to them but to their future children as well.

Kidney function is necessary for life and healthy living. Accordingly, kidney development begins during the fifth week and by the eighth week, the kidneys are functioning. A large percentage of amniotic fluid is urine excreted by the developing fetus.

By the end of the eighth week, the foundations for all the main organ systems are in place and the embryo is clearly distinguished. The head represents about half the embryo size, the neck region is more apparent, and there are distinguishable eyelids.

The Placenta   The *placenta* (from the Greek *plakoenta*, flat cake) is the prenatal life support system and develops during the embryo period. It automatically separates the circulatory systems of the fetus and the mother, so that all exchanges of material in any form must take place across this interface. The placenta is therefore the sole purveyor of all embryo/fetal needs and the sole route for the disposal of all fetal waste. Nutrients, oxygen, and waste are exchanged across the placenta. In this sense, the placenta serves all of the functions provided by the lungs, kidneys, stomach and intestines. The placenta also provides the fetus with the same immunological system as the mother and for about six months after birth, the baby is immune to the same diseases as the mother.

The *umbilical cord* is the link between the fetus and the placenta. Through it passes the fetal blood supply. The umbilical cord contains two umbilical arteries and one umbilical vein. The vein carries oxygenated blood to the fetus and the arteries return deoxygenated blood to the placenta.

At full term, the umbilical cord is about two centimeters (3/4 inch) in diameter and fifty centimeters (twenty inches) long, while the placenta is about fifteen to twenty centimeters (six to ten inches) in diameter, two and one-half to three centimeters (1.18 inches) thick, and weighs from 400 to 600 grams (one pound to one pound, five ounces) (Bobak & Jensen, 1987, pp. 189, 191).

Amniotic Fluid   The *amnion*, a thin, tough, membranous sac lining the inner portion of the uterus, contains the *amniotic fluid*, which is clear, light yellow and recycled about every three hours. At full term, the fetus is immersed in about 1000 milliliters (2.1 quarts) of fluid. Amniotic fluid originates from a number of sources, including fetal urine, which is the significant contributor as the pregnancy progresses. Amniotic fluid is constantly produced, a fact that negates the old wives' tale regarding "dry births," which says that once the "waters break" there is no more fluid and therefore the birth will be a "hard one."

The purpose of the amniotic fluid is to:

1. Protect the fetus from injury, for example, if the mother's abdomen receives a bump
2. Provide the developing fetus with room to grow and move freely
3. Protect the fetus from loss of heat and maintain a relatively constant fetal body temperature
4. Serve as a source of oral fluid for the fetus
5. Act as an excretion-collection system (Bobak & Jensen, 1987, p. 191)

Enveloped in amniotic fluid, the fetus is suspended in its own environmentally controlled growth capsule.

In addition to the functions mentioned, the amniotic fluid has great diagnostic value, enabling diagnosticians to determine the fetus' sex, assess its health and maturity, and make predictions about its growth. (See discussion of amniocentesis later in this chapter.)

Fetal Stage—Nine Weeks to Birth

The fetal period begins with the ninth week and ends at birth or whenever the pregnancy is terminated. The transition from the embryo to the fetal stage is significant, because the fetus is now recognizable as a member of the human race. During the next thirty-two weeks, the *fetus* grows and develops those structures formed during the critical embryo stage. Body size and length increase rapidly. For example, by the ninth week, the head constitutes almost half the fetus size, but by the thirteenth week, fetus length doubles in size and head growth slows so that now the head comprises one-third of the fetal size. At the twelfth week, male and female external genitalia are sufficiently developed to be easily distinguishable. Between sixteen and twenty weeks, the mother often feels fetal movements, known as quickening. By the end of the twentieth week, the fetus is covered with *vernix caseosa*, a greasy, cheese-like substance, and by *lanugo*, a down-like hair. The vernix protects the delicate fetal skin from chapping, drying, and

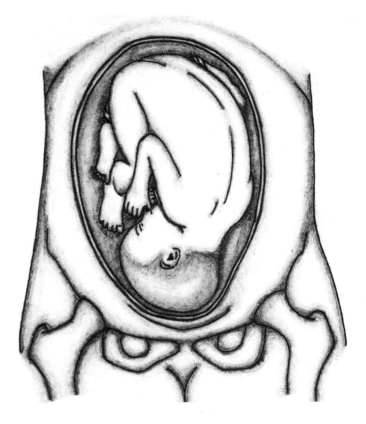

FIGURE 4-8 With the beginning of the fetal period, the fetus is recognizable as a human being. Notice the size of the head and its proportion to the rest of the fetal body. (From Caldwell & Hegner/NURSING ASSISTANT, 5th edition, copyright 1989 by Delmar Publishers Inc.)

hardening as a result of immersion in the amniotic fluid. The lanugo keeps the vernix in place.

By week twenty-two, the fetus is minimally *viable*, meaning it is able to survive—with intensive care—outside the uterus. Fetal survival outside the uterus is dependent on the maturity of the central nervous system for directing rythmic respirations and controlling body temperature, and the maturity of the lungs (Bobak & Jensen, 1987, p. 187). Critical to the proper functioning of the lungs is a substance called *surfactant*, which enables the lungs to remain

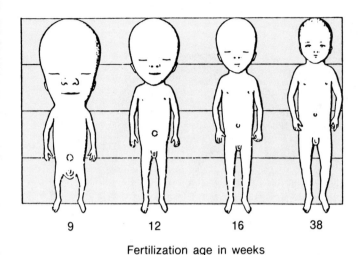

9   12   16   38

Fertilization age in weeks

FIGURE 4-9   Beginning at week nine, the above figure depicts the proportional development of the fetus through week 38. (Used with permission from Neeson & May, *Comprehensive maternity nursing: nursing process and the childbearing family,* copyright 1986 by J.B. Lippincott Co.)

open, not stick together, and permits the easy exchange of oxygen. (Surfactant contains *lecithin*, the same ingredient as in commercial aerosol products designed to prevent food from sticking to pots and frying pans.) The lungs begin to produce surfactant during the twenty-first week.

By the twenty-fourth week, the eyelashes and eyebrows are formed and the eyelids are open. During the twenty-eighth to the thirty-first weeks, the contours of the fetus become rounded because of the accumulation of subcutaneous fat (see Figure 4–8). From weeks thirty-two to thirty-eight the fetus steadily gains weight. By the end of thirty-eight weeks of fetal age, (forty weeks of gestational age), the toenails and fingernails are fully formed and extend beyond the fingertips, both male testes have descended into the scrotum, and the head is larger than any other part of the body. Figure 4–9 shows proportional development during the fetal stage and Figure 4–10 shows growth in size during the fetal period.

Fetuses, about one-fifth actual size. Head hair begins to appear at about 20 weeks. Eyebrows and eyelashes are usually recognizable by 24 weeks, and the eyes open by 26 weeks. Fetuses born prematurely (22 weeks or more) may survive, but intensive care is required. The mean duration of pregnancy is 266 days (38 weeks) from fertilization, with a standard deviation of 12 days. In clinical practice, it is customary to refer to full term as 40 weeks from the first day of the last menstrual period (LMP), assuming that conception occurs 2 weeks after the onset of menses. Thus, when a provider refers to a pregnancy of 20 weeks, the actual age of the festus is only 18 weeks.
(Moore KL: The Developing Human. Philadelphia, WB Saunders, 1982)

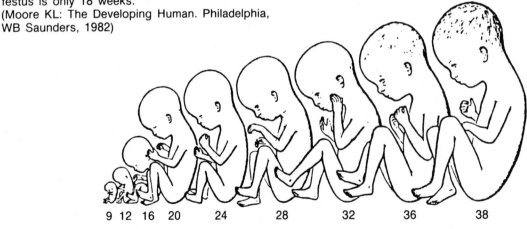

9 12 16 20   24   28   32   36   38

Fertilization age in weeks

FIGURE 4-10   The figure above gives a vivid and visual understanding of the growth of the fetus from weeks 9 to 38. (Used with permission from Neeson & May, *Comprehensive maternity nursing: nursing process and the childbearing family,* copyright 1986 by J.B . Lippincott Co.)

TABLE 4–2

FETAL DEVELOPMENT BY TRIMESTER

First Trimester	Second Trimester	Third Trimester
Period of organ differentiation	Period of continued growth and development of tissue and organs	Period of storage of subcutaneous fat, minerals, iron, vitamins, and calcium, and increasing tissue mass
Most critical period for teratogenic effects		
Fetal membranes appear: a. amnion b. chorion	Skeleton visible on x-ray	Testes descend
Germ layers differentiate: a. ectoderm b. mesoderm c. entoderm	Vernix caseosa forming on skin Lanugo appearing Meconium collecting	Eyelids open
Organs develop	Begins to store iron	Lanugo begins to shed
Sex distinguishable	Eyebrows and eye lashes present	Vernix caseosa decreases on skin
Human appearance	Head and body more proportionate	Immune bodies acquired from mother
Ossification of bones	Skin transparent; face wrinkled	Scalp hair grows
Fragments of nails begin to appear	Hair appears on head	Cartilage develops in nose and ears
Placenta developing	Quickening (fetal movement) felt by mother	Nails grow to tip of fingers and toes
Kidneys able to function	Grows about thirty centimeters (twelve inches) long and 680 grams (one and one half pounds)	All female eggs have completed the first stage of development and are stored in the ovaries
Called *embryo* from first to eighth week; called *fetus* after eighth week to birth	Fetal heart tones detected by fetoscope	
Heart beats sturdily and sends blood throughout the body		Exercises by kicking and stretching
Fetal heart tone may be heard by Doppler effect (the process of detecting change in sound waves—in this case the sound of the heart) by eleven to twelve weeks		Size increases: *Length*—thirty-five centimeters (fourteen inches) to fifty centimeters (twenty inches) *Weight*—1134 grams (two and one half pounds) to 3175–3400 grams (seven to seven and one half pounds)
Size increases from a minute structure to about three and one half inches in length and weighs above one ounce		

Note. Developed by Jacquelyn T. Hartley, Associate Professor of Maternal and Child Nursing, Florida International University.

A PRIMER OF PRENATAL DEVELOPMENT (FETAL AGE)

Month One—Zygote Stage and First Two Weeks of Embryo Stage

Fertilization occurs and implantation is completed. During this month, the embryo undergoes tremendous growth, increasing its weight 8,000 times! (Feinbloom, 1979). Major body systems are forming. The fetus measures about .4 to .5 centimeter (⅛ to ¼ inch), the head is one-third of its total length, and its skin is very light pink. The cardiovascular system is the first system to function, and the tiny, tube-shaped heart with double chambers is beating. The gastrointestinal system—stomach, liver, esophagus, and intestine—are present. Lung buds (swellings), indicators of the developing lungs, are visible as are the beginnings of the eyes and ears. The fetus does not yet respond to stimulation. Developmentally, the first month is a critical one because so many of the vital body organs are forming. This is why it is important for the pregnant woman to avoid drugs, nicotine, alcohol, caffeine, and radiation.

Table 4–2 shows fetal development by trimester.

Month Two—Embryonic Stage

The second month is one of impressive growth, and organ development is almost complete. If you saw the fetus during this month, you would easily recognize it as a human being, but you would see that it is out of proportion, with its head the largest part, totaling about one-half its size. It now weighs about two grams (one-quarter ounce) and measures about 2.5 to 3 centimeters (one inch) long. The heart has valves, is divided into a right and left side and beats regularly at from forty to eighty times a minute. The liver is producing blood cells and by the end of the month, the umbilical cord is fully functioning. The embryo is floating in about one to two teaspoons of amniotic fluid.

Month Three—End of First Trimester

At the beginning of this third month, the entire fetus moves in a jerky manner, but by the end of the month, the movements are more graceful and free flowing, with periods of activity and rest. Reflexes are refined because muscles, nerves, and bones are now working together. A mother is not yet aware of fetal movements because they are not strong enough for her to feel them. The fetus has mastered the swallowing reflex. Some babies are sucking their thumbs while floating serenely in their watery world! The fetal heartbeat can be detected with ultrasound and a fetoscope (a modified stethoscope with a head piece). The kidneys secrete small amounts of urine through the bladder. Tooth buds are formed under the gums. The eyelids form and seal shut to protect the eyes during final development and will reopen during the seventh month. Genitalia are now developed and parents, with the aid of ultrasound, can discover if they have a girl or boy.

Month Four

This is the month mothers can detect fetal movement as the fetus kicks with growing viability in its amniotic fluid. The fetus grows rapidly, about one-eighth of an inch *each day!* The placenta, now fully formed, supplies the fetus with nutrients and oxygen and takes away waste products. Lanugo, the fine, downy hair, begins to grow. The fetus is about 4.5 inches long and weighs about 3.7 ounces.

Month Five

Lanugo covers the baby's body, the eyelids are still closed, and development continues. The fetus now weighs about one pound and measures about one foot. During this month, many fathers enjoy placing their ear on the mother's abdomen to detect the fetal heartbeat. The fetus is settling into a regular prenatal routine of sleep and activity and even has a favorite position!

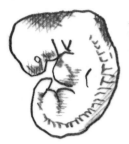

4 WEEKS — FIRST LUNAR MONTH
- Crown to rump length 2.0 mm
- Heart is bulging and begins to pulsate
- Arm and leg buds are present

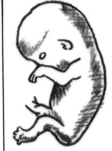

8 WEEKS — SECOND LUNAR MONTH
- Crown to rump length 30.0 mm
- End of embryonic period
- Organogenesis completed
- Facial structures more distinct
- External genitalia present

12 WEEKS — THIRD LUNAR MONTH
- Crown to rump length 3 inches
- Head is one-third of length
- Ossification centers in bones
- Genitalia now distinguishable

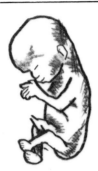

16 WEEKS — FOURTH LUNAR MONTH
- Crown to rump length 6 inches
- Hair present on the head
- Lanugo present on the body
- Ossification permits visualization by x-ray
- Meconium in intestines

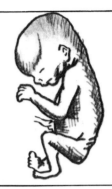

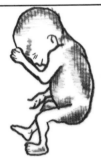

20 WEEKS — FIFTH LUNAR MONTH
- Crown to rump length 10 inches
- Vernix caseosa covers skin
- Fingernails and toenails are distinguishable
- Brown fat deposits in back

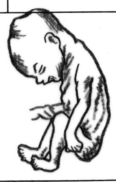

28 WEEKS — SEVENTH LUNAR MONTH
- Crown to rump length 15 inches
- Bone marrow is major source of red blood cells
- Minimal subcutaneous fat
- Deep red, wrinkled skin
- If born, fetus is considered viable but only one in ten survive

32 WEEKS — EIGHTH LUNAR MONTH
- Crown to rump length 17 inches
- Subcutaneous fat deposits
- Iron and minerals stored
- Responds to extrauterine sounds

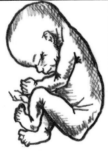

38 WEEKS — TENTH LUNAR MONTH
- Crown to rump length 20 inches
- Vernix and lanugo decreased
- Considered full term
- Muscles well developed
- Testes in scrotal sac

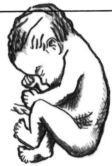

FIGURE 4-11 Prenatal growth from lunar months 1-10 enables you to see the dramatic changes that occur in a very short period of time. These illustrations also help you understand the stages of prenatal growth and at the same time realize what a wondrous process prenatal development is, given all the growth and development that occurs during prenatal life. (Adapted from Lesner/PEDIATRIC NURSING, copyright 1983 by Delmar Publishers Inc.)

Month Six—End of Second Trimester

Lung growth is a very important developmental process during this month. Surfactant begins to cover the lungs. Some babies born during this month are able to survive with heroic medical assistance, and such survivals are becoming more common with the advent of new advanced technology in neonatal intensive care units. Vernix caseosa, a cheese-like substance, covers the fetus' body to protect it from constant immersion in the amniotic fluid. The fetus is now about fourteen inches long and weighs about one and one-quarter pounds.

Month Seven

During this month, the fetus weighs about two and one-half to four and one-half pounds (1100 grams) and is about sixteen inches long. The baby starts storing fat and this accumulation, in combination with overall growth, adds two pounds by the end of the month. Because of the added weight, the fetus' skin color changes from reddish to flesh tone. The fetus begins to shed its lanugo and starts to grow hair. Eyelashes and eyebrows are present and the eyes are now open. Vital life support functions of breathing, swallowing, and temperature regulation are more fully developed. The baby is about two-thirds grown.

Month Eight

By the end of the eighth month, the fetus is about sixteen and one-half to eighteen inches long and weighs about five or six pounds. The fetus has turned in the uterus to the normal head-down position. This is called "presentation" for birth. Some fetuses are positioned with their buttocks down and head up. This is known as a *breech* position. The brain is developing rapidly and the fetus can distinguish light from dark and can hear sounds.

Month Nine to Delivery—Third Trimester

During this month the fetus completes its growth and developmental process. It gains about an ounce a day and by full term (266 days from fertilization and 280 days gestation) will weigh about 7.21 pounds if it is a boy and about 7.12 pounds if it is a girl. Boys tend to be a little longer—19.9 inches—than girls, who measure 19.6 inches. There is virtually no more room to grow, since the fetus occupies all of its mother's uterus! The eyes are normally slate gray, gray, or blue, and their true, permanent color will not be known until several months after birth. Vernix caseosa is still present but in varying amounts. Lanugo has disappeared except for the upper arms and shoulders. All body systems, with the exception of the lungs, are functioning and the fetus is urinating about once an hour.

The baby settles into the pelvis and is ready for birth. This settling occurs about one to two weeks prior to birth for the first-time mother, and at the time of birth for mothers who have had other babies.

At birth, the mother transfers her immune system to the baby and until about six months of age, the infant is immune to the same diseases to which the mother is immune.

FETAL CIRCULATORY SYSTEM

The fetal cardiovascular system is developed in such a way to support intrauterine life and facilitate transition to life after birth. The fetus receives oxygen through the placenta because the lungs do not function as an organ of respiration while the fetus is in the uterus. To meet this situation, fetal circulation utilizes three blood diverting mechanisms, called *shunts*. These shunting systems are the *ductus venosus*, the *foreman ovale* and the *ductus arteriosus*. (See Figure 4–12.) Closure of these special fetal structures after birth is imperative or childhood cardiovascular disorders develop.

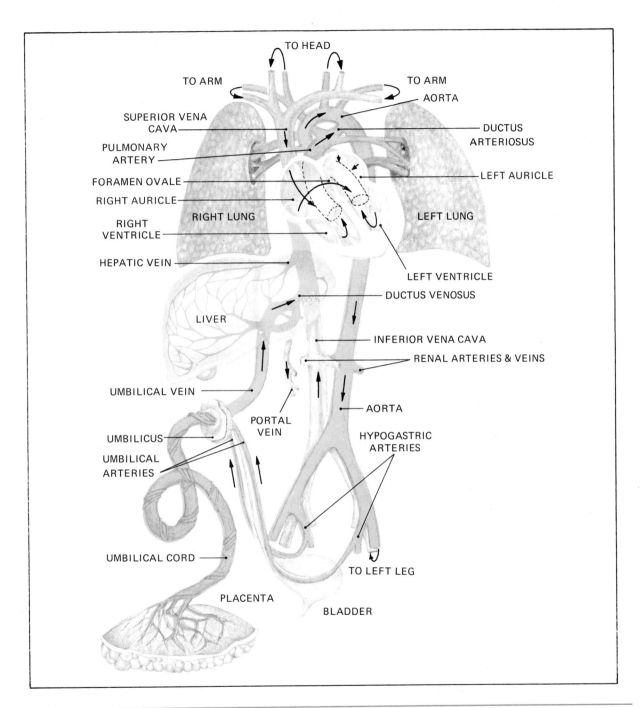

FIGURE 4-12 Fetal circulation is shown above. This figure helps explain how the circulatory system functions in utero and the changes that must occur following birth. (From Anderson/BASIC MATERNAL-NEWBORN NURSING, 5th edition, copyright 1989 by Delmar Publishers Inc.)

Prenatally, oxygenated blood flows up the umbilical cord and through the umbilical vein. Some goes to the liver, while the majority goes through the ductus venosus, the foreman ovale, through the left ventricle of the heart, and to the arms and head. Blood returns from these structures into the right ventricle, where a small amount goes to the lungs, and the rest—the major portion—goes through the ductus arteriosus and supplies the trunk and lower extremities. The deoxygenated blood leaves the fetal body by way of the umbilical arteries where it again arrives at the placenta and is oxygenated.

When the baby is born and commences breathing, the lungs begin to function and placental blood circulation ceases. The fetal blood diverting structures cease to exist and newborn circulation begins.

The fetal circulatory system assures that well-oxygenated blood is supplied to the heart, head, neck, and upper limbs. This circulatory pattern is one of the reasons fetal and, as we will see, infant development occurs from *cephalo* (head) to *caudal* (tail), and from *proximo* (midline) to *distal* (the arms, hands, and fingers).

PRENATAL PERSONALITY DEVELOPMENT

There is a great deal of interest in how prenatal events and experiences, beginning at conception, influence personality development. For example, psychiatrist Frank Lake proposed a theory of development based on the premise that "the behavioral reactions of a pregnant mother affect her fetus in ways which contribute to its perceptions of itself and of its environment in the womb; and these perceptions persist into adult life" (Moss, 1986, p. 52). Specifically, Lake believed such personality behaviors as anxiety, depression, phobias, and psychosomatic and hypochondriac disorders have prenatal origins (Moss, 1986, p. 53).

Lake's theory of maternal behavioral influences on prenatal personality development certainly merits discussion. However, the persistence of these influences throughout life is an interesting, but not widely supported or accepted theory. It

does cause us to consider the possibility of personality development beginning prior to birth. It may well be that, given the increased interest in prenatal development and the early years, more professionals will examine the possibilities involved in Lake's theory.

PRENATAL SENSORY DEVELOPMENT

The sensory abilities of fetuses are well developed. By six or seven weeks of gestation, a fetus will avoid a noxious stimulus. After twenty-four weeks it will respond to sound. Researchers are still uncertain exactly what the fetus hears. The baby is swimming in an aquatic environment, so what she hears is filtered through fluid. Also, the inner ear of the developing child is filled with amniotic fluid, which is different from the external world where the inner ear is filled with air. However, the development of the ability to hear must serve some useful function because development is efficient, not wasteful. Development does not occur only for the sake of development.

The fetus will move to the rhythm of its mother's speech and blink and start at a loud noise. Sensitivity to light develops at about the sixteenth week and by twenty-nine weeks, when a source of light is placed in the uterus, a fetus will open its eyes and search for the source. Toward the end of gestation, the fetus swallows large amounts of amniotic fluid. Compared to adult standards, amniotic fluid does not taste good, but has a bitter, salty quality (Crook, 1987).

The Womb As a Classroom

Many parents and the public are, at long last, giving the fetus her due! Researchers are exploring the frontiers of what the fetus knows and is able to do. As a result, the importance of prenatal abilities and learning are taking on added significance.

In several interesting studies (Kolata, 1984), researchers had mothers read *The Cat in the Hat*, a famous Dr. Seuss book of distinctive rhythm

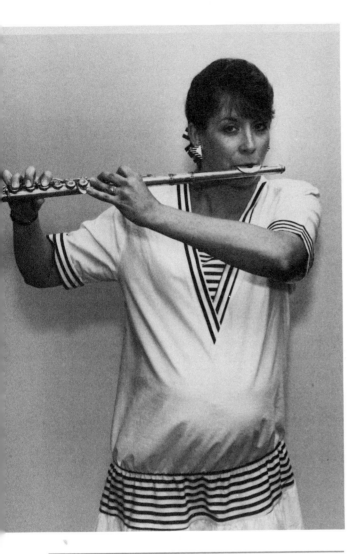

FIGURE 4-13 The idea of prenatal learning has always captivated and intrigued parents and researchers. Today, prenatal learning is receiving renewed attention and more mothers-to-be are exploring such possibilities.

hours. At birth, the babies were provided with a nonnutritive sucking device that enabled them to suck in order to hear *The Cat in the Hat* or *The King, the Mice and the Cheese*, a poem with a very different cadance. The babies' sucking patterns—short bursts, followed by a swallow—indicated they preferred their familiar prenatal story to the unfamiliar one. The researchers also found that when fetuses are read familiar stories, their heart rates decrease, signifying a more restful state. Consequently, prenatal auditory experiences do influence postnatal preferences. Perhaps pregnant mothers who serenade their babies with strains of Mozart, hoping to stimulate enjoyment of classical music after birth, are on to something!

The increasing discovery and acceptance of babies' in utero abilities has a number of practical applications for infant development and care. First, many prenatal intensive care nurseries (see Chapter Five) provide sensory stimulation for premature babies to simulate the prenatal sensory environment. Some nurseries, for example, will play sounds of the mother's heartbeat as a means of soothing the baby.

Second, many parents are learning how to "get in touch" with their babies. For example, at the Prenatal University, founder Rene Van de Carr teaches parents how to talk to their unborn babies with the intended purpose of helping them be "smarter" and happier newborns (Newsweek, 1987). Certainly one of the advantages of such efforts by parents to stimulate their babies in utero is that it begins the process of bonding before birth.

Where all of these discoveries of prenatal abilities will eventually lead fuels speculation and makes child development an exciting field of study. Undoubtedly, attempts to unravel prenatal mysteries will assist our efforts in providing children and mothers optimal pre- and postnatal care. For now, prenatal abilities and their importance, much like the sirens beckoning Ulysses, challenge researchers as one of the most significant and virtually unexplored frontiers of human development.

and cadence, to their children twice a day for the last six and one-half weeks of pregnancy so that by birth they had heard the story for about five

*I*N THE SPOTLIGHT

HOW DO WE KNOW WHAT BABIES KNOW?

With all the research going on in the fields of pre- and postnatal development, it is only normal to ask the question, "How do researchers know what babies know?" This is a good question, with a number of reasonable and plausible answers. One of the measures researchers use to "know" what babies think is through their sucking patterns. For example, in a study of voice preference, researchers De Casper and Fifer (1980) placed earphones over the babies' ears and a nonnutritive nipple was placed in each one's mouth. The nipples were connected to recording equipment. Following an adjustment period, during which the researchers determined the median sucking rate and pattern for each baby, a baseline period was used to determine the median interburst interval (IBI) or time elapsing between the end of one burst of sucking and the beginning of the next.

The infants then were given an opportunity to produce by sucking either their mother's voice or the voice of another infant's mother. A preference for the maternal voice was indicated when an infant produced it more often than the nonmaternal voice. "Preference for the mother's voice was shown by the increase in the proportion of IBIs capable of producing her voice; the median IBIs shifted from their baseline values in a direction that produced the maternal voice more than half the time" (De Casper & Fifer, 1980, p. 1175).

From data gathered in their study, based on the sucking patterns of neonates, the authors concluded: "Thus within the first three days of postnatal development, newborns prefer the human voice, discriminate between speakers, and demonstrate a preference for mothers' voices with only limited maternal exposure" (p. 1176).

FETAL BIOLOGY

Progress in prenatal diagnosis brings about the arrival of fetal biology and the advent of even more daring and innovative practices.

Amniocentesis

Amniocentesis (from amnion + *kentesis* [to prick]) is the procedure whereby the amniotic fluid is sampled at sixteen to seventeen weeks gestation to determine the sex of the fetus and reveal genetic defects or other developmental conditions, such as Down syndrome. Twenty-five milliliters (about an ounce) of amniotic fluid is required for amniocentesis, and at sixteen to seventeen weeks gestation, there is enough fluid available. The amniotic fluid contains, among other things, cells from the developing fetus and these are used in diagnosis. Amniocentesis predicts about seventy problems that lead to birth defects. It also helps doctors monitor fetal development in a diabetic mother, enabling

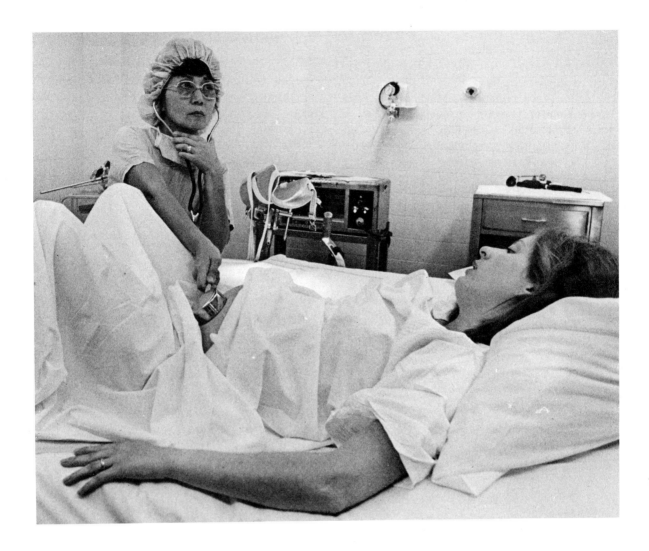

FIGURE 4-14 Fetal biology and fetal surgery are on the frontier of researchers' and medical practitioners' efforts to provide prenatal care to developing fetuses and their mothers. What was once considered impossible is now becoming routine in the treatment and care of the fetus. (From Anderson/BASIC MATERNAL-NEWBORN NURSING, 5th edition, copyright 1989 by Delmar Publishers Inc.)

all involved to determine the best time of birth.

Amniocentesis in late pregnancy can be performed in order to denote fetal lung maturity in the case of a *high-risk pregnancy*—a pregnancy in which the medical and physical history of the parents indicates that the fetus has a great chance of developing physiological or psychological problems after birth—in order to determine the amount of surfactant. This information is useful if a cesarean section or inductment of labor is necessary.

Amniocentesis is the most widely used procedure for the prenatal diagnosis of fetal development. The risk of *spontaneous abortion* as a result of amniocentesis is about one percent.

The use of amniocentesis or "amnio," as it is frequently and often nonchalantly referred to, is viewed by many as an almost routine part of pregnancy procedures. So routine, in fact, that when a woman decides *not* to have amniocentesis, it can cause an outpouring of emotion. In a "Life in the 30s" column in *The New York Times*, Anna Quildlen, thirty-five and pregnant with her third child, wrote that the assumption was that she would have amniocentesis, but, "The reality is I am not. The child is ours for better or for worse." Her decision prompted an unusually large number of letters to the editor, both for and against her decision.

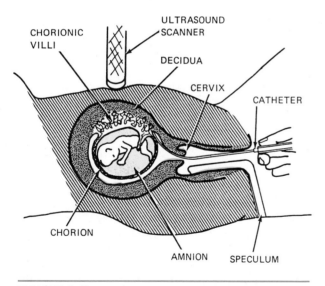

FIGURE 4-15 Chorionic villus sampling is one of the prenatal diagnostic procedures used to help parents and medical personnel make decisions relating to the fetus. (From Anderson/BASIC MATERNAL-NEWBORN NURSING, 5th edition, copyright 1989 by Delmar Publishers Inc.)

Chorionic Villus Sampling (CVS)

In *chorionic villus sampling* (CVS), a fetoscope, guided by ultrasound, is inserted through the cervix and into the uterus where cells are cut (biopsied) from the chorionic villi, the membranous cellular projections that anchor the embryo to the uterus. These villi disappear at about ten weeks. An alternative to amniocentesis, chorionic villus sampling is used to detect chromosomal disorders such as Down syndrome. A primary advantage of this procedure is that it can be performed as early as the eighth week of pregnancy, about eight weeks earlier than amniocentesis, allowing for an earlier, safer abortion if this is the choice of the parents. The risk of spontaneous abortion is about 2 percent. (See Figure 4–15.)

Ultrasound

Ultrasound, also known as *echography* and *sonography,* is essentially the same process and technology used by the Navy to detect submarines. In our case, however, instead of detecting submarines, the obstetrician is assessing fetal development. High-frequency sounds, inaudible to the human ear, are transmitted through the mother's abdomen to the uterus, where they are reflected back by the fetus. Different tissues and organs echo back the ultrasound at different rates. These echoes are converted to electrical impulses and are displayed as the baby's image on a television monitor. (See Figure 4–16.) Echoes are also converted to sound, making it possible to hear the fetus' heartbeat.

Sonography serves many useful purposes, for example, it can:

1. Identify the fetus and confirm pregnancy
2. Monitor fetal growth and determine multiple pregnancies
3. Detect abnormalities—this is particularly valuable in detecting defects in the central nervous system
4. Assist with diagnostic procedures, such as amniocentesis and fetal treatment

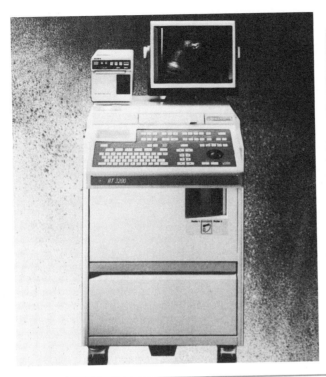
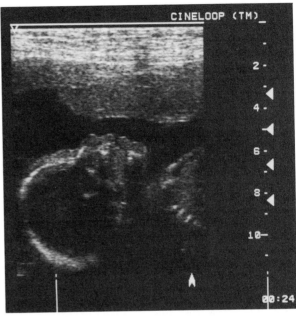

FIGURE 4-16 Ultrasound or sonography is an excellent way for mothers and medical personnel to visualize the fetus. It is an excellent diagnostic tool and is also used to make decisions regarding the status, health, and care of the fetus. (Courtesy of GE Medical Systems)

The National Institutes of Health recommend that "ultrasound examinations performed solely to satisfy the family's desire to know the fetal sex, to view the fetus, to obtain a picture of the fetus should be discouraged. In addition, visualization of the fetus solely for educational or commercial demonstrations without medical benefit to the patient should not be performed" (National Institute of Health, 1984, p. 11).

Fetoscopy

Fetoscopy is a method for directly examining the fetus. The fetoscope used for this procedure is the same one used to aspirate eggs from the ovum. The fetoscope is inserted through the abdomen and into the uterus, enabling the neona-

tologist or other trained practitioner to observe the fetus for abnormalities. Also, with the fetoscope, a small amount of blood is drawn and as well as a sample of fetal skin, which are used to test for genetic diseases.

Alpha-Fetoprotein Test (AFP)

The *alpha-fetoprotein test* (AFP) is conducted by taking samples of the mother's blood to measure levels of alpha-fetoprotein, a substance the fetus excretes into the amniotic fluid, which then enters the mother's bloodstream. Abnormally high levels of the protein indicate possible neural tube defects, such as spina bifida, while abnormally low levels may indicate genetic disorders, such as Down syndrome. This blood protein test is conducted at about sixteen weeks of pregnancy. Results are not conclusive, and suspicious results must be followed up with ultrasound and/or amniocentesis. Critics of this procedure fear it will lead to increased and unnecessary use of amniocentesis.

Percutaneous Umbilical Blood Sampling (PUBS)

Another way of evaluating fetal health is *percutaneous umbilical blood sampling* (PUBS), developed in France in 1983. The procedure involves inserting a fine needle through the mother's abdomen and drawing a sample of fetal blood from a vein in the umbilical cord. This test, which takes about twenty to forty minutes to perform, enables physicians to:

1. Test for many blood disorders, including anemia and sickle-cell anemia
2. Determine possible Rh incompatibility between mother and fetus
3. Perform genetic screening
4. Measure levels of fetal medications
5. Give fetal blood transfusions.

A fetus with Rh positive blood, whose mother has Rh negative blood and Rh positive antibodies, may need blood transfusions to combat the anemia caused by the destruction of its red blood cells.

FETAL MEDICINE

Fetal medicine has come a long way since that day in 1963 when Sir William Liley performed the first successful *intrauterine* blood transfusion for a baby suffering from a severe case of Rh disease. Also, fetal medicine is no longer simply a matter of prenatal diagnosis. With the increasing use of ultrasound, physicians drain blocked bladders, implant tubes to draw off accumulated cephalic fluids, and inject proteins and medicines. Also, open womb procedures, whereby physicians remove the fetus from the uterus, perform fetal surgery (for example,

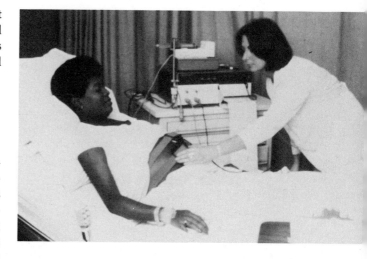

FIGURE 4-17 The use of fetal medicine and surgery enable medical personnel to help fetuses survive and complete their prenatal development. Another consequence of the increased use of technology is that parents are being given more information on which to make decisions regarding the well-being of their fetuses and themselves. (Photo courtesy of Memorial Medical Center of Long Beach, CA)

repairing a hole in the diaphragm between the abdomen and the chest), and return the fetus to the uterus is becoming more common, although not yet commonplace.

FETAL THERAPY— ACCELERATING DEVELOPMENT

Sometimes a pregnant woman may need medical treatment that would adversely affect her unborn baby. Such was the case of Sandra Garcia de Feliciano, who developed cancer during pregnancy and, at seven months, needed radiation treatments. Instead of aborting the fetus or performing a Cesarean section, her doctor, Karlis Adamsons of the University of Puerto Rico School of Medicine, gave her baby treatments of thyroxine, a drug used to treat people with underactive thyroid glands. Thyroxine also speeds prenatal growth in the last trimester of pregnancy. Adamson says that the use of this drug, injected into the womb, accelerates development two or three times. A fetus given a week of thyroxine treatment would develop comparably to a fetus at thirty-four weeks. The one side effect of the treatment is "some" hyperactivity in the children, with no effect on the mothers, because the drug does not cross the placenta (Cornell, 1988).

MEDICAL USE OF FETAL TISSUES

The medical use of fetal tissues has sparked a lively debate about medical technology and the beginnings of life. Increasingly, fetal tissue is being used to treat Parkinson's disease and other nerve disorders. Dr. Ignacio Madrazo, of La Raza Medical Center in Mexico, transplanted brain and adrenal tissue from a thirteen-week-old spontaneously aborted fetus into the brains of two patients suffering from Parkinson's disease. The operation took place within three and one-half hours of the certification of the fetus' death (Madrazo et al., 1988).

Dr. Robert Gale, who treated victims of the Soviet Chernobyl nuclear accident, transplanted fetal liver cells, which generated bone marrow in six of the victims (Lewin, 1987).

Undoubtedly, research will continue to use fetal brain, pancreas and liver tissue to treat Parkinson's disease, Alzheimer's disease, Huntington's chorea, spinal cord injuries, diabetes, leukemia, aplastic anemia, and radiation sickness.

FETUSES' VS WOMEN'S RIGHTS

There is a growing tension between the rights of the unborn fetus and the mother's rights of privacy, bodily integrity, and self-determination. Increasingly, medical personnel and legal experts are securing court orders to override the wishes of women regarding such procedures as caesarean births and treatment of the fetus. Judges are having to decide increasingly complex medical questions and ethical issues that seek to balance the desires of the parents with the risks to the unborn caused by these desires.

Questions regarding how much treatment pregnant women can be forced to undergo for the benefit of their unborn children will become increasingly complex and controversial as treatment procedures become more sophisticated. The halls of justice will be the arena for the battles that will likely ensue regarding the extent to which the rights of the unborn fetus supersede those of the mother.

Fetal rights groups and fetal advocates maintain that the unborn child deserves just as much legal protection as the pregnant woman. They further argue that when a woman endangers her fetus, society must act to protect the fetus. Legal questions are being raised about the appropriateness of prosecuting women for prenatal abuse just as one would if the parent were abusive of a postnatal child.

In a celebrated and much publicized case, Pamela Monson was acquitted of charges related to her allegedly failing to summon medical help when she began to hemorrhage the day her son was born. The prosecutor in the case charged that Mrs. Monson engaged in sexual intercourse against her doctor's orders, took amphetamines, and then began to bleed heavily. Police said she waited six hours before she went to the hospital, endangering the child's life. Mrs. Monson's attorney argued that the statute under which Mrs. Monson was charged was not intended to apply to pregnant women and that the constitutional issue of privacy outweighed the right of the state to act (Chambers, 1987).

What Would You Do?

Mary Hastings is twenty-three years old and has been in labor with her first child for twenty-four hours. Mary comes from a conservative background and while not altogether distrustful of modern medicine, she nonetheless thinks that "less is best," and avoids any medical procedure that she considers intrusive. Mary did not keep her last two appointments for her prenatal checkups because, as she explains it, "I felt fine and I wasn't doing anything I shouldn't, so there wasn't any real need to go."

Mary's doctor advises her that he wants to perform a caesarean section because, he says, "The baby isn't going to come out and it is risky to the baby to wait any longer." Mary still believes she can have a natural delivery and says, "No."

A committee on ethics of The American College of Obstetricians and Gynecologists, in a policy statement, advises that obstetricians refrain from performing procedures unwanted by pregnant women (1987).

Some hospitals, not willing to accept a parent's decision, seek court orders to override the wishes of a pregnant parent, enabling them to perform a caesarean section.

What do you think should happen in Mary's case?

IS THERE A BEST TIME TO BE BORN?

When Julius Caesar cautioned his betrayer, "The fault, dear Brutus, is not in our stars, but in ourselves," was he cautioning Brutus not to justify his actions in the name of astrology or was he missing the point? Does the season of our birth affect our psychic conditions? Apparently so. Winter births produce a significant excess of individuals later diagnosed as schizophrenics. A number of reasons are presented for this seasonal variation: socioeconomic status; the influence of climatic and meterologic conditions on coital and conception rates; maternal dietary deficiencies, which may be more pronounced during winter, increased viral infections during the winter, particularly if the birth takes place in a crowded urban setting; and complications during the neonatal period (Konstantareas, Hauser, Lennox, & Homatidis, 1986). On the other hand, more children with *autism* (a condition of impaired intellectual functioning frequently accompanied by absence of speech) are born in the spring and early summer, with the highest incidence occurring in March (Konstantareas et al., 1986).

PREGNANCY AS A DEVELOPMENTAL PROCESS

Pregnancy is a critical and important experience in the lives of women and men. Expectant parents must face and resolve many psychological issues in order to successfully adapt to parenthood. Four developmental tasks associated with a woman's experience of pregnancy include:

1. Development of an emotional attachment to the fetus
2. Differentiation of self from the fetus
3. Acceptance and resolution of the relationship with her own mother
4. Resolution of dependency issues, for example, with her mother, husband and others (Valentine, 1982)

Interestingly, the developmental tasks for expectant fathers are similar to those of expectant mothers. They are:

1. Acceptance of the pregnancy and attachment to the fetus (father attachment behaviors include buying things for the baby and attending childbirth classes)
2. Evaluation of practical issues, such as financial responsibilities
3. Resolution of dependency issues, for example, with the wife

4. Accepting and resolving relationships with his own father, for example, memories of being fathered and giving up being a son (Valentine, 1982)

During pregnancy, many women and couples want to be involved in decisions relating to child-birth and make their preferences known regarding medicated vs. nonmedicated labor, support person(s) who will be present at delivery, and use of electronic fetal monitoring. There are two kinds of electronic fetal monitoring—external and internal. External monitoring is done with an ultrasound device, about the size of a pack of cigarettes, strapped to the mother's abdomen. With internal monitoring, an electrode is attached to the fetus' scalp and measures the fetal heart rate and strength of the mother's contractions. Routine use of electronic monitoring is controversial for two reasons. First, incorrect interpretations can lead to increases in cesarean births. Second, more attention may be paid to the monitoring process than to the mother's condition and comfort.

LABOR

Labor is the process by which the fetus, placenta, and umbilical cord are discharged from the uterus. It is an intensely personal, frightening, exciting, painful, rewarding, and meaningful experience. For 80 percent of all women, labor begins between the thirty-eighth and forty-second week, with the peak number occurring in week forty. Signs that the body is preparing for labor include:

- Increased vaginal discharge
- The settling of the fetus' head into the pelvis (this is known as *engagement, lightening,* or *dropping*)
- Increases in contractions known as "practice contractions" (also known as Braxton-Hicks contractions, with *false labor* a more intense version of these contractions)
- Increased activity involved in "getting things ready for the baby" and other "nesting" activities
- The softening and thinning of the cervix

There are generally three signs that indicate that labor has begun:

1. Increased bloody-tinged mucus (called a *bloody show*)
2. Rupturing of the sac of amniotic fluid (called "breaking of the waters" and rupturing of the membranes)
3. Regular contractions that, over time, are close, longer, and stronger.

Just as in the discussion of child development we cannot forget the individual child, so, too, in a discussion of pregnancy and labor we cannot overlook the individual woman. Descriptions of the "average" labor signs and experiences help us understand what is involved, but they are always particularized for individual women. The experience of labor for an eighteen-year-old *primigravida* who is giving birth for the first time is different from the experience of a twenty-eight-year-old who has two children. Also, in spite of our attempts to neatly categorize, label, and assign times to certain events such as childbirth, the reality of nature is that most babies will come when they are ready, sometimes with a rapidity that surprises even the mother. The medias carry accounts daily of children being born in taxicabs, shopping centers, and the myriad other places women happen to be when their baby's time comes.

Stages of Labor

First Stage   With the onset of true labor the time has come for the child to be born. The first stage is known as the *beginning of labor* and lasts until the cervix (mouth of the uterus) is thinned out (*effacement*) and dilated to about ten centimeters and wide enough for the fetus' head to pass through. This stage is the longest and lasts anywhere from six to eighteen hours, but can be longer if it is a first birth.

Second Stage   The second stage begins once the cervix is fully dilated to about ten centimeters and

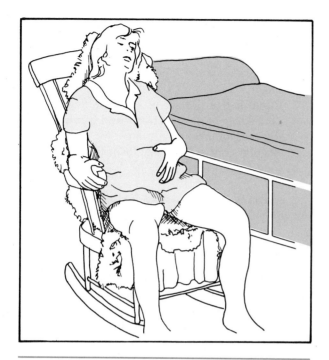

FIGURE 4-18 The experiences of labor and birth are intensely personal, exciting, and rewarding times for parents, families, and the newborn. (From Anderson/ BASIC MATERNAL-NEWBORN NURSING, 5th edition, copyright 1989 by Delmar Publishers Inc.)

ends with the birth of the fetus. This stage lasts about an hour and a half for first-time mothers.

Third Stage Labor is not completed until the placenta or *afterbirth* is discharged. This third stage involves the separation and expulsion of the placenta. This stage lasts anywhere from five minutes to an hour.

Fourth Stage The fourth stage of labor is the first hour of the postnatal period. During this time, the mother's vital signs (blood pressure, pulse, and respiration) are monitored and vaginal bleeding is controlled. Also, mother/infant/father bonding is encouraged and promoted.

BIRTHING PRACTICES

During the nineteenth century, home births were commonplace. However, between 1900 and the 1970s, childbirth was frequently treated as a pathological condition. It was customary to use a combination of drugs (including morphine to induce a "twilight sleep") during the first stage of labor, a general anesthetic during the second stage, and the use of forceps to deliver the baby from the unconscious or semiconscious mother (Eagan, 1985).

But times have changed, and for the better. Many parents are demanding that the medical professions return to them the experience and process of childbirth, enabling them to exercise control over birthing events. This is one reason for the increase in the number of home births and the growth of *midwifery*, the practice of trained and certified persons other than physicians attending at births.

The pendulum of birthing practices has swung back from the impersonal, dehumanizing event it once was to more natural forms of childbirth in more comfortable settings, including birthing centers and the home. Contemporary childbirth procedures place parents, families, and children on the center stage of this important life event and treat it as one of life's rightful and legitimate passages, rather than a medical event. Changes in childbirth practices include:

1. Involvement of parents in pre- and postnatal care decisions
2. The use of birthing rooms in hospitals and maternity centers
3. Home births
4. Participation of fathers, children, and "significant others" in the birthing process
5. Emphasis on infant/mother/father bonding
6. A recognition that all births are not complicated
7. A reexamination of the uses of medication and technology during birth

Generally, the decision about who participates in the birthing process is made by attending per-

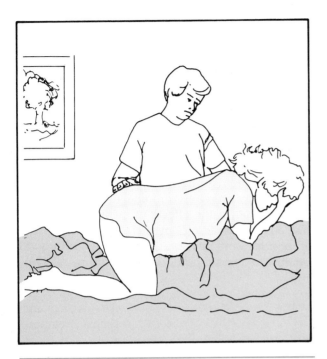

FIGURE 4-19 Today there is much emphasis on preparation for childbirth and spouses, significant others, and families are being involved in the process. (From Anderson/BASIC MATERNAL-NEWBORN NURSING, 5th edition, copyright 1989 by Delmar Publishers Inc.)

sonnel and the family. The presence of children is based on age and maturity. Some hospitals limit children's participation to those ten years of age and older.

Natural Childbirth

In 1933, Grantly Dick-Read published *Natural Childbirth*, which advocates *natural childbirth*. His method stresses preparation for birth in order to eliminate fear, tension, and pain. Emphasis is placed on the physiology of pregnancy, the process of labor, and the ways women can help themselves during the birth process. Read also advocated the use of exercises to help control abdominal breathing during contractions. In his other book, *Childbirth without Fear* (1959), Dick-Read also stressed the importance of a supportive environment throughout labor and delivery.

The Bradley method (1981), designed to help women achieve an unmedicated pregnancy, labor, and delivery, is frequently referred to as partner- or husband-coached childbirth, and uses basically the same procedures as Dick-Read.

An event that had considerable impact on the current childbirth reform movement was the publication by Frederick Leboyer (1975) of his book *Birth without Violence*. The *LeBoyer method* advocates a gentle and humane birth process which includes:

1. Dimming the delivery room lights and talking in soft voices
2. Placing the baby on the mother's stomach immediately following birth with the umbilical cord intact
3. The separation of the umbilical cord only after it has "died"
4. Gentle massaging of the baby
5. Simulation of the baby's prenatal environment by placing her in warm water following birth.

Although research does not support the belief that babies delivered according to the LeBoyer method are "gentler" and developmentally accelerated (Nelson, 1980), the method does involve the father and promotes bonding.

Fernand Lamaze (1970), a French gynecologist, developed a system of "birth without pain." This program, based on behaviorist principles, utilizes exercises and chest breathing to promote a less painful delivery—perhaps one without anesthesia—and to facilitate the mother's assistance in the delivery. The *Lamaze method* stresses techniques for substituting favorable conditioned responses for unfavorable ones and the use of breathing procedures to block pain, a technique known as *psychoprophylaxis*. The American Society for Psychoprophylaxis in Obstetrics (ASPO/Lamaze) is a support group for expectant parents.

Preparation for childbirth should involve a program of parent education that includes nutrition, health, physical and psychological changes, and exercise. Exercise promotes comfort during pregnancy, facilitates the birthing process, and helps to strengthen muscles.

The issue of pain during childbirth is one that is far from settled. First, some women maintain it is unrealistic to promote childbirth as a painless process, just as it would be false to promote an appendectomy as a painless process. Second, pain, the experience of pain, and attitudes toward pain are all subjective, based on attitudes, past experiences, and one's emotional state at a particular time. All people do not have the same reaction to or threshold for pain tolerance. Third, women want to actively participate in the birth of their children and they cannot do this when they are in a "twilight sleep." Fourth is the concern regarding the effects of medication on the neonate.

There are four classifications of drugs used during labor:

1. Drugs used to induce or assist labor
2. Pain relievers (analgesics)
3. Pain eliminators anesthesia
4. Tranquilizers (relaxing agents)

Oxytocin, or *Pitocin*®, is a childbirth drug that has received a great deal of publicity. It was widely used in the 1960s and 1970s to induce labor. The risk involved with this drug is that it can produce powerful uterine contractions and can result in a rupture of the uterus. In 1978, the FDA issued a warning regarding its use in the elective inducement of labor. However, it is useful when used to strengthen contractions during labor.

Almost all drugs given to the mother during labor have some effect on the neonate. Anesthetics used during delivery, for example, affect babies' behaviors in the following ways. Babies of mothers who receive anesthetics do poorer on behavior assessments scales at day one *and* at twenty-eight days than do those babies whose mothers did not receive anesthetics. Babies who performed the poorest of all were born by cesarean section (Muhlen, Pryke, & Wade, 1986). In addition, unmedicated mothers reported their babies to be more

sociable, rewarding, and ready-to-care-for, and they themselves were more responsive to their babies' cries (Murray, Dolby, Nation, & Thomas, 1981).

The implications of childbirth medication for parents and their children are several. First, the ideal use of medication in obstetric practice is to control maternal pain for those mothers who want and need it without affecting the abilities of their babies to adapt to their new world. In this regard, least is probably best. Second, a mother who has had medication during childbirth must recognize that her baby's fussiness or initial unresponsiveness could be due to the effects of medication. Rather than being "turned off" by their baby, they should be positive and encouraging in their efforts to establish a warm, caring, and nurturing relationship.

Water Babies

A Soviet physician, Igor Charkovsky, is a pioneer in underwater or sea births. (See Figure 4–20.) He claims such births are beneficial to the mother by reducing blood loss and reducing pain. He claims subaquatic births ease babies' postnatal stress, and that babies are healthier, stronger, and developmentally advanced. He also reports that four-month-old water babies are capable of swimming several kilometers (Kryukova, 1987). Here is what Charkovsky says about water births:

Since the embryo is surrounded by amniotic fluid, water birth eases postnatal stress. Babies born on land are oppressed by overloads, like space pilots during the first moments after they return to earth. So every minute a baby spends in the water benefits its health. The newborn of a mother who has received special prenatal training can spend five to six hours in the water. This stimulates its blood circulation, cardiovascular system and cerebral metabolism to promote brain activity. It is also possible to cut the umbilical cord as long as two days after birth so that the baby can continue to receive nutritive substances from the placenta. (Kryukova, 1987, p. 22).

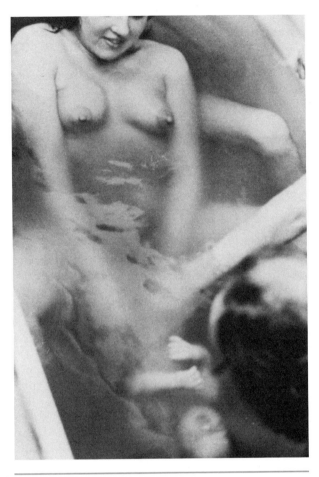

FIGURE 4-20 "Water-babies"—those who experience a water birth—are the objects of a growing amount of attention. (Courtesy of Karil Daniels, Point of View Productions, San Francisco)

Cesarean Births

Of the 3.76 million births in the United States in 1986, 906,000 or 24 percent were born by *cesarean section*, the process of making an incision in the stomach and uterus to deliver the baby (Public Citizen Health Research Group, 1987). (See Figure 4–21.) (Cesarean comes from the Latin *caesus*, "to cut." Tradition has it that Julius Caesar's ancestors and possibly Julius himself were cesarean babies.)

There is a definite paradox associated with cesarean or C-section births. On the one hand, there is a growing public outcry against the routine use of C-sections and their contributions to increasing health costs. This comes at a time when interest in natural childbirth is high and when many parents are searching for ways to simplify the birthing process. The reasons for the increase in C-sections are varied. First, many C-sections are performed as a result of the parents' insistence and are sometimes scheduled for their convenience. Second, the increase in cesarean deliveries is attributed to repeat cesareans by many women who have had a cesarean but who could safely have a vaginal delivery. At one time, the use of a midline incision in a C-section practically precluded a vaginal birth because of the danger that the weakened uterus would rupture during birth. The rule of thumb was, "Once a cesarean, always a cesarean." Today, however, with the use of the "bikini" incision (a low, transverse incision) and changes in obstetric practice, a repeat cesarean is not necessarily the automatic decision it once was. Third, increases in malpractice lawsuits make some doctors more inclined to perform a cesarean section. Fourth, many parents want "perfect" babies and think that a cesarean birth will spare them the rigors of the birth trauma and fifth, sterilization through *tubal ligation* (tying the fallopian tubes) can be performed at the same time.

The U.S. Department of Health and Human Services gives the following reasons for performing a C-section: abnormalities of the mother's birth canal, such as a small pelvis; abnormalities in the position of the fetus, including breech position or large fetal size; and abnormalities in the forces of labor, including infrequent or weak uterine contractions.

The National Institutes of Health (1980) recommend that physicians make a determination as to the need for a cesarean delivery based solely on sound medical judgment and that they should support the patient's right to participate in the decision-making process concerning whether to have a cesarean birth.

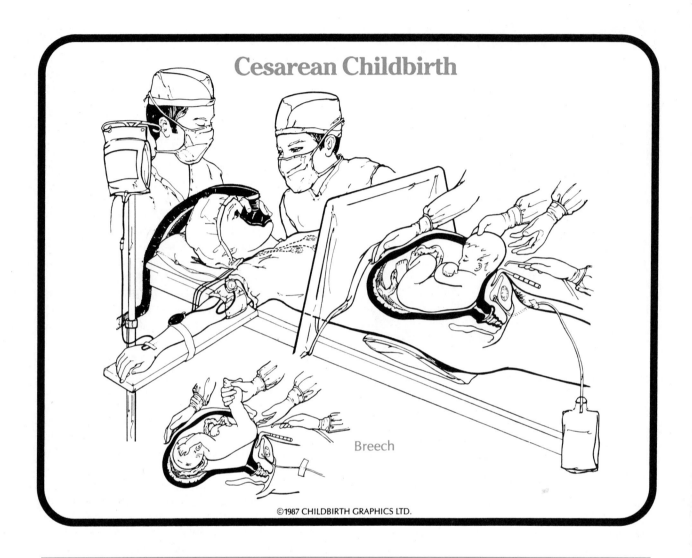

FIGURE 4-21   Cesarean births are the nation's most common kind of surgery. "Wealthy" women are nearly twice as likely as other women to have a Cesarean section. (Illustration courtesy of Childbirth Graphics Ltd., Rochester, New York, © 1987)

Personal Stories

PATRICIA LANIUS—BECOMING A MOTHER

According to Patricia Lanius, "From the moment my pregnancy was confirmed, I started worrying. I worried about such things as:

- Would my baby be all right?
- Would I be a good mother?
- Would my husband Pat be a good father?
- What about those Christmas parties I attended before I knew I was pregnant?
- Would we have enough money?
- Would I stay home or return to work after my baby was born?
- What about changing life-styles?
- Would the infectious diseases I am exposed to as a pharmacist in a large, urban hospital affect my baby?"

"I think we are typical of a large number of modern couples today. Pat was thirty and I was twenty-eight when my pregnancy was confirmed. My mother and father were both twenty-two when I was born. We both have good and well-paying professional jobs. We thought nothing of staying late at work, we ate out a lot, and neither of us knew much about pregnancy, labor, or babies!

"I realized education about parenthood is one of the best ways to alleviate worry and that good prenatal care is essential for a healthy baby, so my first step was to search for a good obstetrician. A general internist I know referred me to a doctor. Fortunately, I liked and respected the doctor he recommended. I felt it was important to have an obstetrician who was "young enough to be progressive, but old enough to be conservative." Also, I wanted one who was willing to take the time to answer my questions without making me feel rushed. Since pregnancy was new to me, I knew I was going to have a lot of questions over nine months!

"The next thing I did was to go to a bookstore and search for books on pregnancy and labor. I wanted books that dealt with what to expect, prenatal development and normal stages of the expectant mother.

"With my obstetrician's approval, I joined an exercise class for expectant mothers at the local hospital. The classes met two days a week, were low-impact, and stressed the importance of proper posture, and sleeping and sitting positions. The program improved my muscle tone and helped with the minor complaints of pregnancy, such as back and leg aches. The class also was great as a support group. *Talking* with other first-time mothers-to-be really helped alleviate many of my worries.

"The childbirth preparation classes that Pat and I attended helped a lot. I chose classes through my obstetrician that were taught by a nurse practitioner. I was able to meet with her before the classes started and she was available at my obstetrician's office to answer my many between-class questions. A tour of the hospital's delivery suites, maternity ward, and nursery was also very helpful.

"As I became more informed and aware of pregnancy, labor, and child care, I relaxed and was able to concentrate on *enjoying* my preparations for parenting, rather than worrying too much about the responsibilities.

"I worked for thirty-nine weeks of gestation and went into labor a week before my due date. Because this was my first child, both my obstetrician and childbirth class instructor stressed that the labor might not move rapidly. I kept in touch with my obstetrician over the phone, so I was able to stay at home where I would be more comfortable. I was relieved that the end of the pregnancy was near, but apprehensive of the actual birth process.

"When my water broke, we were off to the hospital. On admission, I was checked for progress by an obstetric nurse. Although it seemed I had been in labor for a long time, I really hadn't progressed very far. The nurse attached me to a fetal monitor so my baby's heart rate could be measured against the strength of my labor contractions. Pat was with me at all times through labor and delivery. He was a great comfort and help to me. Also, after delivery, he helped me ask all the right questions—'Is our baby all right and does he have all his fingers and toes?'

"After thirty-one hours of labor, a healthy, normal William Andrew, seven pounds, three ounces, and twenty-two inches long, was born. With him in my arms and Pat at my side, we started making phone calls to all our relatives and friends. It was a very emotional time—we were just beginning to realize we were now three. A few days later we all went home to begin our life as a family."

INFLUENCES ON PREGNANCY

Some people, including pregnant women, think their babies' development begins at birth and, until recently, it was not uncommon to assume that the factors that influence development, particularly environmental influences, exercised their influences primarily after birth. With the exception of proper nutrition, there was not much a pregnant woman could do to safeguard the life of her unborn child. Fortunately, today's prospective parents are more informed. We now know that education, good prenatal care, avoiding drugs, and maintaining a healthy body are all important considerations for a healthy pregnancy. However, the problem is still one of education. Not all would-be parents are informed about their roles during the prenatal period.

SURGEON GENERAL'S WARNING: Smoking By Pregnant Women May Result In Fetal Injury, Premature Birth, And Low Birth Weight.

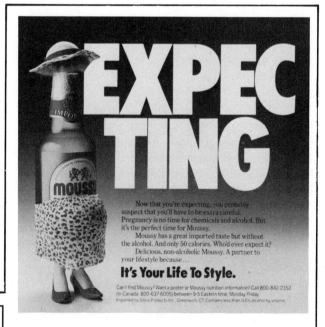

FIGURE 4-22 Today, the public is much more conscious of what constitutes good and bad prenatal health and nutrition. The challenge to everyone is to have all pregnant women follow those guidelines that will benefit them and their fetuses. (Advertisement courtesy of Heidelberg & Associates Advertising Agency)

Unfortunately, some pregnant women don't understand the effects their behaviors have on their developing children. Some think the placenta is a protective barrier designed to keep the child safe and immune to hazards, regardless of their behaviors. Some believe that the fetus, bathed in amniotic fluid, is serenely secure in the womb. For some it is a case of "out of sight, out of mind."

We now know that developing babies are very much affected by what their mothers eat, drink, and do. Many drugs, for example, including recreational and street drugs like cocaine, cross the placenta and affect the baby. The placenta does not form a barrier to cocaine. It enters the fetal bloodstream, addicting the tiny developing child. Cocaine stays in the bloodstream of the fetus longer than it would stay in the bloodstream of an adult, because the fetus' liver lacks the ability to metabolize and excrete it.

Teratogenic Substances

Teratogens are substances that adversely affect the normal growth and development of the fetus. The effects of teratogens are most profound during the critical embryo stage. Many of the effects of teratogens are immediately known. The effects of others may not be known for years. A well-publicized example of the delayed effects of a teratogen is the development of cervical cancer in adolescent females whose mothers took diethylstilbestrol (DES) during pregnancy to combat morning sickness.

On the other hand, there are many agents that may be teratogenic, such as certain pesticides, but for which there is not yet conclusive evidence regarding their influences. The best advice to pregnant women is to avoid, in so far as is possible, those substances that are considered environmental hazards.

Chemicals

As increasing numbers of women enter the work force, some pregnant women will find that their jobs may be hazardous to their health and the health of their babies. Workplace reproductive health hazards are many, and while the effects of some chemicals on reproduction are known, the effects of thousands of others are either not known or little examined. For example, women who work with paint, batteries, typesetting, and stained glass may be exposing their fetuses to the effects of lead, which can cause fetal growth retardation and irregularities. In fact, lead poisoning is a persistent problem in the early childhood years. An estimated 675,000 children between the ages of six months and five years show signs of excessive lead in their system (Annest et al., 1982).

Under a California state law, Proposition 65, citizens must be warned about chemical risks to them, their children, and their unborn children. Workers at a computer chip factory, for example, are cautioned about their being exposed to "chromium, arsenic and lead—known to the State of California to cause cancer and birth defects" (Reinhold, 1988).

Drugs and Pregnancy

Drugs from almost every major pharmacologic classification are capable of crossing the placenta and entering the fetus' circulation (Van Petten, 1976). Pregnant women should take drugs only when absolutely necessary and on the advise of a physician, remember that the use of drugs carries a risk to the developing child, and avoid the use of tobacco and alcohol.

Thalidomide Thalidomide, a drug taken by thousands of women in European countries during the 1960s to counteract the effects of nausea during the early stages of pregnancy, alerted the public and medical professions to the inherent dangers of drugs on prenatal development. Children born to mothers who took thalidomide were born with physical defects, including malformed limbs (for example, a leg missing from the point just above where a knee might have been), with the greatest effects occurring during the critical embryo period. Thalidomide was never approved by the Federal Drug Administration (FDA) for use in the United States. However, it was available in Europe and women on vacation and others living there did take it. The effects of thalidomide on children helped shift the focus of concern away from the comfort of the mother to the physical, mental, and long-term well-being of the unborn fetus.

Accutane—Beauty and the Beast The FDA estimates that in the 1980s, more than 1,000 babies were born with severe birth defects because their mothers took Accutane, a popular anti-acne drug, while they were pregnant (Kolata, 1988). When initially marketed in September, 1982, Accutane was known to cause birth defects, but was nonetheless sold through prescription with a strong warning to female patients regarding its dangers if taken during pregnancy. This is a case where the benefits of the drug—which is the only treatment available for disfiguring acne—are weighed against its harmful consequences. The birth defects caused by Accutane include facial malformations, especially ears that are missing or misplaced below the chin; mental retardation; and heart defects.

A list of commonly used drugs with their possible consequences on in utero development is shown in Table 4–3.

Radiation

To live is to be exposed to radiation from space, the sun, and the earth. Therefore, exposure of the unborn child to some radiation is unavoidable. However, such low doses pose no threat to the developing fetus. What women have to guard against is *excessive* exposure to radiation for themselves and their developing child. The prenatal stage is most sensitive to the effects of radiation between weeks two and nine (Jankowski, 1986). The greatest risk is for women who work in occupations where they are exposed to radiation. The maximum amount of exposure for such workers is set at 5 rems (*roentgen equivalent man*, the radiation dose absorbed by body tissue).

The National Council on Radiation Protection and Measurements (1977) recommends that "during the entire gestation period, the maximum per-

TABLE 4–3

DRUGS AND PREGNANCY	
Drug	Effect
Alcohol	Risk of FAS (Fetal Alcohol Syndrome) increases with average daily maternal alcohol intake.
Amphetamines	Excess of oral clefts in offspring of mothers who took amphetamines in first 56 days from last menstrual period.
Aspirin	Ingestion in late stages of pregnancy is associated with low birth weight, increased incidence of stillbirth and neonatal death, increased length of pregnancy, prolonged labor, increased incidence of antepartum and postpartum bleeding. FDA has issued a strong warning against the use of aspirin during the last trimester of pregnancy.
Caffeine	Excessive intake may influence spontaneous abortion or perinatal mortality.
Nicotine	Increase of early fetal death due to premature delivery, lower birth weight, lower heart rate and breathing.
Diazepam (Valium)	Ingestion in first trimester of pregnancy is associated with frequency of cleft lip with or without cleft palate.

missible dose equivalent to embryo and fetus from occupational exposures of the expectant mother *should* be 0.5 rem" (p. 3). The Nuclear Regulatory Commission (NRC) (1975) recommends that women who are or expect to be pregnant and whose fetus could be exposed to more than 0.5 rem should reduce their exposure, request reassignment, delay having children, or choose to work in their job with full awareness of some small risk to their child. To put all of this in perspective, if a pregnant woman needed an X-ray of her skull for diagnostic purposes, the dose to her fetus would be <0.01 (Jankowski, 1986).

Additionally, pregnant women can do some things to reduce the risks associated with exposure to radiation. They should tell their physician, dentist, or other medical personnel that they are pregnant and discuss any other recent X-ray examinations, make sure protective precautions are taken in the event of an X-ray, and avoid unnecessary X-ray procedures.

Tobacco

Women who smoke give birth to babies with lower birth weight than nonsmokers (Neeson & May, 1986, p. 388). Carbon monoxide from the woman's blood stream crosses the placenta and reduces the amount of oxygen to the fetus, interfering with growth. The best advice to pregnant women who smoke is to stop.

Rh Blood Factor

What is your blood type? There are four major blood types—A, AB, B and O. In addition, almost everyone also has an Rh factor, a protein on the surface of red blood cells. Those that have it are Rh positive, and those that don't, about 10 percent of the population, are Rh negative. If a father is Rh positive and the mother is Rh negative, then there is a fifty-fifty chance that one of the children will have Rh positive blood and therein is the problem. If a woman is Rh negative and her baby is Rh positive, there is the risk that her body will react to the foreign, Rh positive blood cells. The mother's antibodies may attack the baby's blood cells, causing them to break apart. This is called Rh hemolytic disease. The baby could become anemic causing brain damage, or even death.

The first child is usually not affected by the mother's Rh negative blood, because it is only after the mother's and baby's blood have mixed that the mother produces antibodies. Generally during pregnancy, the mother's and baby's blood do not mix. If, however, for some reason the baby's blood enters the mother's bloodstream (this mixing sometimes happens at delivery, during abortions, miscarriages, amniocentesis, chorionic villus sampling, tubal [ectopic] pregnancy, and at delivery), then the mother forms antibodies and her blood is sensitized to the Rh factor. During the second pregnancy, if the baby is also Rh positive, the mother's antibodies attack the baby's blood.

A substance called *Rho immune globulin* (One brand name is RhoGAM [Ortho]) is administered to the mother *before* she has developed antibodies to prevent Rh hemolytic disease. RhoGAM does no good if the mother has developed Rh sensitization. Many physicians give two injections of RhoGAM, one at twenty-eight weeks pregnancy and one within seventy-two hours of delivery.

Rubella

Rubella, or German measles, is a usually mild childhood disease that causes a rash and swollen glands in children. A woman who has not had rubella and contracts it during the first eleven weeks of pregnancy runs an almost 100 percent risk of having her baby contract congenital rubella syndrome (CRS), which causes blindness and heart defects. After the sixteenth week, the risks are almost nonexistent (Miller et al., 1982). A vaccine is available for young girls and women who have not contracted rubella. While there is a negligible risk to the fetus if a pregnant woman is vaccinated against rubella during the first three months, the rubella vaccine is nonetheless a live vaccine and the virus can cross the placenta. The Centers for Disease Control (1987) does not recommend the vaccine for expectant mothers because of the small risk involved. However, at the same time, it sees no reason to interrupt a pregnancy even though a woman was vaccinated within three months of conception.

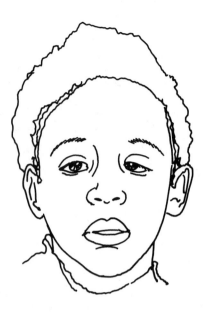

FIGURE 4-23   The effects of FAS (Fetal Alcohol Syndrome) are apparent in all children regardless of heritage. Women who are pregnant should not drink. (Adapted from and used with permission from P.A. McCarthy, "Fetal alcohol syndrome and other alcohol-related birth defects." *Nurse-Practitioner*, January 1983).

TABLE 4–4

RISKS ASSOCIATED WITH MATERNAL ALCOHOL CONSUMPTION	
Two or More Drinks Daily	Risks
Includes: 2 mixed drinks, 1 oz. liquor each 2 glasses of wine, 5 oz. each 2 beers, 12 oz. each	Intrauterine growth retardation Immature motor activity Increased rate of anomalies Decreased muscle tone Poor sucking pressure Increased rate of stillbirths Decreased placental weight
Five or More Drinks on Occasion	Increased risk of structural brain abnormalities
Six or More Drinks Daily	FAS

Note. From P. A. McCarthy, *American Journal of Primary Health Care, 8*, p. 34.

Fetal Alcohol Syndrome (FAS)

Fetal alcohol syndrome consists of four categories of abnormal features. These four categories are:

1. Central nervous system dysfunctions
2. Growth deficiencies, for example, low birth weight
3. Facial abnormalities
4. Mental retardation

Children with FAS are born to mothers who are heavy alcohol users—about six drinks a day.

Table 4–4 shows the effects of various levels of alcohol consumption. The best advice to pregnant women regarding drinking is *"Don't."*

Heroin

Children born to heroin users are small for their gestational age and half are born prematurely. When a pregnant woman uses heroin or cocaine, the drug is carried in her bloodstream and passes directly to the embryo or fetus. The placenta does not form a barrier to these powerful drugs. At birth, the baby suffers central nervous system irritability, respiratory difficulty, insomnia, crying, yawning, and vomiting (Goodfriend, 1956). However, unlike the mother who is psychologically dependent, the baby is not.

Environmental factors are also an issue with pregnant drug users. Quite often the mothers are not providing the best care and nutrition for themselves or their developing children. Consequently, there are other critical interacting and interdependent risk factors impacting prenatal development when pregnant women use drugs. In other words, there are many other environmental and behavioral factors to consider other than drug use.

Caffeine

In 1980, the Food and Drug Administration (FDA) issued a warning that pregnant women should avoid products containing caffeine. There is some evidence connecting heavy coffee consumption and low birth weight (Hogue, 1981). Many drugs (such as some analgesics and cough remedies), sodas, candies, tea, and chocolate contain caffeine.

Maternal Nutrition

Although pregnant women are often advised that they are "eating for two," they should not eat "twice as much." The American College of Obstetricians and Gynecologists recommends that the pregnant woman need only consume about 300 additional calories per day, obtained by eating a variety of wholesome foods.

Maternal Weight Gain It was very common prior to 1970 to restrict the weight gain of pregnant women to twenty pounds or less. In 1983, the recommended weight gain was placed at between twenty-two and twenty-seven pounds (American Academy of Pediatrics and The American College of Obstetricians and Gynecologists, 1983). Low weight gain in pregnancy is associated with a low birth weight. In 1980, one out of five white mothers and one out of four black mothers gained less than twenty-one pounds during the term of their pregnancies. Women at risk for low weight gain

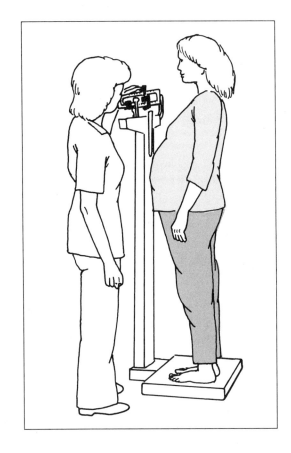

FIGURE 4-24 One of the most positive contributions to prenatal development is good maternal health. Women who want a healthy baby should do all they can to keep themselves healthy. (From Caldwell & Hegner/NURSING ASSISTANT, 5th edition, copyright 1989 by Delmar Publishers Inc.)

during pregnancy include women who have a high weight at the start of pregnancy, smoke, have a low family income, are teenagers or are thirty-five years of age or older, are unmarried, and have less than nine years of schooling (National Center for Health Statistics, 1986), Figure 4–24.

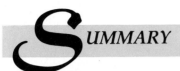

SUMMARY

- Prenatal development consists of three stages: the zygote (conception to two weeks), embryo (three to eight weeks) and fetal (nine weeks to term) stages.
- Pregnancy—the period from conception to birth—is divided into three terms or trimesters.
- During the zygote stage of prenatal development, a rapid period of cell division begins, the blastocyst develops, and implantation occurs. Implantation marks the beginning of pregnancy and represents a critical stage of development.
- Presumptive signs of pregnancy include: a missed menstrual period, excess fatigue, morning sickness, frequent urination, breast tenderness, increased pigmentation of the breast, and quickening. Probable signs of pregnancy include enlargement of the cervix, uterus, and abdomen, and a positive laboratory or over-the-counter pregnancy test result. Positive indicators of pregnancy are fetal movement as detected by a physician, a fetal EKG, a fetal heartbeat, and visualization of the fetus on a sonogram.
- During the embryo period—three to eight weeks—all major organ systems are developed from the three germ layers: the mesoderm, the ectoderm, and the endoderm. This represents the most critical period of prenatal development because any assault on or interruption of the developing organs results in developmental anomalies. Folding begins whereby the embryo is transformed to a "C" shape with distinguishable head and tail.
- The placenta is the fetal life support system and is the sole purveyor of fetal oxygen and nutrition and disposer of fetal wastes. The umbilical cord is the lifeline between the fetus and placenta.
- The amnion contains the amniotic fluid in which the developing fetus grows. The amniotic fluid protects the fetus, helps maintain normal fetal temperature, provides the fetus with room to grow, serves as a source of fetal fluid, and acts as an excretion collection system.
- The fetal period of prenatal development begins with the ninth week when the fetus is recognizable as a human. During this period, the fetus grows and "finishes off" the organ systems differentiated or "laid down" during the embryo period. While the normal development of all the organs is important, respiratory system development is especially critical.
- The fetus has a wide range of sensory abilities. Researchers are beginning to discover the sensory capabilities of the fetus, and along with parents are increasingly interested in the influences these abilities have on pre- and postnatal learning.
- Pregnancy is a critical developmental process for parents, during which they have to resolve many issues relating to themselves, their developing children, and their own parents.
- Physicians use many diagnostic procedures to assess the health, well-being, and developmental status of the fetus. These include amniocentesis, ultrasound, fetoscopy, chorion villus sampling, alpha-fetoprotein testing, and percutaneous umbilical blood sampling.

■ As fetal medicine grows in popularity and sophistication, the rights of the mother and those of her fetus often conflict. Increasingly, legal and ethical issues are raised about whose rights take legal and moral precedence.

■ Labor is the process by which the fetus, placenta, and umbilical cord are expelled from the uterus. Three signs of labor include: a "bloody show," rupturing of the amniotic fluid, and regular contractions. There are four stages to labor; the first is the period from the beginning of contractions to the dilation of the cervix to about ten centimeters; the second stage is the delivery of the baby; the third stage is the delivery of the placenta; and the fourth is the first hour of the postpartum period, during which the mother's condition is monitored and bonding is encouraged.

■ There have been significant changes in childbirth practices over the last two decades. Some of these include giving parents more opportunity to determine how and where their children will be born, and making childbirth less of a medical procedure.

■ Many prospective parents are involved in programs relating to "natural childbirth" as a means of preparing them for a more participatory and less stressful birth experience. Some of the more popular childbirth programs utilize the ideas of Dick-Read, Bradley, Lamaze, and Leboyer.

■ Cesarean births, whereby the baby is delivered through an incision in the mother's abdomen, are increasing. There is not universal agreement that this trend is warranted and necessary.

■ There are many harmful and negative influences on pregnancy. Teratogenic substances—agents that adversely influence prenatal growth and development—should be avoided by the pregnant women. These substances include many chemicals and drugs, tobacco, alcohol, and caffeine. Other factors that can influence the course of prenatal development include diseases, the Rh blood factor, and maternal nutrition.

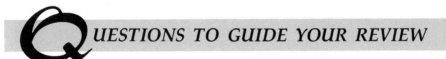

QUESTIONS TO GUIDE YOUR REVIEW

1. What is conception and when does it begin?
2. What are the three stages of prenatal development?
3. What are the different methods for dividing the gestation period?
4. What are the hallmarks of development during the zygote period?
5. What are the presumptive, probable, and positive signs of pregnancy?
6. What are the hallmarks of pregnancy during the embryo stage of development?
7. What body organs develop from the mesoderm, ectoderm and endoderm?
8. What is folding and what does it signify?
9. What are neural tube defects?
10. What are the purposes and functions of the placenta and umbilical cord?
11. What is amniotic fluid and what purposes does it serve?
12. What are the hallmarks of development during the fetal period?
13. What are some indicators that there is prenatal sensory development?
14. How is pregnancy a developmental process for women and men?
15. What are the four stages of labor and what occurs during each?

16. How have birthing practices changed over the past two decades?
17. What is "natural childbirth" and what is its significance?
18. What are teratogenic substances? How do they affect prenatal development?
19. What is Rh hemolytic disease? How does it occur?
20. What is fetal alcohol syndrome?
21. What role does maternal nutrition play in prenatal development?
22. What is amniocentesis and what are its purposes?
23. What are the purposes of ultrasound?
24. What are the differences between CVS and PUBS?
25. What are the major issues in the current controversy regarding mother/fetal rights?

CTIVITIES FOR FURTHER INVOLVEMENT

1. The birth experience is a very powerful one and plays a significant role in the lives of parents and families.
   a. Interview mothers who have just recently given birth. What, for them, are their most memorable and important feelings and impressions about giving birth and the events surrounding it?
   b. What are fathers' experiences of the birth event?
   c. Talk to siblings of newborn children. What are their feelings and impressions about their new brother/sister?
   d. What implications does the information you gathered have for those who work with young children and their families?
   e. Do you think that making the birth experience family-centered is a "good" practice? Why?
2. A great deal is being written about the rights of young children. Indeed, the new frontier of legal rights seems to be the rights of the fetus.
   a. Interview a fetal advocate to determine his or her role and the legal issues involving the fetus.
   b. Do you think that too many rights are being extended to young children? Why? Why not?
   c. Interview two attorneys, one who is a champion of children's rights and one who is a champion of parents' rights. How do their views differ? Which views do you agree most with? Why?
3. Visit a health clinic that specializes in providing care for pregnant women.
   a. What services does the clinic provide?
   b. How do the services provided contribute to good maternal and fetal health?
   c. Why don't all pregnant women who are eligible utilize the services of prenatal clinics?
4. Given the many critical events happening in the lives of prospective parents, and the public need for information and guidance about good prenatal care and practice, pursue the following:

     a. Gather data about the importance of good prenatal care and what constitutes good prenatal care.

     b. Compile a booklet that outlines important guidelines and recommendations.

5. Some people believe that the events of the birth experience influence a child's later emotional growth and development.

     a. Interview pediatricians and obstetricians to determine what they believe.

     b. Why is it that you and others don't remember being born?

6. Review the various procedures for prenatal diagnosis and then visit hospitals specializing in these procedures. Find out how these are performed. Determine any special insights from these people. What new diagnostic procedures are on the horizon?

7. Interview a representative of the National Organization of Women (NOW). What are the issues vis-a-vis fetal rights and women's rights?

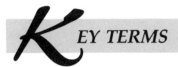

KEY TERMS

Abortion The termination of pregnancy before the viability of the fetus.

Afterbirth Lay term for the placenta and umbilical cord after the birth of the baby.

Alpha-fetoprotein test A procedure for sampling the mother's blood to measure levels of alpha-fetoprotein, a substance the fetus excretes into the amniotic fluid, which then enters the mother's bloodstream.

Amniocentesis The procedure whereby the amniotic fluid is sampled at sixteen to seventeen weeks gestation to determine the sex of the fetus and reveal genetic defects or other developmental conditions, such as Down syndrome.

Amnion A thin, tough, membranous sac containing the amniotic fluid.

Amniotic fluid A clear, light yellow fluid that surrounds the fetus.

Anencephaly The condition in which the fetus is born with a rudimentary brain or no brain at all.

Blastocyst Developmental stage of the fertilized ovum that is a hollow ball of cells.

Breech Refers to the position the fetus presents itself for birth. In this case, the buttocks or shoulders are presented first rather than the head.

Caudal Tail. Development occurs from the head (cephalo) to the caudal.

Cephalo Head. Development occurs from the head to the tail (caudal).

Cesarean section The process of making an incision in the mother's abdomen and uterus for the purpose of delivering a baby.

Chorionic villus sampling (CVS) The process of securing a sample of the chorionic villi, the membranous cellular projections that anchor the embryo to the uterus.

Conception The fusion of the male and female *gametes*, or sex cells.

Critical period A time during which pre- and/or postnatal development is influenced, either positively or negatively, by environmental factors.

Dick-Read method Natural childbirth preparation that centers on eliminating the fear-tension-pain syndrome.

Distal Descriptive of the extremities or outer parts of the body.

Ectoderm Outer layer of germ cells that

give rise to the skin, nails, hair, mouth, eyes, and tooth enamel.

Ectopic Refers to implantation that occurs outside the uterus.

Effacement Thinning out of the cervix during labor.

Embryo The developing child in the third through eighth week of prenatal development.

Embryo stage Weeks three through eight in prenatal development.

Endoderm The inner layer of germ cells that gives rise to internal organs, such as the intestines and glands.

Fetal alcohol syndrome (FAS) Four categories of abnormal features in the fetus caused by excess alcohol consumption during pregnancy.

Fetal stage Prenatal development from the ninth week until birth.

Fetoscopy A method for directly examining the fetus.

Fetus The prenatal child from the ninth week through birth.

Gametes Female and male sex cells.

Gestation The period of time the child is in the uterus.

Human chorionic gonadotrophin (HCG) A hormone that is present following implantation.

Hydrocephaly A condition in which fluid accumulates in the head and that can result in brain damage.

Implantation The process whereby the blastocyst attaches to the uterine wall.

Lamaze method A method of childbirth preparation that emphasizes the use of behaviorist principles and breathing techniques to reduce the pain of childbirth. Also known as psychoprophylaxis.

Lanugo A fine, down-like hair that covers the fetus and keeps the vernix in place.

Leboyer method Birthing technique that eases the newborn's transition to the external world.

Mesoderm The middle layer of germ cells that gives rise to connective tissue, bone, muscle, and blood.

Midwifery The practice of trained and certified persons other than physicians attending at births.

Percutaneous umbilical blood sampling (PUBS) The procedure for drawing a sample of fetal blood from a vein in the umbilical cord.

Placenta The organ that connects the developing child to the mother and provides a system for prenatal nourishment, oxygen, and disposal of carbon dioxide and waste products.

Primigravida A woman giving birth for the first time.

Proximo Characteristic of the process of growth and development from the middle of the body outward toward the extremities.

Quickening The first fetal movement recognized by the mother.

Spina bifida A defect in prenatal development in which the neural tube is left exposed.

Spontaneous abortion An abortion resulting from natural causes. Also known as a miscarriage. An early spontaneous abortion occurs before sixteen weeks gestation. A late abortion is one occurring between sixteen and twenty-four weeks.

Surfactant A substance that enables the lungs to expand, remain open, and not stick together, and permits the easy exchange of oxygen.

Teratogens Substances that adversely affect the normal growth and development of the fetus.

Trimester One of the three periods of pregnancy.

Trophoblast The outer layer of cells of the blastocyst.

Tubal ligation A method of sterilization whereby the fallopian tubes are tied.

Ultrasound Also known as *echography* and *sonography*, is the process of using sound waves to project an image of the fetus.

Umbilical cord The link between the fetus and the placenta; through it passes the blood supply of the fetus. The umbilical cord contains two umbilical arteries and one umbilical vein.

Vernix caseosa A greasy, cheese-like substance that protects the delicate fetal skin from chapping, drying, and hardening as a result of immersion in the amniotic fluid.

Viable Characteristic of a fetus able to survive (with intensive care) outside the uterus. See *Abortion*.

Villi Finger-like projections from the trophoblast that anchor the blastocyst to the uterus.

Zygote The child during the first two weeks of prenatal development.

Zygote stage Also called the *germinal* and *ovum* stage. Includes the first two weeks of prenatal development.

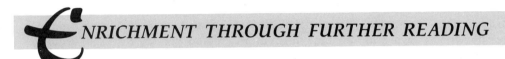

ENRICHMENT THROUGH FURTHER READING

Apple, R. D. (1988). *Mothers and medicine: A social history of infant feeding, 1890–1950.* Madison, WI: University of Wisconsin Press.

> Provides examples of attempts by the food industry and medical establishment to promote baby food rather than breast feeding. Women embraced bottle feeding in part because of their faith in "scientific motherhood." Apple advises women to follow their instincts and not be fooled by advertising.

Colen, B. D. (1987). *Hard choices.* New York: G.P. Putnam.

> Examines the ethical and practical problems caused by advances in neonatology—the care of sick and premature newborns—and genetic engineering, in vitro fertilization, and organ transplants.

Gustaitis, R. and Young, E. (1987). *A time to be born, a time to die: Conflicts and ethics in an intensive care nursery.* Reading, MA: Addison-Wesley.

> A fascinating and interesting look at infants in the intensive care nursery at Stanford University. Also describes the social environment of these units and the attitudes of doctors and nurses.

Kuhse, H., & Singer, P. (1988). *Should the baby live?* New York: Oxford University Press.

> The authors argue that people need to detach themselves from the ideal of the sanctity of human life and seriously consider on practical grounds whether all human life is of equal value. Thought-provoking and challenging reading.

Shelp, E. E. (1986). *Born to die? Deciding the fate of critically ill newborns.* New York: The Free Press.

> Ethicist Shelp argues that parents and their viewpoints and moral convictions must be considered when making decisions about the treatment of newborns.

Sorel, N. C. (1984). *Ever since Eve: Personal reflections on childbirth.* New York: Oxford

University Press.
   A pleasurable and interesting compendium of birthing accounts, experiences, practices, and superstitions.

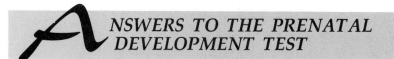

ANSWERS TO THE PRENATAL DEVELOPMENT TEST

1. *False.* Nonstrenuous and "low impact" exercises are beneficial to the mother and developing child. Exercise strengthens muscles, helps condition the body, and promotes a sense of well-being. Many childbirth preparation classes include programs of exercise and breathing. The baby's umbilical cord may wrap around its neck as a result of fetal movement. Physicians and certified birth attendants are trained to deal with such a situation during the birth process.
2. *False.* A missed menstrual period may indicate pregnancy to a woman with regular periods who is trying to become pregnant. A missed period, by itself, is not a positive indicator of pregnancy.
3. *False.* If the child becomes afraid of dogs it will be because she will be taught to be afraid of dogs. Some theorists believe a woman's temperament affects a child prenatally and influences postnatal behavior. Also, a woman's mental state may be the root cause of a *spontaneous abortion.* However, a one-time occurrence, such as depicted in the question, will not influence the child's postnatal behavior.
4. *False.* Cutting down on any bad habit helps. However, the best advice to Nancy would be to stop smoking. Maternal smoking can result in low birth weight, and heavy alcohol consumption can result in fetal alcohol syndrome.
5. *False.* Although many people believe the placenta is a perfect barrier that protects the developing child from all harm, it is not. Many drugs and toxic substances can and do cross the placental barrier between mother and child.
6. *False.* The most critical period of prenatal development is the embryo period (three to eight weeks). It is during this period that the main organ systems are developed.
7. *False.* There is growing concern over the use of diagnostic procedures *specifically* for the reasons indicated. The National Institutes of Health recommend that such uses should be discouraged.
8. *False.* The first child is not affected. The mother develops Rh positive antibodies when her blood and her baby's blood mix. This can happen during the birth process or as a result of a diagnostic procedure or some natural cause. RhoGAM (a brand name) is given to women before they develop Rh antibodies to prevent such formation. The incompatibility of Maria and her husband's blood is not the cause of a hemolytic disease.
9. *False.* Low maternal weight gain is associated with low fetal birth weight. The American Academy of Obstetricians and Gynecologists recommends a weight gain of between twenty-two and twenty-seven pounds.
10. *False.* The birth of the fetus ends the second stage of the four stages of labor. Labor is not complete until the placenta is discharged, the new mother attended to, and bonding has begun.

ANSWER TO "WHAT WOULD YOU DO?"

A committee opinion of The American College of Obstetricians and Gynecologists (1987) provides the following guidelines.

As fetal diagnostic technology and therapy advance, the pregnant woman and obstetrician will be facing an ever increasing number of difficult decisions. Two ethical principles need consideration: 1) autonomy, or the right of the pregnant woman to choose or refuse recommended treatment; and 2) the obligation to promote her well-being as well as that of the fetus.

In addition to respecting the autonomy of the pregnant woman to decide, the committee also reminds its members about "the destructive effects of court orders on the pregnant woman's autonomy and on the physician-patient relationship." The committee goes on to state that to "resort to the courts is almost never justified."

BIBLIOGRAPHY

American Academy of Pediatrics and The American College of Obstetricians and Gynecologists. (1983). *Guidelines for prenatal care.*

The American College of Obstetricians and Gynecologists. (1987, October). Patient choice: Maternal-fetal conflict. *ACOG Committee Opinion*, No. 55. Washington, DC: The American College of Obstetricians and Gynecologists.

Annest, J. L. et al. (1982, May 12). *Blood lead level for persons 6 months to 74 years of age: U.S. 1976–80* (Vital and health statistics). National Center for Health Statistics (Advance Data, No. 79) pp. 1–24.

Bobak, I. M. & Jensen, M. D. (1987). *Essentials of maternity nursing: The nurse and the childbearing family* (2nd ed.). St. Louis: C.V. Mosby.

Bradley, R. (1981). *Husband-coached childbirth* (3rd ed.). New York: Harper & Row.

Centers for Disease Control. (1987). Rubella vaccination during pregnancy. *Morbidity and Mortality Weekly Report, 36*, 460–461.

Chambers, M. (1987, February 27). Case against woman in baby death thrown out. *The New York Times*, p. 5.

Cornell, B. (1988, February 18). Drug speeds development of fetuses in ailing women. *The Miami Herald*, pp. 1, 16A.

Crook, C. (1987). Taste and olfaction. In P. Salipatek & L. Cohen (Eds.). *Handbook of infant perception: Vol 1. From perception to sensation* (pp. 237–264). Orlando: Harcourt Brace Jovanovich.

DeCasper, A. J. & Fifer, W. P. (1980). Of human bonding: Newborns prefer their mothers' voices. *Science, 208*, 1174–1176.

Dick-Read, G. (1959). *Childbirth without fear.* New York: Harper & Row.

Eagan, A. B. (1985, December). Two hundred years of childbirth. *Parents*, p. 188.

Feinbloom, R.I., and The Boston Children's Medical Center. (1979). *Pregnancy, birth and the newborn baby*. New York: Delacorte Press.

Goodfriend, M., Shy, M. A., Klein, M. D. (1956). The effects of maternal narcotic addiction on the newborn. *American Journal of Obstetrics and Gynecology, 71*, 29–36.

Hogue, C. (1981). Coffee consumption in pregnancy. *Lancet, 1*, 554.

Jankowski, C. B. (1986, March). Radiation and pregnancy: Putting the risks in proportion. *American Journal of Nursing, 86*, 260–265.

Kelbanoff, M. A., Koslowe, P. A., Kaslow, R., & Rhoades, G. G. (1985). Epidemiology of vomiting in early pregnancy. *Obstetrics and Gynecology, 66*, 612–616.

Kolata, G. (1984). Studying learning in the womb. *Science, 225*, 302–303.

Kolata, G. (1988, April 22). Anti-acne drug faulted in birth defects. *The New York Times*, p. 1.

Konstantareas, M. M., Hauser, P., Lennox, C., & Homatidis, S. (1986). Season of birth in infantile autism. *Child Psychiatry and Human Development, 17*, 53–65.

Kryukova, N. (1987, June). Child of the sea. *Soviet Life*, pp. 22–25.

Lamaze, F. (1970). *Painless childbirth*. Chicago: Henry Regnery.

LeBoyer, F. (1975). *Birth without violence*. New York: Alfred Knopf.

Lewin, T. (1987, August 16). Medical use of fetal tissue spurs new abortion debate. *The New York Times*, p. 16.

Madrazo, I. et al. (1988). Transplantation of fetal substantia nigra and adrenal medulla to the caudate nucleus in two patients with Parkinson's disease. [Correspondence]. *New England Journal of Medicine, 318*, 51.

Mama, talk to your baby. (1987, November 2). *Newsweek*, p. 75.

McCarthy, P. (1983). *American Journal of Primary Health Care, 8*, 34.

McCarthy, P. A. (January, 1983). Fetal alcohol syndrome and other alcohol-related birth defects. *Nurse-practitioner, 8*, 34. (Inclusive pages 33–34, 37).

Miller, E., Cradock-Watson, J. E., & Pollock, M. (1982). Consequences of confirmed maternal rubella at successive stages of pregnancy. *The Lancet, 2*, 781–784.

Moore, K. L. (1974). *Before we are born*. Philadelphia: Saunders.

Moss, R. C. S. (1986). Frank Lake's maternal-fetal distress syndrome and primal integration workshops—part II. *Pre- and Perinatal Psychology, 1*, 52–53.

Muhlen, L., Pryke, M., & Wade, K. (1986). Effects of type of birth and anaesthetic on neonatal behavioral assessment scale scores. *Australian Psychologist, 21*, 253–270.

Mulinare, J., Cerdero, J., Erickson, D. J., & Berry, R. J. (1988). Periconceptional use of multivitamins and the occurrence of neural tube defects. *JAMA, 260*, 3141–3145.

Murray, A. D., Dolby, R. M., Nation, R. L., & Thomas, D. B. (1981). Effects of epidural anesthesia on newborns and their mothers. *Child Development, 52*, 71–82.

National Center for Health Statistics. (1986, June). *Maternal weight gain and the outcome of pregnancy, United States, 1980* (Vital and Health Statistics, Series 21, No. 44, DHHS Publication No. PHS 86-122.) Washington, DC: Public Health Service.

National Council on Radiation Protection and Measurement. (1977). *Review of NCRP radiation dose limit for embryo and fetus in occupationally exposed women* (NCRP Publication No. 53). Washington, DC: U.S. Government Printing Office.

National Institutes of Health. (1980). *Cesarean childbirth*. National Institutes of Health Consensus Development Conference Summary.

National Institutes of Health. (1984). National Institute of Health Consensus Development Conference Summary. *Diagnostic ultrasound imaging in pregnancy.*

Neeson, J. D., & May, K. A. (1986). *Comprehensive maternity nursing.* Philadelphia: J. B. Lippincott.

Nelson, M. et al. (1980). Randomized clinical trial of the LeBoyer approach to childbirth. *The New England Journal of Medicine, 302,* 655–659.

Post-graduate pharmacist/continuing education drugs and the human fetus, (1981, March). *U.S. Pharmacist, 6,* 44–61.

Public Citizen Health Research Group. (January/February, 1989). C-section rates remain high, but postcesarean vaginal births are rising. *Family planning perspectives, 21,* 36–37.

Reinhold, R. (1988, February 22). New law will warn Californians of chemical risks of modern life. *The New York Times,* pp. 1, 10.

Rosenblith, J. F., & Sims-Knight, J. E. (1985). *In the beginning: development in the first two years.* Monterey, CA: Brooks/Cole.

U.S. Department of Health and Human Services. *Facts About Cesarean Childbirth* N.D.

U.S. Nuclear Regulatory Commission. (1975). *Instruction concerning prenatal radiation exposure* (Regulatory guide 8.13, Rev. 1), pp. 3–4.

Valentine, D. P. (1982). The experience of pregnancy: a developmental process. *Family Relations, 31,* 243–248.

Van Petten, G. (1976). Principles of fetal pharmacology. In J.W. Gooden, J.O. Goden, & G.W. Chance (Eds.), *Perinatal Medicine: The Basic Science Underlying Clinical Practice* (pp. 286–302). Baltimore: Williams & Wilkins.

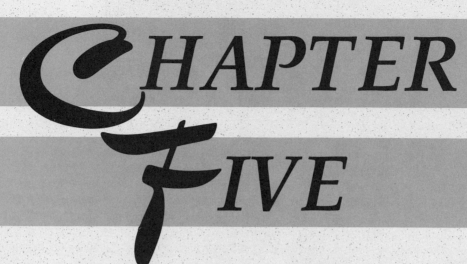

CHAPTER FIVE

The neonate: life's first month

VIGNETTE

INTRODUCTION

FIRST APPEARANCES: WHAT
  DOES THE NEONATE LOOK
  LIKE?

Implications

WHAT'S IN A NAME?

In the Spotlight: High-risk
  Pregnancies—AIDS at Birth

ADJUSTMENTS TO THE NEW
  WORLD

Respiration

Cardiovascular Changes

Hepatic Functions

Gastrointestinal Functions

Kidney Function

Neurological Function

Metabolic Adaptations

Immunologic Adaptations

Behavioral Adaptations

NEONATAL ASSESSMENT

Apgar Scoring System

Brazelton Neonatal Behavioral
  Assessment Scale

Physical Tests and Procedures

In the Spotlight: Circumcision

REFLEXES

Sucking

Tonic Neck Reflex

Moro Reflex

Grasping Reflex (Palmar Grasp)

Plantar Reflex

Walking

Stepping

Crawling

Swimming

Rooting Reflex

Babinski Reflex

Babkin Reflex

Implications

NEONATAL STATES

Implications

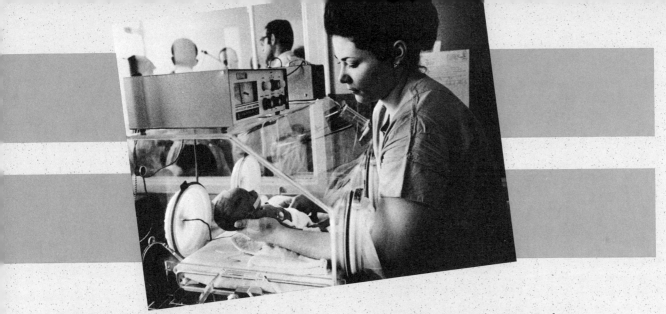

WHAT IS THE NEONATE ABLE
   TO DO?
Vision
Touch and Motion
Kinesthetic Awareness
Imitation
Olfaction
Taste
COGNITIVE DEVELOPMENT
Stages of Cognitive Development
Implications
NEONATAL LEARNING
NEONATES AT RISK
Being Born Too Soon
What is Prematurity?
Life In Neonatal Intensive Care
Personal Story: Meredith Nelson—
   Neonatal Nurse
Parenting the Preemie
In the Spotlight: Is Life at Any
   Cost Worth It?
In the Spotlight: Preventing
   Prematurity
The Developmental Magic of
   Massage
In the Spotlight: Getting in Touch
   with Your Baby
Ecological Influences on Preterm
   Infants

What Would You Do? Infant
   Organ Donations
SOCIAL DEVELOPMENT
Bonding and Attachment
THE INDIVIDUALITY OF
   NEWBORNS
Temperament
PSYCHOSOCIAL DEVELOPMENT
LANGUAGE DEVELOPMENT
CARING FOR THE NEONATE
In the Spotlight: Naming Baby
Breast or Bottle?
SIDS
Responding to Babies' Cries
Soothing Babies
Infant-parent Styles
What to Do with a Colicky Baby
SUMMARY
QUESTIONS TO GUIDE YOUR
   REVIEW
ACTIVITIES FOR FURTHER
   INVOLVEMENT
KEY TERMS
ENRICHMENT THROUGH
   FURTHER READING
ANSWER TO "WHAT WOULD
   YOU DO?"
BIBLIOGRAPHY

ᴜIGNETTE

Anyone looking at three-day-old Hillary Wagner would think she is a normal baby. Hillary weighed seven pounds, two ounces and measured nineteen and one-half inches incumbent length at birth. Her Apgar score was nine at both one and five minutes. If everything else were equal, Hillary could look forward to a life of health and happiness.

But everything else is not equal. Hillary's mother, Kathy, never really considered herself a drug user or anything like those people you see on television being picked up for drug use. Kathy lives in a moderately affluent suburb and enjoys her job as a representative for an import-export firm. Kathy is what is popularly known as a recreational drug user, and it was this flirtation with the forbidden that attracted her to Carlos, her live-in boyfriend. Kathy isn't exactly sure how she contracted AIDS, but her best guess is that it was through her sexual relations with Carlos, who is an intravenous drug user.

Since Kathy has AIDS, a serology blood test was performed on Hillary, and she also tested positive for AIDS. This positive result is not surprising since most antibodies, including HIV, cross the placenta. In effect, when Hillary was tested, it was really a test for her mother.

Because there is no *physical* way to determine if a child is infected with AIDS, Hillary looks normal in every way.

According to Dorothy Thomas, infection control practitioner with Miami Children's Hospital, "Proactive health care for Hillary will include testing her at six to nine months and again at fifteen months to see if her current positive HIV test is indeed positive or a reflection of her mother's positive test. If Hillary's test converts to negative, then there will be no further treatment."

However, as long as Hillary is HIV positive, she will require proactive health care. According to Dorothy, this will include reduced exposure to disease and infection; maintaining Hillary's immune status to keep her as healthy as possible; maintaining Hillary's nutritional status, for example, making sure she gets the iron and protein she needs; and maintaining a home environment conducive to Hillary's growth and development.

Kathy has accepted the fact that since she has AIDS, she will eventually die from it. Her biggest problem now is to try and stay healthy as long as possible so that she can provide for Hillary. "My parents have said that they will take Hillary," says Kathy, "but sometimes I think that the best thing to do is to put her up for adoption. I wish to God that I never had done anything to cause this. As long as it was just me I didn't worry too much, but now I have Hillary to think about too. It's a heavy burden to know that not only have I ruined my life, but maybe my child's life too."

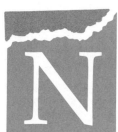

orth Shore Hospital and Medical Center ("When Life Begins," 1986) Wednesday, September 17, 11:47 PM

Labor begins after only thirty-one weeks of pregnancy. Special

team—nurse, doctor, neonatal respiratory therapist—is on alert.

Thursday, September 18, 9:21 AM

Baby is born. Skin: transparent. Hair over body (lanugo). Creases are absent on hands and feet.

Ears lack cartilage. Blood vessels: clearly visible. Posture: stilted and insufficiently flexed. Recoil of elbows and knees: laxed. Color: pink at first, quickly shading to gray. Response to noxious stimuli: slow. Heart rate: fifty beats per minute. Respiration: slow, irregular, three breaths per minute, and grunting. Team is ready.

9:22 AM

Tube is placed in baby's trachea to initiate ventilation—actually artificial breathing.

9:24 AM

Heart rate increases to 110 beats per minute with continued ventilation. Baby's skin temperature closely monitored.

9:28 AM

Baby moved from delivery room to maximum care nursery; placed on mechanical ventilator. Weight is now determined: two pounds, five ounces.

9:29 AM

First blood gas test administered to determine levels of oxygen, carbon dioxide, acid in baby's blood. Possibility of infection assessed. Small blood sample, less than one cubic centimeter, is taken and analyzed.

9:31 AM

Intravenous "drip" is started. Dextrose solution insures hydration for maintenance of blood volume.

9:34 AM

Baby placed in Isolette, a highly sophisticated form of incubator. Temperature and humidity under constant control.

9:35 AM

Baby's heart and respiratory functions now connected to monitors and watched continuously.

9:42 AM

Umbilical catheterization is ordered. Catheters in place; will permit continuous monitoring of baby's oxygen levels, carbon dioxide, acid balance, white cell count, electrolytes.

9:43 AM

Heart rate, pulmonary function, blood pressure, and blood gas continue under constant monitoring. Ventilation carefully controlled; pulmonary function improving. Precautions against infections are implemented. Intravenous dextrose drip maintains blood volume. Baby continues to stabilize. Prognosis is hopeful.

Total time elapsed: twenty-two minutes (pp. 8, 11).

FIRST APPEARANCES: WHAT DOES THE NEONATE LOOK LIKE?

Thanks to the popularity of prepared childbirth classes, many parents are able to get a good look at their newborn baby in the first moments of life. What they see is not what many parents' magazines and television advertisements portray—picture-perfect prodigies—cherubic, cuddly, and charming, attentively anxious to use whatever product they are helping advertise. The nine months of prenatal development in a dark, watery world followed by a hard journey through the birth canal provides parents with a much different looking baby.

Immediately after birth, the neonate may be covered with blood, vernix, amniotic fluid, and may still have *lanugo* (down-like hair) on the back, shoulders, cheeks, and forehead. (See Figure 5–1.) Some parents may be shocked with how their baby's skin looks. It is wrinkled and has the appearance of your hands and fingers after a long swim or a bout with the dinner dishes. The skin is dry in appearance and will remain that way for

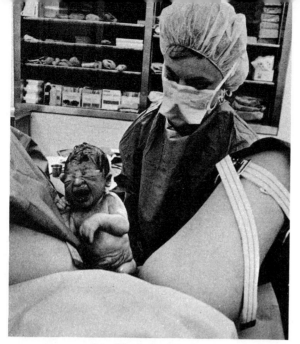

A — The baby is born

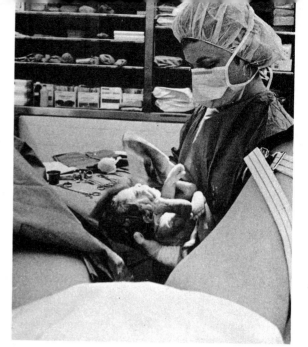

B — He is wiped dry

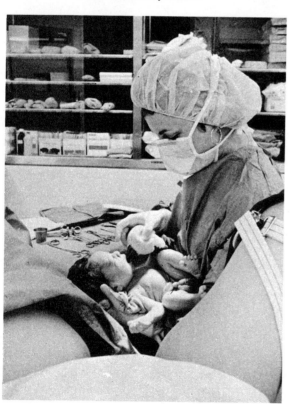

C — Mucus is removed

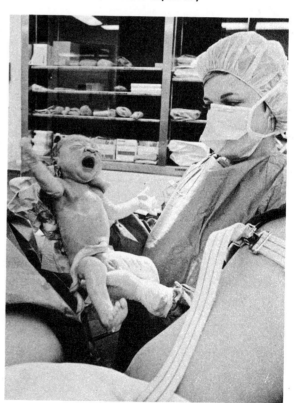

D — Assessment is made

FIGURE 5-1 Newborn babies look very different from the way people think they will. How does this baby look different from the public's view of the newborn? (From Anderson/BASIC MATERNAL-NEWBORN NURSING, copyright 1989 by Delmar Publishers Inc.)

several weeks until the sweat glands begin to function. There may also be red blotches on the forehead and face resulting from ruptured blood vessels caused by the tremendous pressure on the head as it passed through the birth canal. Pimple-like spots called *milia* or milk spots may appear on the nose and cheeks. These indicate blocked sebaceous glands and will disappear in a few days or weeks. (Sometimes parents mistake these for whiteheads and try to squeeze them, but the milia are best left alone.)

Some babies have birthmarks. The most common are the "port wine stains," which are flat, nonelevated, reddish-pink areas just below the skin. The size and shape of these marks are variable, and they do not fade in color, change in shape, or go away. Also fairly common are pale reddish-pink spots found on the eyelids, forehead—"angel's kiss"—and nape of the neck—"stork bite." They are most noticeable when the neonate cries and usually disappear before the second birthday. "Strawberry marks" are raised, rough, dark red areas that mainly appear on the face and head. They may grow before becoming fixed in size and almost always disappear by the end of the primary school years. Dark, bluish areas called "mongolian spots" may be present on the lower back of dark complexioned babies. They occur most frequently in black and Asian babies; they usually disappear in about three to four years. In years past, it was common for parents to think that a birth mark was a sign that they had done something wrong during pregnancy to "mark" their baby.

There may be other marks on the baby as well, caused by the efforts of nurses and physicians to assist in the delivery. For example, there may be some facial bruising caused by the use of forceps; small scalp lacerations may be present due to the attachment of an internal fetal monitor or the collection of capillary blood samples; and a raised red mark may be observable on the body part presented for delivery due to the use of a vacuum extractor.

Babies are born with varying amounts of hair. Some may be almost bald, while others may have a full head of hair. Hair color at birth is not a good predictor of adult hair color as you know from your baby pictures. It is not uncommon for most neonates to lose some of their hair during the first month.

All babies have blue or slate gray eyes at birth, making many brown-eyed parents wonder how such a thing could have happened! And, when babies cry they do so without tears, because it will be several weeks before the tear ducts begin to function. Some babies may have enlarged breasts and may even secrete a tiny amount of milk known as "witches' milk." Also, both boys and girls may have disproportionately large genitals. The swelling of the breasts and the genitalia, the result of prenatal hormones, will gradually subside. Girl babies may have a slight bloody discharge from the vaginal area; this, too, is due to maternal hormones.

Parents are often surprised by their baby's facial appearance. It often is asymmetrical (see Figure 5–2) and has a flattened, "squashed" look with a flattened nose, puffy eyes, and slightly elongated head. This asymmetrical look, called *molding*, occurs because the baby has to traverse through the mother's rather small pelvic opening. To make this passage easier, the baby's skull bones are not fully fused or developed. Instead of being

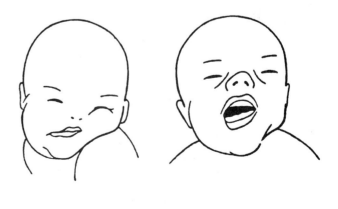

FIGURE 5-2 A baby's face has an asymmetrical appearance.

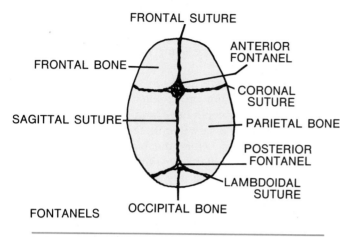

FRONTAL SUTURE

ANTERIOR
FONTANEL

FRONTAL BONE

CORONAL
SUTURE

SAGITTAL SUTURE

PARIETAL BONE

POSTERIOR
FONTANEL

LAMBDOIDAL
SUTURE

FONTANELS   OCCIPITAL BONE

FIGURE 5-3   The head of a newborn baby is flexible so that it can pass through the birth canal. As is shown, children are born with many skull bones, rather than one. These bones are separated by fontanels.

one piece of solid bone, the head consists of several bones connected by cartilage. The bands of connective tissues between small areas are called *sutures* and the larger connecting areas are called *fontanelles*. (See Figure 5–3.) The large fontanelle at the top of the head closes in about eighteen months, and the small fontanelle, located at the back of the head, closes at two months. It is possible to observe the baby's cerebrospinal fluid pulsating through the thin membrane covering the fontanelles. The fontanelles enable the head to "mold" on its passage through the birth canal. Also, the baby's head appears out of proportion to the rest of its body, and it is, comprising about 25 percent of total body size.

At birth, the baby is in a *flexion*, or bent position, resulting from her position in the uterus. (See Figure 5–4.) The baby's chest is rather narrow,

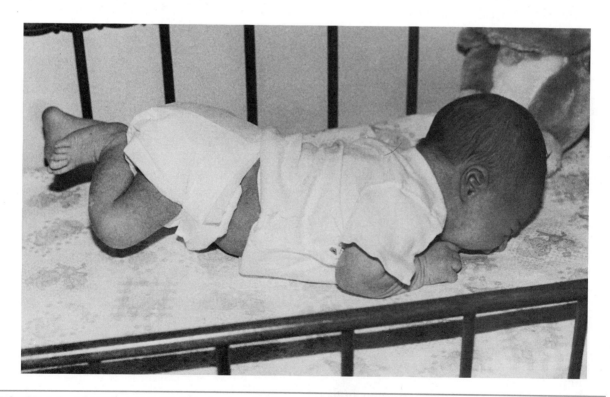

FIGURE 5-4   At birth, a baby is in a bent or flexion position because this is the position she was in during nine months of prenatal development. (From Lesner/PEDIATRIC NURSING, copyright 1983 by Delmar Publishers Inc.)

the abdomen large and protruding, and its short arms and legs are tucked close to the body with the fists tightly clenched.

Implications

A newborn baby has a right to look different from how babies look in advertisements. She has emerged from one world to another where the environments are almost completely different. Parents must be prepared for how their babies will appear and the possibility that they will not be anatomically or neurologically perfect. Your author and his wife were very surprised to find several large red birthmarks on their son's face and legs. Dermatological surgery was performed and now, several years later, the marks are almost impossible to see except in very cold weather. When babies are not perfect, parents need support and counseling to help them know the nature of the problem, how to deal with it, and sources of available help.

WHAT'S IN A NAME?

As you have discovered by now, people who work with young children have names for everything and everything has a name. This is true for the neonatal period as well, so the following terms will help you to be familiar with the terminology of this developmental period.

- *Neonate*—The child in the first month of life. Neonatal comes from the latin *neo* for "new" and *natus* for "born."
- *Neonatal period*—The first twenty-eight days of life.
- *Perinatal*—The period from twenty-nine weeks gestation to twenty-eight days after birth.
- *Postnatal*—The time after birth.
- *Birth age*—The age of the child from the time of delivery from the vaginal opening. In some cultures however, age begins at conception, so the neonate is nine months, or when rounded off, a year old, when she is born!

*I*N THE SPOTLIGHT

HIGH-RISK PREGNANCIES—AIDS AT BIRTH

Acquired immune deficiency syndrome (AIDS) has emerged as one of the leading threats to infants' health. One in sixty-one—almost 2 percent of the babies born in New York City, for example—are born infected with the AIDS antibody (Lambert, 1988). Of the babies that carry the antibody, about 30 percent will develop the disease and many of them will die before age three. Unfortunately, there is frequently a long time lag between initial infection and the appearance of the disease—often up to five years or more. Thanks to new medicines and medical care, many children are able to live longer than they might normally—some until they are eight or nine years old. Mothers who are infected also infect their babies in the womb. In effect, the disease is transmitted maternally from mother to child in utero probably in the twelfth to sixteenth weeks. AIDS is thus a congenital health problem. Many infants infected with AIDS can be identified through facial malformations beginning at five months. They have "box-like" foreheads, noses with predominately flat bridges, small heads and eyes set wide apart (*The New York Times*, 1986).

ADJUSTMENTS TO THE NEW WORLD

After forty weeks of prenatal existence, life in the new world demands many critical, life-saving adjustments. The first month (twenty-eight days) is a particularly critical time for the neonate. Coming from a dark, warm, watery, and protected environment where its needs were constantly met, to another world, which is relatively cold and full of light, sound, and tactile stimulation, requires many important physiological and behavioral adjustments.

Respiration

The ability to breathe is one of the major adjustments the newborn must make to *extrauterine* (outside the womb) life. When you stop and think about it, the ability to breathe places great demands on the neonate. In preparation for breathing, the fetus begins breathing movements during the last month of prenatal development and the lungs are full of amniotic fluid, which helps stretch them and improves their ability to function. Four categories of stimuli contribute to the initiation of respiration in the neonate (Neeson & May, 1986).

1. *Chemical*—A decrease in placental blood flow during labor and the cutting of the umbilical cord lowers oxygen and increases carbon dioxide levels, which in turn stimulate the respiratory center in the brain.
2. *Sensory*—All the visual, auditory, and tactile stimulations associated with birth help initiate respiration.
3. *Thermal*—Cold, caused by the evaporation of amniotic fluid on the skin, is a powerful breathing stimulus.
4. *Mechanical*—Compression of the chest during delivery squeezes about 30 percent of the amniotic fluid from the lungs. As the chest is delivered, chest recoil draws air into the lungs (pp. 987–988).

With the separation of the placenta from the uterus, the neonate is essentially deprived of oxygenated blood and now the lungs must start breathing on their own in order to oxygenate the blood and remove carbon dioxide. About a third of the fluid is expelled at birth and with the first breath, the remaining fluid is drawn back into the lungs where it is quickly absorbed into the system. In normal, healthy babies, the lungs are usually cleared after the first several breaths and at least within the first hour. During delivery, the maternity nurse suctions the nose, mouth, and throat of excess fluid. Normal breathing also usually restores a more pinkish color to the skin and mucous membranes. Respiratory rate for the neonate ranges from thirty to sixty breaths per minute, and during sleep, there are periods of long, regular breathing.

Cardiovascular Changes

As a mother holds, looks at, and admires her baby, several life-and-death events are occurring within the neonate. Three blood-flow detours previously used during fetal life now have to shut down if the baby is to get enough oxygen. Within several hours of birth, the *foramen ovale*, a hole between the two top chambers of the heart, partially closes due to a drop of blood pressure in the right side of the heart and a rise in pressure in the left side. In fetal life, the hole permitted blood to flow in and out of the heart in a simpler, two-step pumping process compared to the four-step postnatal process. The covering over of the foramen ovale by a flap of tissue is similar to the way a door blows shut in the wind. Permanent closure will take several months.

As blood/oxygen levels increase with the first breath, the *ductus arteriosus*, a connection that diverted blood away from the lungs during fetal life, now collapses, permitting maximum blood flow to the lungs. Partial closure occurs within fifteen hours and permanent closure by about the third week. The *ductus venosus*, a blood vessel that diverted blood from the fetal liver, permitting it to get to the heart faster, is closed with the clamping of the umbilical cord.

Sometimes, surgical intervention is necessary to make these critical cardiovascular changes if nature failed to accomplish them. This is the case, for example, with *patent ductus arteriosus,* in which there is a persistent opening in the ductus arteriosus. When serious enough, and when medical management cannot correct the condition, then neonatal surgery is necessary.

Hepatic Functions

At birth, the neonate's liver is immature but still capable of performing many vital functions. However, the neonate has many more red blood cells than it needs because of changes in respiration. The liver breaks down red cells, and one of the products is *bilirubin,* which is eventually excreted. When the liver cannot handle all the breakdown, excess bilirubin results in a yellowish appearance or *physiological jaundice* in the skin and whites of the eyes, a condition that occurs between forty-eight and seventy-two hours after birth. In small amounts, this is normal and occurs in many healthy babies. When jaundice appears during the first twenty-four hours after birth, it is called *pathological jaundice.* It is usually caused by an Rh negative mother who delivers an Rh positive baby. A high concentration of bilirubin, however, can cause brain damage. Customary bilirubin therapy includes placing the neonate, dressed only in a diaper, under ultraviolet light with the eyes covered for protection. The bilirubin on the baby's skin is broken down and excreted.

Gastrointestinal Functions

The neonate's mouth is rather shallow and the tongue is short and wide. These features, together with the strong sucking reflex, ably equip the neonate for the important survival function of feeding. Chubby cheeks are an anatomical feature that invite many comments. They serve two functions. One is to make nursing easier and the other to invite adult attention. This attention is both a survival mechanism and a means of providing interaction. What happens to your cheeks when you suck hard through a straw? They collapse and sucking becomes more difficult. Fat pads on the neonate's cheeks keep them from collapsing and make sucking easier. They are so important that they are usually present even in malnourished children.

The neonate is capable of digesting mother's milk, cow's milk, baby formula, and eliminating waste products. The neonate is able to intake and digest a large quantity of milk in proportion to what an adult is able to consume. An anatomical reason for this is that the stomach readily passes its contents into the intestine. Stomach capacity the first day is about one and one-half to two ounces, but gradually increases to three ounces after three to four days. The stomach empties in anywhere from two to four hours.

The first stool is called *meconium* and is passed in the first twenty-four hours. It is odorless, dark green, and composed of bile, fetal cells, hair, and amniotic fluid. Once feedings begin, the nature of the bowels change, depending on whether the baby is breast or bottle fed. The *transitional stools,* greenish-brown in color, are passed in the first two to three days after feeding begins. After the fourth day, breast-fed babies pass a stool that is golden-yellow, while formula-fed babies have stools that are pale yellow and pasty.

Weight loss of anywhere from 5 to 15 percent in the first four to five days is normal and is the result of urination, limited fluid intake, and a high metabolic rate. With adequate feeding, weight loss stabilizes in one to two weeks, and a weight gain of about one ounce per day is normal, with the average weight gain being about six to eight ounces per week.

Kidney Function

The fetus began urinating in utero during the fourth month. The majority of newborns pass their first urine within twenty-four hours and it is of a dark amber color. As fluid intake increases, the urine becomes clear and light yellow. Frequency of urination can be as high as twenty times a day with normal fluid intake.

Neurological Function

The neonate is capable of a great many physiological and behavioral functions. Nonetheless, the brain is developed to only 25 percent of capacity, and *myelinization*, or production of a sheath around nerve fibers, is incomplete, and will continue to develop over the next two years. This is one of the reasons why sufficient nutrition is so important during this period of critical brain development. The neonate uses her many built-in reflexes for a wide repertoire of behaviors in feeding, survival, and social functions.

Metabolic Adaptations

One of the neonate's most vital metabolic functions is the ability to produce heat and to maintain normal body temperature. Neonates are very prone to heat loss for a number of reasons. First, they have a large surface area in relation to their weight. Second, they don't have a lot of fat to insulate them. And third, they have thin skin and their blood vessels are close to the skin surface. Also, the feeling of cold you feel when you get caught in the rain or step out of a warm shower into a cold bathroom is much the same feeling the neonate experiences when she comes dripping wet into an air-conditioned delivery room. How do you respond when you feel cold? You shiver. However, initially, babies do not shiver and this is one of the reasons they are at risk for losing excess body heat. At birth, the neonate's body temperature is the same or a little higher than the mother's, but because of colder outside air, and because the baby is wet with amniotic fluid, she loses heat rapidly. This is the reason babies are dried, wrapped in warm blankets, and placed in radiant warmers after birth.

The neonate's response to heat loss is primarily two-fold. First is the increased metabolism of *brown fat*, which is only found in infants. Brown fat is stored during the final months of prenatal development. The absence of significant amounts of brown fat in premature babies explains why special efforts must be made to provide for temperature regulation through the use of incubators and radiant heat warmers. The second way babies maintain body temperature is through muscular activity.

All humans have an inborn need to maintain *homeostasis*, a state of balance and equilibrium in our body systems. Your body is unconsciously in a constant state of homeostasis. For example, you shiver to create additional body heat and you perspire to cool down.

The ability of the neonate to maintain stability in her physiological states is a crucial life function. If the neonate cannot maintain or is having difficulty maintaining homeostasis, then help and care are necessary.

Immunologic Adaptations

During the third prenatal trimester, the fetus acquires passive immunity against many bacterial and viral diseases to which its mother developed antibodies. These include diphtheria, poliomyelitis, tetanus, measles, and mumps. The neonate's ability to develop his own immunological system is limited at birth. Breast-fed babies receive additional antibodies from *colostrum*, a substance secreted from the breasts prior to the production of milk.

Behavioral Adaptations

The neonate progresses through three stages or *periods of reactivity* immediately following birth. These wake and sleep states are as follows:

- *Period of Reactivity*—In the first fifteen to thirty minutes following birth, the neonate is alert with periods of vigorous activity. The eyes are open and a strong sucking reflex is present. This period is often used as a time for parent and baby to become acquainted, for bonding to begin, and for initial attempts at breast-feeding.
- *Period of Inactivity*—This quiet phase, characterized by sleep, lasts about two to four hours.
- *Period of Reactivity*—This period last about four

to six hours and is a period characterized by variability in behavioral responses. Bowel sounds increase, meconium may be passed, and the neonate shows increased interest in feeding.

At the end of the first eight hours, the neonate has achieved a state of equilibrium with the successful transition from intrauterine to external environment. The neonate begins to establish its own behavioral cycles based on its behavioral nature and the nature and demands of its environment.

Vital statistics for the *average* neonate are shown in Table 5–1.

TABLE 5–1

AVERAGE NEONATAL VITAL STATISTICS (AT BIRTH)

Height (length)
    Males . . . . .19.9 inches
    Females . . . . .19.6 inches

Weight
    Males . . . . .7.21 pounds
    Females . . . . .7.12 pounds

Temperature . . . . .97.5–99 degrees F
Heart rate (Pulse) . . . . . . .120–160 beats per minute
Head circumference . . . . . .14 inches
Eye color . . . . .Blue or slate gray

NEONATAL ASSESSMENT
Apgar Scoring System

Virginia Apgar, an anesthesiologist, developed her *Apgar scoring system* in 1952 as a means of assessing the neonate's physical condition immediately following birth. The neonate is rated at one minute and five minutes after birth and receives a score of zero to ten. The rating is based on five categories—heart rate, respiratory effort, muscle tone, reflex irritability, and skin color. Table 5–2 shows the Apgar scoring system. The total score is arrived at by totalling the number of points available in each of the five categories. A score of nine or ten is excellent and indicates a healthy newborn. A score of seven or below is cause for concern. The Apgar score provides a gross measure of the neonate's chances of survival.

In addition, neonates' Apgar scores are related to mental and motor scores at eight months as measured by the Bayley Infant Mental and Motor Scales, designed to provide a developmental assessment of psychomotor functions in young children. Neonates with Apgar scores of zero to three have significantly lower eight-month mental and motor scores than neonates with Apgar scores of seven to ten (Serunian & Broman, 1975).

TABLE 5–2

THE APGAR SCORING SYSTEM			
	0	1	2
Heart rate	Absent	Slow (below 100 beats/minute)	Over 100 beats/minute
Respiratory effort	Absent	Slow or irregular	Good crying
Muscle tone	Limp	Some flexion of extremities	Active motion
Response to catheter in anterior nostril (tested after oropharynx is clear)	No response	Grimace	Cough or sneeze
Color	Blue or pale	Body pink, extremities blue	Completely pink

Note. From "The Newborn (Apgar) Scoring System, Reflections and Advice" by V. Apgar, 1966, *Pediatric Clinic of North America, 13*, p. 645.

Brazelton Neonatal Behavioral Assessment Scale

T. Berry Brazelton (1973), a pediatrician, developed an assessment tool to assist in the development of the neonate's behavioral characteristics. The *Brazelton Neonatal Behavioral Assessment Scale* is composed of twenty-seven behavioral items and twenty measures of reflexes that assess the neonate's capabilities. The assessment, which evaluates the neonate's interactions with the examiner and environmental stimuli, is usually done on the third day after delivery and takes about thirty minutes to complete. Brazelton is one of those responsible for educating professionals and the public to the wonderful range of neonatal behaviors and the neonate's role in learning and behavioral adjustments.

The behavioral items of the Brazelton scale are assessed under the following six areas:

1. *Habituation*—the ability of the neonate to diminish a response to repeated stimuli. Habituation is frequently used as an indicator of neonatal learning.
2. *Orientation*—the ability to attend to visual and auditory stimuli.
3. *Motor maturity*—the ability to control and coordinate motor activities.
4. *Self-quieting ability*—the ability of the neonate to use her own resources to quiet and comfort herself.
5. *Social behaviors*—neonates' needs for and responses to cuddling and their frequency of smiling.
6. *Sleep/awake states*—how long the neonate remains in a particular state and how frequently he moves from one to another.

Behavioral assessments of neonates are important for a number of reasons. First, they provide an assessment of a neonate's capabilities, which in turn provides insight into future cognitive and personality development. Second, the results of assessments are important to parents in that they can learn about their individual children's temperaments and how to respond to them. For example, by understanding their children's characteristics and basic personalities/temperaments, parents can respond more appropriately to them as individuals.

Physical Tests and Procedures

Eyes Most states have laws requiring that newborn children's eyes must be treated with an antibiotic ophthalmic ointment or a 1 percent ophthalmic solution of silver nitrate following birth in order to prevent gonococcal infection (the bacterium that causes gonorrhea). Both the ointment and the solution are irritating to the neonate's eyes, and therefore their administration is delayed for several hours in order to allow parents and child unimpaired eye contact.

Vitamin K Injection A prophylactic dose of vitamin K is given to the neonate to prevent hemorrhage, which is a possibility due to the low *prothrombin* level in the first days of life. The potential for hemorrhage is the result of bacteria in the intestines that influence the production of vitamin K, which is necessary for the production of prothrombin.

Phenylketonuria (PKU) About one in 1500 infants are born with an inborn error in metabolism resulting in *phenylketonuria*, the inability to convert the amino acid phenylalanine found in breast milk and most formulas. When untreated, the neonate fails to thrive, followed by central nervous system and mental retardation. The test for phenylketonuria is usually performed twenty-four hours after the initiation of milk feeding, using a blood sample secured from the baby's heel. This "heel stick" procedure is the source of blood for a number of standard diagnostic tests, such as phenylketonuria (PKU) and blood sugar levels of babies whose mothers are diabetic.

*I*N THE SPOTLIGHT

CIRCUMCISION

Not too many years ago, when parents were anticipating the birth of their baby, the major decision they had to make was two names—one for her and one for him. Not any more. Now when parents have a boy, they face a decision about *circumcision* (from the Latin *circumcidere* meaning "to cut around"), the surgical removal of the foreskin (prepuce) from the penis. For most parents during this century, the circumcision of their infant sons was an accepted surgical procedure. In 1970, over 90 percent of boys were circumcised. In 1986, the number had dropped to about 60 percent. What previously was unquestionably accepted is now being challenged as an unnecessary surgical procedure. In fact, in 1975, the American Academy of Pediatrics concluded that there is no absolute medical indication for the routine circumcision of newborns. Some health insurance groups in some states do not pay for circumcision, maintaining that it is medically unnecessary. Critics of routine circumcision charge that it has grown from a religious and cultural practice to a million-dollar industry; that its alleged hygienic benefits are unsupported; its supposed deterrence to masturbation is unsupported; like any surgical procedure it constitutes a risk; and it is akin to child battery and child abuse (no anesthesia is used during the procedure). Interestingly, until recently it was common to think that newborns do not experience pain, even during such surgical procedures as circumcision! This false belief helped contribute to the rather widespread opinion that neonates are poorly developed and capable of very little.

REFLEXES

The neonate is born with an amazing array of innate, unconditioned, involuntary responses called *reflexes*, which constitute the purest form of reaction to external stimuli. Some of these will disappear entirely during the course of development, while others form the basis for coordinated, voluntary movement.

Sucking

The sucking reflex occurs when an object such as a nipple or finger is placed in the neonate's mouth. This reflex has high survival value and changes to voluntary sucking during the second month. A major developmental problem with premature neonates is their inability to suck because of the immaturity of their nervous systems. The feeding reflex, which consists of sucking and swallowing, is developed by thirty-two weeks gestation. When the premature baby does not have a coordinated suck-and-swallow reflex, he is fed through *gavage feeding*, whereby a tube is inserted via the nose or mouth into the stomach and a syringe is used to insert formula through the tube. Drooling is characteristic of very young children because of their immature ability to coordinate the swallowing reflex. This control will gradually develop over the first three months.

Some parents interpret sucking as a sign of hunger even following a feeding. The neonate's need to suck is usually satisfied with a pacifier or soother, a nonnutritive sucking device that will quiet the baby if she is not hungry, but will not pacify her if she is hungry. A pacifier is an effective

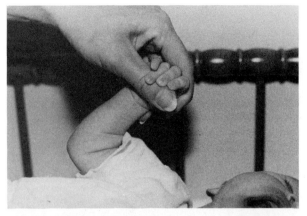

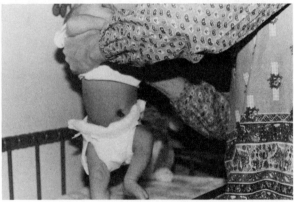

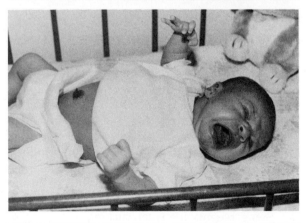

FIGURE 5-5   At birth a baby is capable of many reflexive actions. These reflexive actions (Top: grasping; middle: stepping; bottom: Moro); are used to help diagnose the baby's physiological and neurological status. Reflexive actions also play a role in early intellectual development. (From Lesner/PEDIATRIC NURSING, copyright 1983 by Delmar Publishers Inc.)

way of soothing a baby and has the added benefit of being a self-soothing activity the neonate can perform herself.

The involuntary sucking reflex, although a much-written-about characteristic of infancy, disappears by the end of the first year. However, the continuation of voluntary sucking primarily as a soothing mechanism is observed in people of all ages in many forms, from thumb sucking to pipe smoking to pencil chewing.

Tonic Neck Reflex

When the neonate is lying in the *supine* (face upward) position, she will turn her head to one side and extend the arm and leg on the same side in a "fencing" position, while on the opposite side the arm and leg flex. When in this position, the neonate has an asymmetrical look. The tonic neck reflex helps bring eye and hand into coordination, may be an early sign of handedness (depending to which side she turns), and plays a role in early learning when the baby reaches out to objects. This reflex disappears around the third or fourth month.

Moro Reflex

The Moro reflex, named after the German physician who described it, is also known as the startle reflex. It occurs when the neonate is startled by a loud noise, bright light, or the feeling of a sudden loss of support. The neonate's response is to fling out her arms, open her hands, and bring the arms to an embrace-like position. This reflex is also survival-oriented, helping the neonate and infant grasp the caregiver for protection. The startle reflex disappears at about four months and is replaced by a general startle pattern displayed by anyone who jumps in response to a loud, sudden noise.

Grasping Reflex (Palmar Grasp)

When an alert neonate's palm is stimulated with an object, the fingers curl around and grasp it. The grasp actually strengthens as it is pulled against so that it is often possible to lift the baby so his weight is self-supported, while both hands are grasping the parent's or care-giver's fingers. This powerful reflex is also used to grasp a blanket, bottle, or breast. As most parents can attest, it is difficult, in a gentle way, to take something from a baby who has a firm grasp on it. The grasping reflex is developed as early as the twelfth prenatal week and persists until the fourth to sixth postnatal months. Until the grasping reflex diminishes, the infant will not be able to exercise voluntary control over the opening and closing of her hand.

Plantar Reflex

The grasping reflex is also evident in the toes and is called the plantar grasp. When the balls of the feet are stimulated, the toes will wrap around an object such as a pencil. This reflex disappears around the ninth month, thereby permitting voluntary control over the feet, which is necessary for walking.

Walking

The average age for independent walking is twelve months. However, neonates are born with a walking reflex. When held under the arms, with the feet slightly touching a flat surface, the neonate makes walking motions that give the appearance of walking. This reflex usually disappears in the fifth month.

Stepping

In addition to the walking motion, the neonate also steps. When held under her arms, with her shins and toes against the edge of a surface such as a step, the neonate lifts her foot up, as though placing her foot on the top of the step. This reflex usually lasts about four to eight weeks.

Crawling

When supported on all fours, the neonate makes a crawling motion.

Swimming

The neonate is born with a rather well-coordinated swimming movement. When supported face-down in water, he will attempt to "swim" using the dog paddle. This reflex is usually operative until about five months of age.

Rooting Reflex

The rooting reflex is elicited when the neonate's cheek is touched. In response, the head turns to the touched side, the mouth opens, and the lips move in a sucking motion. This rooting reflex, which disappears in about two to three months, is another example of the survival value of reflexive actions.

Babinski Reflex

When the neonate's foot is stroked from the heel up across the ball, the toes spread out or "fan," and the foot turns or twists. The reflex lasts until about nine to twelve months of age and after this, the same stimulus results in the curling down of the toes.

Babkin Reflex

When the neonate's palms are pressed, she closes her palms, opens her mouth, and turns her head from the side back to the midline.

The neonate is capable of other reflexive responses in addition to those previously outlined. She also blinks, yawns, coughs, sneezes, and draws away from pain. The Brazelton (BNBAS) assesses twenty different reflexes.

Implications

The significance and importance of neonatal reflexive behaviors lies in their survival, protective, and adaptive value within a nurturing and caring environment. The human infant is born designed to survive with care. Blinking to keep light or foreign objects out of the eyes and automatically sucking objects placed in the mouth (the Brazelton assessor places a clean finger in the mouth to determine neurological integration) assures a better opportunity to get nourishment. The neonate and infant adapt certain reflexive actions, especially the sucking reflex, to reflect individual experiences. Infants, for example, differentiate between nutritive and nonnutritive sucking. They also adjust their crying patterns; modify grasp gestures; and adapt to the nature and habits of their child-rearing environments.

The role of reflexes in psychic development, especially those associated with the oral cavity, cannot be overlooked. When the neonate sucks its finger, for example, the mouth and finger may constitute the beginnings of an ego nucleus (Spitz, 1965). In addition, Freud believed that how parents meet children's needs, for example, feeding and weaning, helps shape their personalities.

NEONATAL STATES

If you have ever had the opportunity to observe neonates for a period of time, you have undoubtedly noticed that they behave differently at different times. The particular *state* or behavior of an infant determines how responsive they are— or are not—to a particular stimulus, such as the attention of a care-giver. Likewise, the responses and attention of care-givers are modified by the particular state of a baby. Thus, the states of neonates are important, for they contribute to physical, cognitive, social and emotional development. Peter Wolff (1973) has identified these seven states:

1. *Regular Sleep*—The infant is at full rest, with eyelids closed, facial muscles relaxed, and respiration regular and even.
2. *Irregular Sleep*—Periods of general inactivity vary randomly with periods of stirring and writhing. Grimaces are frequent and include smiling, sneering, frowning, puckering, pouting, precry and cry faces. Rapid eye movements (REM) are detected through the eyelids. Mouth movements including chewing and licking are common. Respiration is irregular and breathing is variable.

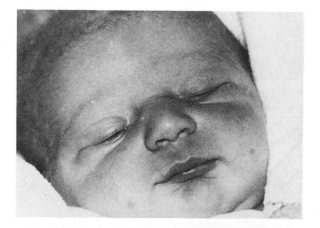
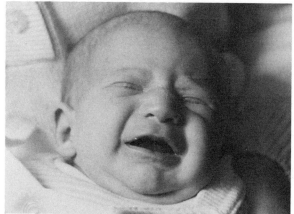
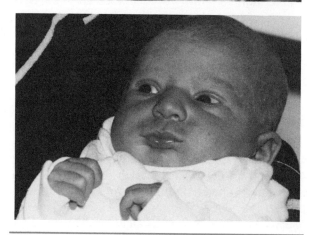

FIGURE 5-6 Neonates assume various states of sleeping, crying and wakefulness. Individual temperament helps determine the nature and extent of these states. (Photos by Kenneth Deitcher, MD)

3. *Periodic Sleep*—Intermediate between regular and irregular sleep, the infant is never completely immobile. Respiratory movements are "periodic," with bursts of rapid, shallow breathing alternating with bursts of deep, slow respiration.

4. *Drowsiness*—The infant is less active than in irregular or periodic sleep, but more active than in regular sleep. Spurts of writhing activity are frequent while the infant is waking up, but rare when she is falling asleep. The eyes open and close intermittently and have a dull, glazed appearance; are not focused; and the eyelids appear to be "heavy."

5. *Alert Inactivity*—The eyes are open and have a bright, shiny appearance and they move together in the horizontal and vertical positions. The infant is relatively inactive and the face is relaxed and does not grimace or smile.

6. *Waking Activity*—There are spurts of diffuse motor activity involving the limbs, trunk, and head. The neonate may make sounds, but does not cry for sustained periods of time. Breathing is irregular and the skin is flushed.

7. *Crying*—The neonate cries with the sound typical of the newborn period. There is vigorous, diffuse motor activity, the face is contracted into a cry grimace and flushed. The eyes are partially opened or tightly closed. During vigorous crying only one in five babies will cry with tears in the first five days.

Implications

Although neonates have identifiable and predictable states as described above, each individual neonate differs from other neonates in her particular state. While it is good to know about the states of babies, it is also important for the parent or care-giver to be attuned to their child's particular states and their ways of responding to the world. Also, the neonate's ability to respond to the world is influenced by the particular state he is in. Caregivers have to learn to "read" these states and act accordingly, making sure they schedule special attention to the baby when he is most attentive, such as during waking activity. Also, the baby who spends much of her time crying or one who tends to sleep a lot will need special attention—the one soothed more often and the other stimulated (but not overstimulated)—more often.

WHAT IS THE NEONATE ABLE TO DO?

Neonates come into the world with a wonderful range of abilities and are ready, willing, and able to learn from and about their environments. Unfortunately over past decades, parents, child development specialists, and researchers have systematically overlooked and ignored, seriously underestimated, and largely understudied the rich repertoire of neonatal abilities. But times have changed. Neonates are now in the spotlights of public interest and research popularity. The neonatal period is now recognized as an extremely important time in the course of human development, and neonates are viewed as competent, social, active and self-regulating individuals. Here is how Lewis Lipsitt (1986), a leading infant researcher, describes the neonate's ability to seek and obtain nourishment in the first hour of life:

> The seeking and obtaining of nourishment, even in the first hour of life, is a most intricate pattern of behavior, a model of complex chains of response and response-induced stimulation in which each elemental response may serve also as a stimulus for the next reaction component. Feeding behavior involves sequencing and coordination of all of the following for the successful passage of the fluid from the nourishing person to the "nourrisson": rooting, mouth opening, grasping of the nipple with the lips, closing of the jaws to touch the buccal cavity, placing of pressure seal around the nipple, dropping of the lower jaw to create suction, tasting of the delivered fluid, determination of whether the taste is "good enough," passing of the fluid to the back of the tongue, followed finally by a series of glottal and swallowing maneuvers (p. 173).

Part of the reason for the discovery of neonatal capabilities lies with public and professionals in all areas of early childhood and child development. Also, the use of modern technology including computers, video cameras, video recorders, and electronic equipment for recording infants' responses, such as heart rate, respiration rate, sucking responses, etc., and the use of mainframe and desktop computers, make it easier to gather and analyze data.

Vision

Eyes, as every lover knows, are wonderful to look at. Parents as lovers of their children are no different. For many of them, it is literally love at first sight. Babies' eyes hold great fascination for mothers and they intuitively attempt to make eye contact with them. This fascination with the eyes plays an extremely important role in bonding, and parents also use their babies' eyes as one measure of their health and responsiveness.

Neonates' eyes are anatomically the same as those of adults, but are about half the size and weight. When neonates emerge from nine months of total darkness to a bright world, they have a strong eyelid closure reflex to keep their eyes covered.

Visual Acuity   As a new mother gazes so fondly and attentively into her baby's eyes, she might assume her baby sees nothing; another mother might think her daughter sees what she sees; while still another might not be sure what her son sees. One thing is for certain, newborn babies can see more than many people think they can see. But how and what they see—in the first year of life, at least—is not how and what you or their mothers see. First, babies' *visual acuity*, the ability to clearly see near and far objects, is not the same as yours. Normal visual acuity is 20/20, the ability to see clearly at twenty feet letters on the Snellen E Chart, the chart to check your vision in the doctor's office. When someone has vision of 20/150, that means she is able to see clearly at twenty feet what a person with 20/20 vision can see clearly at 150 feet. Neonates' visual acuity ranges anywhere from 20/150 to 20/800.

A person who is legally blind has a visual acuity of 20/800. The visual acuity of the young child improves rapidly, however, and by four months it is 20/200, at one year 20/50, and at eighteen months 20/20.

Focal Length   The focal distance of neonates, that distance at which they can focus clearly on an object, is fixed at birth at about seven and one-half to eight inches, so they do not see much detail in their environment unless it is close to them. This is why it is important for mothers and other care-givers to bring themselves and the world to their babies. Parents almost instinctively hold their faces close to their babies' faces when they talk to and nurse them.

Depth Perception   Neonates move their eyes together at one time. However, both eyes do not focus or fixate on the same point, meaning that they do not have binocular vision and won't have it until about eight weeks of age. This lack of coordinated fixation accounts for why neonates tend to have a somewhat cross-eyed appearance. Although babies have binocular vision, they do not have *stereopsis*, or the ability to perceive the relative distance of objects. This ability is developed at about three and one-half months (Haith, 1986).

Form Perception   The ability of neonates to perceive form is innate. And, what is more, they prefer their forms complex. Babies show a decided preference for complex patterns over plain. (See Figure 5–7.) What is perhaps even more significant for parents and care-givers is that from the moment of birth babies, prefer the form, shape, and complexity of the human face more than anything else (Fantz, 1961). (See Figure 5–8.) The implication of this for parents and care-givers is quite clear. *They are the toy their babies prefer*, and they should make sure that during all the routines such as feeding and diapering, and during all the nonroutine activities, such as playing, that babies get an opportunity to see their faces. So, when you offer a baby a choice of things to look at, make sure

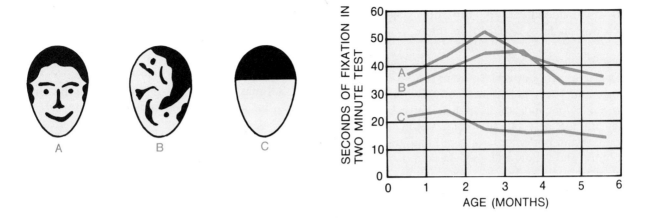

FIGURE 5-7   Babies show a decided preference for complex patterns over plain. (Adapted and used with permission of the *Scientific American Inc.* from an article by Robert Fantz (1961) "The origin of form perception."

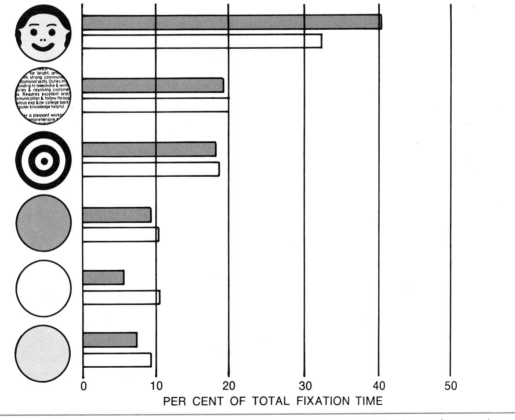

FIGURE 5-8   Contrary to what some mothers and other care-givers might think, babies prefer complex patterns including the human face. So, the very best thing for a baby to look at is the human face. (Adapted and used with permission of the *Scientific American Inc.* from an article by Robert Fantz (1961) "The origin of form perception."

you are included, or you can offer objects that have human faces depicted on them.

Color Vision   Although some parents believe that their babies see the world only in shades of black, white, and gray, this is not so. Newborn babies perceive colors and can distinguish between colors. They immediately put this color vision ability to good use and prefer looking at red and gray, green and gray, and yellow and gray checkerboards rather than plain gray squares (Adams, Maurer, & Davis, 1986). It is as though neonates are biologically programmed to look at color. After all, what good is an ability if it isn't used? However, neonates' color vision is not complete or fully developed. They cannot discriminate blue from gray (Adams, Maurer, & Davis, 1986). The reason for this inability is because the blue color cones, necessary for the discrimination of blue, are not functional until around three months of age (Haith, 1986). Indeed, the baby's color vision, like its entire visual system, is immature in comparison to that of the adult, but develops rapidly over the first two years.

Neonates' rather well-developed visual competencies enable them to learn about their world almost from the moment of birth and explore that world from their parents' arms. They are not passive reactors to serendipitous stimuli, but rather active initiators in exploring their new world. The neonate's ability to see color and detect pattern, form, and shape helps her organize her environment and make sense of the world. This ability is vital and necessary for cognitive development.

Keep in mind that vision is not necessarily only a process of looking at something. *Seeing* also involves emotions and affective experiences. From this perspective, *seeing* is an apperceptive process. For, as Spitz (1965, p. 65) so correctly points out, the nursing baby lying in his mother's arms sees his mother's face *and* feels the nipple in his mouth *and* derives pleasure from nourishment. Also, the baby would hear his mother talking to him and would be aware of her breathing, warmth, etc. Many of our visual experiences are overlaid by other experiences and sensations.

Touch and Motion

We no longer think of the infant as a bundle of helplessness. As Reisman (1987) says, "They are born with some exquisitely tuned sensory abilities. Although sight is still fuzzy and hearing muted, the neonate is equipped with a sense of touch that accurately homes in on the source of its meals, a sense of motion that triggers reflexes to protect it from falls, and a sense of its body parts that allows the infant to mold its body comfortably to that of its caretakers" (p. 265).

Kinesthetic Awareness

Kinesthesis is the sense of body movement and position in space. Neonates demonstrate they have this sense and put it to good use as well. For instance, when crying babies are given kinesthetic stimulation by being picked up and carried on their parents' shoulders, rocked, and patted, they cry less and are more alert. Apparently they find this position more soothing, enjoyable, and can see more of their environment.

Imitation

Shortly after birth, neonates can discriminate and imitate happy, sad, and surprised facial expressions (see Figure 5–9), indicating an innate ability to compare the sensory information of a visually perceived expression with the feedback of the movements involved in matching that expression (Field, Woodsen, Greenberg, & Cohen, 1982). The developmental significance of such ability may be that it is the starting point of infant psychological development (Meltzoff & Moore, 1983).

Olfaction

Neonates have a rather remarkably developed sense of smell from birth. Reactions to odors include facial expressions, increased body movements, and increased respiratory activity. In addition, there is every indication that neonates have

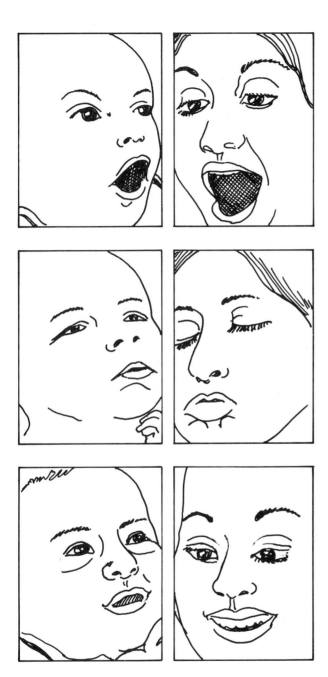

FIGURE 5-9 Part of a baby's remarkable repertory of behaviors is the ability to imitate parental or care-givers' facial gestures. Such abilities have important implications for early learning.

innate preferences for particular olfactory stimuli (Crook, 1987).

At three days neonates can respond to the odors of asafetida (strong garlic odor), lavender, and valerian (an herb with a strong odor) (Self, Horowitz, & Paden, 1972). Although they have the ability to detect odors, they don't seem to have a preference for particular odors, with one major exception—they like the smell of their mothers. By the end of the first week of life, a neonate can tell the difference between her mother and a stranger, a feat we can all agree requires rather fine olfactory discrimination, and from a research perspective has ecological significance. When presented with the breast pad of her nursing mother, a neonate will turn her head significantly more to that pad than she will to the breast pad of an unfamiliar nursing mother (McFarlane, 1978).

Taste

From birth, the neonate not only tastes, but discriminates between the four primary taste sensations: sweet, sour, salty, and bitter. This ability to discriminate between tastes, just as adults do, shows a preference for "good"-tasting food and a rejection of "bad"-tasting food. Neonates prefer a sweet fluid as demonstrated by their willingness to suck harder to get it (Nowlis & Kessen, 1976). Furthermore, while sucking a sweet fluid, babies' sucking rates decline, leading one researcher to conclude that this indicates a "savoring" of the "pleasure of sensation" between sucks (Lipsitt, 1977).

In addition, they can discriminate between intensities of these fluids. Affectively, neonates prefer sweet fluids over other fluids. This innate preference for sweet is even more marked for females and heavier children (Crook, 1987). In fact, neonates are capable of discriminating small differences between the sweetness of fluids. In the neonate, when taste stimulations are not dominated by fluid flow, such as in laboratory tests, then she will reject sour, salt, and bitter. However, during feeding, fluid in the mouth is a very powerful tactile stimulant and the infant will ingest fluids that are bitter or salty (Crook, 1987). This helps explain why babies will ingest formula accidentally prepared with salt rather than a sweetener.

Significance of Taste—The Sweet Tooth   The innate preference of the neonate for sweet tastes serves the purpose of promoting food intake. The sweet taste is a powerful stimulus to sucking. Even a slight increase in the sweetness of an infant's formula produces increased sucking rhythms (Crook, 1979). The taste preferences learned over the developing years—the infant's likes and dislikes—play significant roles in development relating to current and future health and well-being. Figure 5–10 shows "that newborns with no prior taste experience respond differently to sour and bitter stimuli, demonstrating that they can discriminate among these taste qualities as well as make a more general sweet versus nonsweet distinction" (Rosenstein & Oster, 1988).

COGNITIVE DEVELOPMENT

In Chapter Two we discussed Piaget's theory of cognitive development. His theory is the standard in discussions of infant intellectual development. Piaget's theory was known in Europe long before it became popular and widely applied in the United States. During the last thirty years, researchers all over the world have refined his theory. Educators are constantly seeking ways to apply his ideas to parenting, preschool settings, and elementary classrooms.

Piaget was trained as a biologist, and many of his ideas have their basis in biological theory. Biological theory suggests, for example, that the physical structure of an organism changes and adapts to environmental conditions and circumstances. Piaget believed the same process helps promote intellectual development. He used the term *scheme* to describe the cognitive structures or units of knowledge that change and adapt as a result of experiences and maturation.

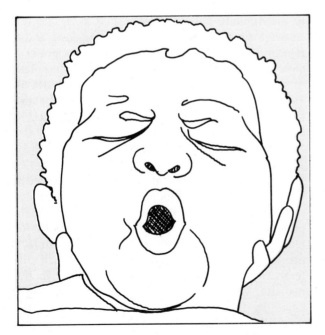 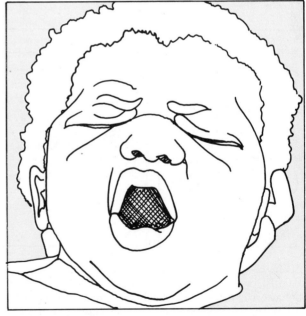

FIGURE 5-10   Newborn babies have the ability to differentiate between different tastes.

The first schemes are the *sensorimotor schemes.* At birth, infants do not know that there are objects in the world. Also, according to Piaget, infants do not have internalized thought processes or "thoughts of the mind." Rather, infants come to know their world by acting on it through their senses and motor actions.

Infants *construct* (as opposed to absorb) schemes using their innate sensorimotor reflexive actions. Sucking is an innate sensorimotor scheme. This scheme involves turning the head to the source of nourishment, closing the lips around the nipple, sucking, and swallowing. All these actions are the behavioral manifestations of the sucking scheme. As an infant matures, and in conjunction with sucking experiences, this basic sensorimotor scheme *adapts* to include anticipatory sucking movements and nonnutritive sucking, such as sucking a pacifier or blanket.

New schemes are constructed or created through the processes of *assimilation* and *accommodation.* Piaget believed children are active con-

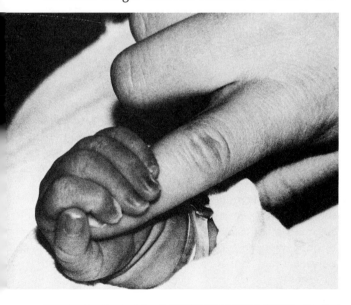

FIGURE 5-11 It is important for neonates to have opportunities to interact sensorially with their environments. Such interactions contribute to physical, social and intellectual development. (Photo by Kenneth Deitcher, MD)

structors of intelligence, assimilating or taking in new experiences and accommodating or changing existing schemes to fit new information. He thought that infants are constantly in a quest for equilibrium. *Equilibrium* is a balance between assimilation and accommodation, between new experiences and old ideas, between what the world is really like and a person's view of the world. In this sense, humans are programmed to develop their intelligence through active involvement in the environment.

Sensorimotor schemes help infants learn new ways of interacting with the world. These new ways of interacting promote cognitive development. One infant sensorimotor scheme, for example, is grasping. At birth, the grasping reflex consists of closing the fingers around an object placed in the hand. Through experiences and maturation, this basic reflexive grasping acting becomes coordinated with looking, opening the hand, retracting the fingers, and grasping. In this sense, the scheme develops from a pure, reflexive action to an intentional grasping action. As the infant matures, and in response to experiences, the grasping scheme is combined with a releasing scheme, which leads to the delightful activity of grasping and releasing things.

Infants begin life with only reflexive motor actions. These are used to satisfy biological needs. By using these reflexive actions on the environment and in response to specific environmental conditions, the reflexive actions are modified and *adaptations* to the environment occur. Patterns of adaptive behavior are used to initiate more activity, which leads to more adaptive behavior, which in turn leads to more schemes.

Infants are not capable of engaging in reflective action, which is mentally representing and manipulating objects. The first stages of intellectual growth occur through the senses and innate reflexive actions. As the infant continually engages in reflexive action, behavior becomes more predictable. The baby demonstrates instances of "knowing" how to do certain things. The first sensorimotor actions become the basis for later *adaptive* behaviors, which are more organized. The reflexive motor action of sucking is adapted to many instances of nonnutritive sucking through which the neonate explores objects. In this way, a scheme or model is developed about the objects sucked. These early schemes are the foundation for cognitive development. The neonate builds a foundation on which the accomplishments of the infant are built. Accomplishments accumulate from one stage of intellectual development to another. In this way, the actions and scheme development of the neonate help give meaning and order to environmental objects, people, and events.

Stages of Cognitive Development

The sensorimotor stage of intellectual development consists of six stages, as shown in Table 5–3.

Stage One   During this reflexive action stage, neonates suck and grasp everything. They are literally ruled by reflexive action and are not in control of their behavior. Through the practice of these reflexive actions, however, infants assimilate, accommodate, and build schemes. While in the reflexive stage, an infant cannot perform a mental act; rather, all acts take place through the basic reflexive actions. Freedom from complete dependence on reflexive actions comes with maturation and development of schemes. Reflexive responses to objects are undifferentiated and infants respond the same way to everything. Objects are assimilated through reflexive actions and infants accommodate to the environment as a result of experiences with solid objects.

During Stage One, infants are totally self-centered and do not differentiate between themselves and the external world. Indeed, infants are not "aware" that external objects exist, but treat them as part of themselves.

Implications

Because infants must create their own intelligence by interacting with the environment, it is important for care-givers to provide many objects to suck, feel, grasp, and look at. Piaget believed that activity and the child's quest for equilibrium between the old and new, the known and the unknown, fuel the process of intellectual development through assimilation and accommodation. Consequently, a rich social and physical environment plays a major role in intellectual development by creating disequilibrium.

A rich social environment depends in part on how care-givers and parents interact with infants. Care-givers are the best toys infants have, and there is no substitute for an attentive care-giver. There is no substitute for spending time with infants. Infants need positive and stimulating human environments.

Although Piaget believed the environment plays a role in development, the environment does not determine intelligence. The active child in an enriched environment assimilates and accommodates. Care-givers have to provide for, encourage, and be a part of this interaction. Meeting infants' basic trust needs is also important, since they will accommodate more in an environment they can trust.

NEONATAL LEARNING

That neonates can learn is no longer questioned but rather widely accepted as a given fact, as evidenced by both classical and operant conditioning. Lipsitt and Kaye (1964) conditioned neonates to expect food on the presentation of a tone. In a combination of both classical and operant conditioning, neonates were rewarded with a sugar solution every time they turned their heads and then gradually learned to turn their heads at the sound of a bell (Papousek, 1967). Another example of and evidence for neonatal learning is that neonates *habituate*, that is, they become accustomed to certain stimuli such as odor, sight, taste, and sound, and no longer respond to them. For example, if you repeatedly present a neonate with the sound of a voice saying, "Hello, baby," the baby will gradually stop responding to the voice. However, when a *new* voice says "Hello, baby,"

TABLE 5–3

	STAGES OF INTELLECTUAL DEVELOPMENT	
Stage	Age	Cognitive Development and Behavior
I. Reflexive action	Birth to one month	1. Infant engages in the reflexive actions of sucking, grasping, crying, rooting, and swallowing. 2. Reflexes are modified and become more efficient as a result of experiences, e.g., infant learns how much sucking is required to result in nourishment. 3. Reflexive schemes become adaptive to the environment. 4. Little or no tolerance for frustration or delayed gratification.
II. Primary circular reactions	One to four months	1. Acquired adaptations are formed. 2. Reflexive actions are gradually replaced by voluntary actions. 3. Beginning of understanding of causality evidenced when infant tries to repeat action that prompted response from care-giver. 4. Circular reactions result in modification of existing schemes.
III. Secondary circular reactions	Four to eight months	1. Infants increase responses to people and objects. 2. Intentional activities increase. Infant able to initiate activities. 3. Beginning of object permanency.
IV. Coordination of secondary schemes	Eight to twelve months	1. Increased deliberation and purposefulness in responding to stimulus. 2. First clear signs of developing intelligence. 3. Continued development of object permanency. 4. Actively searches for hidden objects. 5. Comprehends meanings of simple words.
V. Experimentation (tertiary circular reactions)	Twelve to eighteen months	1. Active experimentation begins, as evidenced through trial and error. 2. Toddler spends much time "experimenting" with objects to see what happens. Toddler is literally a little scientist. Insatiable curiosity. 3. Toddler differentiates self from objects. 4. Realizes that "out of sight" is not "out of reach." 5. Can find hidden objects in first location hidden. 6. Beginning of understanding of space, time, and causality of spatial and temporal relationships.
VI. Representational intelligence (intention of means)	Eighteen to twenty-four months	1. Mental combinations evidenced by thinking before doing. Development of cause/effect relationships. 2. Representational intelligence begins. That is, the toddler is able to mentally represent objects. 3. Engages in imitative behavior, which is increasingly symbolic. 4. Beginnings of sense of time. 5. Aware of object permanence regardless of the number of invisible placements. 6. Searches for an object in several places. 7. Egocentric in thought and behavior.

Note. From *Education and Development of Infants, Toddlers, and Preschoolers* (p. 48) by G. S. Morrison, 1988, Glenview, IL: Scott, Foresman.

and she responds, it is an indication that she was habituated to the previous voice. This habituating ability has been and is the basis for many experiments and is used in the Brazelton Neonatal Behavior Assessment Scale to assess normal development.

Habituation plays an important role in a neonate's life because it allows her to become used to sounds, smells, and visual stimuli that otherwise might interfere with her growth and development. In addition, habituation means that a baby will tolerate more and will therefore likely place fewer demands on her care-giver. A child reared in a noisy environment, for example, soon learns to tune out the noises of television, meal preparation, and family living, and contentedly sleep through it all.

NEONATES AT RISK
Being Born Too Soon

Many babies—as many as seven out of 100—are born before their time. Being born too soon means that the baby is underdeveloped—premature and often underweight. The high-risk neonate is one who is more susceptible to illness and death than the neonate who is not at risk. There are a number of factors that cause a baby to be born prematurely. These include (Simon, 1983):

- Mother's age—younger than seventeen or over thirty-five at time of conception
- Mother's weight—underweight for height at start of pregnancy
- Mother's social background—little education and/or low income
- Previous preterm births—one preterm birth increases the odds of another to 1:4; two preterm births increases the odds still further to 1:2.

- Uterine abnormality—about three women in 100 have a uterine abnormality.

- Existing diseases—high blood pressure, heart, kidney, or liver diseases

- Multiple births—about half of all multiple births are preterm. (This has implications for infertile parents who seek medical help. Frequently, women who take fertility drugs conceive twins or triplets, and, in embryo transplants, more than one embryo is transplanted.)

- Placental abruption—the separation of the placenta from the walls of the uterus during pregnancy
- Incompetent cervix—a condition in which the cervix opens too soon, permitting an early delivery
- Infections—veneral diseases, German measles, vaginal infections, and kidney infections
- Weight loss or inadequate weight gain during pregnancy
- Life-style factors—drinking, smoking and use of drugs
- Strenuous physical work
- Stress

As noted, the age of the mother at the time of conception is frequently cited as a cause of prematurity. The young mother (seventeen years old and under) and the older mother (over thirty-five years old) are often placed in this at-risk age category. However, the contention that age per se causes prematurity, especially in older women, comes at a time when medical technology and educational support groups are providing for more reproductive freedom than at any time in history. While some research supports the contention that older women are at increased risk for delivering a low birth weight and preterm baby, (Forman, Meirik, & Berendes, 1984), other research (Barkan & Bracken, 1987) indicates that it is not age per se that attributes to the increased risk of a low birth weight or preterm delivery in older women. Rather, previous health and the reproductive history of the mother also must be taken into consideration. Many professional men and women delay childbearing in order to devote more time and effort to their careers. It may well be that

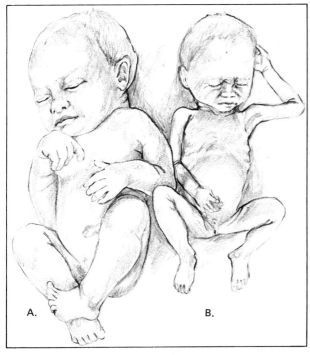

A. FULL-TERM BABY   B. PREMATURE BABY

FIGURE 5-12 A neonate whose gestational age is less than 38 weeks is preterm. Those neonates who are small for gestational age and who are underweight are developmentally at risk. (From Anderson/BASIC MATERNAL-NEWBORN NURSING, copyright 1989 by Delmar Publishers Inc.)

these older parents, who are highly educated and who are more in tune to the need for prenatal care, may as a result offset risks thought to be associated with prematurity and age of the mother.

What is sometimes overlooked is that the premature neonate must also make the same adjustments from uterine to extrauterine life as the full-term infant. However, she has to do it with less developed—really inadequately developed—body systems. Because of this, some of the survival problems facing preterm infants include:

- *Respiratory problems*—These result because of inadequate surfactant, leading to the inability of the lungs to easily fill with air, and the failure of the ductus arteriosus to close or to close completely, resulting in increased respiratory effort and higher oxygen use. *Apnea*, or the cessation of breathing for twenty to thirty seconds, is frequently a complication found in the premature neonate.

- *Body temperature maintenance*—Heat loss in the premature neonate is a critical problem for a number of reasons. First, there is a higher ratio of body surface to body weight than in the full-term infant. This means the neonate is not able to produce the heat it needs to replace the heat it loses. Second, the premature neonate has little insulation in the form of subcutaneous fat, which is another reason for the rapid loss of body heat. Subcutaneous fat develops in the last two to three months of intrauterine life. If the baby is born early, he is deprived of this aspect of development.

- *Digestive problems*—Because of the immaturity of the digestive system and small stomach capacity, the premature neonate is unable to ingest and absorb the calories and nutrients it needs for growth. Also, the sucking reflex is poorly developed in the preterm neonate, which limits its ability to intake nutrition orally.

What is Prematurity?

When we refer to prematurity, maturity means *functional capacity*, or the degree to which the neonate/infant's organs are able to adapt to the

---

Preterm (premature)—neonate born before 37-weeks gestation (conception to 37 weeks)
Term—neonate born between 38 and 42-weeks gestation (start of week 38 through week 42)
Postterm—neonate born after 42-weeks gestation (start of week 43)

FIGURE 5-13 Classifications of neonates by gestational age.

demands of extrauterine life. Consequently, gestational age—the length of time the fetus develops in the womb—is a better determiner of neonatal maturity than is birth weight. "Preterm" is up to thirty-seven weeks, "term" is thirty-eight to forty-one weeks, and "postterm" is after forty-two weeks.

(See Figure 5–13.) A *premature* infant, then, is one born before the completion of the thirty-seventh week of gestation, regardless of weight. However at birth, neonates are classified according to the data shown in Figure 5–14. An infant classified as T-AGA, for example, is one whose weight and

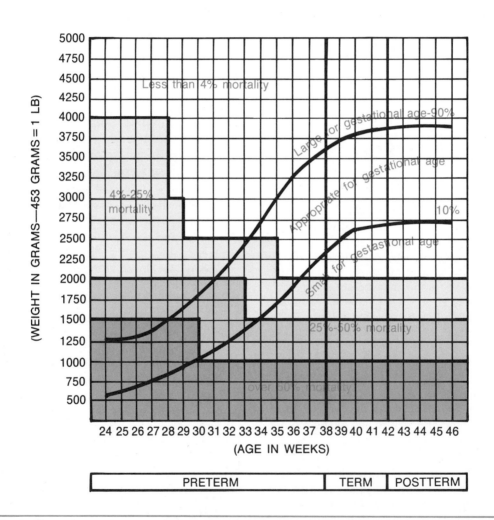

FIGURE 5-14 The relationship between gestational age, weight and mortality is an important and significant one for neonates. Prematurity is a significant cause of infant mortality. (Adapted and used with permission of C.V. Mosby. From *Nursing care of infants and children*, by Whaley and Wong (1987). p. 306.)

development is appropriate for her gestational age. Thus when taken together, gestational age and birth weight are the two best determiners of neonatal maturity and mortality risk. Figure 5–14 shows the relationship of weight and gestational age between the tenth and ninetieth percentile. A neonate whose weight is appropriate for gestational age (AGA) has grown at a normal rate regardless of the time of birth—preterm, term, or postterm. Figure 5–14 also shows the relationship of weight and gestational age to mortality. Notice that children who are small for gestational age and who are preterm have a 50 percent mortality rate.

Life in Neonatal Intensive Care

Neonatology became a medical specialty in 1960. The founder of the field was Pierre-Constantin Budin, a French physician who invented the incubator for premature babies. To promote public attention and support, he displayed it at the Berlin Exposition of 1896. He "borrowed" premature infants, which he put in the incubator. In 1933 at the Chicago World Fair, his exhibit was very popular, and the first incubator was used at Chicago's Michael Reese Hospital. As late as 1963, the art and science of rescuing premature babies was not advanced enough even to save Jack and Jacqueline Kennedy's three-pound son, Patrick. Today, however, parents of premature babies have reason to be much more optimistic. With advances in medical technology, even two-pound babies, born at twenty-seven weeks gestation may have an 80 percent chance of living.

Because of an immature respiratory system and the lack of surfactant, a premature baby's fight for life begins when she is placed on a Constant Positive-Pressure Ventilation Machine (CPPV), also referred to as a ventilator. The ventilator is both a boon and a blessing. While it can save the baby's life by providing oxygen and keeping enough air pressure in the lungs to keep them from collapsing, it can also cause irreparable harm. While some children fight off the effects of the ventilator, others

die because of bursting blood vessels. Others can go through life with breathing difficulties resembling a bad case of emphysema due to scarring of the lung tissue.

Dehydration is also a problem for the premature neonate, who requires intravenous feeding to restore fluids to dried-out tissue. A complication of intravenous feeding and medication is that the baby's veins can collapse from overuse. Since a premature baby is not large to begin with, where to put a tube can create a problem—sometimes there is no more room. When this happens, surgery is performed and a "deep line" feeding tube is inserted.

Since the mother's immune system is passed along to her child during the last trimester of pregnancy, a neonate born too early does not have an immune system and therefore is subject to diseases and sickness. Contracting infectious diseases, while a concern for all neonates, is a life-and-death matter for the premature neonate. For this reason, parents and health care professionals who visit and care for premature babies must scrub their hands and arms with antiseptic soap and don a hospital gown. Although parents are encouraged to touch their babies, finding a place to touch is oftentimes difficult because of tubes and lines.

Because of their immature livers, many premature neonates have abnormal liver function. The resulting neonatal jaundice is from a build-up of bilirubin in the bloodstream. When this occurs, the neonate is placed under "bili lights" similar to flourescent lights that give off light at a wavelength that speeds up the breakdown of bilirubin. During this treatment, the neonate wears eye patches to protect his eyes from the light.

Since the sucking reflex is not mature in many premature babies, it is difficult for them to suck. Some can nurse at their mother's breast; others from a small bottle. When an infant is too weak to breast-feed, the mother's milk is pumped, frozen, and used as needed. Others too weak to nurse from breast or bottle are fed intravenously or via the gavage method.

*P*ersonal *S*tories

MEREDITH NELSON—NEONATAL NURSE

Some of the questions that run through the minds of parents who have a child admitted to an intensive care nursery are, "What is the matter with my baby?"; "Will my baby die?"; and "Will my baby be deformed or retarded?" Whether the child is premature, small for gestational age, full term, or born with congenital defects, it is a tremendous upset to the parent's picture of a normal, healthy baby. Transferring the infant to a special care nursery or to another facility increases the parents' anxiety level, may hinder their reception of effective nursing intervention, and may also delay the bonding process. The parents are often fearful of the dying infant and therefore remain distant, hesitating to bond to this new life, a life that needs them now more than ever. The neonatal nurse is the link between the parent and the infant in fostering this vital connection.

It is important for parents to maintain close contact with their infant and to know that their infant is receiving the necessary care. It is also important for parents to realize and understand that their nurturing and tender loving care is greatly needed. The stroking and touching that a parent provides is very different from that of the nurse, no matter how gentle.

The transfer of ill babies to a special care nursery intensifies emotions, thereby increasing the need for a comprehensive approach that is developmentally appropriate for the infant's condition. The severity of the illness directs the actions of the nurse. There is an abundance of machinery and life support equipment that can be in contact with the infant. The nurses are constantly providing care and allowing only small rest periods when the infants are in critical condition. There is a high amount of auditory stimulation, such as the sounds of alarms and conversations. These things in and of themselves may overstimulate the infant.

The parents of sick newborns feel very detached. They may express the feeling that it doesn't seem like its their baby with all the tubes and wires. When an infant's condition is serious, the parents can still be involved in her care. The infant can listen to their voices, and many times it has a very soothing effect. In utero, the infant was hearing the muffled version, now things are clearer and the infant recognizes these familiar sounds. This is very important with regard to neurological development, and the nurse can assist by encouraging parents to talk to their infant. It is helpful for the parents to make a tape recording of their voices, including the noise their pet makes! This can be played when the parents are unable to visit. Small music boxes are also helpful.

Many parents still feel distant. The nurse can encourage parents to stroke their infant and hold his tiny hand. Applying lotion to available skin surface areas is a wonderful opportunity for parents to have contact with their baby when he is

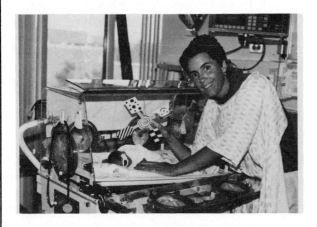

FIGURE 5-15 Meredith Nelson uses her knowledge of child development to help her in her daily work with premature neonates and their families.

unable to be held or rocked. The nurse must remember that the infant and his illness limit the stimulation he is able to receive.

As the infant's illness or disease improves, the parents and the infant are able to tolerate a little more. The parents can change the diapers and may even give the baby a sponge bath. They are usually very excited to help in these tasks.

The lighting in many special care nurseries tends to be very bright. If at all possible, dimming the lights at the infant's bed is very soothing. The baby has been in the dark for nine months! Reducing the intensity of light also simulates night and day to the infants, thereby creating a more home-like atmosphere. When it is not possible to turn off some of the lights, there are some things the nurse can do to decrease the lighting intensity. There is filter paper available that can be cut into "sunglasses" and "sunvisors" for the infants. If this is unavailable, draping a sheet over the crib or infant warmer is helpful. Placing a pillowcase over the top of the isolette (incubator) also inhibits the light from entering the infant's little "home." The nurse must remember to allow enough room to visualize and assess the infant's color and condition.

Mobiles are a common item found on the cribs of many normal, healthy babies. A sick infant need not be deprived of this. The nurse can start by making a mobile out of small pieces of paper attached to tongue depressors and suspended above the infant's bed. The designs should not be too busy in detail. Infants tend to focus on the sharp contrast within the picture; black squares on white paper, a picture of a face, a picture showing motion. Again, the key is "moderation."

Rest is very important in an infant's life because of its importance in the child's growth and development. The baby should be encouraged into a wake-sleep routine. By doing this, the infant is more rested and alert during his wakeful periods. The nurse should attempt to provide her care in clusters. Monitoring vital signs, diaper changes, repositioning, dressing changes, chest physiotherapy and suctioning, and bathing can be done a few at a time rather than doing one thing per hour. This clustered care allows the baby to rest for possibly two to three hours if his condition permits. The nurse can place a sign on the bed stating "NAP TIME: DO NOT DISTURB—unless you check with my nurse first!"

Considering all the extra stimulation a baby feels, hears, and sees in a special care nursery, she needs to have a sense of security. Positioning the infant on her abdomen is very natural. Sometimes you, as the nurse, may need to help the infant achieve this by placing her knees and arms in a flexed position underneath her. If an infant is unable to be positioned on her abdomen because of equipment or surgical dressing, the nurse can still maintain her sense of security by the use of rolls. A small roll should be placed under her shoulders and neck. The next roll

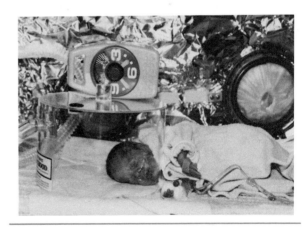

FIGURE 5-16 In neonatal nurseries, many adaptations are made to provide for the developmental needs of the neonates. Here, Meredith Nelson modified breathing equipment, enabling the neonate to use a pacifier to satisfy her need to suck.

should be placed under her knees next to her buttocks so that the hips and knees are flexed. Lastly, a roll is placed on either side of the infant, bringing her arms inward.

Sucking is an innate reflex that is one of the infant's basic needs. When a baby is on a ventilator/respirator with an oral endotracheal tube in place, the nurse may notice the infant sucking on the tube. You may wonder how you can provide a proper sucking experience with all this equipment in her mouth. Using a pair of scissors, make a notch for the ETT to fit in the pacifier. (See Figure 5–16.)

When the infant is not on a ventilator, but is receiving formula through an oral or nasal gastric tube, she should be held during feeding time. To provide a "normal" feeding time, the nurse or parent can hold the infant while the formula is being delivered, and she can be offered the pacifier on which to suck. The infant believes her sucking and feeling of fullness is all her doing. The nurse may need to check with the physician as to when the infant may be bottle fed. When that is allowed, the infant should be offered the bottle first and, if she tires, the remainder can be given through a tube. The important thing is to provide the infant with this experience while, at the same time, facilitating parental bonding.

Utilizing a care plan, developed by the infant's primary nurse, is essential. This may take the form of a twenty-four-hour schedule at the infant's bedside, showing naptimes, feeding times, and times for blood drawing and special procedures. Posting the infant's schedule may help redirect care to allow for rest periods and preventing sensory overload. The nurse may also see a need to obtain the advice of occupational, physical, and play therapists. These experts should include the parents in their therapies so the parents can use these techniques when playing with the infant, both in the nursery and when the baby goes home.

By now you have realized that the parents' role in their infant's care has a great effect on his future development. The parents and the nursing staff, working together from the moment of birth, are a vital part of the infant's growth and development, and this cooperative effort should continue through hospitalization, discharge, and home care. [See discussion of Maureen Reilly in Chapter One.]

When caring for the premature infant, all of the previously mentioned interventions may be used. The nurse and the parents must take into consideration the number of weeks or months the baby was premature. This tiny infant does not have a sucking reflex until she is approximately thirty-three to thirty-five weeks gestation. The parents must also understand that as the infant develops, she will be lagging slightly behind. When other children are sitting up at the age of six to seven months, the premature infant will need that number of months plus the amount of time she was premature. This is also true for fine and gross motor skills as well as other developmental milestones. The premature infant will usually catch up developmentally to other children by the time she is two years of age.

Parenting the Preemie

Parenting the premature neonate/infant is frequently more demanding, disappointing, exhausting, and unrewarding than parenting the normal neonate. There are a number of reasons for this.

The preemie is not like other neonates and therefore does not meet parents' expectations about what their baby should be like. (See Figure 5–17.) He is hard to care for because he does not have a fully developed sucking response; requires more frequent feedings; is not as responsive as a normal

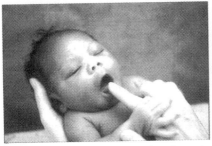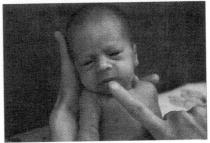

A full-term baby (left), has normal sucking reflex. A healthy baby, but born six weeks premature, responds minimally.

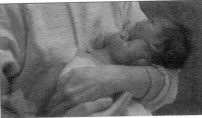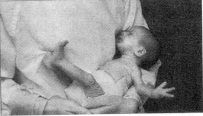

The full-term baby appears receptive, eager to interact; Preemie stiffens, pushes away.

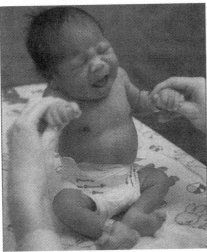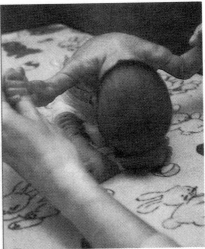

The full-term baby can hold his head up; The preemie can't, obscuring eye contact.

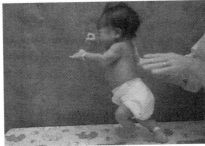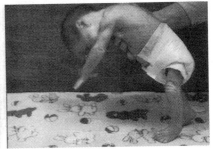

The full-term baby tries to walk when held; The preemie appeears fragile, incompetent.

FIGURE 5-17 Parenting the preemie can be a traumatic and trying experience for new parents. Part of a plan for providing good care for the preemie includes support and training for parents. (From *Psychology Today* in an article entitled "Preemie Perils," September 1986. Used with permission.)

neonate (that is, he does not mold himself to the care-giver's embrace); startles more; and is more difficult to soothe. Parents of premature babies are oftentimes full of doubt about the reasons for their baby's prematurity and their ability to care for him or her. If the baby is in the hospital for a long time, then the parent may not bond to the baby or may have difficulty bonding. Indifference results.

Also, as more premature babies' lives are saved, tens of thousands of parents are thrust into a different parenting mode, whether they like it or not. Frequently their parenting roles demand from them tasks and responsibilities not bargained for in their view of parenting, nor demanded of other parents. These nerve-wracking and also rewarding demands frequently include constant monitoring of the baby's heart rate and respiration, and resuscitating a limp baby whose breathing has stopped. According to the FDA, about 45,000 apnea monitors (devices to monitor the baby's breathing) are in use, and about 12,000–15,000 are sold each year. However, even the best technology won't be a substitute for informed and wise prenatal care.

How Can You Tell When Your Baby Is Ready for Interaction?   (Wheeler-Liston, 1986, pp. 4–5)

- He will have a soft, relaxed facial expression.
- His relaxed (not floppy) limbs will appear to reach out to you.
- He will turn toward your voice without any of the signs of stress that follow.
- He will show an ability to look at your face and listen to your voice without any of the signs of overstimulation that follow.

How Can You Tell When Your Baby Is Overstimulated?

- She has uncoordinated eye movements.
- She changes color; becomes pale or flushed.
- She looks "worried"; may frown or grimace.
- She may seem to be looking *through* you, with eyes fixed and staring.
- She hiccups, gags, or spits up (sometimes, but not always, unrelated to feedings).
- Her muscle tone changes: she may become limp or floppy; or may become stiff with extended limbs and fingers.
- She may have lots of startles or tremors.

What Coping Strategies Do Babies Use When Overstimulated?

- Avoiding eye contact (this breaks the intensity of a gaze for them).
- Sneezing or yawning (this gives them time out).
- Bracing hand, legs, or back against the side of the crib (this stabilizes them).
- Postural change—babies dislike being on their backs, and they love their sense of balance, so they may extend their arms and legs to help get into a side-lying position.
- Sucking on hands or fingers or lips (sucking is a powerful soother).
- Holding on to something with one or both hands—your finger, one of the tubes, clothes, their own hands (this also stabilizes and calms them).
- Getting into a drowsy or light sleep state to shut out stimulation.

*I*N THE SPOTLIGHT

IS LIFE AT ANY COST WORTH IT?

Should we push technology to the limits to save a life? Children with birth defects are being saved with dramatic new medical techniques. But what about the long range effects on the children and families? What about the impairments and effects of such miracles? What about the future costs to families who have to provide special food, care, and equipment for their children? Should babies be saved so that they can lead lives of pain and handicaps? And what about the cost? Oftentimes, medical care for premature neonates and infants can cost $1,500 a day and more.

Society is willing to pay the cost for prolonging and maintaining life at any price because of the sanctity of human life. But more people are starting to challenge whether this is acceptable, given future suffering and consequences.

On the other hand, some people challenge the notion that parents should be allowed to wash their hands of their premature infants or turn their backs on a child who will require a great deal of money and care. Also, who decides between the use of ordinary care and extraordinary care to save a child's life?

*I*N THE SPOTLIGHT

PREVENTING PREMATURITY

Many major industrial employers across the United States are finding that it is much more economical to help their employees prevent prematurity than it is to pay the high cost of medical bills, which can run as high as one million dollars for the care of a single baby (Freudenheim, 1988). Consequently, companies like Oster/Sunbeam in Milwaukee, Wisconsin, are developing education and care programs designed to help employees prevent prematurity. These special programs include classes every two weeks for pregnant employees and their spouses on company premises and on company time. Classes include topics relating to nutrition and complications of pregnancy. The educators are professors from Northwestern Louisiana University, Shreveport, and neonatal specialists from Memphis State University. At Oster/Sunbeam's two locations in Louisiana and Mississippi, all employees are encouraged to consult a doctor early in their pregnancies. Prior to 1986, the number of premature births averaged six a year, with an average cost to the company of $25,000–$30,000 per maternity case. Since the inception of the program in 1986, employees are averaging one premature birth per year overall. According to Kevin M. Breese, Director of Employee Relations at Oster/Sunbeam (1988), "The biggest accomplishment is that we were successful in having pregnant women make contact with their doctors as soon as they knew they were pregnant. As an employer, we want to work in liaison with our employees to get women to see their doctors as soon as they know they are pregnant." Companies are viewing their involvement in prenatal care as a way of reducing their insurance costs and addressing other social problems, such as school attrition, infant mortality, and inadequate medical care for families.

The Developmental Magic of Massage

Think for a minute about what love would be like without touch. We all love to be touched in the right ways and for the right reasons. Infants are no different. In fact, touch in the lives of neonates and infants has positive effects on growth and development. We have known for a long time that a lack of love and affection and the absence of touch retards physical and emotional growth. The pioneering work of Harry Harlow (1962), for example, demonstrated that infant monkeys, who were well-cared-for and fed, but deprived of physical contact, exhibited fear, withdrawal, and an inability to establish social and sexual relations. Current research with nonhumans—especially rats—indicates that they positively benefit from closeness to and licking by their mothers. Sensory stimulation is particularly important for premature infants, since "birth before term deprives the infant of the regulatory influence of maternal biorhythms and the tactile, kinesthetic, and auditory stimulation that characterizes the intrauterine environment" (Rose, Schmidt, Riese, & Bridger, 1980). Recent research by Shanberg and Field (1987) reveals that massage for premature infants has dramatic, positive, and long-lasting benefits. Whereas many premature nurseries and ICU units have a minimal touch rule, now it appears as though this will change. Shanberg and Field conducted a study in which extremely premature/low-birth-weight neonates received tactile/kinesthetic stimulation for three fifteen-minute periods during three consecutive hours per day for a ten-day period. The routine consisted of head, neck, limb, and back with arm and leg exercises. Results of such stimulation were dramatic:

1. The stimulated infants averaged a 47 percent greater weight gain a day than did the control group.
2. The stimulated infants spent more time awake and active.
3. The stimulated infants showed more mature

habituation, orientation, motor, and range-of-state behaviors on the Brazelton assessment scale.
4. The stimulated infants were discharged six days earlier than the control infants. Also, from economic, public policy, and political perspectives, the earlier discharges saved $3,000 per child in hospital costs.

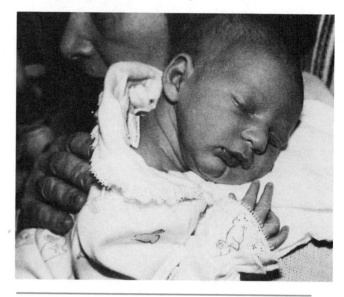

FIGURE 5-18 Touching can contribute positively to development. Also, many parents are discovering the positive effects of touching for all neonates and infants. (Photo by Kenneth Deitcher, MD)

Touch and touching are important for other reasons as well—they provide infants with tactile information and therefore help them learn about their world, in addition to being a source of comfort and solace. As infants grow into toddlerhood, being able to touch a parent or care-giver prior to and after ventures out into the world is a comforting reassurance. A loving pat, a hug, and a kiss are also signs and reassurances that children are liked and loved. Such touching and demonstrations of affection are necessary for girls *and* boys in order for them to develop the feelings of security so necessary for the development of independence. The security of touch that children need is often

IN THE SPOTLIGHT

GETTING IN TOUCH WITH YOUR BABY

Baby massage is growing in popularity. Many towns across America have at least one program for helping parents—usually mothers—learn how to rub their babies the right way. Baby massage is not to be confused with the stereotypical pounding of flesh, grunting, and groaning seen in films and television. Rather, it is stroking, gentle pressing, rubbing, and communicating through touch.

Baby massage provides parents the opportunity to more fully enjoy their children. It is also a great way for hesitant parents to develop a closer relationship with their babies. Some parents and professionals think there are other benefits as well. They believe it stimulates the mind, improves alertness, helps develop other senses, and promotes general relaxation in infants.

The current emphasis on the importance of touch in the lives of young children has spawned the growth of baby massage programs whereby parents learn the ancient art and practice of massage. Baby massage is used by many mothers in many parts of the world, and the practice is slowly growing in the United States. Following is a lovely and enchanting glimpse of how one young Indian mother in Calcutta massaged her baby (Lapierre, 1985).

> Stephan Kovalski continued on his way, observing everything about him. Before reaching the fountain, his eyes were suddenly attracted by the beauty of one young mother swathed in a red sari, sitting in the alleyway, her back firmly upright, with a baby placed on her outstretched legs. The infant was naked, with only an amulet on a thin cord around his waist. He was a chubby child who did not appear to be suffering from malnutrition. There was a strange flame in the way mother and child looked at each other, as if they were talking to each other with their eyes. Captivated, Kovalski put down his bucket. The young woman had just poured a few drops of mustard oil onto her palms and was beginning to massage the little body in her lap. Skillful, intelligent, attentive, her hands moved up and down, actuated by a rhythm as discreet as it was inflexible. Working in turn like waves, they set out from the baby's flanks, crossed his chest, climbed back up to the opposite shoulder. At the end of the movement, her little finger slid under the child's neck. Then she pivoted him onto his side. Stretching out his arms, she massaged delicately one after another, singing to him as she did so ancient songs about the loves of the god Krishna or some legend that stemmed from the depths of epic ages. Then she took hold of his little hands and kneaded them with her thumb as if to stimulate the blood flow from the palms to their extremities. Thus, his stomach, legs, heels, the soles of his feet, his head, the nape of his neck, his face, nostrils, back, and buttocks were successfully caressed and vitalized by those supple, dancing fingers. The massage concluded with a series of yogic exercises. The mother crossed her son's arms over his chest several times in succession to free his back, his rib cage, his breathing. Eventually it was the legs' turn to be raised, opened, and closed over his stomach to induce the opening and complete relaxation of the pelvis. The child gurgled in sheer bliss (pp. 81–82).

Tiffany Field, an expert in prenatal development and one of the modern pioneers in the therapeutic benefits of baby massage, believes that the best stroke to use with infants "is gentle, firm and slow. If the touch is too light, it can overstimulate and even irritate the infant." (Goleman, 1988).

supplemented through a favorite blanket or teddy bear. There is nothing wrong with such security objects as long as parents are not themselves content with this being the child's only source of touch and security.

Ecological Influences on Preterm Infants

The importance of parents, siblings and caregivers, and the experiences of family interactions cannot be underestimated as to their power to influence and direct the development of young children. Today, development is considered a *transactional* process based on *bidirectional* influences between the developing child and the care-giving environment. The influence of this transactional process is dramatically illustrated in the following longitudinal study. In an analysis of the developmental progress of *healthy*, low-birth-weight (1300 grams or two pounds, fourteen ounces) and preterm (thirty-two weeks) babies from birth to age five, Crnic and Greenberg (1987) concluded that "generally healthy preterms with very low birth weights are not significantly different from their full term counterparts at age five across a range of variables describing their cognitive and behavioral competence." They also add that "although preterms and full terms were essentially equivalent in their competency by age five, it appears they took very different routes to this goal." In addition, "early maternal interactive behavior, maternal attitudes, the home environment, and family functioning may assist more competent functioning by preterm children by age five." They conclude that even though the familial environment and interactions are important in the lives of all children, for children of high-risk birth status, "early interaction and family factors assume a more important role within the developmental process." The researchers also believe that "the dynamic process of parent-child interactions within specific contexts and over time appears to compensate in some form for the early detrimental influence of

being born too small and too soon," and, "it may be that these early familial and interaction factors serve as a self-righting mechanism given the presence of a specific birth risk, as our sample of preterm children appear to be quite competent at age five." The researchers are quick to point out that the population consisted of healthy babies who did not encounter many of the medical complications that so often accompany prematurity and low birth weight.

A parents' group, Parent Care (University of Utah Medical Center, Room 2A210, 50 North Medical Drive, Salt Lake City, Utah 84132) acts as a source of information and support to parents whose children required neonatal intensive care.

The "Big Four" handicaps of prematurity are: cerebral palsy, mental retardation, visual problems, and hearing problems. In a recent follow-up study of 218 low-birth-weight babies (Elliman, Bryan, & Elliman, 1986) eleven had cerebral palsy, seven had developmental delays, three had severe hearing impairments, and one had visual impairment. In addition, SGA children were shorter and lighter than the normal population.

Although the survival rate for preterm and low-birth-weight babies is increasing, there frequently remain for some children long-term consequences of being born early, one of which is difficulty with school achievement. The prospects for future school success are not good. In a longitudinal study of the school performance of children with birth weights of 1000 grams or less (one pound, four ounces), Nickel (1982) and his colleagues concluded that "one of the most striking findings of our study group was the number of very-low-birth-weight children who required or still require a special educational program and the failure of those children in regular classes to achieve as expected levels. Only seven of the twenty-five study children are currently achieving at or above grade level. Three of those seven children have previously been in full-day special education programs, two in learning disability classes and one in a class for the visually impaired.

What Would You Do?

Infant Organ Donations

In a widely publicized case, the parents of an unborn child diagnosed as having anencephaly (see Chapter Four) wanted the baby's normal organs donated immediately at birth, rather than keeping the child alive for a few days on a respirator until she was officially declared brain dead. Brain death is difficult to determine in infants who have no cerebral cortex. In addition, there is no accepted definition of brain death in infants less than seven days old (Blakeslee, 1987).

If you were the parent of an unborn anacephalic child, what would you want to happen to your child?

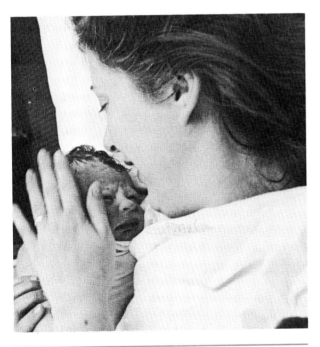

FIGURE 5-19 Bonding and attachment are important developmental processes and contribute to social and emotional development. Parents and other care-givers are emphasizing how they can help facilitate both these processes. (From Anderson/BASIC MATERNAL-NEWBORN NURSING, copyright 1989 by Delmar Publishers Inc.)

SOCIAL DEVELOPMENT

Social relationships begin at birth and are evident in the daily interactions between neonates and their parents and care-givers. Babies are social beings with a repertoire of behaviors they use to initiate and facilitate social interactions. *Social behaviors* are used to begin and maintain a relationship with others. Regardless of their temperament, all babies are capable of social interactions and benefit from interactions with others.

Crying is the neonate's primary social behavior. It attracts the parent and promotes a social interaction of some type and duration, depending on the skill and awareness of the particular parent or care-giver. Merely meeting the basic needs of a baby in a perfunctory manner is not sufficient to form a firm base for social development. Parents and other care-givers must react to babies with enthusiasm, attentiveness, and concern for them as unique *persons*.

Another social skill exhibited by babies is their imitative behavior. As was previously pointed out, they have abilities to mimic the facial expressions and gestures of adults. When a mother sticks out her tongue at a baby, after a few repetitions the baby will also stick out her tongue. This imitative behavior is satisfying to the infant. The mother is also pleased by this interactive "game." This is precisely the point. The imitative behavior is pleasant for both persons of the dyad. They continue to interact for the sake of interaction, which in turn promotes more social interaction. Social relations develop from social interactions.

Bonding and Attachment

Bonding and attachment play major roles in the development of social and emotional relationships. *Bonding* is the process by which parents and or other care-givers become emotionally attached or bonded to infants. It is the development of a close, personal, affective relationship. *Attachment* is the emotional tie between the infant and the parents or other primary care-givers. As such, it is a unique relationship between two people that is specific and endures through time (Klaus and Kennell, 1982, p. 2). Bonding and attachment are not synonymous terms or processes. Bonding is the early mother-to-infant affection, while attachment is the slowly developing infant-to-mother affection (Myers, 1987, p. 224).

Attachment behaviors serve the purpose of getting and maintaining proximity and form the bases for the enduring relationship of attachment. Care-giver attachment behaviors include kissing, fondling, caressing, holding, touching, embracing, eye contact, and looking at the face. Neonate and infant attachment behaviors include crying, sucking, eye contact, babbling, and general body movements. Later, attachment behaviors will include following, clinging, and calling.

Touching is the first physical encounter parents have with their children and is one of the principal means of developing attachment. Touching includes such contact as massaging and palmar stroking, which is a rubbing or massaging with the palms of the hands. Most parents almost intuitively engage in some kind of massage while diapering and bathing their babies. Now, however, instructors and books are teaching the fine art of massage to parents who want to get in touch with their babies.

Eye contact is also an important attachment behavior. Most new parents are visually attentive to their babies and hold them so they can have direct eye contact. Perhaps you have seen parents almost instinctively hold their faces about eight to twelve inches from their babies' faces.

Adult speech has a special fascination for babies. Interestingly enough, given the choice between listening to music or listening to the human voice, babies prefer the human voice. Also, babies move their bodies in rhythmic ways in response to the human voice. Babies' body movements and parents' speech synchronize with each other. As a mother talks to her baby, a behavioral response is triggered in the baby, which in turn stimulates a response in the mother, resulting in a "waltz" of attention and attachment.

Attachment and attention go hand in hand. For the neonate, what is important is not so much who provides the attention—although we would hope that it would be provided by the parents—but that the baby receives the attention and affection necessary for his physical and emotional growth and development.

Fathers and Attachment Fathers are "in" in child development circles. Many fathers have always played important roles in child rearing and have engaged in shared and participatory parenting. Today, however, there is an increased emphasis on ways to encourage fathers to become even more involved in child rearing. Fathers who feed, diaper, bathe, and engage in other care-giving activities demonstrate increased bonding behaviors such as holding, talking, and looking. Child development professionals can encourage fathers to participate in all facets of care-giving.

Child care programs can conduct training programs that will help fathers gain the skills and confidence they need to assume their rightful places as coparents in rearing responsible children.

Michael Lamb, a leading authority on fathering and child development, maintains there is no biologically-based sex difference in responsiveness to infants, and that fathers can be as responsive to babies as mothers. Nevertheless, custom and practice provides mothers with a larger role in child rearing, which necessitates the further encouragement of fathers to be involved in the parenting process.

Children can and do form attachments to their fathers. They and their fathers should be encouraged to develop such relationships.

Sensitive Periods for Attachment Marshall Klaus and John Kennell (1982), pediatricians and researchers, popularized the "sensitive period" view of maternal-infant bonding. According to their theory, bonding of infant and mother occurs within minutes and hours after birth through close skin contact. This belief popularized the concept of "love at first touch." It also encourages expectant parents to believe that if they don't have physical contact with their babies immediately after birth they will "fail to bond." Their theory further maintains that failure to bond early results in a later breakdown in the mother-child relationship and may even contribute to child abuse.

Follow-up studies of the Kennell and Klaus research do not support their theory (Gold, 1983). There is not universal agreement about the existence, length, and duration of a sensitive period for bonding, although the fascination with and belief in early bonding remains strong. The early bonding idea has had a beneficial effect on childbirth and hospital maternity practices. This is reflected in an increase of natural childbirth practices, family-centered births, a general humanizing of childbirth practices, and the inclusion in the fourth stage of labor and delivery of an opportunity for baby and parents to bond.

The idea of early attachment has also promoted an increase in the popularity and practice of breast-feeding, which is seen as one way of initiating and maintaining early contact. The return to breast-feeding would seem, on the surface at least, a reaffirmation of Freudian theory (see Chapter Two), which emphasizes oral gratification. Freud believed that feeding promotes attachment, and that when too many people feed a baby, he fails to attach and, therefore, fails to learn how to love.

Early parent-child contact is only one of many constellations of behaviors that influence attachment. Attachment is a developmental process that occurs over time and within a social environment. Factors involved include the quality and nature of the infant-parent relationship, basic nutrition and health care, the quality of the child-rearing environment, economic factors, and the time, opportunity, and desire for effective parent-child interaction. While early contact is desirable and should be encouraged, the practice by itself is no substitute for effective parenting across the life cycle.

THE INDIVIDUALITY OF NEWBORNS

Temperament

As most parents will attest, their baby is different from every other baby, including its brothers and sisters. This uniqueness is not confined solely to the physical realm, but includes the *temperament*—the child's individual behavioral characteristics, and how the child approaches and reacts to life, situations, and people.

A baby's temperament, what she is like, helps determine her personality. This development occurs as a result of the interplay between particular temperamental characteristics and the environment. In a classic study, Thomas, Chess, and Birch (1970) identified nine characteristics of temperament:

1. Level and extent of motor activity
2. Rhythm and regularity of functions, such as eating, sleeping, regulation, and wakefulness
3. Degree of acceptance or rejection of a new person or experience
4. Adaptability to changes in the environment
5. Sensitivity to stimuli
6. Intensity or energy level of responses
7. General mood, for example, pleasant or cranky, friendly or unfriendly
8. Distractibility from an activity
9. Attention span and persistence in an activity.

Using these nine characteristics, the researchers identified three classes or general types of children according to their temperament characteristics. These types are: the "easy" child, the "slow-to-warm-up" child, and the "difficult" child. Easy children present few problems in care and training. They are positive in mood, regular in body functions, have a low or moderate intensity of reaction, and show adaptability and a positive approach to new situations. Easy babies have regular eating habits, smile a lot, are cheerful, and respond quickly to the parents.

Slow-to-warm-up children have a low activity level, are slow to adapt, withdraw from a first exposure to new stimuli, are somewhat negative in mood and respond with a low intensity. Slow-to-warm-up babies take more time to adapt to new situations, are quiet in nature, and may even be viewed as passive. They are hard to interact with and as a result, a parent may lose interest in them.

A new parent with a slow-to-warm-up baby may feel defeated because her baby does not readily respond to her.

Difficult children are irregular in body functions, tense in their reactions, tend to withdraw from new stimuli, are slow to adapt to changes in the environment, and are generally negative in mood. Difficult babies are the most difficult to parent because they are so fussy. When presented with a new situation, they become upset and cry. Parents of difficult babies have to be understanding of the kind of child they have. They will have to invest extra time and energy in providing good, constant care in order to get their babies' lives off to a good start and provide a supportive environment for good developmental growth.

PSYCHOSOCIAL DEVELOPMENT

In Chapter Two we discussed Erik Erikson's theory of psychosocial development. According to Erikson, ego development occurs within and in response to social institutions, including family and school. Erikson's theory has eight stages or "ego qualities" which occur throughout the human life span.

The first of these stages, Basic Trust vs. Basic Mistrust, begins at birth and lasts until about eighteen months to two years. For Erikson (1963) basic trust means that "one has learned to rely on the sameness and continuity of the outer providers, but also that one may trust oneself and the capacity of one's organs to cope with urges" (p. 249). The key for children developing a pattern of trust or mistrust is the "sensitive care of the baby's individual needs and a firm sense of personal trustworthiness within the trusted framework of their culture's life style" (p. 249). Basic trust occurs when children are reared in an environment of love, warmth, and support. An environment of trust also reduces the opportunity for conflict between children, parents, and other care-givers.

LANGUAGE DEVELOPMENT

Language development begins at birth with the neonate's first cry. Crying represents the first form of vocal communication between baby and mother. Indeed, the first cry signals and reassures parents that their baby is alive and able to cry. Although crying cannot be called language, it is prespeech vocalization and is important for the beginning of language. Crying is common in infants, who may cry from 7 to 22 percent of the time. There are distinct phases of a baby's cry: a short cry, a rest period, intake of breath, another rest, and another short cry. The amount of time between the phases distinguishes one cry from another. Babies' cries have different meanings, as most parents know. One cry signals hunger, another anger, and another pain (Wolff, 1971). Crying then is the neonate's primary means for expressing and communicating basic needs and states.

Parents and others must not consider crying a negative act and should avoid responding to it in negative ways. Crying is a signal that merits response. The parent should respond to crying and investigate the conditions that may cause it. Wolff found that inexperienced mothers responded differently to the cries of babies from experienced mothers. Experienced mothers, for example, responded to the hunger cry by also checking for a wet diaper, and they tended to ignore the hunger cry if the baby had just been fed.

CARING FOR THE NEONATE

All newborn babies require love, care, and protection for their health, welfare, and normal growth and development. In life's first month, they must make many new adjustments and responses to their new world. For children of poor parents, in urban and rural areas especially, this is a critical and difficult time. As many as 10 percent suffer from *failure to thrive (FTT)*, a condition without a diagnosed medical cause, characterized by underdevelopment and lethargy. Some reasons given for FTT are child-related, such as being small for developmental age, general sickness, and temperamental difficulty. Other perhaps more significant reasons relate to the care-giving environment and include social isolation of parents, lack of child-rearing support systems, and large families (Bithoney & Newberger, 1987). The parental need for support and information regarding child rearing is therefore a critical priority, especially in the early days, months, and years. For many children, life is full of pleasant, growth-producing experiences. For others, ordinary life can be more deadly than the deepest jungle.

*I*N THE SPOTLIGHT

NAMING BABY

When a baby is born, others usually ask three questions of the parents: "Is it a boy or girl?", "How much does he/she weigh?", and "What's her/his name?" Quite often parents have the name picked out for the baby before birth, and as is evident from the vignettes, a firstborn son is frequently named after the father. Cultural influences are powerful determiners of what a baby's name will be, as shown in Table 5–4. Names reflect the ethnic background of the persons bestowing the names.

TABLE 5–4

NAMES FOR CHILDREN AND THEIR CULTURAL BASIS

Here is a sampling of names from the pre-school/kindergarten rosters of five South Florida schools or day-care centers.

Duhart's Day Care Center in Liberty City, where all the children are black:	*Conchita Espinosa Academy* in Sweetwater, where most children are Cuban-American:	*Temple Beth Sholom Foundation School* in Miami Beach, where most children are reform Jewish:	*Summit Private School* in Fort Lauderdale, where most children are Anglo:	*Hope Pre School Day-Care* in North Miami Beach, where most children are Haitian-American:
	Cassandra Alicia	Avi	Ashley	Apple
Bloneva	Elizabeth Luisa	David	Jared	Cindy
Devphan	Francisco Steven	Hannah	Jason	Farrah
Ladarius	Gabriella Maria	Jonah	Jennifer	Gregory
Larquasha	Jonathan Xavier	Joseph	Jesse	Natasha
Lévod	Nicole Juana	Noah	Michelle	Rodney
Shunteria	Osvaldo Richard	Rachel	Nicole	Shirley
Tykema	Stephanie Maria	Samuel	Sean	Stephanie
Tyshika	William Jose	Sarah		Watson
Vavakia				

Note. From "What's a Name?" by Debbie Sontag, May 25, 1989, *The Miami Herald*, p. 1F.

Breast or Bottle?

Today there is a great deal more interest in and support for breast-feeding than there was a decade or two ago. Much of this support has come from women's groups and the American Academy of Pediatrics (1982), which recommends that all mothers attempt to breast-feed their babies. There are a number of compelling reasons for breast-feeding babies.

1. Mother's milk contains nutrients necessary for optimal infant growth and development. Although commercial formulas try to simulate breast milk, there is really no substitute for the real thing.
2. Breast milk has immune properties that protect the neonate from both viral and bacterial infections. This protection includes diarrhea, which is a serious health problem for infants, especially in third world countries.
3. Breast milk is agreeable to babies.
4. Mother's milk is sanitary and there is little, if any, contamination. Sanitation in infant feeding is a serious concern especially in third world countries where safe water supplies may be unavailable.
5. Breast-feeding can enhance the mother-infant bond.
6. Breast-fed infants are more "in charge," since unlike a bottle-fed baby, they are not encouraged to drink all the formula in the bottle.

Frequently, the economy of breastfeeding is cited as an advantage—after all, it is free. However, the cost of formula and mother's milk are about the same when the added nutritional intake to support the mother's lactation is taken into consideration.

For mothers who breast-feed, however, there are three important considerations. First, they must have an adequate caloric and fluid intake to support breast-feeding. For example, mothers need to drink a lot of fluids and must maintain an adequate supply of calcium by eating and drinking dairy products or using a calcium supplement. Second,

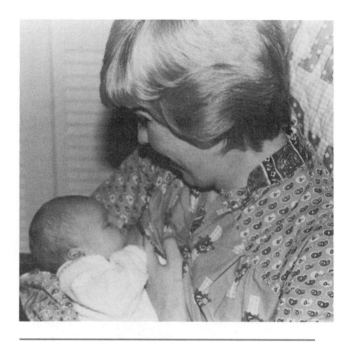

FIGURE 5-20 Breast feeding is now very popular and contributes to the optimal development of infants' physical and social development. (From Anderson/BASIC MATERNAL-NEWBORN NURSING, copyright 1989 by Delmar Publishers Inc.)

nursing mothers must be cautious about the effects birth control pills, caffeine, nicotine, and other drugs have on their babies. Nursing babies may be the unintended recipients of medication or other substances secreted through their mother's milk. Also, birth control medication will interfere with the production of milk. Third, the breast-fed baby's taste preferences are influenced by her mother's diet. Consequently, the greater taste experiences gained by a nursing infant will make it easier to wean her than the bottle-fed baby (Crook, 1987). Learning as a result of breast-feeding would then seem to play a powerful role in the development of food and flavor preferences and aversions beginning at birth.

Breast-feeding, supplemented with vitamin D, fluoride, and iron, meets the total nutritional needs of the neonate and the infant until about five or six months of age (Owen, 1980, p. 38).

Two obstacles that seem to prevent new mothers from making a positive decision about breast-feeding their babies are a lack of knowledge regarding the benefits of breast-feeding for babies, and views about the personal, social, and physical inconveniences of breast-feeding. Therefore, programs designed to inform prospective and new parents about breast-feeding would do well to stress the positive benefits breast-feeding has for babies, to address parents' concerns about personal inconveniences, and help parents see how they can manage and overcome such inconveniences (Baranowski, Rassin, Richardson, Brown, & Bee, 1986). There are many support agencies that help parents with breast-feeding. One of these, the La Leche League International (9696 Minneapolis Ave., P.O. Box 1209, Franklin Park, IL) holds monthly meetings for mothers in all parts of the United States.

SIDS

Sudden Infant Death Syndrome (SIDS), also known as crib death, is one of the more perplexing causes of death in infants and occurs in about one to three per thousand live births. SIDS is of unknown origin and is defined as sudden and unexpected death without an adequate medical cause. Most SIDS deaths occur at night while the infant is asleep on its stomach. Siblings of SIDS infants are more at risk than other children. (See Figure 5–21.) Another group at risk for SIDS are those infants who have suffered *infantile apnea;* they have stopped breathing and have been brought back to life. These two groups usually require home apnea monitoring.

Responding to Babies' Cries

Mothers and pregnant women who have not had children (nulliparous) seem to be "predisposed" to correctly understand infants' cries and what they "mean" better than single women or married women without children (Adachi & Okada, 1985).

Factors	Occurrence
Incidence	2 to 3:1000 live births
Peak age	3 to 4 months, 90% occur by 6 months
Sex	Higher percentage of males affected
Time of death	Always during sleep
Time of year	Increased incidence in winter
Racial	Greater incidence in nonwhites
Socioeconomic	Increased occurrence in lower socioeconomic class
Birth	Higher incidence in: Premature infants Multiple births Neonates with low Apgar scores Infants with central nervous system disturbances
Feeding habits	Not significant, breast-feeding does not prevent SIDS
Siblings	Five times greater incidence

FIGURE 5-21 SIDS or sudden infant death snydrome as a cause of infant death concerns all parents. Researchers continue to search for its cause and for ways to prevent its occurrence.

Babies' crying serves many useful functions and it should not be viewed or reacted to negatively by parents and care-givers. This is easier said than done in everyday life, especially when parents are upset and tired, inexperienced, or indifferent. Nevertheless, early parent-neonate interaction patterns are established around such major child care issues as crying, feeding, and sleeping. As Lester (1985) points out, crying provides an opportunity for positive social interaction, and when positively responded to, rewards parents in two ways. The crying ceases and this, in turn, creates the possibility for playful interactions.

Parents tune into this channel [crying], learn to understand what their infant is trying to say (how to read their baby) through the rhythm and other qualities of the cry, and establish the foundation

of a communications system. Parents learn to mod-
ulate and manage their infant's crying by supplying
verbal and nonverbal feedback, which in itself is
rhythmic, establishing early cycles of social interaction. In soothing an infant, we introduce cadence
and patterning to our voices; we use rocking,
walking, music, sucking on a pacifier—all forms
of rhythmic stimulation that establish the temporal
patterning of social interaction (Lester, 1985, p. 7).

Crying serves the following useful functions:

1. Promotes contact with the care-giver.
2. Plays a role in physiological processes by
   increasing pulmonary capacity, generating
   heat, contributing to thermoregulation, and
   signals the care-giver of hunger or stress.
3. Cessation of crying often leads to alertness,
   which serves to regulate input from the environment and promote stimulus intake.
4. Acts as a defensive response by signaling and
   leading to stimulus rejection (Lester, 1985,
   p. 9).

Soothing Babies

All parents and care-givers are faced with how
to soothe a crying baby. Indeed, the effectiveness
of parents and care-givers is often judged by their
ability to soothe a fussy baby. Two methods for
soothing that are effective are the application of
continuous and monotonous stimulation and
rhythmic stimulation. Wrapping—also known as
bundling and swaddling—in a soft blanket provides continuous tactile stimulation, and rocking
and mild jiggling provide rhythmic stimulation
(Reisman, 1987).

Korner and Thoman (1972) found that movement *and* the act of lifting the infant from a supine
(lying down) position to upright at the shoulder
was more effective than lifting to the horizontal
position and cuddling. Many parents seem to intuitively know that motion soothes a fussy baby
and use many methods to provide movement from
walking to rocking to taking the baby for a ride
in the car. Incidently, with regard to rocking, a

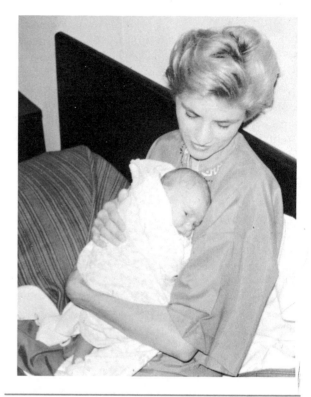

FIGURE 5-22 All parents—at one time or another—
indeed on many occasions, have had to soothe a crying
baby. Motion and soft sounds are two things that are
beneficial in determining what will soothe a baby best.
(From Anderson/BASIC MATERNAL-NEWBORN NURSING,
copyright 1989 by Delmar Publishers Inc.)

high amplitude—five inches or more—and a high
frequency work best (Pederson & TerVrught, 1973).
So, if you are going to rock a baby to soothe it,
rock away!

However, soothing a crying baby is one thing
and putting a baby to sleep for the sake of putting
it to sleep is quite another matter. Babies need
periods of quiet alertness in order to receive the
stimulation necessary for emotional, physical, and
intellectual development. Neither a care-giver nor
a parent should have as one of their primary goals
a constantly sleeping baby. Holding a baby in the
upright, over-the-shoulder position other than just

to soothe him is important, for it gives him an optimal opportunity to scan his environment. Other effective soothing procedures include the use of a pacifier, since babies usually require and want more sucking than feeding provides, and soft sounds, such as the mother's voice and music.

Good maternal care contributes to attachment. Such care is characterized by a quality of responsiveness and sensitivity to the infant as a person. Alan Sroufe (1978) offers the following advice about the care-giver role in promoting attachment:

> Good maternal care involves responding to the infant's signals promptly and effectively. When, during face-to-face interaction the infant turns his head away, signaling that he needs less stimulation, the sensitive care-giver relaxes and waits. Not until the baby signals his readiness does she reengage him. When the infant cries, the sensitive care-giver responds promptly, and effectively puts an end to the infant's distress. When the baby seeks contact, the sensitive care-giver responds warmly and affectionately, teaching the infant that his signals are effective. The sensitive care-giver provides smooth transitions and meshes her (or his) stimulation or assistance with the infant's behavior. She does not thrust interaction on an unresponsive infant. Sensitivity requires that the mother respond to the individual needs and nature of her infant. This is why sensitive care generally promotes healthy emotional development in vastly different babies (p. 57).

Neonate/Care-giver Styles

The interplay between temperament and environment plays a role in personality development. Consequently, care-givers need to consider the nature of this interaction for children in their care. For example, the easy child who adapts readily to various child-rearing styles may have difficulty adapting to an authoritative-restrictive parenting style after previously adapting to a laissez-faire style, characterized by freedom and independence.

Parents with a difficult child may intuitively treat the child in an authoritative, restrictive, and punitive manner. When parents are inconsistent, impatient, or punitive in their handling of their children, however, their children are more likely to react negatively than other children.

One key to good child rearing with the slow-to-warm-up child is to allow him to develop at his own pace. This does not mean leaving the child alone to do whatever he wants to do. He needs encouragement and support—not pushing—to participate in new activities.

The importance of developing a match between a child's temperament and the parent/care-giver's child-rearing style cannot be overemphasized. This is particularly true in child care programs. In this sense, parenting is a process that extends beyond the natural parents to include all those who care and provide services to infants. It is reasonable to expect that all who are part of this parenting cluster will accommodate their behavior to account for infants' basic temperaments.

What to Do with a Colicky Baby

Between 7 and 23 percent of babies under three months suffer from *colic*, characterized by pain and cramping of the stomach accompanied by loud, incessant, inconsolable crying that can last for hours and usually occurs early in the evening. The cause or causes of colic are not really known, but some suspected reasons are: too rapid feeding, swallowing of excess air, inadequate burping, excess gas production in the lower intestines where it is trapped, an immature nervous system, irregular sleep-wake patterns, and sensitivity to cow's milk. While colicky babies continue to thrive and colic is not considered a life-threatening or major ailment, it can and does have an intense impact on mother/parent/family-child relationships. Colic can disrupt daily and nightly routines, leaving parents physically and emotionally fatigued, with feelings of anger, frustration, and inadequacy.

The best remedy for colic, if indeed there is one, is vestibular stimulation. Parents try everything from rocking to walking to mild jiggling to placing their baby in a baby carrier strapped to the top of a clothes dryer, to buying such products as *Sleep Tight*, which consists of a 3.5 pound vibration unit that attaches to the springs of the baby's crib, and a sound unit that simulates sounds passing a closed car window at fifty-five miles per hour. *Sleep Tight* was tested in the Infant Colic Research Project supported by the National Institute of Child Health and Human Development, and reduced the colic symptoms in fifty-eight of sixty infants ("Invention Eases," 1988). Other remedies include a hot water bottle filled with warm water and placed on the baby's abdomen, lying the baby on her stomach on a lambskin rug, and gentle massage of the stomach. Fortunately for colicky babies and their parents, after about three months the incidence of colic decreases.

In any interactions with and while caring for their infant, parents should avoid overstimulating him. They should be responsive to their infant's temperament and states, taking their leads from their baby. When the baby is sleeping, they should allow him to sleep, and when he is awake and alert, they should "read" his signals, so that the relationship is enjoyable for everyone.

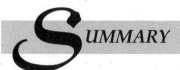

SUMMARY

- At birth, babies look different from what their parents might expect. A baby may be covered with blood, have hair covering her body (lanugo) and her skin may be wrinkled. Some babies have birthmarks as well as marks associated with delivery. A baby's face may have a flat and squashed look, called molding. Fontanelles enable the head to accommodate passage through the birth canal.
- Acquired immune deficiency syndrome, or AIDS, is emerging as one of the leading threats to neonatal health.
- The neonate begins breathing movements prior to life. Four categories of stimuli contribute to the initiation of respiration: chemical, sensory, thermal, and mechanical.
- Life-threatening and life-saving cardiovascular changes occur shortly after birth. The foramen ovale closes, the ductus arteriosus collapses, and the ductus venosus is closed with the clamping of the umbilical cord. These changes in blood flow enable the neonate to make the transition to extrauterine life.
- The presence of excess bilirubin can cause jaundice. Therapy includes placing the neonate under ultraviolet light.
- The neonate is capable of ingesting nourishment and eliminating waste. Although the neonate is capable of many neurological functions, the brain is only 25 percent developed, underscoring the importance of nutrition early in life. An important neonatal metabolic function is the ability to produce heat and maintain body temperature. Immediately after birth, the neonate passes through states of reactivity, inactivity, and reactivity.
- Virginia Apgar developed a scale for assessing the physical conditions of neonates immediately following birth.
- T. Berry Brazelton developed the Brazelton Neonatal Behavioral Assessment Scale, which assesses twenty-seven behavioral items and twenty reflex measures.
- Routine medical procedures following delivery include placing solution or ointment in the eyes, an injection of vitamin K, and a test for PKU.

■ Neonates demonstrate a wide range of reflexes. These include: sucking, tonic neck, Moro, grasping, plantar, stepping, walking, crawling, swimming, rooting, Babinski, and Babkin. Reflexes have protective, survival, and adaptive value.

■ Neonates are capable of a wide range of behaviors. Child development professionals, parents, and the public are increasingly recognizing and understanding many of these remarkable abilities. Neonatal visual acuity is between 20/150 and 20/800 at birth, but rapidly improves to a normal 20/20 at eighteen months. Babies can see forms, and they like the shape and complexity of the human face better than other forms. Neonates can see color and prefer looking at colored patterns of red/gray, green/gray and yellow/gray. Babies are quite proficient at imitating the facial expressions of their parents and care-givers. Neonates also have a well-developed sense of taste and smell.

■ Neonates are in the sensorimotor stage of cognitive development and are actively involved in constructing their intelligence. Through assimilation, accommodation, and equilibrium, neonates develop sensorimotor schemes that help them interact with and learn about the world. Neonates are in Stage One—the reflexive action stage—of intellectual development.

■ Evidence of neonates' abilities to learn is provided through reinforcement and habituation studies.

■ Approximately one of every fourteen babies is born before they are ready. Many factors contribute to prematurity, including the mother's age, weight, social background, stress, trauma, and type of prenatal care. Premature neonates face many obstacles, including respiratory difficulties, body temperature maintenance, and digestive problems.

■ Technology, such as the constant positive pressure ventilation machine, makes it possible to save premature infants, but also causes harm that may be with a child for a lifetime. Dehydration, the lack of an immune system, and immature organs all create life-threatening problems for preemies.

■ Parents of premature neonates have a difficult time in their parenting roles and need help and support to successfully meet the many demands placed on them.

■ Many legal, economic, and ethical issues are associated with helping to save infants born before their time.

■ Massage has a positive therapeutic effect on premature neonates and is being used to promote development and reduce hospitalization costs.

■ Crying is the beginning of language development and represents the first communication between parent and child.

■ Social relationships begin at birth and babies have a variety of social skills, such as crying and imitative behavior.

■ Bonding enables parents and care-givers to become emotionally attached to children. Attachment is the emotional tie that exists between parents and children. Bonding behaviors used by adults include touching, eye contact, speech, and attention. Although their is much interest in the idea of early parent-infant bonding, there is not universal agreement that it is as deterministic as previously thought.

■ Every child has individual behavioral characteristics or ways of responding to the world and to people. Based on these behavioral characteristics, researchers have identified three classes of children: easy, slow-to-warm-up, and difficult.

■ The first stage of Erikson's psychosocial stages of development, Basic Trust vs. Mistrust, begins at birth and ends at eighteen months. Basic trust develops when children are reared in a context of love, warmth, and support.

■ As many as 10 percent of newborn children will suffer from failure to thrive (FTT), a condition associated with health, parental, and environmental conditions.

■ There are six compelling reasons for encouraging mothers to breast-feed their babies. These include the nutritional and immune properties of breast milk; the fact that it is sanitary and agreeable to babies; the fact that babies are in charge of their own feeding; and that it enhances bonding. Mothers must eat enough to support milk production and should avoid medications.

■ Babies' crying serves many useful functions, including the initiation of positive social interactions. It also increases pulmonary capacity, leads to periods of alertness, and acts as a defensive response.

■ The application of continuous stimulation, such as wrapping and rhythmic stimulation, are two effective ways to soothe a baby. It is important for parents to develop a parenting style that "fits" their child's temperament.

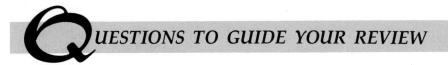

QUESTIONS TO GUIDE YOUR REVIEW

1. What do newborn children look like? Why is their appearance different from what parents often expect?
2. Why do newborn babies look the way they do?
3. Why do babies' heads look molded after birth? What makes this molding possible?
4. What respiratory adjustments must neonates make to their new world?
5. What cardiovascular changes take place in the neonate shortly after birth?
6. What is jaundice and why do neonates have it? How is jaundice treated?
7. What metabolic adaptations does the neonate make at birth?
8. What are the purposes of "periods of reactivity?"
9. What is the Apgar scale? Is it possible for a baby to have a score of 10?
10. What is the Brazelton Neonatal Behavioral Assessment Scale?
11. What physical tests and procedures are conducted immediately after birth and why are they important?
12. What are the primary reflexive actions babies are born with? What are their purposes and why are they important?
13. What are the neonatal states that Wolff describes?
14. Why are children born prematurely?
15. What are some of the procedures to help premature infants survive? What are the ethical issues surrounding the care of premature infants?
16. Why do premature neonates have difficulty making adjustments to extrauterine life?
17. What ecological influences impact on the neonate?
18. Why is massage important and what positive therapeutic affect does it have on premature infants?

19. How does language development occur in the first month of life?
20. What is circumcision and what is the controversy surrounding its routine practice?
21. What visual abilities do neonates possess and what are their implications for normal development?
22. What sensory abilities do neonates have? What role do sensory abilities play in development?
23. What are sensorimotor schemes? How do neonates begin the process of cognitive development?
24. What are the six stages of cognitive development in the sensorimotor period?
25. What social abilities does the neonate possess? What purposes do they serve?
26. What are attachment and bonding? Are they important? Why?
27. What is temperament? How are the temperaments of babies different? What implications do temperaments have for parenting?
28. What can parents do to promote basic trust in their children?
29. Why should mothers try to breast-feed their babies?
30. What are the advantages of mother's milk to babies?
31. What is SIDS?
32. What are the best ways for parents to soothe a fussy baby?
33. What purposes does crying serve? How should parents respond to babies' cries?

 CTIVITIES FOR FURTHER INVOLVEMENT

1. Abortion is an issue and topic that is very much in the news and on the minds of the American public.
    a. Develop a list of topics showing the pros and cons of abortion. Try to be unbiased in presenting both points of view.
    b. Invite speakers from both pro- and anti-abortion groups to speak to your class.
2. What implications does fetal surgery have for parents? Children?
    a. Invite a fetal surgeon and a neonatal specialist to address your class regarding advances in their fields. Emphasize the demands placed on parents regarding choices and the impact of those choices on their families' lives.
    b. Comment on the statement: "Parents should be satisfied with the children that are born to them, they shouldn't fool around with nature."
3. Caring for a newborn baby is not always an easy task for many first-time parents.
    a. Develop a pamphlet that provides new parents with tips or guidelines for caring for their new baby.
    b. One area new parents frequently have difficulty with is getting their baby on a schedule. Ask experienced parents for their advice to new parents about developing and maintaining a feeding and sleeping schedule for their babies.
4. Talk to mothers who are nursing and those who are not nursing their newborn babies.
    a. Identify the reasons new mothers give for nursing and not nursing their new babies.

  b. Identify the problems, pleasures, and advantages encountered by both groups.
  c. Identify the newest products, such as nipples and bottles, used in bottle feeding.
5. Bonding and attachment are very important topics in child development and parenting.
  a. What behaviors, such as feeding and comforting, can parents do that will help them bond with their baby?
  b. What are some of the variables that affect and influence bonding and attachment? What can parents and others do to counteract those variables that may interfere with bonding and attachment?
  c. What behaviors in particular can mothers and others do to help fathers engage in bonding and attachment behaviors?

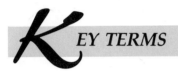

KEY TERMS

Accommodation Changing schemes to fit new knowledge.

Adaptation The processes of assimilation and accommodation.

Apgar scoring system A scale for assessing the physical state of neonates following birth.

Apnea The cessation of breathing.

Assimilation Fitting or adding new knowledge into already existing schemes of reality.

Attachment The emotional tie between the infant and the parents or other primary care-givers. As such, it is a unique relationship between two people that is specific and endures through time.

Bilirubin A bile pigment produced by the breakdown of hemoglobin.

Bonding The process by which parents and other care-givers become emotionally attached to infants. The development of a close, personal, affective relationship.

Brazelton Neonatal Behavioral Assessment Scale A scale composed of twenty-seven behavioral items and twenty measures of reflexes that assess neonatal capabilities.

Circumcision From the Latin *circumcidere*, meaning "to cut around." The surgical removal of the foreskin (prepuce) from the penis.

Colostrum A substance secreted from the breasts prior to the production of milk.

Constructivism The process of continually organizing, structuring, and restructuring experiences into existing schemes of thought.

Ductus arteriosus A connection that diverts blood away from the lungs during fetal life.

Ductus venosus A blood vessel that diverts blood from the fetal liver.

Equilibrium A balance between assimilation and accommodation, between new experiences and old ideas, between what the world is really like and a person's view of the world.

Extrauterine Descriptive of life outside the womb.

Failure to thrive (FTT) A condition without a diagnosed medical cause, characterized by underdevelopment and lethargy.

Flexion The bent position of the neonate as a result of its position in utero.

Fontanelle Wide areas of membranous tissue at the juncture of the sutures on the top of the neonate's head.

Foramen ovale The hole between the top

two chambers of the neonate's heart that partially closes a few hours after birth.

Gavage feeding Method by which a tube is inserted via the nose or mouth into the stomach and a syringe is used to insert formula through the tube.

Habituation The process whereby infants become accustomed to certain stimuli, such as odor, sight, taste and sound, and, as a result, no longer respond to them.

Kinesthesis The sense of body movement and position in space.

Lanugo A fine, down-like hair present on the skin of neonates.

Meconium The first stool passed by the neonate.

Milia "Milk spots" or tiny spots that appear on the cheeks, chin, and nose of neonates.

Myelinization Production of a sheath around nerve fibers.

Patent ductus arteriosus A persistent opening in the neonatal ductus arteriosus. When serious enough and when medical management cannot correct the condition, then neonatal surgery is necessary.

Pathological jaundice Jaundice that appears in the first twenty-four hours after birth. Usually caused by an Rh negative mother who delivers an Rh positive baby.

Phenylketonuria (PKU) The inability to convert the amino acid phenylalanine found in breast milk and most formulas. When untreated, the neonate fails to thrive, followed by central nervous system and mental retardation.

Physiological jaundice A yellowish appearance of the skin and whites of the eyes that may occur between forty-eight and seventy-two hours after birth.

Premature Characteristic of an infant born before the completion of the thirty-seventh week of gestation, regardless of weight.

Reflex The purest form of reaction to an external stimulus.

Scheme The cognitive structures or units of knowledge that change and adapt as a result of experiences and maturation.

Sensorimotor schemes The first schemes of intelligence.

Stereopsis The ability to perceive the relative distance of objects.

Supine Lying in a face-up position.

Sutures Bands of connective tissue between the bones on the top of the head.

Temperament Infants' unique individual behavioral characteristics and how they approach and react to life, situations, and people.

Visual acuity The ability to see clearly near and far objects. Normal visual acuity is 20/20.

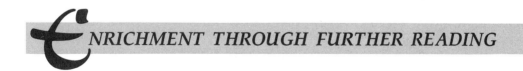

ENRICHMENT THROUGH FURTHER READING

Eiger, M. S., & Olds, Sally Wendkos. (1987). *The complete book of breastfeeding.* New York: Workman.

    An excellent guide to everything parents need to know about breast-feeding their baby.

Gustaitis, R., & Young, E. W. D. *A time to be born, a time to die: Conflicts and ethics in an intensive care nursery.* Reading, MA: Addison-Wesley.

    Matters relating to life and death are almost routine in today's intensive care nurseries.

This book examines the decisions made in these nurseries and how they affect families, infants, and medical personnel.

Maurer, D., & Maurer, C. (1988). *The world of the newborn.* New York: Basic Books.
The Maurers attempt to make the reader understand what the world looks like to infants. They begin by taking readers inside the womb and helping them understand that the adult's world is vastly different from that of infants.

Nance, S. (1982). *Premature babies.* New York: Arbor House.
Written by mothers who have coped with the stresses, challenges, and joys of caring for their premature infants. Covers all aspects of "preemie care."

Pfister, F. R., & Griesemer, B. (1983). *The littlest baby: A handbook for parents of premature children.* Englewood Cliffs, NJ: Prentice-Hall.
A fascinating story of Falecia Pfister who weighed less than two pounds at birth and spent the first three and one-half months of her life in an intensive care nursery.

Weissbluth, M. (1984). *Crybabies, coping with colic: What to do when baby won't stop crying.* New York: Arbor House.
An interesting blend of medical research and practical suggestions on how to deal with colic. Useful discussion of drug treatment for colic.

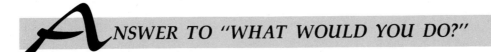

ANSWER TO "WHAT WOULD YOU DO?"

The controversy surrounding what a parent can and cannot do is fueled by two factors; first, growing numbers of parents who want to derive some meaning from the heart-breaking experience of having a baby with anencephaly, and second, the shortage of available organs for the very young.

Some of the ethical issues involved in a decision of any kind are these:

1. Is it morally defensible to prolong human life for the sole purpose of providing organs? A related issue is whether or not medical technology and skill should be used to prolong life for the sole purpose of finding organ recipients.
2. As presented in the ethical dilemma, the issue of when "death" has occurred in neonates is still unresolved.
3. For some people, the specter of human organ farms is already on the horizon. They maintain such practices demean human life and will lead to all kinds of abuses including selling organs to the highest bidders. *Ectogenesis* is the growth and development of a fetus outside its mother's womb during the period when it would normally be in the womb.

Many of the decisions about what is and what is not permissible in terms of human life and organ donations are dependent upon state law. Consequently, for the definitive answer to "What Would You Do?," you should consult the laws and court decisions of your particular state. For example, in the state of Florida, F.S. 1987, ch. 732.912, states that "any of the following persons may give all or any part of the decedent's body. . . . (a) the spouse of the decedent; (b) an adult son or daughter of the decedent; (c) either parent of the decedent; (d) an adult brother or sister of the decedent; and, (e) a guardian of the person of the decedent at the time of his death." In addition, a Florida case, *John F. Kennedy Hospital v. Bludworth*, 452 So.2d 921 (Fla. 1984),

> . . . concluded that a decision by parents supported by competent medical advice that their young child suffers from a permanent, incurable, and irreversible physical or mental defect likely to soon result in the child's death should ordinarily be sufficient without court approval. The court pointed out, however, that although judicial intervention need not be solicited as a matter of course, the courts must always be open to hear these matters on request of the family, guardian, affected medical personnel, or the state. It acknowledged that in cases where doubt exists or where there is a lack of concurrence among the family, physicians, and the hospital, or where an affected party simply desires a judicial order, then the court must be available to consider the matter (pp. 925–926).

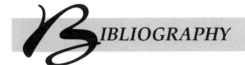

BIBLIOGRAPHY

Adachi, T., & Okada, H. (1985). Acoustic properties of infant cries and maternal perception. *Tohoku Psychologica Folia, 44,* 51–58.

Adams, R., Maurer, D. & Davis, M. (1986). Newborns' discrimination of chromatic from achromatic stimuli. *Journal of Experimental Child Psychology, 41,* 267–281.

AIDS infants malformed. (1986, August 12). *The New York Times.*

American Academy of Pediatrics. (1982). Promotion of breast feeding. *Pediatrics, 69,* 654–660.

Apgar, V. (1966). The newborn (Apgar) scoring system, reflections and advice. *Pediatric Clinic of North America, 13,* 645.

Baranowski, T., Rassin, D., Richardson, C. J., Brown, J., & Bee, D. (1986). Attitudes toward breastfeeding. *Developmental and Behavioral Pediatrics, 7,* 367–372.

Barkan, S. E., & Bracken, M. B. (1987). Delayed childbearing: No evidence for the increased risk of low birth weight and preterm delivery. *American Journal of Epidemiology, 125,* 101–109.

Bithoney, W. G., & Newberger, E. H. (1987). Child and family attributes of failure to thrive. *Developmental and Behavioral Pediatrics, 8,* 32–36.

Blakeslee, S. (1987, December 14). New attention focused on infant organ donors. *The New York Times,* p. 18.

Brazelton, T. B. (1973). *The neonatal behavioral assessment scale.* Philadelphia: J.B. Lippincott.

Breese, K. M. Director of Employee Relations, Oster/Sunbeam. (1988, July 13). Telephone conversation with the author.

Crnic, K., & Greenberg, M. (1987, April). *Early family predictors of developmental and social competence of risk and normal children at age five.* Paper presented at the bienniel meeting of the Society for Research in Child Development, Baltimore, MD.

Crook, C. (1979). The organization and control of infant sucking. In H. Reese & L. P. Lipsitt (Eds.), *Advances in child development and behavior:* Vol. 14 (pp. 209–251). New York: Academic Press.

Crook, C. (1987). Taste and olfaction. In P. Salapatek & L. Cohen (Eds.), *Handbook of infant perception: Vol. 1. From sensation to perception* (pp. 237–264). Orlando: Harcourt Brace Jovanovich.

Elliman, A. M., Bryan, E. M., & Elliman, A. D. (1986). Low birth weight babies at 3 years of age. *Child Care, Health and Development, 12,* 287–311.

Erikson, E. (1963). *Childhood and society.* New York: Norton.

Fantz, R. (1961). The origin of form perception. *Scientific American, 204,* 66–72.

Field, T., Woodsen, R., Greenberg, R., & Cohen, D. (1982). Discrimination and imitation of facial expressions by neonates. *Science, 218,* 179–181.

Forman, M. R., Meirik, O., & Berendes, H. W. (1984). Delayed childrearing in Sweden. *JAMA, 252:* 3135–61.

Freudenheim, M. (1988, December 28). In pursuit of the punctual baby. *The New York Times,* p. 25.

Gold, S. (1983). Parent-infant bonding: Another look. *Child Development, 54,* 1355–1382.

Goleman, D. (1988, February 2). The experience of touch: Research points to a critical role. *The New York Times,* pp. 17 and 20.

Haith, M. (1986). Sensory and perceptual processes in early infancy. *The Journal of Pediatrics, 109,* 158–171.

Harlow, H. F., & Harlow, M. K. (1962). Social deprivation in monkeys. *Scientific American, 207,* 136–144.

Invention eases colic symptoms. (1988, January–February). *Children Today, 17,* 2.

Klaus, M. H., & Kennell, J. H. (1982). *Parent-infant bonding* (2nd ed.). St. Louis: C. V. Mosby.

Korner, A. F., & Thoman, E. B. (1972). The relative efficacy of contact and vestibular-proprioceptive stimulation in soothing neonates. *Child Development, 43,* 443–453.

Lamb, M. E. (1981). *The role of the father in child development* (2nd ed.). New York: John Wiley.

Lambert, B. (1988, January 13). One in 61 babies in New York has AIDS antibodies, study says. *The New York Times,* p. 1.

Lapierre, D. (1985). *The city of joy.* Garden City, NY: Doubleday.

Lester, B. M. (1985). There's more to crying than meets the ear. In B. M. Lester and Boukydis, C. F. Z. (Eds.) *Infant crying* (pp. 1–27). New York: Plenum Press.

Lipsitt, L. P. (1977). Taste in human neonates: Its effects on sucking and heart rate. In J. M. Weiffenbach (Ed.), *Taste and development: The genesis of sweet preference* (pp. 125–140). Bethesda, MD: National Institutes of Health. (HEW [NIH] 77–1068).

Lipsitt, L. P. (1986). Learning in infancy: Cognitive development in babies. *The Journal of Pediatrics, 109,* 173.

Lipsitt, L. P., & Kaye, H. (1964). Conditioned sucking in the human newborn. *Psychometric Science, 1,* 29–30.

McFarlane, A. (1978). What a baby knows. *Human Nature, 1,* 74–81.

Meltzoff, A., & Moore, K. M. (1983). Newborn infants imitate adult facial gestures. *Child Development, 54,* 703–709.

Morrison, G. S. (1988). *Education and development of infants, toddlers and preschoolers.* Glenview, IL: Scott, Foresman.

Myers, B. J. (1987). Mother-infant bonding as a critical period. In M. H. Bornstein (Ed.), *Sensitive periods in development: Interdisciplinary perspectives.* Hillsdale, NJ: Lawrence Erlbaum.

Neeson, J. D., & May, K. A. (1986). *Comprehensive maternity nursing.* Philadelphia: J.B. Lippincott.

Nickel, R. E., Forrest, B. C., & Lamson, F. N. (1982). School performance of children with birth weights of 1,000 g or less. *American Journal of Disabled Children, 136,* 105–110.

Nowlis, G. H., & Kessen, W. (1976). Human newborns differentiate differing concentrations of sucrose and glucose. *Science, 191,* 865.

Owen, A. L. (1980). *Feeding guide: A nutritional guide for the maturing infant.* Bloomfield, NJ: Health Learning Systems.

Papousek, H. A. (1967). Conditioning during early postnatal development. In Y. Brackbill & G. B. Thompson (Eds.), *Behavior in infancy and early childhood.* New York: Free Press.

Pederson, D., & TerVrught, D. (1973). The influence of amplitude and frequency of vestibular stimulation on the activity of two-month-old infants. *Child Development, 44,* 122–128.

Reisman, J. E. (1987). Touch, motion and proprioception. In P. Salapatek & L. Cohen (Eds.), *Handbook of infant perception: Vol. 1. From sensation to perception.* (pp. 265–303). Orlando: Harcourt Brace Jovanovich.

Rose, S., Schmidt, K., Riese, M., & Bridger, W. (1980). Effects of prematurity and early intervention on responsivity to tactile stimuli: A comparison of preterm and full-term infants. *Child Development, 51,* 416–425.

Rosenstein, D., & Oster, H. (1988). Differential facial responses to four basic tastes in newborns. *Child Development, 59,* 1562.

Self, P. A., Horowitz, F. D., & Paden, L. Y. (1972). Olfaction in newborn infants. *Developmental Psychology, 7,* 349–363.

Serunian, S. A., & Broman, S. H. (1975). Relationship of Apgar scores and Bayley mental and motor scores. *Child Development, 46,* 699.

Shanberg, S. M., & Field, T. M. (1987). Sensory deprivation stress and supplemental stimulation in the rat pup and preterm human neonate. *Child Development, 58,* 1431–1447.

Simon, N. (1983). Preventing prematurity. *Parents, Vol.58, Sept.)* pp. 74–79.

Sontag, D. What's a name? (1989, May 25). *The Miami Herald,* p. 1F.

Spitz, R. A. (1965). *The first year of life.* New York: International Universities Press.

Sroufe, A. L. (1978). Attachment and the roots of competence. *Human Nature, 1,* 57.

Thomas, A., Chess, S., & Birch, T. (1970). The origin of personality. *Scientific American, 223,* 102–109.

Whaley, L. F., & Wong, D. L. (1985). *Essentials of pediatric nursing* (2nd ed.). St. Louis: C.V. Mosby.

Whaley, L. F., & Wong, D. L. (1987). *Nursing care of infants and children.* St. Louis: C.V. Mosby.

Wheeler-Liston, C. (1986). *Parents and preemies: Nurturing the preemie.* Dallas: Touchpoints.

When life begins at two pounds. (1986, Fall). *Portraits* (Health and Wellness Publication). Miami, FL: North Shore Hospital and Medical Center.

Wolff, P. (1971). Mother-infant relations at birth. In J. G. Howels (Ed.), *Modern perspectives in international child psychiatry* (pp. 20–97). New York: Brunner/Mazel.

Wolff, P. (1973). The classification of states. In J. L. Stone, H. T. Smith, & L. B. Murphy (Eds.), *The competent infant* (pp. 269–272). New York: Basic Books.

CHAPTER SIX

Infancy: life's first year

◆

VIGNETTE
INTRODUCTION
CHANGING VIEWS OF INFANCY
In the Spotlight: Brian's Weekly
  Schedule
THE IMPORTANCE OF INFANCY
MODELS OF DEVELOPMENT
PHYSICAL DEVELOPMENT
Height and Weight
Dental Development
Motor Development
In the Spotlight: Is Beauty in the
  Eye of the Beholder?
Visual Development
Taste and Smell in Infancy
Touch and Motion
INTELLECTUAL DEVELOPMENT
Stage II (One to Four Months)
Stage III (Four to Eight Months)
Stage IV (Eight to Twelve Months)
Important Concepts
LANGUAGE DEVELOPMENT
Behaviorism

Heredity
Cognitive Development
Biology
Environmental Influences
Social Interactions
In the Spotlight: Motherese
The Emergence of Language
Communication: Games Infants
  Play
ATTACHMENT
Stages of Attachment
The Importance of Attachment
Multiple Attachments
The Quality of Attachment
Maternal Responsiveness and
  Attachment
Want a Happy Baby?—Be Happy!
Fathers and Attachment
NUTRITION
The Importance of Nutrition in the
  Early Years
The Nutritional Needs of Infants
Caloric Intake

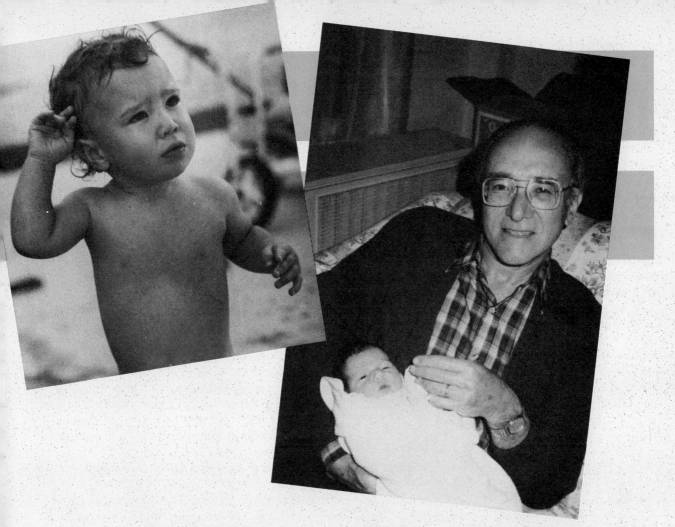

When to Introduce Solid Foods
Nutritional Supplements
Bottle Mouth
PARENTING THE INFANT
In the Spotlight: Dr. Spock—
  Common Sense and Parenting
In the Spotlight: Where Should
  Baby Sleep?
CARING FOR THE INFANT
Safety
Childproofing the Home
Immunizations
STRANGER ANXIETY
What Would You Do?
CHILD CARE FOR INFANTS

What Constitutes Quality Infant Care?
Accreditation
In the Spotlight: Is Child Care
  Good for Infants?
SUMMARY
QUESTIONS TO GUIDE YOUR
  REVIEW
ACTIVITIES FOR FURTHER
  INVOLVEMENT
KEY TERMS
ENRICHMENT THROUGH
  FURTHER READING
ANSWER TO "WHAT WOULD
  YOU DO?"
BIBLIOGRAPHY

⊍IGNETTE

At birth, Joseph Prebianca Jr. weighed seven pounds, nine ounces and was 21 3/4 inches long. His mother, Leslie, was in labor thirty-eight hours. As Leslie explains it, "I went into labor at 9 AM while I was at work. I spotted so I thought I was in labor. I went to the doctor and was only dilated one centimeter, so he told me to go home. Friday I went back to the doctor and I was still only dilated to one centimeter. So he told me to go home and walk around. I went home and walked around for about six hours, hoping I could speed things up. Finally at 2:30 AM on Saturday, I went back and I was still at one centimeter. They don't admit you to the hospital until you are dilated to four centimeters, but since I had been in labor so long, they admitted me. They gave me an epidural block at 8:30 AM and then at 11:00 AM they gave me pitocin to speed the contractions. The baby wouldn't crown, so the doctor had to crown him with his hands. Then all of a sudden, Joey was born. It was really long. I'm glad I didn't have to have a caesarean, because we wanted to have as natural a birth as possible."

Joey is a healthy baby. "The only problem he has had was umbilical granuloma, a tumor like mass on the umbilical area," says Leslie. "After Joey was born, I kept drenching his cord with alcohol like they told me to, and the doctor told me it would dry up, but it didn't. When the cord comes off the internal part organs are supposed to be healed, too. I was afraid that he would have trouble. It kept getting worse and started to drain a little. That's when I took him to the doctor and said, 'This doesn't look right to me.' He sent me to a specialist, and he gave Joey a local anesthesia and removed it. They did a biopsy and there wasn't any intestinal tissue in it. Now, it is healed and is fine."

Leslie breast-fed Joey and weaned him at the end of the fourth month. "He nursed so much I made too much milk. I had to wean him. I was uncomfortable all the time."

"It was hard to get Joey on a schedule," explains Leslie. "Now he is fine, but in the be-ginning, we had a lot of trouble. In fact, it was almost four months until we got things straight-ened out. For the first three months, he slept in a bassinet in our room. Then I put him in the bassinet in his room and then at four months I put him in his crib. But he wouldn't sleep. He'd start crying and I would have to get up and go sleep in his room. I would say to my husband, 'Bye, Honey' and go to Joey's room. Our love life was going down the tubes. I knew we had to do something, so one night we just decided to let him cry. He cried for two nights and that was it. From then on he has slept by himself. He's eleven months now and he sleeps thirteen hours a night. I put him to bed at 8 PM and he wakes up at about 7:30 AM. I give him a bottle and he goes back to sleep for another hour. It's great this way. By then we are dressed, have had breakfast, and I'm ready for him. The next baby I have I'm going to put in the crib in his own room right from the beginning. I've learned my lesson."

"When we first had Joey, we were always going places and doing things. It was hard for us to put him on a schedule and harder for us to keep a schedule. Everything kept throwing him off at the beginning. My mom told me, 'If you let him run you, he will. If that happens, it's over.' My doctor also said to me, 'Look, you have to put him on a schedule.' So I made up my mind and put him on a schedule and I keep him on a schedule. He's a happy baby, and so are we now.

"My husband works hard so I can stay home with Joey. I'm lucky. But, I think we're all better off because I can be with Joey during these form-ative years. My friend sends her little girl, who is the same age as Joey, to a day-care center. Some-times I babysit for her and she wants to be held all the time. She is afraid to do anything. Joey's not afraid to go away from me because he knows I'm here when he wants me. I think it's because he gets the love and attention he needs from me. If he was in a child care center all day, I don't think he would get the attention he should.

"At the end of the first month, I started him

on a little formula. After I weaned him at four months, we had to try three different formulas before we found one that agreed with him. He's on Isomil, a soy-based formula, and he's doing fine."

"Rather than follow a rigid feeding schedule, my doctor said, 'Give him what he wants,' and I do. The doctor said that he doesn't need vitamins, so I don't give him any. The only thing he gets is fluoride in his water. We all drink bottled water because we don't think the local water is good for us. Also, Joey gave up his pacifier at seven months. One day he just didn't want it so I threw it away and he hasn't asked for it since."

Leslie and Joey began going to a "Mommy and Me" class at eight months. "They teach us how to do things with our babies, such as how to substitute one activity for another, so that we don't have to say 'No' all the time. The experience is good for Joey, too, since it gives him a chance to be with other kids."

Joey was between the seventy-fifth and one-hundredth percentiles for normal height and weight. His weight and height for the first year are:

HEIGHT AND WEIGHT CHART FOR JOEY PREBIANCA IN THE FIRST YEAR		
Age	Weight	Height
2 weeks	7 pounds, 14 ounces	21¾ inches
8 weeks	11 pounds, 11 ounces	23 inches
3 months	17 pounds, 6 ounces	24¾ inches
5 months	18 pounds, 9 ounces	26¾ inches
6 months	20 pounds, 6 ounces	28¼ inches
9 months	23½ pounds	30¾ inches
1 year	26 pounds	31 inches

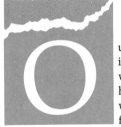

Our knowledge of infancy was in its infancy twenty years ago, but what we have learned since then has dramatically changed the way we perceive and treat infants. We now know that infants are capable of some very sophisticated cognitive acts and have learned all the rudimentary skills of social interaction at a very young age. They make eye contact; use social expressions, such as smiling; understand the rules of conversational turn-taking; and are interactive partners with parents, care-givers, and peers. They can discriminate emotional states in others, they can themselves express emotion, and they are subject to different mood states.

Today, the study of infancy is in its early childhood, and what we have learned makes significant differences in the rearing of infants. Now they are treated as interesting, sophisticated, and impressionable human beings with minds of their own that need careful nurturing and enrichment.

Unfortunately, some adults have gone overboard in seeking to hasten the development of infants into miniature adults.

Many more questions need to be answered before the study of infancy reaches maturity, but basically, I expect we will increasingly see that the infant is a very sophisticated perceiver of the world, with very sensitive social and emotional qualities and impressive intellectual abilities (Field, 1987).

CHANGING VIEWS OF INFANCY

Oftentimes, much of what we believe about children is based on what we think of them as infants. And, particular views of infants depend very much on political, social, and economic conditions. Children are literally products of the times. Today, as our opening introduction indicates, infancy is very much on the center stage in the play of life. This infatuation with infancy and researchers' optimism as they probe the abilities and memories of infants, hoping to discover even more remarkable beings, did not always exist. Shakespeare, for example, in his play *As You Like It*, cast infants in a much different role and portrayed them as "mewling and puking in the nurse's arms." This was not a very complimentary or encouraging portrait and, fortunately for infants and ourselves, quite different from our view of infancy today. However, as recently as a decade or two ago, infancy was often considered a time in which very little occurred:

> For a long time it was thought that in the early weeks of life a baby's senses were not yet capable of taking in any information from the outside world, so that to all intents and purposes he was blind and deaf. Unable to move much either, he seemed a picture of psychological incompetence, of confusion and disorganization. Only the regularity of his experience, provided principally by his parent, was thought to bring order to the baby's mind. Until that was achieved, all he could do was feed and sleep (Schaffer, 1977, p. 27).

Happily, because of our recognition of the importance of infancy as a period of development worthy of study in its own right, neither parents nor infants will need to be constrained and limited by such a narrow view of young children.

Yet, on the other hand, infancy is a precarious time of life, and in many developing countries, 10 percent of all children die before reaching their first year of life (Pollitt, 1988). In 1980, the United Nations General Assembly adopted a resolution that called for the reduction of infant mortality in all countries to fifty per 1,000 live births by the year 2000. To meet this challenge, The United Nations Children's Fund (UNICEF) and the World Health Organization (WHO) have adopted a program to combat infant mortality. This program includes growth monitoring; oral rehydration for infants with severe diarrhea; promotion of breastfeeding; immunization against measles, poliomyelitis, diptheria, pertussis, tetanus, and tuberculosis; female literacy; family planning; and food supplementation (Pollitt, 1988).

TABLE 6–1

DEADLY DISPARITIES (INFANT MORTALITY RATES IN 1986 CALCULATED AS DEATHS IN THE FIRST YEAR PER 1,000 BIRTHS. BOTH RACIAL GROUPS INCLUDE HISPANIC PEOPLE.)

City	Total	White	Black
Boston	13.9	8.4	23.0
Chicago	16.6	10.7	22.9
Dallas	11.8	9.8	16.0
Detroit	20.3	9.7	24.0
District of Columbia	21.1	n.a.	24.0
Indianapolis	14.2	10.7	24.6
Los Angeles	10.1	8.0	21.2
Memphis	15.8	10.7	18.4
New Orleans	15.5	12.5	16.8
New York City	12.4	11.2	15.5
San Diego	9.4	8.7	14.3
United States	**10.4**	**8.9**	**18.0**

TABLE 6–2

INFANT MORTALITY COMPARING THE UNITED STATES AND OTHER DEVELOPED AND UNDERDEVELOPED COUNTRIES

Country	Infant Mortality Rate*
India	104.0
China	44.0
Argentina	35.3
USSR	25.0
Austria	10.3
United States	10.0
Australia	9.8
United Kingdom	9.5
West Germany	8.6
Denmark	8.4
France	8.0
Canada	7.9
Switzerland	6.8
Finland	5.8

* Infant deaths per 1,000 live births.
Note. From "1988 World Population Data Sheet," April 1988, Population Reference Bureau.

The infant mortality rate, the ratio of deaths per thousand live births, is considered a barometer of a nation's interest in and dedication to infants. The United States government, under President Jimmy Carter, set a national goal on reducing infant deaths to nine per 1,000 by the 1990s. Our nation still has a long way to go to reach this commitment. In 1982, the infant mortality rate was 11.2, in 1983, 10.9, in 1984, 10.7, and in 1985, 10.6, the lowest level in the nation's history. In spite of this progress, the infant mortality rate for black children is *twice* that of white children. Table 6–1 shows the rate of infant mortality by major cities for whites and blacks. The leading cause of infant mortality is low birth weight, which can be attributed in part to poor maternal prenatal care.

Also, when compared to other developed countries of the world, the United States does not fare well in its rate of infant mortality, as shown in Table 6–2.

Then, too, there is another, freshly-minted side of the infancy coin. Parents view their job of child rearing and parenting with more fervor and determination than ever. They are goal-directed and look to professional who they think have all the answers. Parents want knowledge about how to bring up bright and successful children. This boom in interest has in turn caused a boom in the publishing business. It is common to see books on bookstore shelves with such titles as *Give Your Child a Superior Mind*, and *Infant Success–Future Success*.

*I*N THE SPOTLIGHT

BRIAN'S WEEKLY SCHEDULE

Nine-month-old Brian Weisbard has a full week of activities, all designed to help him become smarter and brighter.

Monday: "Baby and Me" program at the local junior college.
Tuesday: Neighborhood play group consisting of infants, toddlers, and their mothers who live in the same condominium complex.
Wednesday: Kiddie Kraft classes at the local YWCA, where Brian explores with materials designed to enhance his creativity.
Thursday: Tomboree classes held at a local shopping center.
Friday: Shopping and various outings with his mother or baby sitter.
Saturday: Family day, during which Brian's father makes a special effort to "do things together."
Sunday: Brunch with his parents in the morning and a visit to his paternal grandparents in the afternoon.

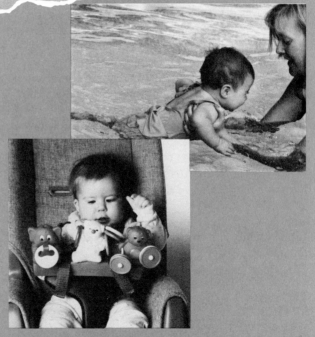

FIGURE 6-1 Today, many parents are more goal directed for themselves and their young children. In this sense, infant's lives reflect those of their parents. Also, what happens in parent's and infant's lives reflect changes occurring in society.

THE IMPORTANCE OF INFANCY

"We are primarily learning animals; we need a long period of dependent and flexible childhood to provide time for the cultural transmission that makes us human. If we matured and began to fend for ourselves as early as most other mammals, we would never develop the mental capacity that our neotenic brain permits" (Gould, 1982, p. 12).

The study of infancy is important for a number of reasons. First, along with the neonatal period, it is the beginning of life outside the womb, and is traditionally viewed by professionals, writers, and artists as the first of the many stages of human development. In this sense, it is the first step in the long and wondrous journey across the life span. As such it also provides a remarkable opportunity to study the postnatal origins and progress of physical and psychological development. Second, it is a period of rapid and dynamic developmental growth. As we will see, many important milestones occur in the first year of life, and infancy is a year of many "firsts"—the first smile, the first word, and toward the end of the infancy period, first steps. Third, infancy is viewed as a "sensitive" time for development, during which babies learn to "trust" or "mistrust" the world and begin the processes of cognitive and language development. Furthermore, although the human infant is remarkable and competent at birth, unlike many other animals of creation, children have to continue many developmental processes and "finish off" their development before they can achieve their full potential.

MODELS OF DEVELOPMENT

There are a number of ways people can and do look at and explain development, and account for variations in individual development. The *status quo model* (sometimes referred to as the medical model) maintains that the status of the child—who and what she is—remains stable over time because the environment has very little influence on development. A second model, the *environmental model*, maintains that development is primarily influenced and affected by environmental factors. A third model is the *interactional model*, which asserts that both what children are like—their basic constitution—and their environment play a role in development. A good child, for example, reared in a good environment will turn out better than a good child reared in a "bad" environment. The *transactional model*, is more widely accepted and is the one ascribed to in this book. It is based on the premise that contact between the developing child and the environment is a transaction in which each is influenced by the other. Variations in the environment and variations in the child's response to and interaction with that environment continually transact with each other, so that the child's behavior and the environment are both changed. A child smiles at her care-giver and this smile in turn elicits a smile from the care-giver, which in turn produces a change in the child's behavior. She now smiles *and* moves her arms and legs, inviting further changes in the care-giving environment. This transactive model emphasizes several basic assumptions regarding infancy: the infant is competent, active, and a social being.

PHYSICAL DEVELOPMENT

Human babies are born "early." There is an elegant and logical explanation for this. If all human development necessary for survival took place prior to birth, babies would be too big to pass through their mothers' pelvic openings. The baby's brain for example, is only one-fourth (23 percent) of its adult size at birth, and develops to about 80 percent of its adult size by age two. Babies are born while their brains are still immature and in the process of developing. Since much of human development takes place after birth, this explains in part why it takes years for growing children to become independent and able to care for themselves. This long period of dependency, however, gives humans the opportunity and time they need to develop to their fullest potential so that they can achieve remarkable things.

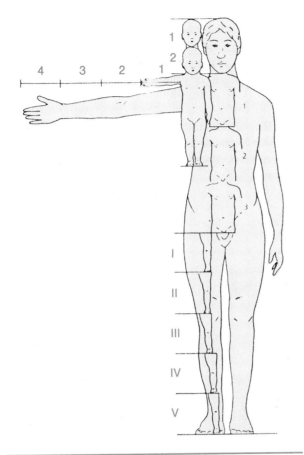

FIGURE 6-2 The proportional development of humans from infancy to adult is illustrated by the 2-3-4-5 principle. Viewed in this way, we can see how much development must occur in order to achieve adult proportions. (Used with permission of Alfred A. Knopf. From Fritz Kahn (1971). Man in structure and function.)

All you need to do to fully and finally realize that infants are not miniature adults is to observe them closely. They are out of proportion to adults, as shown in Figure 6–2. In order to achieve adult proportions, infants develop according to the two-three-four-five rule. The head will double in size, the trunk will triple in size, the arms will grow four times in length and the legs will increase to five times their infant length.

This long period of dependency is one of the things that makes humans unique among animals.

However, it also accounts for the vulnerability of the human infant and, in some measure, for the high infant mortality rate when prenatal care is lacking and when postnatal care is minimal or indifferent.

Height and Weight

Height and weight growth for humans is progressive toward their genetic potential and is dependent on such factors as nutrition, health, and socioeconomic status. Average heights and weights for children through five years are shown in Tables 6–3 and 6–4. (As you study these figures, keep in mind that averages are just that—averages.) The average is not some ideal toward which development is aimed; rather, it is the "middle ground" of development. Parents' interest in normal growth

TABLE 6–3

AVERAGE (FIFTIETH PERCENTILE) HEIGHT NORMS FOR MALE AND FEMALE INFANTS, TODDLERS, AND PRESCHOOLERS IN THE UNITED STATES				
	Males		Females	
Age	Centimeters	Inches	Centimeters	Inches
Birth	50.5	19.9	49.9	19.6
1 month	54.6	21.5	53.3	21.1
3 months	61.1	24.1	59.5	23.4
6 months	67.8	26.7	65.9	25.9
9 months	72.3	28.5	70.4	27.7
1 year	76.1	30.0	74.3	29.3
1½ years	82.4	32.4	80.9	31.9
2 years	87.6	34.5	86.5	34.1
2½ years	92.3	36.3	91.3	35.9
3 years	96.5	38.0	95.6	37.6
3½ years	99.1	39.0	97.9	38.5
4 years	102.9	40.5	101.6	40.0
4½ years	106.6	42.0	105.0	41.3
5 years	109.9	43.3	108.4	42.7

Note. From "Physical Growth: National Center for Health Statistics Percentiles" by P.V.V. Hamill, T.A. Drizd, R.B. Reed, C.L. Johnson, A.F. Roche, and W.M. Moore, 1979, The American Journal of Clinical Nutrition, 32, pp. 607–629.

and development are understandable and valid. However, when assessing a child's growth, everything about that child must be taken into consideration—health, sex, nutrition, and parents' size and stature. For example, Andrew Lanius (son of Pat and Patte, who you read about in Chapter Four), at seven months is consistently in the twenty-fifth percentile for height and weight, which appears to be normal for him. Some children will not grow as expected because of individual growth patterns that are normal for them. Within a context of good physical and emotional care, infants will achieve the level of development that is normal for them. The point is that an infant can be very normal without being "normal."

Normal weight gain for the infant is to double its birth weight by four months and triple it by twelve months. This works out to an average gain of one to two pounds per month the first year.

TABLE 6-4

AVERAGE (FIFTIETH PERCENTILE) WEIGHT NORMS FOR MALE AND FEMALE INFANTS, TODDLERS, AND PRESCHOOLERS IN THE UNITED STATES				
	Males		Females	
Age	Kilograms	Pounds	Kilograms	Pounds
Birth	3.27	7.21	3.23	7.12
1 month	4.29	9.46	3.98	8.77
3 months	5.98	13.18	5.40	11.90
6 months	7.85	17.30	7.21	15.89
9 months	9.18	20.24	8.56	18.87
1 year	10.15	22.38	9.53	21.01
1½ years	11.47	25.29	10.82	23.85
2 years	12.59	27.76	11.90	26.23
2½ years	13.67	30.14	12.93	28.45
3 years	14.69	32.39	13.93	30.71
3½ years	15.68	34.57	15.07	33.22
4 years	16.69	36.80	15.96	35.19
4½ years	17.69	39.00	16.81	36.98
5 years	18.67	41.16	17.66	38.94

Note. From "Physical Growth: National Center for Health Statistics Percentiles" by P.V.V. Hamill, T.A. Drizd, R.B. Reed, C.L. Johnson, A.F. Roche, and W.M. Morre, 1979, *The American Journal of Clinical Nutrition, 32*, pp. 607–629.

Dental Development

Teeth are made of calcium phosphate and are much harder than bone. The first tooth (lower incisor) emerges or erupts on the front of the lower jaw at about six months and other teeth erupt as shown in Figure 6-4. Again, the average has to be balanced with individual children, some of whom are born with teeth, while others may not have teeth for several months after what is considered "normal."

Humans have two sets of teeth. The first set is called baby, "milk," primary, or *deciduous* (meaning to "fall out") teeth and consists of twenty teeth. Most children have all their deciduous teeth by thirty to thirty-three months. The second set

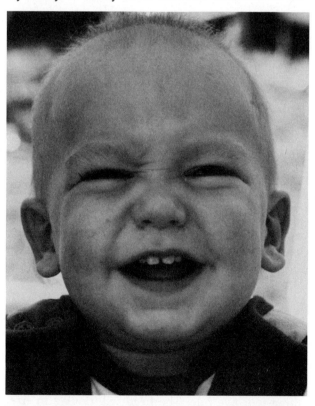

FIGURE 6-3 When infants are teething, they are frequently cranky, and cry from the pain and irritation of the erupting teeth. However, the discomfort of teething can be relieved by providing objects to "gum," e.g., refrigerated teething rings and teething biscuits.

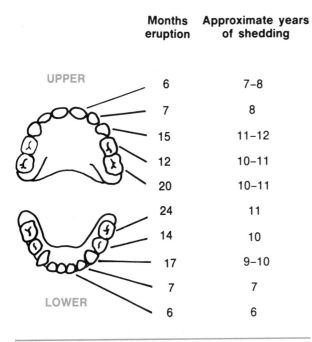

	Months eruption	Approximate years of shedding
UPPER	6	7–8
	7	8
	15	11–12
	12	10–11
	20	10–11
	24	11
	14	10
	17	9–10
	7	7
LOWER	6	6

FIGURE 6-4 The eruption of the deciduous or primary teeth occurs in an orderly pattern and according to the times shown.

of teeth, the permanent or secondary set, consists of thirty-two teeth. Figure 6–4 shows the eruption order of deciduous teeth.

Dental development brings about several changes in the young child. First, teeth fill out the jaws and give the infant an "older" look. Second, with teeth, infants are able to join the rest of the human race in chewing their food.

Motor Development

The importance of motor development cannot be overemphasized, for it pervades all of infant behavior and development. Accomplishments based on motor development contribute to intellectual development, for example, the active infant modifying her grasping reflex. Motor development also contributes to social development when the smiling infant attracts his mother. Human development and motor development are inherently entwined, and when motor development is deficient it can

have a pronounced influence on the rest of development. For example, an infant with cerebral palsy, in which the tone and control of the muscles are affected, benefits from physical and occupational therapy to promote voluntary and smooth muscle movement.

Motor Development Guidelines The following motor development principles are helpful guidelines in understanding infant development:

1. Motor development is sequential, and the sequences for development of motor behaviors and skills are the same for all infants. (See Tables 6–5 and 6–6.) Some motor behaviors

TABLE 6-5

GROSS MOTOR MILESTONES OF THE FIRST YEAR		
Accomplishment	Age at which 90 Percent of Infants Accomplish	Age range of Accomplishment
On stomach—head up 45°	2½ months	birth–2½ months
On stomach—head up 90°	3¼ months	1–3¼ months
Sits—head steady	4¼ months	1½–4¼ months
On stomach—chest with arm support	4½ months	2–4½ months
Rolls over	4¾ months	2–4¾ months
Bears some weight on legs	7¾ months	3–7¾ months
Sits without support	7¾ months	4¾–7¾ months
Stands holding on	10 months	5–10 months
Pulls self to stand	10 months	6–10 months
Gets to sitting position	11 months	6–11 months
Walks holding on to furniture	12¾ months	7½–12¾ months
Stands momentarily	13 months	9–13 months
Stands alone well	13¾ months	9¾–13¾ months
Stoops and recovers	14¼ months	10½–14¼ months
Walks well	14¼ months	11–14¼ months

Note. From "The Newly Abbreviated and Revised Denver Developmental Screening Test," by W.K. Frankenburg, A.W. Fandal, W. Sciarillo, and D. Burgess, 1982, *The Journal of Pediatrics, 99,* pp. 995-999.

TABLE 6–6

FINE MOTOR MILESTONES OF THE FIRST YEAR

Accomplishment	Age at Which 90 Percent of Infants Accomplish	Age Range of Accomplishment
Follows past midline	2½ months	birth–2½ months
Hands together	3½ months	1½–3½ months
Grasps rattle	4½ months	2½–4½ months
Reaches for object	5 months	3–5 months
Passes cube from hand to hand	7½ months	4½–7½ months
Sits, looks for yarn	7½ months	4½–7½ months
Thumb-finger grasp	10½ months	7¼–10½ months
Bangs two cubes held in hands	12¼ months	7–12¼ months
Neat pincer grasp	14½ months	9½–14½ months

Note. From "The Newly Abbreviated and Revised Denver Developmental Screening Test" by W.K. Frankenburg, A.W. Fandal, W. Sciarillo, and D. Burgess, 1982, *The Journal of Pediatrics, 99,* pp. 995–999.

occur simultaneously, such as reaching for an object and rolling over, but infants cannot pull themselves to a standing position before they can sit with support.

2. The age ranges in which infants accomplish motor tasks vary from infant to infant, as is evident from Tables 6–5 and 6–6. Part of the variability in age ranges has to do with maturation, which is controlled by such factors as heredity, environment, and nutrition. Muscles, nerves, and the skeletal system must develop to the point where a particular motor activity is possible.

3. Maturation of the motor system proceeds from gross activities to fine motor coordination. When learning to reach for objects, for example, the infant sweeps toward an object with her whole arm. Gradually this gross reaching behavior is replaced by a more specific reaching and grasping movement. When given a new toy, the young infant expresses delight by shaking all over, kicking legs, and waving arms. The older infant, on the other hand, expresses pleasure over a new toy by smiling and reaching.

4. Motor movement, like physical development, proceeds from the head to the lower parts of the body. This is called *cephalocaudal development* (from the Greek *kephale,* "head" and the Latin *cauda,* "tail"). This principle implies that the head is the most developed structure at birth, and the feet, the least. Infants hold their heads erect before they sit and they sit before they walk.

5. Motor development and physical development proceed from the *proximal,* or central part of the body, to the *distal,* or parts of the body at the extremities. Consequently, infants control arm movements before they control finger movements.

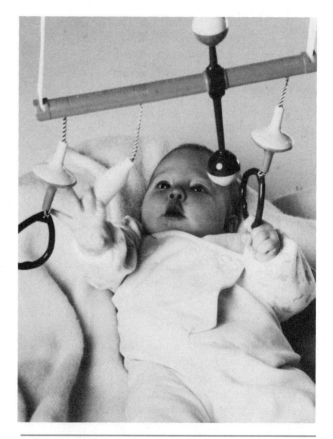

FIGURE 6-5 Physical & motor development proceeds from proximal to distal. This crib toy is an aid the baby can use to practice and refine his arm (large motor) and finger (small motor) movements.

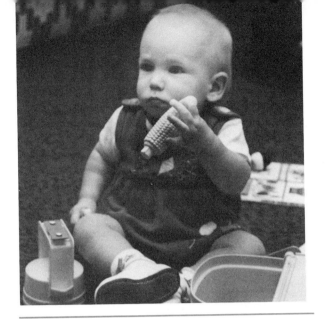

FIGURE 6-6 While babies are born into the world with a grasping reflex, this disappears at around four months and is replaced by voluntary grasping. Grasping enables the infant to pick up and manipulate objects which contributes to sensory input which thus contributes to cognitive development.

Crawling and Creeping Between four and seven months, infants can hold their heads and chests off the floor. They are still not able to get their stomachs off the floor, but they use their arms to pull and legs to push. The result is *crawling*.

Creeping begins between nine and eleven months. This is possible when infants can support themselves on their hands and knees. Creeping occurs by alternating arm and leg movements. Infants prefer this method of locomotion even during the beginning-to-walk stage, which is not too far in the developmental future. Creeping enables infants to cover a lot of territory at a pace parents often find hard to match!

Grasping Figure 6–7 shows the development of grasping skills through the first year. The use of the hands in grasping objects is important because the hands are themselves a source of sensory input *and* the means whereby the infant provides herself with rich sensory input.

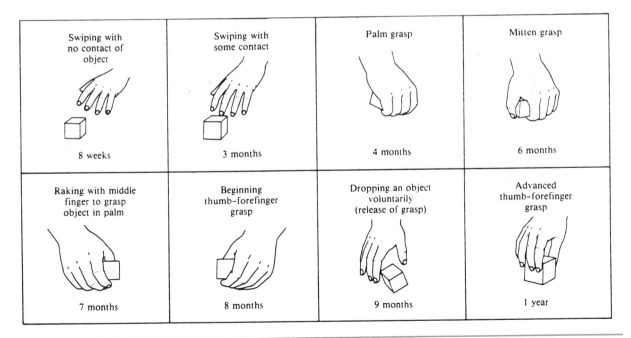

FIGURE 6-7 Hand use and grasping ability is stage related and progresses as shown. (Adapted from and used with permission by Holt, Rinehart & Winston, Inc. From Lisa Barclay (1985). *Infant development*, p. 189—development of hand use during the first year.)

Depth Perception Most infants have the ability to discriminate depth at the time of crawling (Gibson & Walk, 1960). Researchers used a "visual cliff" (as shown in Figure 6–8) to ascertain whether or not infants would crawl from one area, over the "cliff," to another designed to give the perception of depth. They would not, thus indicating their ability to perceive depth.

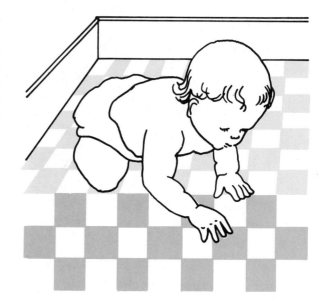

FIGURE 6-8 Infants reluctance to crawl "over the edge" of the visual cliff is evidence of their ability to perceive depth.

*I*N THE SPOTLIGHT

IS BEAUTY IN THE EYE OF THE BEHOLDER?

How often have you admired an attractive person, only to have a friend huffily reply that "beauty is in the eye of the beholder"? You probably nodded in agreement reluctantly and went on about your business. But is it really true that each of us has our own standards of attractiveness and that standards of attractiveness are learned by exposure to cultural norms? Perhaps not, and we have infant research to thank for challenging such ordinary, daily assumptions. Infants look longer at attractive faces (as judged by adult standards), are capable of discriminating between attractive faces and unattractive faces, and show a preference for attractive faces (Langlois et al., 1987). There are several reasons for this built-in preference for attractiveness. First, attractive faces may be more curved, less angular, and more vertically symmetrical, features which are attractive to infants. Second, attractive faces may have better defined features than unattractive ones. So, the next time someone introduces a discussion about beauty, you can impress them with your knowledge of beauty from an infant's point of view.

Visual Development

In comparison with the rest of the body, the size of the eye changes relatively little after birth. While the body as a whole increases about twenty times, the eye only undergoes a two- to three-fold increase from birth to adulthood, and most of this occurs in the first two years of life (Hicky & Peduzzi, 1987).

The young infant is sensitive to a much lower and perhaps much more restricted range of spatial frequencies than the adult visual system. Also, the range of contrasts to which infants are sensitive are quite restricted at birth, but grows steadily in the first year and a half. Young infants' ability to detect contrasts, however (for example, skin versus hair), is sufficient for them to detect many such intensity gradients in the environment (Banks & Dannemiller, 1987). Infants' vision is best suited for perceiving objects in the immediate environment rather than in the distant visual environment. As they develop, infants' ability to see objects at a distance and small objects up close increases. Figure 6–9 shows the development of visual acuity in the early months of infancy. Adults often assume infants can see better than they are able to see. Figure 6–9 dramatically depicts what infants can see.

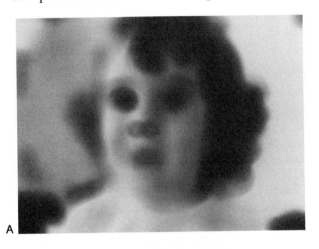

A

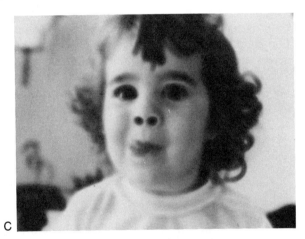

C

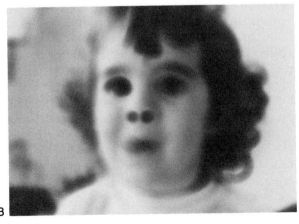

B

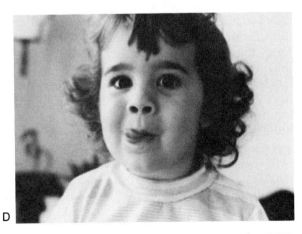

D

FIGURE 6-9 **What the infant sees at (A) one, (B) two, (C) three months, and (D) full eye development is shown by these photographs. Infants' visual acuity increases over three months to the point where they can recognize their sibling or parent.**

What Colors Do Infants Like? I'm sure that like most people, you have a favorite color. What might surprise you is that even though color preference is highly subjective, and even though color preferences often change with fashion trends, there are nonetheless certain color preferences in adults and children that are similar across cultures. Adults have a preference for "focal colors," which are "central exemplars of a color category," for example, a "pure" green rather than shades of green such as blue-green or yellow-green. Also, adults prefer blue and red over other colors. Infants' color preferences are the same as adults. They prefer red and blue over green and yellow. This adult-like preference for focal colors, and for red and blue, is in place at four months of age (Teller & Bornstein, 1987). When parents and other caregivers select colors for children's clothes and environmental accessories, consideration should certainly be given to reds and blues. And, regardless of what colors are selected, the "purest" should be the top choice.

Taste and Smell in Infancy

Taste and smell preferences in infants are basically the same as those preferences for neonates discussed in Chapter Five. Infants who are breastfed can recognize the odor of their mother's breast. In research conducted with one-month-old infants, MacFarlane (1977) found that infants spend more time facing or looking at their mother's breast pad than the breast pads worn by mothers of other infants. This indicates that infants not only discriminate between mothers' odors, but actually prefer their own mother's odor (MacFarlane, 1977).

The taste preferences of a breast-fed baby are influenced by her mother's diet. Consequently, the greater taste experiences gained by a nursing infant will make it easier to wean her than the bottle-fed baby (Crook, 1987). Learning, then, would seem to play a powerful role in the development of food and flavor preferences and aversions.

Touch and Motion

We no longer think of infants as bundles of helplessness. As Reisman (1987) says, "They are born with some exquisitely tuned sensory abilities. Although sight is still fuzzy and hearing muted, the neonate is equipped with a sense of touch that accurately homes in on the source of its meals, a sense of motion that triggers reflexes to protect it from falls, and a sense of its body parts that allows the infant to mold its body comfortably to that of its caretakers" (p. 265).

INTELLECTUAL DEVELOPMENT

Intellectual development during infancy is a continuation of processes initiated in Stage I of sensorimotor intelligence during the neonatal period.

Stage II (One to Four Months)

The milestone of this stage is the modification of the reflexive actions of Stage I. Sensorimotor behaviors not previously present in the infant begin to appear: habitual thumb sucking (which indicates hand-mouth coordination), tracking of moving objects with the eyes, and moving the head toward sounds (which indicates the beginnings of the recognition of causality). Infants begin to direct their own behavior rather than being totally dependent on reflexive actions. The first steps of intellectual development have begun.

Primary circular reactions begin during Stage II. A circular response occurs when an infant's actions cause a reaction in the infant or in another person that prompts the infant to try to repeat the original action. The circular reaction is similar to a stimulus-response, cause-and-effect relationship.

Piaget classified three kinds of circular reactions: primary, secondary, and tertiary. The *primary circular reaction* characteristic of Stage II is indicated when infants use their bodies to initiate and repeat many actions such as thumb sucking, leg kicking, and staring at the hands for extended periods of time because of the pleasure it brings. These reactions are called "primary" because they are reactions involving the infant's own body. An infant's behavior, by chance or accident, leads to a pleasurable or interesting result. The infant attempts to repeat the action. When the sequence is repeated a number of times, the behavior becomes habit.

Implications for Care-givers Care-givers can continue to provide many interesting and varied activities that provide a context for the infant to grasp, manipulate, and look. Crib mobiles and objects hung within the infant's reach promote and support eye-object and eye-hand coordination. Speaking, singing, and playing records promote aural stimulation. Infants can be held or placed so they can look at sources of sound.

Stage III (Four to Eight Months)

Piaget called this stage the stage of "making interesting things last." Infants manipulate objects, which indicates the ability to coordinate vision and the tactile senses. An infant reproduces events with intention or with the purpose of sustaining and repeating acts. These actions become goal-directed and the infant repeats acts that are interesting to him to her.

The intellectual milestone of this stage is the beginning of *object permanence*. When infants in Stages I and II cannot see an object, it literally does not exist for them. It is a case of "out of sight, out of mind." During the latter part of Stage III, however, there is a growing awareness that when things are out of sight they do not cease to exist.

Secondary circular reactions begin during this stage. These reactions are characterized by the infants' repeating an action with the purpose of getting the same response from an object or person. They will repeatedly shake a rattle, for example, in order to repeat the sound. Repetitiveness is a characteristic of all circular reactions. The name "secondary" implies that the reaction is elicited from a secondary source rather than from the infant. The infant interacts with people and objects

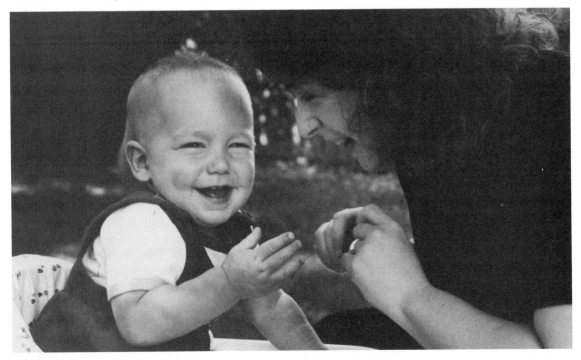

FIGURE 6-10 As an adult you know that an object maintains its identity when it changes location. Infants do not. Piaget maintained that for infants, objects are images that disappear as soon as they vanish and emerge for no apparent reason.

to make interesting sight, sounds, and events last. When the infant is given an object, he or she will explore it using all available schemes, such as mouthing, hitting, and banging. Should one of these schemes produce an interesting result, the infant will continue using the scheme to elicit the same response. This explains why Piaget gave this stage its name. Imitation becomes increasingly intentional as a means of prolonging an interest.

Implications for Care-givers Care-givers can continue to provide objects for infants to grasp and manipulate. Place objects on strings or elastic and hang them over the crib and play area at the infant's level so they can strike them and participate in repetitive actions. However, these objects should be removed when infants begin to turn over, sit up, and stand. Activities that involve imitation are also good. Vocalization games are simple, effective activities in which the care-giver verbalizes and performs actions, the infant responds, and the care-giver, in turn, responds to the infant.

Stage IV (Eight to Twelve Months)

During this stage, the infant uses means to attain ends. Infants move objects out of the way (means) to get another object (end). The shape and size of objects become stabilized concepts for the infant. Infants begin to search for hidden objects, although not always in the places hidden, which indicates a growing understanding of object permanence. Infants become aware that objects cause actions.

Implications for Care-givers Care-givers can play hide-and-seek games with infants by hiding objects under a blanket or diaper. Provide activities that encourage ends and means, such as push and pull toys. Placing a pillow in front of an object the infant wants, for example, will encourage the infant to crawl around the pillow or move it to get the object.

Important Concepts

In summary, there are several important concepts to keep in your developing scheme about infants' intellectual development.

1. The ages of the sensorimotor stage are only approximate. Care-givers should avoid treating the age ranges Piaget specified for the stages of intellectual development as though they were etched in stone. The behavior and developmental progress children demonstrate give a clearer understanding of their intellectual development. Sensorimotor schemes are internal and are manifested in the actions of the infant. These schemes are in infants' heads but operate and are observable through sensorimotor actions. This explains why Piaget named the first stage of intellectual development "sensorimotor."
2. Infants do not "think" like adults. They know their world by acting or operating on it with action-based schemes, such as sucking, grasping, pulling, shaking, listening, and looking. Infants think as they move and observe objects and people.
3. Infants, like all humans, are actively involved in developing or *constructing* their own intelligence. Activity plays an important role in intellectual development. As infants act, they are stimulated mentally, which leads to the development of schemes. The infant's primary way of learning about the world is by interacting in and with it. Sensorimotor involvement establishes a foundation for future learning. Consequently, physical handicaps that restrict the child from being actively involved in the environment have implications for learning as well as for parenting and child care practices. Care-givers must bring activities to handicapped infants, adapt activities to their ability levels, and make special efforts to see that they are not excluded in any way from appropriate activities.
4. Parents and care-givers need to provide the environment and opportunity for infants to

use their reflexive actions, which are modified during the first weeks of life. This is especially important since, as we have discussed, these are two important conditions for intellectual development. Reflexive actions form the basis for assimilation and accommodation, enabling the development of cognitive structures. Infants construct the world of objects through their experiences with it. Care-givers must assure that infants have experiences that will enable them to do a good job of intellectual construction.

5. At birth, infants do not know that there are objects in the world, and, in this sense, have no knowledge of the external world. They do not and cannot differentiate between who they are and the external world. For all practical purposes, the infant *is* the world. All external objects are acted on through sucking, grasping, and looking. It is precisely this acting on the world that enables infants to construct schemes of the world.

6. The concept of causality, or cause-and-effect, does not exist at birth. An infant's concept of causality begins to evolve only through acting on the environment.

7. As infants and toddlers move from one stage of intellectual development to another, the previous stage is not replaced by the new. Rather, later stages develop out of earlier ones. Schemes developed in Stage I are incorporated into and improved on by the schemes constructed in Stage II. So it is with all stages of intellectual development.

Unlike the child whom some think is biologically driven to "mature," the child Piaget describes is driven by physical and mental activity. The implications for parenting and care-giving are clear. The neonate and infant need many and varied opportunities to act on objects and interact with people, because the development of intelligence is dependent on the mental actions that these behaviors promote.

LANGUAGE DEVELOPMENT

"Da-da"—"ma-ma." How sweet these sounds are to the ears of all parents who for months have been encouraging their infants to make them, and have with eager anticipation awaited their utterance. For most parents, these sounds are auditory proof that their children are participating in that most remarkable and wonderful process of language development. As is all language, these words are learned by children regardless of their status in life, and represent one of the most remarkable intellectual accomplishments they will ever participate in. How does the infant go from the utterances, words, and sentences of his parents to producing his own understandable words and sentences? While everyone agrees that children develop language, that is the end of the agreement. There is much disagreement concerning *how* they develop language.

Behaviorism

One popularly held view of language development is that language is acquired through associations resulting from stimulus-response learning. Thus, learning theorists see language acquisition resulting when parents and the environment reward children's language efforts. Parents, for example, reward children for their first sounds by talking to them and making sounds in response to the children's sounds. First words are reinforced in the same way with parents (and others) constantly praising and encouraging. Modeling and imitation also play important roles in this view of language acquisition. (See "Social Learning Theory," Chapter Two.) Children imitate the sounds, words, sentences, and grammar they hear modeled by other children and adults.

While behaviorist ideas help explain much of what humans do, including language acquisition, they are too simplistic to fully and accurately explain the marvelous and wondrous process by which children become possessors and users of language. For example, the behaviorist view cannot account for *novelty* and *generativity*, two characteristics that you and everyone else exhibit every day. Generativity is the ability of children to generate words and sentences without first having heard or previously learned them. Think for a moment what language would be like if all the words and sentences you used had to be learned first through the process of reinforcement. What would life be like in a child care program if children learned only those words you rewarded? What would your language be like if you could only speak those words, phrases, and sentences taught to you by others!

Think also about the novelty factor. You have the ability to generate a sentence that no one but you has ever heard. For example, "The purple pelican eats all he can," is a new and novel sentence for me. Without the novelty factor, which behaviorist approaches to language learning cannot explain, language would be dull indeed.

While researchers are continually expanding their understanding of language development, much remains for us still to learn. And, although we don't know all we would like to know, the current view of language acquisition suggests that heredity, biology, maturation, cognitive development, the environment, and social interactions are all important and involved.

Heredity

Heredity plays a role in language development in a number of ways. First, humans have the respiratory and laryngeal systems that make rapid and efficient vocal communication possible. Second, humans are born with a brain that makes language possible. The left hemisphere is the center for speech and phonetic analysis, and is the brain's main language center. But the left hemisphere does not have exclusive responsibility for the language process. The right hemisphere plays a role in our understanding of speech intonations, enabling us to distinguish between declarative, imperative, and interrogative sentences. Without a brain enabling us to process, language as we know it would be impossible.

Third, "nativist" and "innatist" theories of language development maintain that the human *ability* to learn language is innate. In addition, Chomsky (1965) maintains that children have an innate *language acquisition device*, or *LAD*, which naturally helps them learn language. The LAD guides or directs children in their language development.

Chomsky's theory is based on the premise that the language children hear from others is the input data to the LAD. Accordingly, children receive little or no formal instruction about the language rules that underlie adult language performance. Rather, each individual child is exposed to utterances within the context of events and circumstances in her own environment. From such language utterances, the LAD helps children learn language. As a result, the child has not only the innate ability, but the LAD, which enables her to learn basic syntax—the rules of language construction. While the existence of the LAD seems plausible and helps explain in an understandable way how language develops, one caveat is in order. To date, there is no research data to confirm the existence of a LAD.

Cognitive Development

While cognitive development is imbedded in the idea of an LAD, it is also illustrated by the "waiting room" concept of language acquisition (Slobin, 1982). According to this theory, children use whatever linguistic means are at their disposal while "waiting" to master adult forms of word usage. For example, the young child has in his language repertoire a number of locational terms to use while he is waiting to use more complex terms, such as "between." When an object is placed between two objects, for example, a child might say it is "inside" or "beside" them. It is only after the child has cognitively "figured out" what is semantically involved in the use of "between" that she uses it correctly and it "exits from the waiting room." Consequently, all words and expressions have their own "waiting rooms" while the child figures out their appropriate meaning and use.

Biology

Biology plays a role in language development in the form of maturation. Thus language develops according to a definite sequence and a definite time schedule. Children are literally programmed to learn language, and there are sensitive periods for learning language at which time children learn language better than at any other time.

Another instance of the role of biology is the babbling play of infants, which constitutes a necessary and innately determined play behavior that establishes the neuromuscular skills and control necessary for human speech (Lieberman, 1984). Thus babbling contributes to speech production, so the next time you and an infant are babbling back and forth, you can do it without guilt, knowing that there is more to it than mutual entertainment.

Environmental Influences

It seems obvious to say that in order to learn language, the child must hear language, and we often take this for granted. But let's take the case of Genie, a modern day "wild child" (Curtiss, 1977). During her early days, Genie had minimal human contact and her father and brother barked at her like dogs instead of using human language. She did not have an opportunity to learn language until she was thirteen and one-half years old. Even after prolonged treatment and care, Genie remained basically language deficient and conversationally incompetent.

Social Interactions

Parents and other care-givers play major roles in the development of language by being conversational partners with infants. Parent-child interactions can precipitate many rich and rewarding conversations. The key is for all involved with infants to treat them as individuals capable of participating in the process of language. For example, mothers who believe their babies are potentially communicative partners talk to them in

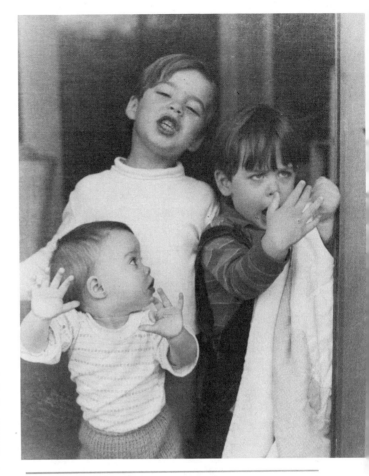

FIGURE 6-11 Infants are very social individuals and are born with tools for social development such as smiling, crying, language and movement. Infants enjoy being around adults, siblings and other children. The friendliness of babies is determined in part by the friendliness of their families. So, if you want a friendly baby, be friendly!

ways that serve to strengthen that belief and make it come true. The fact that mothers talk in predictable ways about recurring events undoubtedly helps children structure their world, segment events, distinguish different types of activities, and anticipate future events (Snow, 1979). It is the role of such communicative acts between adults and children that leads one language theorist (Bruner, 1983) to maintain that a *language acquisition support sys-*

tem, or *LASS*, helps children learn language "formats," enabling them to understand the rudiments of language usage long before they themselves can use language. Thus the LASS complements the LAD. According to Bruner, "In a word, it is the interaction between the LAD and the LASS that makes it possible for the infant to enter the linguistic community—and, at the same time, the culture to which the language gives access" (p. 19).

*I*N THE SPOTLIGHT

MOTHERESE

Many recent research studies have demonstrated that mothers and other care-givers talk to infants and toddlers differently from the way adults talk to each other. This distinctive way of adapting everyday speech to young children is called *motherese* (Newport, Gleitman, & Gleitman, 1977). Characteristics of motherese include the following:

1. The sentences are short, averaging just over four words per sentence with babies. As children become older, the length of sentences mothers use also becomes longer. Mothers' conversations with their children are short and sweet.
2. The sentences are highly intelligible. When talking to their children, mothers tend not to slur or mumble their words. This may be because mothers speak more slowly to their children.
3. The sentences are "unswervingly well formed," that is, they are grammatical sentences.
4. The sentences are mainly imperative and questions, such as "Give Mommie the ball" and "Do you want more juice?" Since mothers can't exchange a great deal of information with their children, their utterances are such that they direct their children's actions.
5. Mothers use *deictic* sentences in which referents ("here," "that," "there") are used to stand for objects or people: "Here's your bottle." "That's your baby doll." "There's your doggie."
6. Mothers *expand* or provide an adult version of their children's communication. When a child points at a baby doll on a chair, the mother may respond by saying, "Yes, the baby doll is on the table."
7. Mother's sentences involve repetitions. "The ball, bring Mommie the ball. Yes, go get the ball . . . the ball . . . go get the ball."

Not everyone agrees that Motherese makes sentence structure more apparent to children and it may be that the claims for the role of Motherese in language development are exaggerated. They believe that some Motherese is undoubtedly important for all children's language development, but just as doses of vitamins contribute little to improved health, so, too, mothers who use Motherese all the time may be saying more than necessary for language development. (Scarborough & Wyckoff, 1986).

However, talking with children using Motherese is fun for all involved and certainly the interaction contributes to more than language development.

The Emergence of Language

Language development is stage-related. The rate of development through these stages varies for individual children, but the stages apply to all children, regardless of culture. There are literally hundreds of languages (some estimates range as high as three thousand) used by different cultures in the world. Children of one culture master the same language patterns as children from another culture who speak a different language. This universal sequence of language development occurs in spite of different environments and child-rearing patterns. This sameness of language development is one of the reasons given as evidence for the innateness of language development.

Table 6–7 illustrates receptive (capable of receiving) and expressive (to communicate) language and its *normal* development in infants.

Smiling   The social smile infants develop in the second month is a powerful signal, and serves to attract attention and promote social interaction with the care-giver. In this sense, smiling is a form of communication. It promotes reciprocal communication—usually speech in the care-giver—and consequently plays a role in language development.

Cooing   Cooing is a positive, noncrying vocalization. Cooing is usually pleasant, a sign that the infant is not distressed. Cooing can be stimulated by social interaction, speech, and toys.

Babbling   Babbling is a combination of a consonant and a vowel repeated over and over again, such as "babababa." Babbling helps strengthen the tongue, throat, and lips. Care-givers may respond to infants by repeating the babbling sounds as a sign of approval and to develop a sense of conversation between infant and care-giver. At this stage, it is the attention and reinforcement that count as much as the actual conversation. Imitating the cooing and babbling of infants is a good game to play with them, and one from which care-givers also derive pleasure.

"Ma-ma" and "Da-da"   "Ma-ma" and "da-da" are sounds that are natural and easy for infants to make. All infants make these sounds, regardless of culture, although these parental names are common in many cultures and languages, including French and Japanese (deVilliers & deVilliers, 1979). Infants make many sounds not needed in the language being learned. Through hearing, use, and reinforcement over time, only those sounds used in the language are retained.

First Word   At about one year, the first word is spoken and the symbolic functioning of words begins. Words are essentially labels for things, and

TABLE 6–7

LANGUAGE DEVELOPMENT IN INFANTS

Age	Receptive	Expressive
Birth	Startle reflex	Crying
1½ months		Social smile
3 months		Cooing
4 months	Orients to voice	
5 months	Orients to bell (looks to side)	"Ah-goo" Razzing
6 months		Babbling
7 months	Orients to bell (looks to side, then up)	"Da-da" and "ma-ma" (used inappropriately)
8 months		
9 months	Gestures	"Da-da" and "ma-ma" (used appropriately)
10 months	Orients to bell (turns directly toward bell)	
11 months		One word
12 months	One-step command (with gestures)	Two words

Note. From "Linguistic and Auditory Milestones during the First Two Years of Life" by A.J. Capute and P.J. Accardo, 1987, *Clinical Pediatrics, 17* (11), pp. 847–853.

infants need help in the labeling process. Care-givers can help in several ways. First, they can verbally label objects through naming and conversation. For example, they can say to the infant, "Here is your cup. The cup is red. Can you say 'cup'?" Second, words that describe action are learned best when accompanied by the action. The word "drink," for example, is learned best when the infant is drinking. "I bet Hector wants a drink! Let's drink from your cup. You like to drink from the cup, don't you?"

From the first cries at birth, the infant begins the process of language development. Language is one of the most essential of all human abilities. All care-givers must do all they can to empower children with the ability to learn and use language to its fullest. This empowerment begins in the first year of life.

Communication: Games Infants Play

Of course, infants communicate with their care-givers in many ways other than through spoken language. For example, infants are very adept at "playing games" with their care-givers. These infant-parent games have a few, simple rules such as turn-taking and repetition of game roles (for example, the parent builds the tower and the infant knocks it down). Infants use many nonlinguistic communication cues, such as prolonged waiting for the adult to take their turn, glancing from partner to game object, showing, offering, and giving the partner the game object, and repeating their own or the partner's turn. Infants as young as nine months old understand the nature of such games and are able to regulate these games by "requesting," through sound and signals, their partners to participate (Ross & Lollis, 1987).

These abilities to communicate increase with age and experience, and infants' knowledge of and skill with language attest to their remarkable capacities.

ATTACHMENT
Stages of Attachment

John Bowlby, a pioneer in the articulation of attachment theory, proposes four phases or stages in the development of attachment, as shown in Table 6–8. Bowlby believes that during Stage 1, infants use basic reflexive actions and crying to initiate interactions. During this stage, the ability

TABLE 6–8

BOWLBY'S STAGES OF ATTACHMENT		
Stage	Age	Behavior
1	Birth to 8 weeks	Infant responds to and attends to any person—parent, care-giver—that is nearby. Looks at and listens to person(s).
2	8 weeks to 6 months	Infant discriminates between familiar people—parents and care-giver—and unfamiliar people. Is more responsive; smiles and vocalizes more to familiar people than to unfamiliar people.
3	6 months to the 2nd and 3rd year	Infant/toddler maintains contact or stays near attached person(s)—parent, care-giver—by creeping to, walking to, and following person(s). Also uses vocal signals—crying and words—to maintain contact.
4	3 years and older	Toddler or preschooler engages in the "formation of goal-corrected partnerships" with the attachment figures. Child plans how to get parents and care-givers to change their behavior to conform to child's wishes.

Note. From *Attachment* (pp. 266–267) by J. Bowlby, 1969, New York: Basic Books.

to discriminate one care-giver from another is absent and, according to Bowlby, it is the attention received that is important, not who provides it.

The Importance of Attachment

We can talk about attachment all we want, but sooner or later we have to ask what purpose attachment serves. Attachment plays a role in the development of competence. As Sroufe (1978) so eloquently states,

> The infant who uses the care-giver as a base for moving into the world, and as a haven when threatened or distressed, develops motor skills and a sense of himself as effective. In sharing his play with his care-giver at a distance, the infant evolves a new way of maintaining contact while operating independently. The infant is free to invest himself in challenging the environment because he is confident that he can maintain his tie with his caregiver even while he is widening his world (p. 52).

Multiple Attachments

Increased use of child care programs inevitably raises questions concerning infant attachment. Parents are concerned that their children will not attach to them. Worse yet, they fear that their babies will develop an attachment bond with their care-givers rather than with them. They need not be so anxious. Research to date indicates that "both across cultures and within the broader culture in American society, children experiencing early day care form primary bonds with their parents, just as home-reared children do. Further, there is no evidence that day care 'dilutes' or 'weakens' attachment bonds that have been previously established" (Farber & Egeland, 1982).

Care-givers and early childhood educators must realize that parents may need help in forming the primary bond with their children. Furthermore, the quality of the care-giving program, be it baby-sitting, family child care at home, or a child care center, should be high, so that parents will be

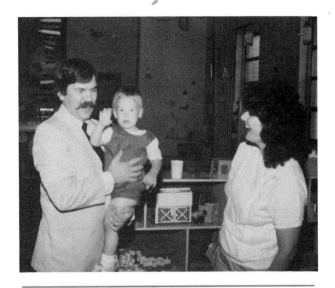

FIGURE 6-12 The language development of infants is facilitated by all who participate in infant care. Infants can and should be part of and involved in the conversations of their caregivers.

supported in their roles as primary care-givers for their children.

Children can and do attach to more than one person, and there can be more than one attachment at a time. Infants attach to parents as the primary care-givers as well as to a surrogate. The latter attachments are not of equal value. Infants show a preference for the primary care-giver, usually the mother. Parents should not only engage in attachment behaviors with their infants, they should select child care programs that employ care-givers who understand the importance of the care-giver's role and function in attachment.

It is natural and desirable for child care workers to form attachments with infants. It is not at all uncommon for care-givers to have feelings of loss when "their" infants leave their care and go to the toddler room. One care-giver said, "I've gone home many nights and cried about losing my infants to another teacher." Better by far for a care-giver and infant to have a relationship that the care-giver can cry about when the attachment must physically and emotionally end, than to have a care-giver indifferent to the importance of attachments and the need to let go.

Surrogate care-givers should handle the weaning of infants from their care with compassion, understanding, and concern for the well-being of all parties involved, especially the child. The transition from home to a child care setting can occur gradually, a little at a time over a period of time. Likewise, the transition from infant room to toddler program can be done a little at a time, with the infant spending an hour or two in the toddler room and then returning to the infant room. In this way, a gradual transition results with opportunities to create an attachment to the new care-giver while "breaking away" from the attached care-giver.

Good child care programs help mothers maintain their primary attachments to their infants in many ways. The staff keeps parents well informed about infants' accomplishments. Parents should be allowed to "discover" and participate in infants' developmental milestones. A care-giver, for example, might tell a mother that today her son showed signs of wanting to take his first step by himself. The care-giver thereby allows the mother to be the first person to experience the joy of this accomplishment. The mother may then report to the center the next day that her son took his first step at home the night before.

Some perceptive mothers initiate a supportive parent–care-giver relationship. One mother explained it this way: "Almost every morning I told the teachers at the child care center that if my son did anything great during the day, such as say his first word or take his first step, not to tell me about it because I wanted to be the first to know."

The Quality of Attachment

The quality of infant-parent attachment varies according to the relationship that exists between them. A primary method of assessing the quality of parent-child attachment is the "Strange Situation," developed by Mary Ainsworth and her colleagues (1978). The Strange Situation consists of observing and recording children's reactions to several events: a novel situation, separation from their mothers, reunion with their mothers, and reactions to a stranger. Based on their reactions and behaviors in these situations, children are classified into one of three groups. These groups are illustrated in Table 6–9.

It is important for care-givers to know and recognize different classifications of attachment so that they can inform parents and help them engage in the specific behaviors that will promote the growth of secure attachments.

Maternal Responsiveness and Attachment

Over the first year of life, many mothers change in their responsiveness to their babies' cues. These changes are associated with the baby's characteristics, maternal attitudes, and the social environment (Crockenberg & McCluskey, 1986). Mothers

TABLE 6–9

INDIVIDUAL DIFFERENCES IN ATTACHMENT BEHAVIORS	
Attachment Classification	Behavioral Characteristics
Group A: Anxious-Avoidant	Avoids contact with mother after separation. Ignores attempts of mother to initiate interaction.
Group B: Secure	Presence of mother supports exploration and facilitates return to exploration after separation.
Group C: Anxious-Resistant	Resists contact with mother during reunion. Is not comforted by the presence of the mother after separation. Lack of exploration prior to separation.

Note. From *Patterns of Attachment* by M. Ainsworth, M. Blehar, E. Waters, and S. Wall, 1978, Hillsdale, NJ: Lawrence Erlbaum Associates.

with irritable babies are less responsive to them at twelve months than they were at three months, indicating that infant temperament has an impact on the care-giver. Furthermore, mothers with generally unresponsive attitudes who have irritable babies are particularly unresponsive to them. Maternal unresponsiveness in turn has implications relating to the security of infant-maternal attachment. One way to help the children of unresponsive parents is through support services enabling parents to improve their parenting skills. While there is not much parents can do to change their baby's temperament, they can lower the stress of parenting by developing a network of supportive people. Women who report high levels of support from spouses, parents, and friends before the birth of their child report greater confidence as parents and feel less depressed three months after delivery (Cutrona & Troutman, 1986).

Want a Happy Baby?—Be Happy!

How many times have you experienced an increased sense of happiness when you were around someone who was happy? The same is true for infants. In Chapter Five, we discussed neonates' abilities to imitate the facial expressions of adults. Infants are even better at it. As early as ten weeks, infants can respond differently to three maternal affect expressions—joy, anger, and sadness—when the presentation is simultaneously facial and vocal (Haviland & Lelwica, 1987). Infants not only respond with an emotional expression, but more importantly, they also respond with the same emotional state as was modeled for them. The implications for parenting are clear. Mothers—and others—can control with their own expressions the expressions and emotional states of their babies. Happiness is contagious.

Fathers and Parenting

Fathers play important roles in the care, nurturing and development of their children. For the past decade and continuing to the present time, feminists, child development professionals, early childhood educators and the media are urging men

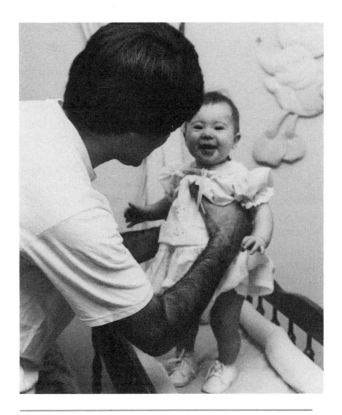

FIGURE 6-13 Fathers are fascinated by their babies. They like to look at, hold, touch, and care for them. Father's interactions with their infants tends to be more physical and their play more rough. Today, the range of fathers' involvements with their young children is increasing.

to be more involved with their children. In particular, men are encouraged to assume and share in many of the traditional "mothering" responsibilities associated with child care and rearing. It is interesting to note however, that fathers' involvements with their children are consistent over time in the early childhood years. There is a high degree of stability in the extent to which fathers are involved with their infants and the degree to which they are involved with them four years later. In this regard, as in many other situations, past behavior is an excellent predictor of future behavior. (Bailey, 1987). Furthermore, just as we know that "telling is not teaching" in school settings, the same holds true for efforts to enhance and increase men's involvements in parenting activities and responsibilities. Simply telling, exhorting and advocating men to assume roles associated with "new fathers" is not sufficient, for attitudes toward women is one of the key factors for involvement of men in parenting activities. (Bailey, 1987). We must therefore direct our efforts toward developing in males in the early years and across the life span those attitudes that will result in effective fathering and coparenting.

One of the reasons for mothers to play a larger role in child-rearing functions may be due to maternal "gatekeeping." According to this hypothesis, certain maternal characteristics and attributes mediate the frequency of a father's involvement with his children. For the most part, the frequency of paternal involvement is based on maternal satisfaction with the father's involvement, the child's age; maternal attitudes of the importance of the father's involvement, and marital satisfaction (DeLuccie, 1989).

NUTRITION
The Importance of Nutrition in the Early Years

On the one hand, most people take nutrition in infancy for granted, and assume that children are well fed and nourished. On the other hand, nightly news broadcasts show graphic and disheartening photos of poverty- and famine-stricken children, photos that act as chilling reminders that all children are not well-cared-for and fed. As we discussed in Chapter Four, there are certain critical periods when maternal nutrition has an impact on fetal development. Likewise, there are critical periods early in life when children are particularly vulnerable to *undernourishment* (a condition resulting from an insufficient amount of food of nutritional value) and *malnourishment* (a condition resulting from the lack of a specific component,

TABLE 6–10

EFFECT OF UNDERNUTRITION ON INFANT BEHAVIOR			
Investigator	Site	Age at Assessment	Behavior Impairment
Lester	Guatemala	1 year	Diminished orienting response
Als et al.	USA	first 10 days	Poor motoric processes; low social responsiveness
Brazelton et al.	Guatemala	1 month	Poor motoric processes; poor at eliciting social responses; lethargic; difficult to arouse
Mora et al	Colombia	15 days	Irritability
Herrera et al.			Poor frustration tolerance; slow visual habituation*
Chavez and Martinez	Mexico	1 year	Frequent crying; clinging; high dependency
		18 months	Low activity; infrequent playing
Rush et al.	USA	1 year	Short duration of play; slow visual habituation
Zeskind and Ramey	USA	3 years	Withdrawn; anxious*
Graves	India, Nepal	1–2 years	Reduced exploration

* These studies also showed significant effects on measured intelligence at age 3.
Note. From "Undernutrition and Child Behavior: What Behaviors Should We Measure and How Should We Measure Them?" by D. Barrett, 1987, in J. Dubbing (Ed.), *Early Nutrition and Later Development* (p. 94), London: Academic Press.

such as protein, necessary for proper growth). Also, because of their immature organ systems and small body size, children are very susceptible to the effects of poor nutrition. Children who are at risk for malnutrition are usually vulnerable to accompanying factors, such as poor housing, poverty, parental unemployment, and poor education. What are the consequences for children who are undernourished in the early years?

Based on Sinisterra's series of studies of children in Cali, Columbia (1987, p. 222), he concluded that children who have chronic nutritional and other health deficits have many retarded psychological characteristics and capabilities. While some retarded developmental characteristics are remediable, and some malnourished children, were able to "catch up" with their neighborhood peers as a result of nutritional *and* educational intervention, they were still behind the "standard" of well-nourished and economically well-to-do children. Table 6–10 shows the results of recent research studies that identify the effects of undernutrition on infant behavior.

Whereas a decade or two ago we thought that the effects of early malnutrition were irreversible, we now know that this is not true. Children who are undernourished in the early years can and do benefit from nutritional, health care, and educational programs (McKay, Sinisterra, McKay, Gomez, & Lloreda, 1978). While such interventions can narrow the cognitive gap between undernourished children and their more advantaged peers, the gap is never closed. This has three implications. First, every effort should be made to provide all children early in life with the nutrition they need for healthy growth and development. Second, intervention programs that help undernourished children "catch up" are worth it, regardless of whether or not the gap is closed. Third, such programs should start as early as possible so that children may receive maximum benefits.

The Nutritional Needs of Infants

Most parents are concerned about meeting the nutritional requirements for their young children. The "ideal" nutrition program for the neonate and infant is breast-feeding by a well-nourished and healthy mother. However, this is not always possible for a number of reasons. First, the mother may not want or be able to breast-feed her baby, her milk supply may not be sufficient for her baby, or she may not be healthy enough to provide her baby with the necessary nutritional requirements.

Today, more than half of all new mothers breast-feed their babies. This growth in the popularity of breast-feeding is attributed to educational programs that stress its benefits to parents and children, the feminist movement and its consciousness raising of women and men, and the recognition that mother's milk is the best food available for children. This reality is also reflected in the fact that commercially prepared formula is designed to duplicate mother's milk as closely as possible. Breast pumps also enable mothers who want to return to work to provide their children with breast milk when they can't be available for a feeding.

Caloric Intake

Keep in mind that the infant triples her birth weight in the first year. This relatively rapid weight

TABLE 6–11

SCHEDULE FOR INTRODUCTION OF SOLID FOODS

0–4 months:	Breast milk or commercially prepared routine infant formula only
4–6 months:	Addition of an iron-fortified cereal (mixed with breast milk or routine formula, not cow's milk)
5–7 months:	Addition of strained or pureed fruits or vegetables and unsweetened fruit juice (by cup)
6–8 months:	Addition of single-ingredient table foods (potatoes, rice, pasta, bread), single-ingredient desserts (puddings, junkets, custards), and "finger foods" (zwieback, teething biscuits, graham crackers, toast)

Note. From *Parent's Guide to Infant Nutrition* (p. 41), 1986, Evansville, IN: Provided courtesy Mead Johnson Nutritionals.

gain requires substantial daily caloric intake, amounting to about fifty calories per pound of body weight. Think what would happen to you if you ate at the same rate!

Infants also have to eat many times a day because of their small stomach capacity. Neonates and young infants may eat as many as six to nine times a day. With growth, the number of meals decreases, so that by the end of the first year, most infants are eating three meals a day consisting of milk and solids. (See Table 6–11.)

When to Introduce Solid Foods

Historically, solid foods were introduced to children at a much earlier age than they are today. Some parents want to introduce solid foods almost immediately. The American Academy of Pediatrics Committee on Nutrition, on the other hand, recommends that solid foods be introduced at between four and six months. There are a number

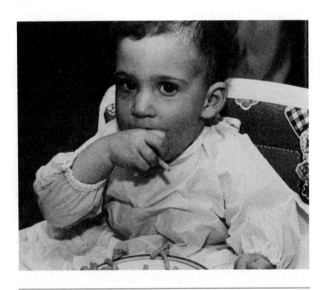

FIGURE 6-14 Finger foods provide the opportunity for infants to be involved in self-feeding and to experience new foods. Mealtimes and all feeding experiences should be as calm and pleasant as possible. (Photo by Kenneth Deitcher, MD.)

of reasons for their recommendation. First, babies need more iron and minerals than their mother's breast milk or formula supplies. Second, during this time babies lose their "extrusion reflex," which assists them in sucking but which makes them push food out of their mouths. Third, babies usually have their first teeth by six months, and fourth, they are mature enough to signal that they don't want any more food. Not everyone agrees that children should be put on solid food during the first year or that the process of weaning should be started at six months. The La Leche League, in particular, emphasizes that all children are individuals and that the perfect food for the first year of life is breast milk. Table 6–11 shows a schedule for the introduction of solid foods.

The current emphasis on breast-feeding would seem to be an unconscious reaffirmation of Freudian theory that infant hunger and oral gratification are necessary for healthy psychic development. Freud also believed that if too many individuals fed a particular child, the child would not attach and, therefore, would not learn to love.

Nutritional Supplements

Generally, infants are given oral supplements of vitamins and iron beginning at birth, but starting no later than the fourth to sixth months. This is the time that infants start to deplete their own storehouse of iron, so a supplement is necessary. Also, a fluoride supplement greatly reduces the incidence of dental caries (decay). The amount of fluoride in the local water supply, if any, determines the amount prescribed as a supplement. Only about half the communities in the United States have a fluoridated water supply.

"Variety" and "natural" are two words used to describe today's food fare for infants. Parents can pick from a wide selection of foods from ready-to-feed formulas to gourmet dessert selections. The natural trend in baby foods is a result of the public's desire for foods that are "natural." Today, baby foods are free of salt, sugar, color, and additives.

Bottle Mouth

Bottle mouth is tooth decay caused by letting children nurse for too long on a bottle, putting a too-sweet liquid (sugar water and soda) in the bottle, and putting the baby to bed or to sleep with a bottle. The American Dental Association recommends not putting the child to sleep with anything but water in the bottle.

PARENTING THE INFANT

During every stage of development, children exhibit particular characteristics that have implications for parenting and care-giving. Parents need to know what children are like in general and the individual characteristics of each of their children. What is involved in the effective parenting of infants? Some of the basics include (Weider & Greenspan, 1987):

Primary maternal functions
1. The ability to provide physical care and protection.
2. The ability to read an infant's signals of pleasure and displeasure.
3. An emotional capacity for attachment between mother and infant.

Secondary maternal functions
1. The ability to discern a child's changing developmental needs.
2. The capacity to respond promptly, effectively, and emphatically to the child's signals.

Although these basic guidelines may seem elementary and based on common sense, knowing about them is much easier than always being able to do them, especially in the face of many of the stresses influencing contemporary parent-child relationships.

*I*N THE SPOTLIGHT

DR. SPOCK—COMMON SENSE AND PARENTING

Most adults like to think of themselves as capable of dealing with most situations that arise. Becoming a parent, however, oftentimes has a way of changing people's perspectives on many things. With many decisions regarding parenting, it is not uncommon for parents to ask, "What should I do?" For millions of parents, the answer to this question has been the reassuring response of Dr. Spock, one of America's best-known names in baby care: "Don't be afraid to trust your own common sense." In fact, trusting oneself has been the recurring theme of parenting for nearly half a century—from 1945, when *The Common Sense Book of Baby and Child Care* was first published—to the present. The advice hasn't changed over the years:

You know more than you think you do. Soon you're going to have a baby. Maybe you have one already. You're happy and excited, but you haven't had much experience, you wonder whether you are going to know how to do a good job. Lately you have been listening more carefully to your friends and relatives when they talk about bringing up a child. You've begun to read articles by experts in the magazines and newspapers. After the baby is born, the doctors and nurses will begin to give you instructions too. Sometimes it sounds like a complicated business. You find out all the vitamins a baby needs and all the immunizations. One mother tells you that egg should be given early because of its iron, and another says that egg should be delayed to avoid allergy. You hear that a baby is easily spoiled by being picked up too much but also that a baby must be cuddled plenty; that fairy tales make children nervous, and that fairy tales are a wholesome outlet.

Don't take too seriously all that the neighbors say. Don't be overawed by what the experts say. Don't be afraid to trust your own common sense. Bringing up your child won't be a complicated job if you take it easy, trust your own instincts and follow the directions your doctor gives you. We know for a fact that the natural loving care that kindly parents give their children is a hundred times more valuable than their knowing how to pin a diaper on just right or how to make formula expertly (Spock & Rothenberg, 1985, p. 1).

The impact of Spock's message to the parents of America was significant in four ways. First, it liberated them from the rigid and prescriptive, behaviorist-based child-rearing advice in vogue during the first half of the twentieth century. It is to this prescriptive rigidity that Spock gives the back of his hand. (See Chapter Two for behaviorist ideas.) For their part, parents welcomed the liberator with open arms. They were happy to have someone who spoke calmly and confidently to them in nondogmatic and nonthreatening terms. It was like having a grandfather available to dispense wise and wondrous advice.

Second, there was a price to pay for this liberation. What about the parents who were not confident in their abilities and who were filled with doubt about the soundness of their common sense? The answer, as you might expect, is self-doubt, which leads to blame. If the leniency advocated by Spock didn't work, and if children didn't grow up as they should or, worse yet, if they grew up wrong, then it was easy to point the finger of blame at parents. Common sense is a two-edged sword. It was easy for parents to be filled with self-doubt and guilt about the trauma they caused their children because of common sense.

Third, the leniency advocated by Spock was the bedrock and foundation of permissive parenting. For as Spock advises, "Better to make a few mistakes from being natural than to do everything letter-perfect out of a feeling of worry" (p. 2). Parents could relax and be themselves while letting their children be themselves.

Fourth, Spock's book and its fatherly, confident tone was the first extended presentation of Freudian advice in the popular literature on child rearing (Sommerville, 1982, p. 224). Although Freud isn't mentioned, he is nevertheless there in discussions of demand feeding and toilet training, where Spock advises that children should become trained of their own free will, with no pressure from parents.

*I*N THE SPOTLIGHT

WHERE SHOULD BABY SLEEP?

In at least 44 percent of societies around the globe, mother and infant share a bed. No other society seems to prefer the American practice of having the baby sleep in a separate room (Konner, 1989). A majority of the infants (55 percent) reared in the United States are never in bed with their parents, and only 8 percent frequently stay with their parents a full night, Figure 6–15.

But, where should a baby sleep? It depends on whose advice you listen to. Dr. Spock advises parents to have their infants sleep in a separate room. The La Leche League, an organization designed to promote breast-feeding, encourages bed-sharing. Also, an increasing number of parents are allowing their children to share their beds with them (Konner, 1989). Although many pediatricians oppose bed-sharing, the decision as to where an infant sleeps will probably be based on what parents believe is best for them and their children at the time.

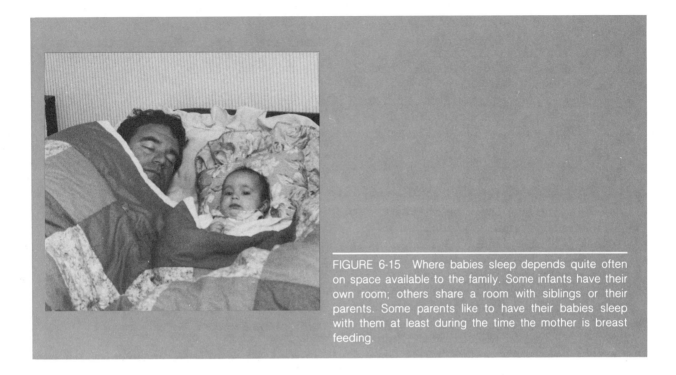

FIGURE 6-15 Where babies sleep depends quite often on space available to the family. Some infants have their own room; others share a room with siblings or their parents. Some parents like to have their babies sleep with them at least during the time the mother is breast feeding.

CARING FOR THE INFANT

Safety

Parents must continuously be alert to the situations and events that would compromise the health and safety of their infants. Again, parents may do certain things with and for their infants without realizing the inherent dangers involved in matters of routine care. For example, pacifiers are rather routinely used as self-soothers. However, they can be a source of injuries. Pacifiers should be of one piece, so that nipple and handle do not separate, and they should not contain rattles or other objects. Infants have choked to death on objects contained in broken pacifiers. Also, parents should not tie a string on the pacifier and hang it around the infant's neck. The string may tangle around the infant's neck and cause strangulation.

Childproofing the Home

Providing a home for children is not enough. That home must be a safe place for the infant to grow. Parents have to be proactive in their efforts to provide such an environment. Likewise, caregivers in child care homes and centers must also make every effort to provide for children's safety. Following are some of the things that all adults can do:

1. Keep small appliances unplugged and out of the baby's reach.
2. Avoid using hot curling irons, etc. near young children.
3. Don't set hot pots, pans, and liquids where the baby can reach them. When cooking, turn pot handles to the back of the stove.
4. Put plants out of the baby's reach. Many houseplants are poisonous, check which ones in your house are and get rid of them.
5. Don't store or keep plastic bags. Any time plastic bags are in the home, keep them out of the reach of all children.
6. Keep knives, scissors, and all sharp items such as pencils out of the baby's reach.
7. A baby can pull a tablecloth and everything

on it down on himself, so don't use one when this is likely to happen.

8. Make sure baby's crib meets the safety standards set by the Consumer Product Safety Commission (CPSC). These include spacing of slates, height of crib sides, and the size of the crib mattress. Prior to such standards, cribs were involved in more infant deaths than any other product.

9. Try to imagine that you are an infant. Get down on the floor and see for yourself what dangers await the unwary child—small objects on the floor, a hot heating register or radiator, or an uncovered wall outlet.

10. Lock all doors to areas to which you don't want the child to have access, such as laundry rooms, garages, and basements.

11. Use gates at the top and bottom of stairs. Make sure the gates meet the standards of the CPSC.

12. Never leave a baby unattended. They can fall off of a changing table in the blink of an eye, and can drown in a bathtub in the time it takes to answer the telephone.

13. Do not leave side rails down on the crib.

14. Toys should be chosen with care. Toys with removable small parts (such as eyes and ears on some dolls) should not be given to small children (infants).

Adults are responsible for children's safety. It is unreasonable to expect any young child to assume responsibility for her own safety.

Immunizations

Immunizations are an important prophylactic procedure in the lives of young children. Table 6–13 outlines the immunization schedule normally followed for infants and children.

STRANGER ANXIETY

During the first year, some babies demonstrate an anxiety or fear of strangers. This may occur at four or five months in some babies and in others,

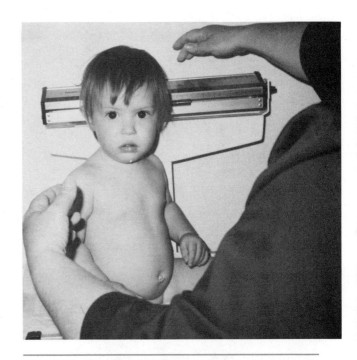

FIGURE 6-16 Part of all infants' care should be regular well-baby visits to a pediatrician and the protection that comes from immunization to childhood diseases.

TABLE 6–12

IMMUNIZATION SCHEDULE FOR INFANTS AND CHILDREN	
Age	Recommended Type of Immunization
2 months	DPT (diphtheria-pertussis [whooping cough] tetanus and oral polio vaccine (OPV)
4 months	DPT, OPV
6 months	DPT
12 months	Tuberculin skin test
15 months	Measles, rubella, mumps
18 months	DPT, OPV (booster)
24 months	Hemophilus influenzae type b (Hib disease)
4–6 years	DPT, OPV (booster)
14–16 years	Adult DT

later or not at all. When a stranger approaches, the infant will cling to the parent, cry, and show a general displeasure. A child develops an attitude toward and concept of "strangers" (for quite often, the stranger is the grandparent!) based on the parents' attitudes and reactions. Parents can greet strangers with smiles, friendly verbal acknowledgements, and generally let the child know that the stranger is "okay." A trusting attachment between parent and child helps children and their parents make the transition from this stage to one of accepting comfortable relationships between themselves and others.

The first year is a year full of tremendous growth and effort on the part of infants. They expend tremendous amounts of energy. Many of their behaviors advent their growing independence and ability. They reach for a brightly colored rattle, crawl determinately after a red ring or favorite toy placed just outside their reach, scream with delight, open their mouths wide for the next spoonful of cereal, and look intently at the face of whoever is repeating their many sounds.

What Would You Do?

Miriam Armbruster and her husband, Daniel, live with their six-month-old daughter, Debbie, in a third-floor condominium apartment. Miriam and Daniel are anxious for Debbie to learn how to walk. They believe that a walker will not only help Debbie learn to walk, but it will also help her learn to walk faster. The Armbrusters also believe a walker will help Debbie get around their apartment better.

Miriam knows you are taking a course in child development and therefore thinks you are a good person to ask for advice. Miriam wants to know if there is any particular brand or style of walker that is better than another. She also wants to know if you think Debbie is too young for a walker. What do you tell Miriam and Daniel?

CHILD CARE FOR INFANTS

Today, with the growing numbers of working mothers and two-career families, more and more infants are being cared for by baby-sitters, relatives, and care-givers in child care programs. Consequently, the parent team today includes more than mother/father/child. It now includes other care-givers as well, making parenting the responsibility of many others.

What Constitutes Quality Infant Care?

All who provide care for infants must recognize that the nature of that care and the environment in which it occurs should be appropriate to them *as infants*. Too often infants are treated as toddlers and preschoolers. Some infant care has been perfunctory at best, with care-givers having the attitude that infants are too young and immature to understand or need much attention other than feeding and diapering. Rather, infant care-givers should have special training that enables them to have an understanding of and provide for the special needs of infants. Following are some guidelines that will enable infant care-givers to provide a developmentally appropriate and nurturing environment.

- Infants need a flexible, safe, healthy, aesthetically pleasing, and protective environment in which care-givers are attuned to them and respond to their individual needs in developmentally appropriate ways.
- Infants need care-givers who use the many routines of feeding, diapering, bathing, and comforting as opportunities to demonstrate affection and to communicate and positively interact with them.
- Infants need care-givers who know them, are involved with them, and view them as worthy individuals. This implies that care-givers are knowledgeable in infant and child care, and are willing to provide infants with a continuous and affectionate relationship. The intelligence

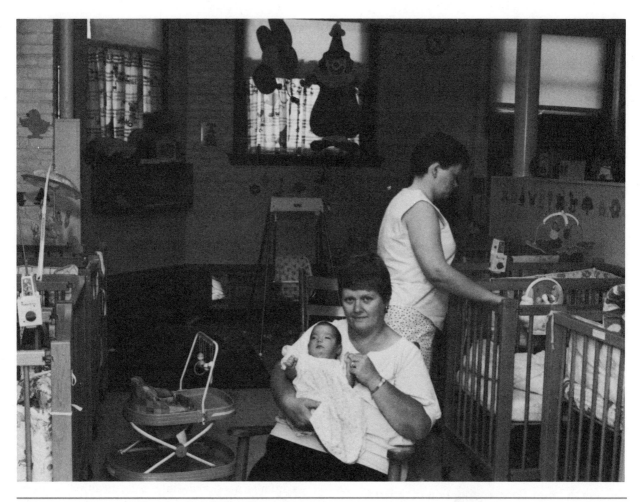

FIGURE 6-17 The care provided for infants outside the home should be appropriate to them as infants. Caregivers should be knowledgeable of infant development; do their best for infants; and support parents in their roles as the primary caregivers of their children.

and knowledge of the care-givers creates the climate for good infant care.

■ Infants need programs and curricula designed specifically for them. This includes the room arrangement, center/home organization, and materials. The program of infant care should be cognitively and emotionally enriching.

■ Infants need programs and care-givers who will work with their parents in providing them the information, emotional support, and prac-tical advice they need to meet the demands of modern parenting.

■ Infants need opportunities to interact with oth-ers. Infants' social development includes more than providing them toys with which to play. The child care environment includes other chil-dren and adults, and infants must be given opportunities to effectively interact with them. Thus, one role of care-givers is to facilitate the social interaction of infants with others.

Accreditation

The National Association for the Education of Young Children, a national child advocacy and professional support organization, accredits or certifies child care programs that meet their professional standards. They provide guidelines and procedures for agencies and centers to follow in order to assure that young children have quality child care.

Several issues are involved in infant child care. They are quality, stability, and accessibility. Quality child care is staffed by knowledgeable, sensible, skilled, and emotionally supportive care-givers who understand infants. Infants—indeed all children—need stable child care that includes care by the same care-giver over a period of time. And, infants and their parents need access to quality child care. Unfortunately, there is more demand for quality child care than there are quality programs.

*I*N THE SPOTLIGHT

IS CHILD CARE GOOD FOR INFANTS?

More women are entering the work force for several reasons: economic necessity and the desire for a career. As a result, more children at earlier ages are being placed in infant child care. While most parents feel they don't have a choice, many privately and publicly wonder, "Is leaving my baby at a center all day good for him?" Until the present time, little, if any, evidence existed proving that early infant care outside the home was harmful to children. Some early childhood experts expressed their doubts about substitute care for very young children. In his book, *The First Three Years of Life*, Burton White (1985) said that "full-time substitute care for babies under three years of age, and especially for those only a few months of age, does not seem to be in the best interest of babies" (p. 267). Generally, however, such cautionary admonitions have been ignored, mainly because of economic necessity and careers.

However, there is now a growing debate about how much child care is good for children and the effects it has on them. The controversy associated with infant care was brought to a boil with the research revelation that "twenty or more hours of such care [nonmaternal] per week were associated with significantly in-

creased risk of the development of insecure infant-mother attachment relationships (Belsky & Rovine, 1988, p. 164).

The fallout over this research is significant and vociferous. Belsky and Rovine were quick to add that the attributes of the mother, the characteristics of individual children, and the nature of the care arrangements form a "complex ecology" that has to be more fully understood and researched. Nonetheless, there are many objections to their conclusions. Some of these are (Lewis, 1988):

1. Questioning whether or not the use of the strange situation to determine the nature of maternal-infant attachment, as Belsky and Rovine did, is comparable to what happens in an infant care program.
2. Raising the possibility that since many working mothers are single parent mothers, this may be a factor in the differences in children's attachment.
3. The real possibility that differences in children's attachments may be unrelated to working or being in infant care.
4. Questioning the significance the differences in attachment behaviors has for children and their parents.

5. The need to consider the nature and quality of the relationship between the infant and the nonmaternal care-giver. It may be that this attachment relationship is stronger and offsets any insecurity in the infant-mother attachment relationship.

It is likely and altogether appropriate that the debate over the effects of infant care on children and their parents will continue. As it does, those who are responsible for caring for the nation's infants will be challenged to provide *quality* care and to support parents in their roles as the primary care-givers of their children.

Summary

■ Our knowledge and understanding of infants has changed over the last several decades. Previously, infants were viewed as capable of very little, and were literally thought to be psychosocially incompetent, with care-givers being the primary sources of their experiences. Today, infants are viewed as possessing very remarkable social, emotional, and intellectual abilities.

■ Infancy is a precarious time of life and the infant mortality rate (the ratio of the number of infant deaths per 1000 live births) is very high in many third world countries. The United States has set as its goal an infant mortality rate of nine per 1000, which it has yet to achieve. On the other hand, many parents of advantaged children are goal directed and seek ways to enhance their children's development. Some early childhood educators and child development professionals caution such parents against "pushing" their children.

■ Infancy is viewed as an important time in life for several reasons: it is the beginning of postnatal development, it is a period of rapid growth, it is a sensitive period of development, and it is a period in which infants "finish off" their development.

■ A number of models can be used to help explain child development, including the status quo, the environmental, the interactional, and the transactional models. The transactional model emphasizes the transactions between children and their environment, and the influences each has on the other.

■ Human infants are born "early" and therefore, unlike many other animals, a great deal of development occurs after birth. In order to reach adult proportions, infants develop according to the two-three-four-five rule.

■ Motor development plays an important role in infants' physical, social and intellectual development. Motor development is sequential, proceeds from gross to fine, is cephalocaudal, and proceeds from the proximal to the distal.

■ Infants' eyes will undergo a two- to three-fold increase in size to reach adult proportions. Infants can see objects in their immediate environment better than at a distance, and prefer focal colors of red and blue.

■ Two of the best methods for soothing a fussy baby are continuous stimulation such as wrapping, and motion through jiggling and rocking. Parents should respond in caring ways to infants' cries.

■ Modification of basic reflexive actions occurs during Stage II of intellectual development. Also, primary circular reactions begin. Stage III is known as the stage of "making interesting things last"; object permanence begins to develop, and secondary circular reactions begin. During Stage IV, infants use means to attain ends.

■ The ages of sensorimotor intelligence are only approximate; infants do not think like adults; infants construct their own intelligence; parents and other care-givers must provide an environment in which infants can construct their own knowledge; knowledge of causality develops over time; and subsequent stages of intellectual development build on previous ones.

■ Behaviorism helps explain many of the ways in which children acquire language. Heredity plays a role in language development through physical structures and a brain that makes language possible. Nativists believe language development is innate. Two theories that help to explain language development are the LAD (Language Acquisition Device) and the LASS (Language Acquisition Support System). Biology, the environment, and social interactions also play a role in language development.

■ Language development begins with crying and progresses through smiling, cooing, babbling, "Ma-ma," "Da-da," and then to first words. Infants also communicate with gestures and through games.

■ John Bowlby's theory of attachment has six stages. During Stage One, infants use basic reflexive actions and crying to initiate attachment interactions. Secure attachment helps children develop a sense of confidence and provide support for independence. Young children can and do develop more than one attachment at a time. The Strange Situation is a method researchers use to ascertain the quality of child-parent attachment.

■ Infant temperament plays a role in infant-parent attachment. Developing a support system is an excellent way for parents to lower the stress of parenting. If parents want a happy child, they should be happy themselves.

■ Nutrition plays an important role throughout the early years. Young children are particularly vulnerable to undernourishment and malnourishment. Children who have chronic nutrition and other health deficits have many retarded psychological characteristics and capabilities. Intervention programs that assist undernourished children in "catching up" are worth it, regardless of whether or not the gap is closed. Nutrition education and enhancement programs should start as early as possible so that children may receive a program's maximum benefits.

■ The "ideal" nutrition program for neonates and infants is breast-feeding by a well-nourished and healthy mother. Today, more than half of all new mothers breast-feed their babies. The infant triples her birth weight in the first year. This relatively rapid weight gain requires substantial daily caloric intake, amounting to about fifty calories per pound of body weight.

■ Today, solid foods are introduced to children later than they were when you and your parents were children. The American Academy of Pediatrics Committee on Nutrition, on the other hand, recommends that solid foods be introduced between four and six months. Young children's nutritional needs are also supplemented by vitamins and minerals.

■ Effective parenting includes care and protection; the ability to read infants' signals; an emotional capacity for attachment; the ability to respond to children's developmental needs; and the ability to respond to children's signals.

■ Parents and other care-givers must provide for the safety of children by childproofing homes and child care settings.

■ Child care for infants should be appropriate to them as infants. Infants need care-givers who know about and care for them. They need an environment that is safe and aesthetically pleasing, and curricula and programs designed specifically for them.

■ There is currently a great deal of controversy in the early childhood and child development fields about whether or not more than twenty hours of nonmaternal child care per week is good for infants.

QUESTIONS TO GUIDE YOUR REVIEW

1. How have views of infancy changed over the last several decades?
2. What is the infant mortality rate? Has the infant mortality rate in the United States increased or decreased over the last decade? Is the infant mortality rate in the United States as low as it should be? Why?
3. In what ways is infancy an important time of development?
4. Why is the transactional model preferred for explaining child development?
5. Why are humans born "early"?
6. What is the two-three-four-five rule and how does it help explain physical development?
7. Can a child be outside the "average" ranges for normal development and yet be developing normally? Why? How?
8. Why does motor development play an important role in infant development?
9. What motor development guidelines help explain infant development?
10. What are the highlights of infant motor development?
11. What colors do infants prefer? Why?
12. What is the significance of infants' abilities to experience through their senses?
13. What are the best ways to soothe a fussy baby?
14. What is a primary circular reaction? How does it contribute to intellectual development?
15. Why is Stage III of intellectual development called the stage of "making interesting things happen"?
16. Do infants "think" like adults? How do they think?
17. Can behaviorism fully explain the process of language development? Why?
18. How do the LASS and LAD contribute to language development?
19. On what basis do people argue for an innate theory of language development?
20. What is the sequence of language development during the first year?
21. How do the games infants play contribute to their language development?
22. What effects do malnourishment and undernourishment have on young children's development?

23. When and how should solid foods be introduced to infants?
24. What primary and secondary functions do good parents provide children?
25. How has Dr. Spock influenced child rearing?
26. What specific things can parents and care-givers do to provide for children's safety in the home and child care center?
27. What immunizations should children have?
28. What constitutes quality child care?
29. What qualities should good care-givers have?
30. Is child care harmful to infants?

ACTIVITIES FOR FURTHER INVOLVEMENT

1. Stimulation plays a major role in cognitive and social development.
   a. What can parents and care-givers do to promote and enhance the play activity of infants?
   b. How do interpersonal relations affect the play interactions and stimulation of infants?
   c. React to the following: "Parents and care-givers need to *allow children to play.*"
2. The role of infants' temperaments is an important consideration in parenting and care-giving.
   a. Interview parents and have them describe their babies' temperaments.
   b. How did parents respond differently to their babies' temperaments?
   c. What specific influences do babies' temperaments have on parenting interactions?
3. Nutrition is an important consideration in the lives of parents and children.
   a. Interview parents of various ages and cultures to determine the differences in the way they feed and wean their infants.
   b. What are the cultural differences in feeding infants?
   c. How can feeding be a learning experience for both infants and parents?
4. Child rearing is no easy task for parents.
   a. How do changing societal standards influence how today's parents rear their infants as compared to how your parents reared you when you were an infant?
   b. Interview parents to determine how they parent their infants. Based on the information you gathered, what advice would you have for parents, based on your knowledge of child development?
5. Language plays an important role in the lives of children and their families.
   a. Observe two infants, first at six months and again at about eleven months. How does their language development differ?
   b. Find evidence to support the biological and behaviorist theories of language development.
   c. What would you tell a parent who asks you for advice about how to enhance the language development of her nine-month-old son?

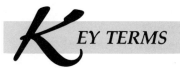

KEY TERMS

Cephalocaudal development (From the Greek *kephale*, "head" and the Latin *cauda*, "tail.") Used to describe development as progressing from the head to the feet.

Deciduous Descriptive of the first set of baby, "milk," or primary teeth.

Distal Descriptive of the extremities of the body.

Environmental model Developmental model that maintains that development is primarily influenced and affected by environmental factors.

Interactional model Developmental model that asserts that what children are like—their basic constitution—*and* their environment play a role in development.

LAD Language acquisition device.

LASS Language acquisition support system.

Malnourishment A condition resulting from the lack of a specific component, such as protein, necessary for proper growth.

Object permanence The understanding that objects exist apart and separate from the individual.

Primary circular reactions Displayed when infants use their bodies to initiate and re-peat many actions such as thumb sucking, leg kicking, and staring at the hands for extended periods of time because of the pleasure it brings. These reactions are called "primary" because they are reactions involving the infant's own body.

Proximal Descriptive of the parts of the body along the midline.

Secondary circular reactions Characterized by the infant's repeating an action with the purpose of getting the same response from an object or person. The name "secondary" implies that the reaction is elicited from a secondary source rather than from the infant.

Status quo model Sometimes referred to as the medical model. Maintains that who and what the child is remains stable over time because the environment has very little influence on development.

Transactional model Developmental model based on the premise that contact between the developing child and the environment is a transaction in which each is influenced by the other.

Undernourishment A condition resulting from an insufficient amount of food.

ENRICHMENT THROUGH FURTHER READING

Bloomgarden, D. (1983). *Stimulation activities age birth to five years*, reprint no. 19. Washington, D.C.: Peace Corps, Information, Collection, and Exchange.

This is a collection of stimulation activities that encourage children's physical and mental growth. The activities were field-tested with children in the Jamaican National Day Care Program. Emphasis is placed on activities that can be supported with low-cost or scrap materials.

Leach, P. (1983). *Babyhood* (2nd ed.). New York: Alfred A. Knopf.

This is a very thorough and comprehensive book, packed with useful information for parents and other care-givers. Leach gives the what and why of development during the first two years (three-quarters of the book is devoted to the first year). She also has a very refreshing attitude about being practical and realistic in the tasks of child rearing.

Lief, N. R.(1982). *The first year of life: A guide for parenting.* New York: Dodd, Mead. The major purpose of this book is to provide parents with practical information about child rearing. Each of the twelve chapters deals with a month of infant development in the first year of life. Much of the content comes from discussions about child development between parents and staff of the New York Junior League's Early Childhood Development Center. The format and content make for interesting reading and provide sound parenting information.

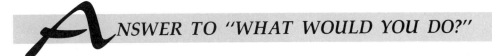

ANSWER TO "WHAT WOULD YOU DO?"

Baby Walkers: All Fall Down

How many times have you seen a baby in a baby walker? Probably many times, but how safe are they? Not very safe at all. In fact they are downright dangerous. So, if you advised Mrs. Armbruster not to buy a baby walker, you gave her good advice. The Consumer Product Safety Commission reports that in one year alone, 24,000 walker-related injuries were serious enough to require medical treatment.

Also, many parents use children's walkers in the belief that they will help their children walk earlier. This is not the case, however. In fact, just the opposite may be true! One study with twins revealed that children who don't use a walker learn to walk slightly earlier than those who do (Lang, 1986). So, the next time a friend or relative anticipates buying a walker for their baby, or a Mrs. Armbruster asks you for advice, you should, in a nice way, tell them about the hazards involved.

BIBLIOGRAPHY

Ainsworth, M., Blehar, M., Waters, E., & Wall, S. (1978). *Patterns of Attachment.* Lawrence Erlbaum.

Bailey, W.T. (1987). Infancy to age five: Predicting fathers' involvement. Paper presented at the biennial meeting of the Society for Research in Child Development, Baltimore, April 23–26, 1987.

Banks, M.S., & Dannemiller, J. L. (1987). Infant visual psychophysics. In P. Salapatek & L. Cohen (Eds.), *Handbook of infant perception: Vol. 1. From sensation to perception* (pp. 115–184). Orlando: Harcourt Brace Jovanovich.

Barclay, L. (1985). *Infant development.* New York: CBS College.

Barrett, D. (1987). Undernutrition and child behavior: What behaviors should we measure and how should we measure them? In J. Dobbing (Ed.), *Early nutrition and later development.* London: Academic Press.

Belsky, J., & Rovine, M. J. (1988). Non-maternal care in the first year of life and the security of infant-parent attachment. *Child Development, 59,* 157–167.

Bowlby, J. (1969). *Attachment.* New York: Basic Books.

Bruner, J. S. (1983). *Child's talk: Learning to use language.* New York: W. W. Norton.

Capute, A.J., & Accardo, P.J. (1987). Linguistic and auditory milestones during the first two years of life. *Clinical Pediatrics, 17* (11), 847–853.

Chomsky, N. (1965). *Aspects of the theory of syntax.* Cambridge, MA: MIT Press.

Crockenberg, S., & McCluskey, K. (1986). Change in maternal behavior during the baby's first year of life. *Child Development, 57,* 746–753.

Crook, C. (1987). Taste and olfaction. In P. Salapatek & L. Cohen (Eds.), *Handbook of infant perception: Vol. 1. From sensation to perception* (pp. 237–264). Orlando: Harcourt Brace Jovanovich.

Curtiss, S. (1977). *Genie: A psycholinguistic study of a modern day "wild child."* New York: Academic Press.

Cutrona, C. E. & Troutman, B. R. (1986). *Child Development, 57,* 1507–1518.

DeLuccie, M. (1989). Mothers as gatekeepers: A model of maternal mediators of father involvement. Paper presented at the biennial meeting of the Society for Research in Child Development, Kansas City, MO.

de Villiers, J.G., & de Villiers, P.A. (1979). *Early Language.* Cambridge, MA: Harvard University Press.

Farber, E. A., & Egeland, B. (1982) Developmental consequences of out-of-home care for infants in a low-income population. In E. F. Zigler & E. W. Gordon (Eds.), *Day care: Scientific and social policy issues.* (pp. 102–125). Boston: Auburn House.

Field, T. (1987). Baby research comes of age. *Psychology Today, 21,* 46.

Frankenburg, W. K., Fandal, A.W., Sciarillo, W., & Burgess, D. (1981). The newly abbreviated and revised Denver Developmental Screening Test. *The Journal of Pediatrics, 99,* 995–999.

Gibson, E. J., & Walk, R. D. (1960). The visual cliff. *Scientific American, 202,* 64–71.

Goldstein, B.E. (1984). *Sensation and perception* (2nd ed.). Belmont, CA: Wadsworth.

Gould, S.J. (1982). Human babies as embryos. In Jay Belsky (Ed.), *In the beginning: Readings in infancy.* New York: Columbia University Press.

Hamill, P. V. V., Drizd, T. A., Reed, R. B., Johnson, C. L., Roche, A. F., & Moore, W. M. (1979). Physical growth: National center for health statistics percentiles. *The American Journal of Clinical Nutrition, 32,* 607–629.

Haviland, J. M., & Lelwica, M. (1987). The induced affect response: Ten-week-old infants' responses to three emotional expressions. *Developmental Psychology, 23,* 97–104.

Hicky, T. L., & Peduzzi, J. D. (1987). Structure and development of the visual system. In P. Salapatek & L. Cohen (Eds.), *Handbook of infant perception: Vol. 1. From sensation to perception* (pp. 1–42). Orlando: Harcourt Brace Jovanovich.

Kahn, F. (1943, 1971). *Man in structure and function.* New York: Alfred A. Knopf.

Konner, M. (1989, January 8). Where should baby sleep? *The New York Times Magazine,* pp. 39–40.

Lamb, M. E. (1981). *The role of the father in child development* (2nd ed.). New York: John Wiley.

Lang, S. S. (1986). Tots on wheels. (1986, July–August). *American Health,* p. 86.

Langlois, J. H., Roggman, L. A., Cassey, R.J., Ritter, J. M., Rieser-Danner, L. A., & Jenkins, V. Y. (1987). Infant preferences for attractive faces: Rudiments of a stereotype?" *Developmental Psychology, 23,* 363–369.

Lewis, M. (1988). Infant concern. *Working Parents, 5,* 14–15.

Lieberman, P. (1984). *Biology and the evolution of language.* Cambridge, MA: Harvard University Press.

MacFarlane, A. (1977). *The psychology of childbirth.* Cambridge, MA: Harvard University Press.

McKay, H., Sinisterra, L., McKay, A., Gomez, H., & Lloreda, P. (1978). Improving cognitive ability in chronically deprived children. *Science, 200,* 270–278.

Newport, E. L., Gleitman, H., & Gleitman, L. (1977). Mother, I'd rather do it myself: Some effects and non-effects of maternal speech style, in C. E. Snow & C. A. Ferguson (Eds.), *Talking to children: Language input and acquisition* (pp. 112–129). Cambridge, England: Cambridge University Press.

1988 world population data sheet. (1988, April) Washington, DC: Population Reference Bureau.

Parent's Guide to Infant Nutrition. (1986). Evansville, IN: Mead, Johnson.

Pollitt, E. (1988, Winter). A child survival and developmental revolution: GOBI-FFF. *SRCD Newsletter,* p. 4.

Reisman, J. E. (1987). Touch, motion and proprioception. In P. Salapatek & L. Cohen (Eds.), *Handbook of infant perception: Vol. 1. From sensation to perception* (pp. 265–303). Orlando: Harcourt Brace Jovanovich.

Ross, H. S., & Lollis, S.P. (1987). Communication within infant social games. *Developmental Psychology, 23,* 241–248.

Scarborough, H., & Wyckoff, J. (1986). Mother, I'd still rather do it myself: some further non-effects of "Motherese." *Journal of Child Language, 13,* 431–437.

Schaffer, R. (1977). *Mothering.* Cambridge, MA: Harvard University Press.

Sinisterra, L. (1987). Studies on poverty, human growth and development: The Cali experience. In J. Dobbing (Ed.), *Early nutrition and later achievement.* London: Academic Press.

Slobin, D. I. (1982). Universal and particular in the acquisition of language. In E. Wanner & L. R. Gleitman (Eds.), *Language acquisition: The state of the art* (pp. 128–170). Cambridge, England: Cambridge University Press.

Snow, C. (1979). Talking and playing with babies: The role of ideologies in child rearing. In M. Bullowa (Ed.), *Before speech: The beginning of interpersonal communication* (pp. 269–288). Cambridge, England: Cambridge University Press.

Sommerville, J. (1982). *The rise and fall of childhood.* Beverly Hills, CA: Sage Publications.

Spock, B., & Rothenberg, M.B. (1985). *Baby and child care.* New York: E. P. Dutton.

Sroufe, L.A. (1978, October). Attachment and the roots of competence. *Human Nature, 1,* 52.

Teller, D. Y., & Bornstein, M. H. Infant color vision and color perception. In P. Salapatek and L. Cohen (Eds.), *Handbook of infant perception: Vol. 1. From sensation to perception* (pp. 185–263). Orlando: Harcourt Brace Jovanovich.

White, B. (1985). *The first three years of life.* Englewood Cliffs, NJ: Prentice-Hall.

Wieder, S., & Greenspan, S. I., (1987). Staffing process, and structure of the clinical infant development program. In S. I. Greenspan et al. (Eds.), *Infants in multirisk families* (p. 11). Madison, CT: International Universities Press.

CHAPTER SEVEN

The toddler: exploration and independence

VIGNETTE
INTRODUCTION
PHYSICAL DEVELOPMENT
Dental Development
MOTOR DEVELOPMENT
Everybody Loves a Ball Game
Fine Motor Skills
Handedness
PERCEPTUAL DEVELOPMENT
Sensory Development
INDEPENDENCE
SAFETY
NUTRITION
Implications for Parents
TOILET TRAINING
INTELLECTUAL DEVELOPMENT
Stage V: Experimentation (Twelve to Eighteen Months)
Stage VI: Representational Intelligence (Eighteen Months to Two Years)

LANGUAGE DEVELOPMENT
Reinforcement and Language Acquisition
Experiences and Language Development
First Words
Holophrasic Speech
Symbolic Representation
Vocabulary Development
Telegraphic Speech
Negatives
"Motherese"
Of LAD and LASS
Games Children Play (and Adults, Too!)
Implications for Parents
Language Learning and Schooling
PSYCHOSOCIAL DEVELOPMENT
DEVELOPMENTAL MILESTONES
Walking
Toilet Training

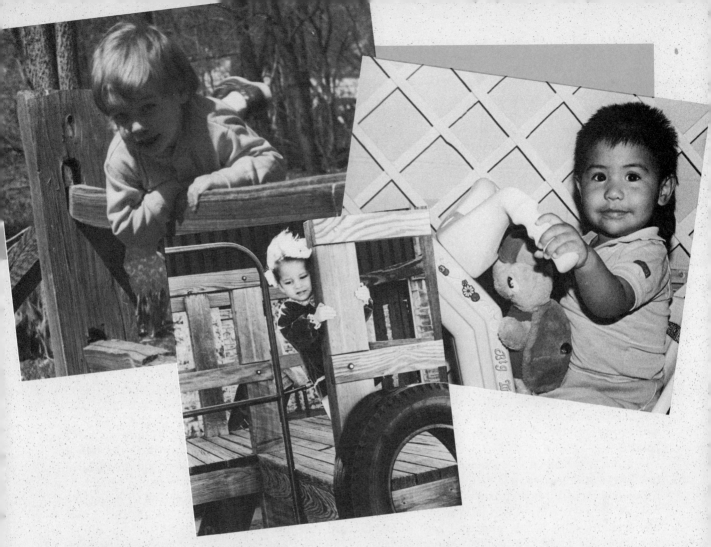

PARENTING THE TODDLER
Activity
Love and Affection
Independence
Making Choices
Self-help Activities
Childproofing the Environment
In the Spotlight: Superbaby
In the Spotlight: Playtime with a
  Purpose
What Would You Do?
TODDLER CHILD CARE
The Environment
Curriculum

Care-givers
Child Care and Social Policy
SUMMARY
QUESTIONS TO GUIDE YOUR
  REVIEW
ACTIVITIES FOR FURTHER
  INVOLVEMENT
KEY TERMS
ENRICHMENT THROUGH
  FURTHER READING
ANSWER TO "WHAT WOULD
  YOU DO?"
BIBLIOGRAPHY

⌣IGNETTE

Jan Johnson is twenty-nine years old and illiterate. She cannot read and write. Jan is also HIV positive. She doesn't know how she became HIV positive and doesn't believe she is. She shows none of the AIDS symptoms.

Jan and her three children, Nicole, three months, Fama, three years, and Nicky, four years, now live at the Inner City Rescue Mission, a shelter for homeless women and their children. Previously they lived at Advocates for Victims, another shelter, but because Jan could not get along with the residents there, she and the children were sent to Inner City, where they have resided for five months.

Almost a year ago, Jan's husband left with all the family's money so Jan, pregnant and with the two children, had no place to stay. The police picked her up for vagrancy and she was then sent to Advocates for Victims. Jan has no support from her family, which consists of her mother, a sister and brother. She does not know where her husband is.

Fama is described as a "brat" by Evelyn, the family's case worker as well as by the other shelter residents. Fama throws tantrums when she does not get her own way, which is most of the time. She screams, falls on the floor, and goes through a number of body contortions. Fama has also learned at the early age of three that regardless of what she tells her mother, her mother will believe her, whether or not what she says is true.

Evelyn acknowledges that since Fama has been living at the shelter she does not throw quite as many tantrums. "We're working on the discipline, mostly by talking to Jan and trying to help her learn how not to give in to Fama all the time. But Fama, she's real smart. Now she's learned to throw her tantrums when nobody else is around!"

However, Evelyn describes Fama as a "sickly" child. And, there is good reason for this description.

Fama is HIV positive and subject to many infections. She does not, however, have any AIDS symptoms.

Fama attends an inner-city day care center. She and other children at the Shelter are transported to and from the day care center each day by the city's bus service. Since it is against the Federal Privacy Act to disclose any information without the parent's permission, the day care staff does not know Fama is HIV positive.

Despite everything, Fama is, according to Evelyn, "a very lovable girl." Evelyn says, "She doesn't know she has a problem. She responds to loving and hugging and all of the other things to which a three-year-old girl would respond. Most of the children here do. It is not till later that you see the anger and other symptoms. And," Evelyn continues, "the children here, they respond to the love of the staff. After they have been here for awhile, they feel more secure. I think it's because the mothers have to stay with their children and can't leave them. Also, there are no drugs, alcohol or fighting here. So the kids really benefit from being with their mothers more and by being here."

"However," Evelyn is quick to add, "shelters are not the most ideal places for the adults or children, but for some children it gives them a feeling of security for the time they are here. Our shelter is a little different, for we're trying to get these women to live on their own. We hope we can do this with Jan. We are looking for an apartment for her now. Her greatest disability is her inability to read.

"I have a lot of hope for the whole family. Fama is real bright and if she can stay healthy, she should get along. But you never know what will happen."

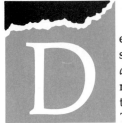

Developmentally and socially, many significant things occur during *toddlerhood*, the period from twelve months through thirty-six months, the second and third years of life. Two developmental processes—unassisted walking and rapid language development—put their stamp on the toddler years and indelibly mark them as unique. Unassisted walking, which for most children occurs between the twelfth and fifteenth months, enables the toddler to demonstrate one of his most unique, endearing, distinguishing, and from a parent's point of view, exasperating characteristics—autonomous mobility and behavioral independence.

Toddlers also participate in another momentous milestone, rapid and significant language development, which enables them to begin to verbally express their autonomy. Who hasn't seen that defiant look with the out-thrust lower lip and heard a determined toddler express her favorite word—"NO!"?

Psychosocially, toddlers are ready to go on from being dependent on others to becoming independent and autonomous. Contemporaneous to the drive for independence is the differentiation of self from others and separation from parents and other care-givers. Assuming that parents and other care-givers have fulfilled infants' basic trust needs, they are then ready to experience fully the achievements of autonomy without doubt and shame.

PHYSICAL DEVELOPMENT

During the toddler years, children will add about eight inches to their height and gain about ten pounds. The remarkable and rather dramatic height and weight gains of infancy are not repeated in the toddler years. Rather, the growth pattern is more steady and even. In this regard, physical development during the toddler years is significant, because the steady growth rate is more suited to

the physical skills they need for the physical activities characteristic of these years. Table 7–1 shows the weight and height averages for toddlers. Table 7–2 shows the *average* annual weight and height gain for toddlers.

The height and weight gains for toddlers as shown in Tables 7–1 and 7–2, can be misleading to someone not accustomed to caring for toddlers. Individually, there is a wide variation in their physical appearance. There are a number of reasons for this. First, some children who were small at birth may be continuing to "catch up" with developmental norms. Second, height is controlled by heredity. At age two, girls have reached 53 percent of their adult height and boys have reached 50 percent. For example, if a boy at age two is 34.5 inches—the norm for that age, then his adult height may be 5 feet, 7 ½ inches. However, if genetically he is to be six feet tall, then more than likely as a toddler, he is three feet tall. A few inches in the toddler years make a big difference later in life!

TABLE 7–1

AVERAGE WEIGHT AND HEIGHT FOR TODDLERS

	Weight (Pounds)		Height (Inches)	
Age (years)	Males	Females	Males	Females
1	22.4	21.0	30.0	29.3
2	27.8	26.2	34.5	34.1

TABLE 7–2

AVERAGE ANNUAL WEIGHT AND HEIGHT GAIN FOR TODDLERS

	Males		Females	
Age (years)	Weight (pounds)	Height (inches)	Weight (pounds)	Height (inches)
1–2	5.4	4.5	5.2	4.8
2–3	4.6	3.5	4.5	3.5

One toddler characteristic is that they no longer look like babies. Many have lost their "chubby" appearance and are starting to "slim down" because of decreasing fat tissue. This slimming down is developmentally significant, because it enables the toddler to engage in motor activities such as walking, running and climbing. While some people believe that toddlers are miniature adults, look closely and you will see that this is not so. The body proportions of toddlers are dramatically different from those of adults. At two years of age, a toddler's head is one-fourth her body size. What is the proportion of your head to body size? About one-tenth! Additionally, a toddler's chest and stomach are about the same size. However, as she grows to adulthood, her chest becomes larger in comparison with her abdomen. These developmental proportions are in keeping with the two-three-four-five rule discussed in Chapter Six.

Dental Development

Dental development, which began in infancy, continues throughout development, Figure 7–1. While there is great individual variation in the ages at which toddlers "cut" their teeth, the sequence of eruption is fairly regular. By thirty months (refer back to Figure 6–4), children have their full set of twenty primary teeth.

Good dental hygiene begins in infancy and should continue in toddlerhood with regular brushing and flossing. In addition, good nutrition, which includes balanced meals and a limit on sugary snacks that contribute to decay, also forms a basis for good dental health.

Children can have their own toothbrushes from the time the first tooth emerges, and brushing teeth should be a regular part of the child's routine—in the morning, after meals and snacks, and before bedtime. Toddlers can continually assume a major role in brushing their own teeth. The parent/caregiver should provide a soft, child-sized toothbrush and toothpaste. The toddler can wet her own toothbrush, help put the paste on the brush and assist in brushing all the teeth, not just the front ones. This is then followed by rinsing the mouth. Parents

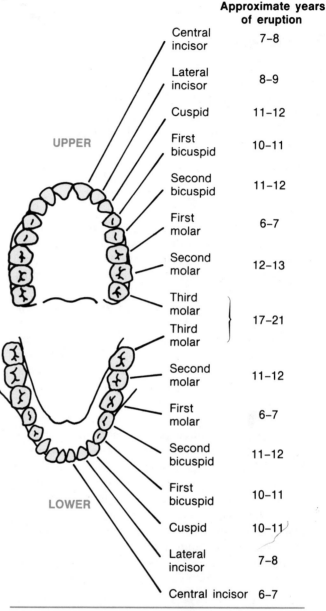

	Approximate years of eruption
Central incisor	7–8
Lateral incisor	8–9
Cuspid	11–12
First bicuspid	10–11
Second bicuspid	11–12
First molar	6–7
Second molar	12–13
Third molar	
Third molar	17–21
Second molar	11–12
First molar	6–7
Second bicuspid	11–12
First bicuspid	10–11
Cuspid	10–11
Lateral incisor	7–8
Central incisor	6–7

UPPER

LOWER

FIGURE 7-1 The permanent teeth begin to erupt at about six years of age. (Adapted from and used with permission of C.V. Mosby, from Whaley and Wong, *Nursing care of infants and children*, 2nd edition, 1983.

should also floss their children's teeth. What is important is the development of the routine and habit of brushing, and instilling the concept that dental hygiene is important.

MOTOR DEVELOPMENT

Motor development plays a significant role in toddlers' lives because it enables them to be autonomous and contributes to their independence. Toddlers spend much of their time practicing and expanding their ever-emerging motor skills by walking, running, climbing, and kicking.

Walking is one of the major motor accomplishments of the toddler years. Although for the average child walking begins at about twelve months, some children walk earlier, while others walk later—it all depends. If a child is a good creeper, this form of locomotion may serve his purposes for a while longer. Also, a toddler of normal weight may walk sooner than an obese child, and girls tend to walk sooner than boys.

When children are delayed in the development of motor skills, then parents and care-givers should seek help and advice from the public school system, public health clinics, or other agencies such as the March of Dimes. Many child care programs are also familiar with referral agencies that can provide assistance.

The beginning walker has an unmistakable stance—feet pointing outward and spread wide apart, with knees flexed for stability and balance. Sometimes beginning walkers are up on tiptoes because they have not yet learned to lower their heels. It is common for beginning walkers to lunge, totter, and fall. Part of the problem with balance has to do with learning the nuances of a new skill; part has to do with body proportions. Remember that the toddler's head is one-quarter of his body size, so he is naturally unbalanced. With maturation and practice, the toddler's walk becomes more balanced, the feet are positioned more closely together, and the knees are less flexed. Also by age two, the typical heel-toe placement of walking provides a much smoother gait, and the toes are pointed more in the direction of the walk. By age three, walking is so automatic that little attention

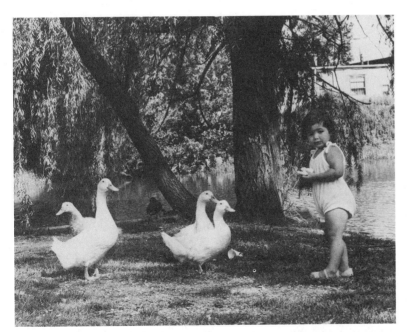
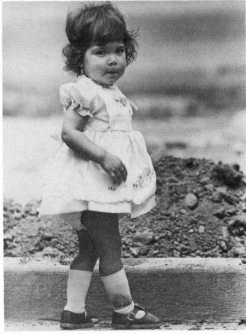

FIGURE 7-2 Walking enables toddlers to become explorers of their world. All early walkers share common characteristics—feet apart, turned outward and knees slightly flexed. When toddlers have mastered walking, then they develop the gross motor skills for running and climbing.

must be paid to it, and by age four, the pre-schooler's stride and gait resemble that of the adult.

Have you ever watched an adult and a toddler walk together? The toddler's step is about half that of her parents. Between eighteen and twenty-four months the rate of walking is about 170 steps per minute, as compared with 140 for a briskly walking adult (Espenschade and Eckert, 1980, p. 137). So if a toddler has a parent who insists that she keep up, she has to double her gate to do so!

Other motor activities of the toddler period include running, jumping, and climbing. What adults consider running begins at about age two. Toddlers are not able to run well for a number of reasons. First, they still have difficulty balancing themselves and second, they are unable to start and stop quickly.

Jumping usually begins with jumping off low objects. The first jump is with one foot first and the landing is usually on the heel. Later, the child jumps with both feet together, and when two- and three-year-old children jump off steps, their arms are usually behind them in a wing-like fashion.

Infants and toddlers begin climbing stairs by going up on all fours. Then, by two years of age, toddlers go up one foot at a time—foot to foot. Then at about three years, they learn to advance one foot over the other as adults do. Toddlers can usually descend stairs unassisted by about age two and a-half. The smooth foot-over-foot descent is achieved by age four.

Everybody Loves a Ball Game

Balls are an important part of play and sport in the United States as well as most other countries of the world. Children and their parents naturally use balls as a means of encouraging participation in play activities. For toddlers, balls should be soft and about the size of a volley ball. Toddlers' first efforts at catching are passive, and adults should gently throw the ball to them so that they can catch it. Toddlers also enjoy throwing small balls, but it is not until age four that they are able to assume the sideways stance and body weight transfer necessary for distance throwing.

At age two, young children can hit a ball from a baseball tee, and as they grow older, many want to emulate the hitting action of ball players they see on television. And many toddlers at age two can enjoy kicking games and are able to make contact with a ball using a kicking motion. Only by age four, however, will they have mastered the full skill of kicking by utilizing a back swing of the foot or kicking from full stride.

For young children in the toddler years, as well as older children and adults, movement is an essential feature of life and one which contributes to all areas of development. Physical activities involving gross motor movements enable toddlers to interact with people and objects in their world. Such activities need to be supported and encouraged by parents and care-givers.

Fine Motor Skills

Gross motor skills seem to play a larger role in the early life of children than do fine motor skills. One reason for this is that gross motor skills develop first and are easier for children to master. Nonetheless, *fine motor skills*, those dependent on the small muscle development of the hands and fingers, also play an important role in children's lives and development. They enable toddlers to hold objects such as crayons, pencils, spoons, and cup handles, and to engage in many pleasurable and self-help activities involving their use.

One of the results of fine motor development is artistic expression. By two years, many toddlers hold a crayon or magic marker, not like adults, but with the thumb on one side and fingers on the other. With this accomplishment and the proper supply of paper, toddlers are ready to freely express themselves. As they do, their artistic endeavors progress through age-related stages (Kellog, 1970):

- Placement stage—two to three years. Children experiment by placing their scribbles on paper.
- Shape Stage—three years. Children make basic shapes such as circles, squares/rectangles, triangles, x's, and crosses.
- Design Stage—three and one-half years. Children combine shapes to make abstract designs.

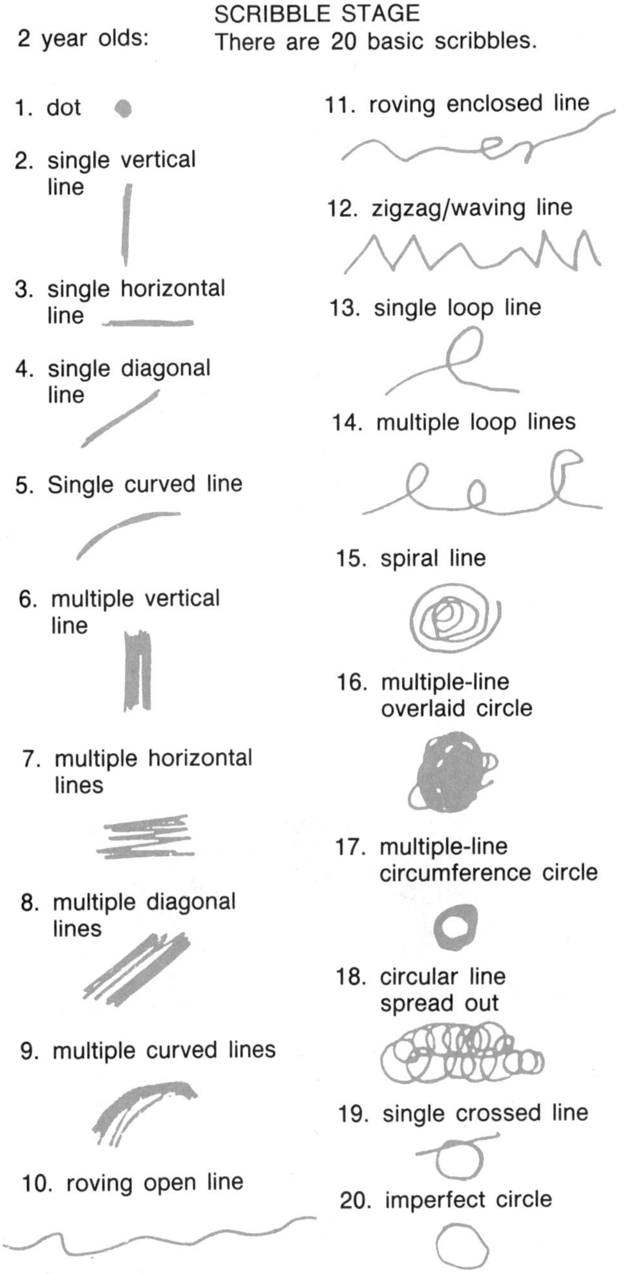

SCRIBBLE STAGE

2 year olds: There are 20 basic scribbles.

1. dot ●
2. single vertical line
3. single horizontal line
4. single diagonal line
5. Single curved line
6. multiple vertical line
7. multiple horizontal lines
8. multiple diagonal lines
9. multiple curved lines
10. roving open line
11. roving enclosed line
12. zigzag/waving line
13. single loop line
14. multiple loop lines
15. spiral line
16. multiple-line overlaid circle
17. multiple-line circumference circle
18. circular line spread out
19. single crossed line
20. imperfect circle

FIGURE 7-3 Toddlers hold crayons, pencils and markers first with their fist and later with their thumb and fingers. Toddlers like to "scribble." The 20 basic scribbles are shown. (From Schirmmacher/ART AND CREATIVE DEVELOPMENT FOR YOUNG CHILDREN, copyright 1988 by Delmar Publishers Inc.)

■ Pictorial Stage—four and five years. At this stage children draw pictures of people, buildings, and animals. As children grow older, their drawings become more representational and detailed.

Handedness

A preference for *handedness* begins in infancy and is present by six months, with most infants demonstrating a right hand-use preference for reaching and manipulating objects (Michel, Ovrut, & Harkins, 1985). It is not surprising, therefore, that by about the age of two, toddlers show a preference for one hand over the other in most tasks. Like adults, 90 percent of toddlers will be right-handed, while 10 percent will prefer their left. *Handedness* is related to *dominance*, the preference for one side of the body over the other. People who are right-handed kick with their right foot and prefer using their right eye and right ear. Left handedness is familial, meaning that it is more frequent in families in which one or more of the parents is left-handed (Longstreth, 1980). However, a genetic model is not sufficient to explain all instances of left-handedness, and practice probably also plays a role. In former times, it was customary for teachers or parents to try to change children's handedness from left to right. Although it is a right-hand world, children should be allowed to determine their own preferences. However, a child who can't seem to develop a preference can be mildly encouraged to use his right hand.

PERCEPTUAL DEVELOPMENT
Sensory Development

Toddlers' sensory organs become increasingly well developed and, as all those familiar with toddlers know, they use them to actively and vigorously explore the world. This innate basis of sensory learning is one reason many educational programs such as the Montessori system emphasize learning through sensory involvement (See Chapter Nine). Toddlers not only visually examine but orally explore every object they can get in their hands. In addition, any object the toddler explores has to withstand rigorous and vigorous shaking and banging.

INDEPENDENCE

The toddler years are characterized by growing independence. Toddlers are anxious to engage in many self-help activities, such as feeding and dressing themselves. They should be encouraged to assist with activities and help themselves as much as is practically possible for care-givers and parents. Toddlers are dependent and independent, both at the same time. They are trying to become independent but need parent and care-giver assistance to achieve this goal. The help and support toddlers need is that which affirms and recognizes their importance as individuals and their right to

independence. They must be permitted and have opportunities to make choices and accomplish tasks by themselves. Achievement leads to autonomy and feelings of positive self-worth.

SAFETY

Safety during the toddler years is an important consideration for all care-givers. Toddlers are so intent on pursuing their own purposes and using their growing abilities that they are unaware of many of the hazards and perils that await them. They lack the common sense and self-awareness that many adults think they possess. On the contrary, adults are the keepers of young children. Toddlers concentrate on doing things and will climb up on, out of, and into anything they can. Many care-givers mistakenly think they can control toddlers merely by saying "No." This, of course, does not work, and is why parents and other care-givers must "childproof" toddlers' environments and be ever-vigilant in supervision. (See "Parenting the Toddler.")

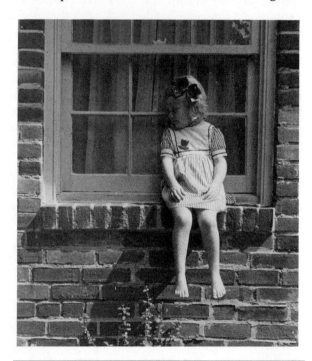

FIGURE 7-4 All young children are at risk for accidents. Parents and other caregivers must provide for toddlers' safety by providing an environment that is as accident free as possible.

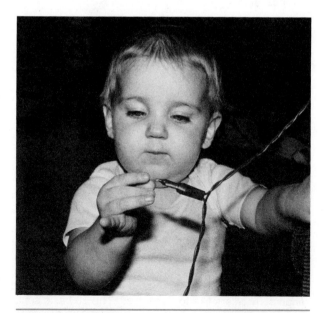

FIGURE 7-5 Clearly, toddlers must be protected from dangerous situations such as this one.

NUTRITION

As we indicated in Chapter Six, children's eating habits are influenced in the early years. This is the time for care-givers to avoid excessive use of salt, sugar, and other sweets. Also, toddlers are easily influenced in their food preferences by parents' food preferences. So, one way to encourage toddlers in good nutrition is for parents to practice it themselves! Toddlerhood is a time when children develop and demonstrate strong taste preferences. It is not uncommon for them to instantaneously spit food out as soon as they have tasted it, much to the exasperation of parents.

Toddlers also tend to eat less than infants simply because they are not growing as fast. This helps explain why toddlers are known as picky eaters.

As a result of their quest for independence and control, toddlers want to feed themselves. Self-feeding is not only a sign of autonomy, but also of increasing fine motor coordination, which enables them to pick up foods and eating utensils. However, to anyone who has witnessed toddlers' involvements at self-feeding, including their many near misses as they attempt to put food in their mouths and accompanying spills as they learn to drink, it is apparent that they are far from fully coordinated.

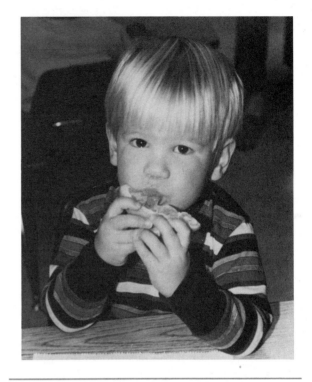

FIGURE 7-6 Toddlers like to be in control and feed themselves. Playing with food is part of the self-feeding process. However, there are limits which parents need to set—e.g., "food on the floor is too hard to clean up." Parents can facilitate the self-feeding process by providing the right eating utensils.

*I*MPLICATIONS FOR PARENTS

Autonomy and independence should be encouraged at all levels of development. Parents can encourage toddlers' independence by allowing them, as much as possible, to feed themselves. Giving children finger foods is one way to allow them to happily and nutritiously help themselves in feeding. Also, by placing a small amount of liquid in a cup with handles on both sides, toddlers are able to drink by themselves. Sometimes parents want to use a straw to teach toddlers to drink, but this is not advisable, since it is too difficult a coordination task for the child.

Food asphyxiation, or choking on food, is a leading cause of accidental death in young children. The primary reasons for this are inappropriate foods being given to young children, and a lack of adequate supervision during feeding. Some inappropriate foods are those that are round and/or cylindrical and therefore easily *aspirated* or inhaled. Some of these include peanuts, hot dogs, popcorn, raisins, grapes, and round candies. Many round foods such as hot dogs can be cut into pieces, making them acceptable for toddlers. As a general rule of thumb, parents with children under four should exercise prudence in the finger foods they provide and should cautiously monitor their children's eating.

TOILET TRAINING

Toilet training, or *toilet learning* as it is increasingly called, is largely a matter of physical readiness and is best accomplished beginning at about age two. Control of the anal and urethral sphincter muscles is not possible until the complete myelination of the spinal cord, which occurs between eighteen and twenty-four months. Also, controlling urine elimination depends on an increase in bladder capacity. By about fourteen to eighteen months, the toddler can go about two hours between voidings. In addition, toddlers must be able to accomplish a number of self-help activities in order to confidently be a participant in this important process. For example, they must be able to pull pants up and down and go to the potty chair.

Toilet training involves timing, patience, preparing the environment, establishing routines, and modeling. Since modeling plays an important role in toilet training, parents should not hesitate to allow their children to imitate them in their toileting habits.

Americans in general are more anxious to toilet train their children than are parents in many other countries. Also, when parents are impatient to resume their careers, or when a child care program or preschool won't enroll children unless they are toilet trained, there is a tendency to attempt to accelerate the training process. However, as a general rule of thumb, later works better than earlier.

Toilet training also involves a partnership between the child and the parent and others who care for the child. With so many children in child care centers, parents and other care-givers must

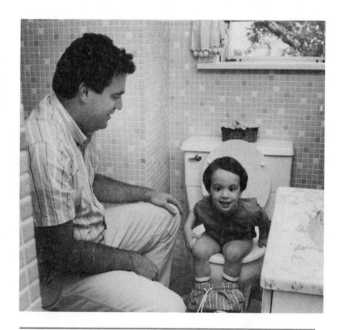

FIGURE 7-7   Toilet training—the process of helping children gain control over elimination—is not the quick and easy process some parents or caregivers think it should be. Many factors are involved in toilet training such as physical and emotional readiness.

work cooperatively with each other to ascertain the time and method for training.

Additionally, parents and other care-givers must avoid being punitive, negative, and nasty to their children while toilet training. Parents need to demonstrate support for and patience with their children. It may be tempting to exclaim in frustration while changing a soiled child, "Aren't you ever going to learn to go to the bathroom by yourself like other children do?" However, it would be more supportive of the child's efforts and his self-esteem to say, "Everyone has accidents. Let's get cleaned up so you can get back to building your tower."

INTELLECTUAL DEVELOPMENT

Toddler intellectual development covers the last two stages of sensorimotor intellectual development: Stage V, Experimentation (also referred to as Tertiary Circular Reactions) and Stage VI, Representational Intelligence (also known as Symbolic Intelligence). (See Chapter Two for additional information on these two stages.)

Stage V: Experimentation (Twelve to Eighteen Months)

Stage V, from twelve to eighteen months, is the stage of experimentation. Toddlers experiment with objects to solve problems. This experimentation is characteristic of intelligence that involves *tertiary circular reactions*, in which toddlers repeat actions and modify behaviors over and over to see what will happen. This repetition helps develop an understanding of cause-and-effect relationships and leads to the discovery of new relationships through exploration and experimentation. Here is Piaget's observation of Laurent, the "experimenter":

Laurent is lying on his back but nevertheless resumes his experiments of the day before. He grasps in succession a celluloid swan, a box, etc., stretches out his arm and lets them fall. He distinctly varies the position of the fall. Sometimes he stretches out his arm vertically, sometimes he holds it obliquely, in front of or behind his eyes, etc. When the object falls in a new position (for example, on his pillow), he lets it fall two or three times more on the same place, as though to study a spatial relation; then he modifies the situation. At a certain moment the swan falls near his mouth; now he does not suck it (even though this object habitually serves this purpose), but drops it three times more while merely making the gesture of opening his mouth (p. 269).

Mobility increases the opportunities for experimentation and new experiences. Toddlers, therefore, act on their environment with a higher frequency than do infants. They learn by the effects their actions have on objects and the environment. Through such experimentation, toddlers learn the consequences of their behavior and cause-and-effect relationships.

Object Permanence The development of object permanence continues during this stage. The child who has acquired *object permanence* knows that objects occupy space, have an existence of their own, and continue to exist even when not seen. You know that a ball hidden under a diaper still exists as a ball. Infants do not. Much of what we as adults take for granted as common sense is not common sense for the infant and toddler. Caregivers must constantly keep in mind that the thought processes of adults are not the thought processes of children.

The beginning of understanding object permanence begins in sensorimotor Stage IV. Awareness of object permanence continues to develop in Stage V. Toddlers are not confused by a change of location when an object is moved. They will search for an object in the last place hidden. But during this stage, toddlers still have to see the object being hidden. They do not yet have object permanence to the extent that they know an object is hidden without seeing it hidden.

Implications for Care-givers In addition to the suggestions provided for Stage V in Chapter Two, this stage has several implications for care-givers. First, all three stages involving circular reactions have a great deal of significance for children. As indicated in Chapter Two, a circular reaction is the repetition of a sensorimotor action. The activity is the context for learning. These sensorimotor acts are necessary for and facilitate adaptation (the end product of assimilation and accommodation). Circular reactions serve to increase the range and kinds of experiences of the very young. The breadth of experiences all children have is critical, because it increases opportunities for assimilation, accommodation, and scheme development. A broader range of experiences with which to adapt is more conducive to intellectual development than a narrow range.

Second, if, as Piaget and others maintain, activity is the context for intellectual development, then care-givers are the ones who must provide the context for the activity. Care-givers are the ones who control the environment in which children have opportunities to engage in sensorimotor acts.

Stage VI: Representational Intelligence (Eighteen Months to Two Years)

Stage VI, from eighteen months to two years, is the stage of symbolic representation. Representation occurs when toddlers can visualize events internally. They can maintain mental images of objects not present. Representational thought enables toddlers to solve problems internally, without having to always solve them in a sensorimotor way through experimentation and trial and error. Representation enables toddlers to more accurately predict cause-and-effect relationships.

During this stage, true object permanence develops. This reflects the toddler's representational intelligence. Toddlers cannot only search for hidden objects, they can now search for objects in the last place hidden. More importantly, they can search for objects they did not actually see hidden. The toddler is liberated, in a small way, from relying only on perceptions.

Object permanence also includes person permanence, and toddlers know their care-givers exist even when absent. The development of object permanence is a signficant achievement. Table 7–3 summarizes the development of object permanence in the sensorimotor stage.

Once they have achieved object permanence, toddlers understand the rudiments of property *identity*, that is, that objects have an identity of their own and exist when the toddler is not present. Later, as preschoolers in the preoperational stage of intellectual development, they will learn other properties of identity, for example, that when clay is rolled out in a long piece, it is still clay. Having achieved property identity, toddlers begin to understand the properties of objects.

Representational thought is evidenced by the pretend play that is characteristic of this stage. Toddlers' representational thought does not necessarily match with the real world and their representations of things are not necessarily others' representations. This accounts for a toddler's ability to have other objects stand for almost anything. A wooden block is a car. A rag doll is a fairy princess. This type of play is also known as *symbolic play* and becomes more elaborate and complex in the preoperational period.

There is a considerable difference, then, between the Stage I infant and the Stage VI toddler. Through the process of assimilation and accommodation, children have developed many schemes of the world. These schemes help them distinguish many objects and animals. They know that a ball is not a cat and that their mother is different from other mothers.

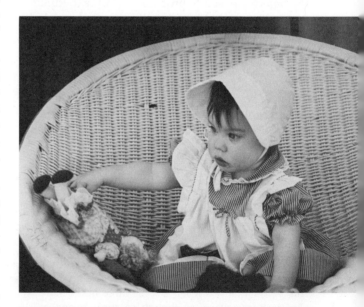

FIGURE 7-8 In symbolic play, anything a child chooses can stand for something else. The important thing is the play, which is the context for physical, social and cognitive development. For toddlers, play is an end in itself.

TABLE 7–3

		THE DEVELOPMENT OF OBJECT PERMANENCE

Stage	Age (Months)	Level of Object Permanence
I	0–1	Infants do not differentiate objects from themselves. They look only at what is in their field of vision.
II	1–4	Infants still do not differentiate objects from themselves. They are able to follow an object and will look at the point where it was last hidden. Infants begin to coordinate seeing and hearing, but there is no visual or manual search for hidden objects.
III	4–8	Infants search for objects that have vanished from their grasp. They will search for a partially hidden object, but not a completely hidden object.
IV	8–12	Infants will search actively for completely hidden objects. When an object is moved from one hidden place to another, infants will look for the object in the first place hidden.
V	12–18	Toddlers in Stage V will search for an object in the last place they saw it hidden. They will, for example, watch the care-giver hide a ball under a blanket and then in a box, and they will then look for the ball in the box. They have no problem with this task as long as they have actually seen the object being hidden. At this stage, however, they cannot account for what Piaget called "invisible displacements."
		Piaget put a potato in a box, placed a rug over the box, and turned the box upside down, leaving the potato hidden by the rug. When he brought the box out from under the rug, his daughter, Jacquiline, looked for the potato in the box; "it did not occur to her to raise the rug in order to find the potato underneath."
VI	18–24	Toddlers achieve object permanence. They realize objects exist apart from themselves and that the objects can move in space. This cognitive achievement is possible because toddlers are now capable of forming mental representations.
		Piaget wrote the following about Jacqueline at nineteen-and-a-half months: "Jacqueline watches me when I put a coin in my hand, then put my hand under a coverlet. I withdraw my hand closed, Jacqueline opens it, then searches under the coverlet until she finds the object. I take back the coin at once, put it in my hand, and then slip my closed hand under a cushion situated at the other side (on her left and no longer on her right); Jacqueline immediately searches for the object under the cushion."*

* Piaget, J. (1954). *The Construction of Reality in the Child* (M. Cook, Trans.). New York: Basic Books, pp. 68, 79.
Note. Adapted from *Piaget for Educators: A Multimedia Program* (p. 19) by R. B. Sund, 1975, Columbus, OH: Charles E. Merrill.

Stage VI children are no longer dominated and controlled by reflexive actions as are infants. The Stage VI child is capable of symbolic thought and is ready to manipulate the environment by use of symbols through language. The toddler is ready to enter the world of preoperational intelligence.

The child entering the preoperational stage is also different in another way. Sensorimotor children do not distinguish between themselves and external objects; preoperational children can. This intellectual distinguishing between self and others, and self and objects, plays a role in the child's discovery of self. As children are able to distinguish themselves from others, they are able to understand themselves as persons.

Implications for Care-givers Since toddlers now have object permanence, they may become more upset by missing a favorite toy or parent. The obvious way to solve this with toys is to make sure the child has the toy present. A better way is to keep toddlers involved in a wide range of activities and not provide a chance for them to dwell on the missing item or person.

Care-givers should keep in mind that children's thoughts are not adult thoughts and that the way children see or represent things is not like adults. Therefore, care-givers should not emphasize "right" answers as much as they should emphasize helping children have meaningful experiences, which will enable them to discover the right answers through the process of living and maturation. The idea that children don't think as adults is one of the best reasons for making education child centered rather than adult centered.

LANGUAGE DEVELOPMENT

Toddlers are active, and that activity is evident in their incessant exploration and in their growing ability to master and use language. They are busy physically operating on the world and participating in the process of language acquisition. The sequence of language development during the toddler years is shown in Table 7–4.

TABLE 7–4

THE SEQUENCE OF TODDLER LANGUAGE DEVELOPMENT	
Age (months)	Language Milestone
10	Babbling—"Da-da"/"Ma-ma"
11	One word
12	Two words
14	Three words
15	Four to six words
15	Immature jargoning
18	Seven to twenty words
18	Mature jargoning
18	Says name of one body part
21	Says name of three body parts
21	Two-word combination
23	Names five body parts
24	Fifty words
24	Two-word sentences (nouns, or pronoun inappropriately, and verb)
24	Pronouns (I, me, you, etc., inappropriately)

Note. From "Linguistic and Auditory Milestones During the First Two Years of Life: A Language Inventory for the Practitioner" by A. J. Capute & P. J. Accardo, November 1978, *Clinical Pediatrics, 17,* pp. 847–853.

Reinforcement and Language Acquisition

Earlier, in Chapter Six, we discussed language development in infancy and the roles of nativist and behaviorist theories. At the time, it was stated that while reinforcement plays a role in language development, it is not sufficient to fully explain the totality of development. Adults do, however, help children learn language through *socially mediated reinforcement,* in the form of such behaviors as attention, praise, and compliance with requests (Whitehurst and Valdez-Menchaca, 1988). In this regard, social feedback is important to language learning. Adults, by their words and actions—by what they do and say to children—provide an environment that is conducive to language learning. This being the case then, as you might expect, children adopt the language usage of their parents. This is particularly evident in learning the names of things. For example, parents who do not know the specific names for dogs or flowers will simply call them "flowers" and "dogs," while parents who know more specific names (like "collie" and "rose") will use them, and so will their children (Macnamara, 1982, p. 49).

Experiences and Language Development

Children can talk about the things they see, touch, taste, and smell, so there is a great need to provide children with sensory experiences of all kinds in order to give them things to talk about.

First Words

Although the process of language development begins at the moment of birth, parents usually don't think of language as beginning until children say their first word. "At about a year children produce their first understandable words, often reduplicated syllables like mama, dada, or papa, or single consonant-vowel syllables like da for dog or ba for baby. For some children babbling ceases when the first words appear, but other children continue to produce long babbled sentences even when their intelligible vocabulary grows" (de Villiers & de Villiers, 1979, pp.19–20).

The first words of children are just that, first words. What are these first words? Children talk about people—dada, papa, mama, mommie, and baby (referring to themselves); animals—dog, cat, kitty; vehicles—car, truck, boat, train; toys—ball, block, book, doll; food—juice, milk, cookie, bread, drink; body parts—eye, nose, mouth, ear; clothing and household articles—hat, shoe, spoon, clock;

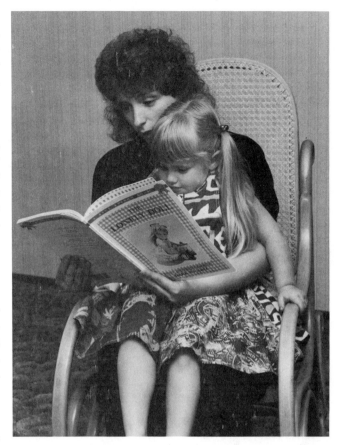

FIGURE 7-9 Language is a process that develops from birth. Parents create an environment for language experiences like this one and facilitate toddlers' early literacy development.

greeting terms—hi, bye, night-night; and a few words for actions—up, no more, off. Interestingly enough, the first words of children today are remarkably similar to those of children fifty years ago (Clark, 1983, p. 798).

Holophrasic Speech

Children are remarkable communicators without words. If they are fortunate and have attentive parents and care-givers, they are skilled communicators, using gestures, facial expressions, sound intonations, pointing, and reaching to make their desires known and get what they want. Pointing at an object and saying, "uh-uh-uh" is the same as saying, "I want the rattle" or "Help me get the rattle." Usually care-givers will respond by saying, "Do you want the rattle? I'll get it for you. Here it is!" One of the attributes of an attentive care-giver is the ability to read children's signs and signals, anticipating their desires even though no words are spoken.

The ability to communicate progresses from "sign language" and sounds to the use of single words. Toddlers are skilled at using single words to name objects, to let others know what they want, and to express emotions. One word, in essence, does the work of a whole sentence. These single-word sentences are called *holophrases*.

The one-word sentences children use are primarily *referential* (used primarily to label objects, such as "doll"), or *expressive* (communicating personal desires or levels of social interaction, such as "bye-bye" and "kiss"). The extent to which children use these two functions of language depends in large measure on the care-giver, as the de Villiers (1979) have pointed out:

> The referral-expressive dimension is clearly a continuum, and most children have both types of words in their early vocabulary, but the classification reflects the predominate use to which the child put language in the early one-word stage. To some extent the child's early use of language reflects his mother's verbal style. Mothers who spend most of their time pointing out objects and their properties tend to have referential children; mothers who use language mainly to direct their child's behavior tend to have expressive children. (p. 39).

Symbolic Representation

Two significant developmental events occur at about the age of two. First is the development of symbolic representation. Representation occurs when something—a mental image, a word—is used to stand for something else not present. A toy may stand for a tricycle, a baby doll may represent a real person. Words become signifiers of things—ball, block, blanket.

This ability frees children from the here and now, from acting on concrete objects present only in the immediate environment. It enables their thoughts to range over the full span of time—past and present—and permits them to remember and project thoughts into the future. "Things no longer need to be present for the child to act on them. In this sense, the ability to represent eventually liberates the child from the immediate present. He can imagine things that are both spatially and temporally separate from himself. It may therefore be said that the use of mental representation permits the child to transcend the constraints of space and time" (Ginsburg & Opper, 1979, p. 78).

The use of mental symbols also enables the child to participate in two processes that are characteristic of the early years: symbolic play, and the beginning of the use of words and sentences to express meanings and make references. Piaget refers to the use of symbolic representation as the *semiotic* function.

Vocabulary Development

The second significant achievement that occurs at about age two is the development of a fifty-word vocabulary and the use of two-word sentences. This vocabulary development and the ability to combine words mark the beginning of rapid language development.

Telegraphic Speech

You have undoubtedly heard a toddler say something like, "Go out" in response to a suggestion such as, "Let's go outside." Perhaps you've said, "Is your juice all gone?" and the toddler responded, "Juice gone." These two-word sentences are called *telegraphic speech*. They are the same kind of sentences you would use if you wrote a telegram. The sentences are primarily made up of nouns and verbs. Generally, they do not use prepositions, articles, conjunctions, and auxiliary verbs.

Once children have their fifty-or-more-word vocabularies, what do they do with them? They do what you and I do, they use them in sentences. The telegraphic speech of infants and their first sentences are governed by two classes of "pivot grammar." In the first class, which occurs most frequently, the first word is a "pivot" or "fixed" word, and the other word is called an "open" word, which pivots around the first word. Almost always, the pivot words are words that occur in the first position and the second words almost always occur in *that* position. Thus, a $P + O$ would be "Patte run." The second class, which occurs less frequently, is the $O + P$ construction in which the O word is one generally found in the O position of a $P + O$ sentence. A $P + O$ sentence would be "Push it." These early sentences can be further categorized according to the relations expressed by each and shown in Table 7–5.

Negatives

Quick! What is the toddler's favorite word? If you guessed "No", you are absolutely right. When young children use negatives, they first add "No" to the beginning of a word or sentence, for example

TABLE 7–5

RELATIONS EXPRESSED IN CHILDREN'S FIRST SENTENCES	
Relation	Example
1. Agent and action	"Mail come"
2. Action and object	"Want more"
3. Agent and object	"Patte lunch"
4. Modifier and head	"Pretty boat"
5. Negation and X (where X is a variable)	"No wash"
6. X and dative	"Throw Daddy"
7. Introducer and X	"There book"
8. X and locative	"Baby room"

Note. From *A First Language* (p. 114) by R. Brown, 1973, Cambridge, MA: Harvard University Press.

"No food." As their sentences become longer, they still put "No" first, for example, "No put hat on." Later, they place negatives appropriately between subject and verb, for example, "I no want milk."

When children move beyond the use of the one-word expression "No," the use of negations progresses through a series of meanings (Bloom, 1970). The first meaning conveys nonexistence, such as "no juice" and "no hat," meaning that the juice is all gone and the hat isn't present. The next level of negation is rejection. "No go out" is the rejection of the offer to go outside. Then the use of "no" progresses to the denial of something the child believes to be untrue. If offered a carrot stick under the pretense it is candy, the child will reply, "No candy."

"Motherese"

One thing most mothers do is talk to their young children differently from the way they talk to adults. They adapt their speech so they communicate in a distinctive way called *motherese* (Newport, Gleitman, & Gleitman, 1977). Review the characteristics of motherese outlined in Chapter Six in order to appreciate the role of these in language development. Mothers' language interactions with their toddlers are much the same as mothers' language interactions with infants.

Of LAD and LASS

In our discussion of infant language development in Chapter Six, you were introduced to the concepts of LAD and LASS. The LAD is the language acquisition device children use to learn language and the LASS is the language support system that supports the LAD. The LASS supports the development of language in four ways:

1. Parents and other care-givers help children learn basic language formats and rules by the way they interact linguistically with their children, for example, through the use of "motherese" and game playing (which follows).

2. Adults encourage and model vocabulary and phrases relating to various means of communication. In this sense, the child learns how to signal her focus of attention and her requests for assistance—that she wants her favorite stuffed animal—long before she has mastered all the words to adequately communicate such intentions.

3. Many parent-child activities have routinized formats that are rich resources for language learning. They include many pretend activities and routines for how to do things, from getting dressed to being securely fastened in the car seat.

4. Within the context of routinized formats, opportunities for many other language activities naturally occur, including naming and requesting (Bruner, 1983, pp. 40–42).

Games Children Play (And Adults, Too!)

"Pat-a-cake, pat-a-cake, Baker man—bake me a cake as fast as you can. . . ." I'll bet you have either played this game with a baby or have heard a mother play a similar game with her baby. Babies give parents and other care-givers all kinds of excuses to do fun things that they might not otherwise do! And, besides being fun, games and game playing play an important role in children's language development:

1. They provide some of the first occasions for the systematic use of language between adult and child.

2. The formats of many language games have certain "rules" that the participants follow and, in this sense, games are "language-like."

3. Games involve another language-like feature—they involve turn-taking.

4. Games are pleasurable and the process of pleasurable game-playing keeps the process of language learning going also (Bruner, 1983, pp. 45–46).

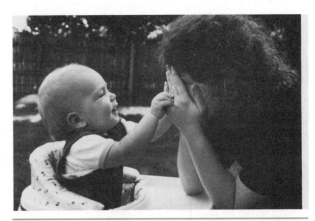

FIGURE 7-10   Through play with persons and objects, toddlers learn about their world and themselves.

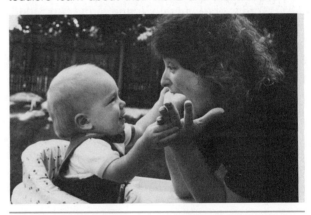

FIGURE 7-11   Adults should let toddlers set the direction of play and should avoid controlling its intent and purpose.

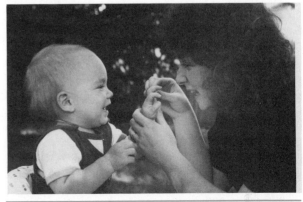

FIGURE 7-12   Toddlers enjoy and readily participate in parent/caregiver-initiated games.

Implications for Parents

Care-givers must attune themselves to children's developing language style and abilities. As children develop in their ability to use language, care-givers can "mirror" that language back, adapting their way of talking to children in accordance with their growing use of language. Communicating with children provides a rich linguistic environment for children to learn language. Language that is short, direct, and grammatically correct supports children's efforts at language development. The care-giver's expansion of what the child says is also helpful.

P.S. Dale (1976), a researcher of children's language, says that "the child can talk about only what he knows" (p. 157). Care-givers need to provide children with a wide range of experiences so they can build a knowledge base. Walks, encounters with other children and adults, field trips, and vicarious experiences through reading and film all provide children with things to talk about. The other half of the equation, of course, is that children need care-givers who will talk with them and provide opportunities for conversation. Having an opportunity to talk is as important as having something about which to talk.

Children's first words are the names of things. Parents and care-givers can teach children the names of things directly ("This is a ball") or indirectly ("Tell me what this is"). They can label, putting the name of the object on the objects: "chair." They can use the names of things in the conversation with children, "This is a shoe; let's put your shoe on." The important thing to remember is that children need to know the names of things if they are going to refer to them and talk about them.

Since children's first words are words for things, and since Piaget believes children need a mental representation of an object to match a name to it, it makes sense to give children experiences with real objects to lay the foundation for knowing the objects' names. Experiences with balls, dogs, pots, dolls, and other everyday items will provide the basis for developing mental representations to which names can then be attached. On the other hand, a child whose environment lacks opportunities for experiences with real objects will have fewer mental representations and consequently a more limited vocabulary.

Given the biological propensity for language development and the tremendous ability of children to learn language on their own, even under the most difficult circumstances, there may be a tendency for parents and care-givers to treat language development with benign neglect and not do much to assist children with language acquisition. This approach is unfortunate and does a great disservice to children. The ability of children to teach themselves language flourishes best in a cooperative and supportive environment.

Success in school is marked by how well children know and use language. Children who know the names of things, who can express themselves well, who can talk to the teacher, who understand the language of schooling, are children who, for the most part, will do well in school and life.

Language allows humans to do what no other creatures of creation can do. The abilities to express emotions, recall past experiences, ask questions, make thoughts known, and intimately share hopes and dreams with others are all unique capacities rendered possible by language. Language development affects future learning and life success. People are frequently judged by the sophistication of their language and the impressions their language conveys to others. Language helps define and express the "humanness" of individuals. It is the responsibility of parents, care-givers, and teachers to help children develop this most remarkable of human abilities so they can express their humanness throughout their lives.

Language Learning and Schooling

Middle-class Americans place an emphasis on language development. They help their children learn the names for things and are interested in helping them know the answers to things. Many read to their children from a very early age. Early language development and use are considered high priorities and essential to school and life success. Indeed, the ability to demonstrate precocity with language—knowing the names for many things, engaging interactively in fluent conversations with others, and familiarity with books—is a passport to school success. On the other hand, the child of a teenage parent, who comes to school knowing some words for things and with limited conversational abilities, is at risk for failure.

Also, an American Indian child who has a good grasp of language but who has been taught to be silent out of respect for others is also at risk without a sensitive and culturally aware teacher. All children who enter school with what are perceived as language deficiencies will fail unless they have caring teachers and administrators who are committed to their success.

PSYCHOSOCIAL DEVELOPMENT

The toddler years are perhaps the most critical in the formation of personality. This is due in part to children's changing behavioral patterns, from one of dependence to one of independence and autonomy. During this time, toddlers make major advances in becoming individuals.

In Chapter Six we discussed infants' psychosocial development involving basic trust and mistrust, based on the psychosocial theory of Erik Erikson. Psychosocial development results from the interaction between maturational processes, such as biological needs, and the social forces encountered in everyday living. Socialization provides the context for conflict and crisis resolution throughout eight stages of life. Social and emotional maturity develop as a result of children's abilities to resolve the psychosocial conflicts of each stage. The interaction of children's needs and drives with the environment and care-giver demands (or lack of them) shapes, and to a large degree, determines personality.

Stage One—Oral-sensory (Trust vs. Mistrust) Stage One begins at birth and ends at eighteen months to two years. The primary psychosocial conflict during this stage is the development of trust or mistrust as a result of interactions with parents and other care-givers. Through daily involvements with adults who are consistent and continuous sources of care, toddlers develop a sense of trust in people and the perception that the world is a good place in which to live.

Stage Two—Muscular-anal (Autonomy vs. Shame) This stage begins at eighteen to twenty-four months and continues until age three. During this stage, toddlers develop feelings of autonomy or shame. Toddlers develop autonomy in part through the control of their physical behavior. Autonomy is not a sudden occurrence, but rather a developmental process that occurs across the life span. A toddler is independent one day and very dependent the next. She may demonstrate more autonomy in one setting than in another and at one task than another. Parents and other care-givers can help children develop autonomy by assessing children's autonomy and promoting its development. Jeffrey may need more of his mother's time and personal attention in order to encourage him to do things for himself. Jennifer, on the other hand, may need only occasional help and encouragement.

DEVELOPMENTAL MILESTONES

Major maturational milestones achieved during this stage are walking and control of elimination. These developmental processes provide the context in which children develop feelings of shame or autonomy.

Walking

As anyone who has provided care for toddlers knows, they like to get into everything and do everything for themselves. They have a basic need to do and to be involved. Parents and care-givers sometimes respond to this natural state by being restrictive, punitive, and overprotective. They try to impose their wills on toddlers. Such care-giver behaviors are antithetical to the development of autonomy. Common sense dictates that toddlers should not be allowed to do everything they want to do. But care-givers need to accommodate their views of acceptable behavior to the needs of the very young in order to meet the toddler's quest for autonomy.

Toddlers want and need to explore their environment and to test the limits of their physical abilities. They should be given the opportunity. Shame and a sense of doubt result from not being allowed to deal effectively with the world.

Toilet Training

The second milestone of this stage is toilet training. This time of life can be difficult and has the potential for creating anxiety in care-givers and parents. Care-givers need to avoid shaming children ("Terri has been toilet-trained for two months, and she's younger than you" or, "When are you going to learn to go in the toilet like a big boy?"). Training toddlers in nonpunitive ways when they are ready helps them develop feelings that they have control over their own behavior.

Sigmund Freud believed that when parents are too strict, over demanding, and punitive in the process of toilet training, children develop "anal" personalities. Adult manifestations of an anal personality, according to Freud, are an overemphasis on neatness, punctuality, and cleanliness.

PARENTING THE TODDLER

Activity

"Where do they get all that energy?" Any parent or other care-giver who has tried to keep up with a toddler has breathlessly asked that question many times. And if the truth be known, they probably, in exhaustion, have said something like, "Andrew, aren't you ready for your nap by now?" Without a doubt, toddlers are tremendously active individuals. Toddlers, like all children, are active in the process of converting their experiences into

physical, cognitive, and linguistic abilities. Activity is part of "human nature." Activity is the normal pattern of toddler development, and to devise means for their inactivity is both pointless and harmful. Because of this innate drive for activity, then, toddlers need many interesting things to do. They need new experiences that involve them in motor, cognitive, and sensory activities. They need toys and materials that are sensorially stimulating with which to play, on which to operate, and from which to learn. All of this can and should occur within a safe and stimulating (but not overstimulating) environment.

Love and Affection

Toddlers need love and affection. They not only need to receive it but must be allowed and encouraged to demonstrate it. This getting and giving affection is the basis for a trusting relationship and the child's ability to learn how to trust and be trusted. Also, many acts of affection—touching, kissing, hugging—in addition to being signals of attachment are also assurances that the toddler needs to leave and explore her environment, safe in the knowledge and understanding that there is affection and support whenever she returns.

Independence

The two-year-old is striving for independence, but she does not have the sophisticated social, communicative, or cognitive skills of the adult. In actions and words—usually with a loud "NO!"—toddlers appear and sound negative. Toes get stepped on, things get knocked over, and a single purpose determination to do things produces frequent and frustrating encounters.

Part of the process of a toddler becoming an independent individual involves the way parents encourage—or suppress—this natural tendency and desire, and how toddlers themselves manage the process of "letting go," even at the tender age of two.

Making Choices

Toddlers need to make choices, not universal choices, but limited choices, such as what clothing to wear. Parents need to "give in" to toddlers and let them have their way when it is appropriate and when health and safety are not issues. However, toddlerhood is a notorious time for tantrums and giving in to a child who is throwing a tantrum is not one of the times to let him have his way. Parents and other care-givers will have to arrange the environment so the toddler can have her own way. At the same time, household rules and routines are wonderful ways to provide the toddler with the physical safety and emotional security she needs while providing a framework within which to become her own person.

Self-help Activities

Parents should do things that help the toddler be independent. For example, they should provide clothing that enables the toddler to help dress herself. They should let the toddler feed himself, but provide a context in which this can happen, such as a high chair with a feeding tray, and have paper towels and other cleaning materials on hand.

Toddlers have many endearing qualities that make them the individuals they are. Toddlers are curious, energetic, eager, independent, and inquisitive. Parents need to focus on these qualities and help children become the best they can be.

Childproofing the Environment

Home

1. Remove throw rugs so toddlers don't trip.
2. Put breakable objects out of toddlers' reach. This may mean storing away antiques and family heirlooms for several years.
3. Cover electrical wall outlets with special covers.
4. Remove electrical cords. Toddlers love to pull on electrical cords, and the lamps or appliances can be pulled down.
5. Install gates in hallways and stairs. Make sure gates are federally approved so the toddlers cannot get their heads stuck, causing strangulation.
6. Take knobs off stoves so toddlers can't turn on burners.
7. Purchase medicines and cleaners that have childproof caps.
8. Store all medicines and cleaning agents out of toddlers' reach. Move all toxic chemicals from low cabinets to high ones. Even items like mouthwash should be put in a safe place.
9. Place safety locks on bathroom doors—the kind that can be opened from the outside. More than once toddlers have locked themselves in the bathroom.
10. Cushion sharp corners of tables and counters with foam rubber and tape. Cotton balls can also be used to cushion corners.
11. If there are older children in the home who use toys with small parts, beads, etc., have them use these when the toddler is not present or in an area where the toddler can't get them.
12. When cooking, turn all pot handles to the back of the stove.
13. Because of toxic fumes, avoid using cleaning fluids while children are present.
14. Place guards over the hot water faucets in bathrooms so toddlers can't turn them on unless supervised.
15. Keep wastebaskets on top of furniture (desks). Toddlers can fall over and in them.
16. Keep the doors to the washer and dryer closed at all times.
17. Keep all plastic bags, including garbage bags, stored in a safe place. Better yet, use paper bags for garbage.
18. Shorten cords on drapes. If there are loops on the cords, cut them.
19. Immediately wipe up any spilled liquid from the floor.
20. Keep the toilet lid down.

Center

1. Cover toddler-area floors with carpeting or mats.
2. Make sure storage shelves are well anchored and won't tip over. Store things so children cannot pull heavy objects off the shelves and onto themselves.

3. Use only equipment and materials that are safe—no sharp edges and broken materials.
4. Store all medicines in locked cabinets.
5. If there are any sharp corners, cushion them with foam rubber and tape.
6. Keep doors closed or install gates so toddlers can't wander off.
7. Fence all play areas.

*I*N THE SPOTLIGHT

SUPERBABY

Superbabies are in. Many parents have never been more enthused or motivated about doing all they can as early as they can to assure that their children become the best and the brightest. One of the earliest advocates of teaching children at an early age is Glenn Doman of the Better Baby Institute, who maintains that every parent can rear a better baby. The Better Baby Institute, located in Philadelphia, is operated by the Institute for the Advancement of Human Potential. Parents pay $490 to enroll in a seven-day seminar on "How to Multiply Your Baby's Intelligence" (Traub, 1986). Here parents are inculcated with "Cardinal Facts for Making Any Baby into a Superb Human Being." Cardinal fact #6 states that "our individual genetic potential is that of Leonardo, Shakespeare, Mozart, Michelangelo, Edison, and Einstein." Doman believes that all children are linguistic geniuses as evidenced by the fact that they master a language in a few short years. He maintains that if children can learn to speak, they can learn to read (Henig, 1988). And teaching parents how to teach their children to read at an early age is one of the things the Better Baby Institute promotes.

Giving baby a sound mind is only one-half of many parents' equation for rearing a superior child. They, like the ancient Greeks, believe that success involves a sound mind in a sound body. Consequently, the physical fitness craze is not just for adults. It has also hit the early years. Many parents are working out with their children. Infants and toddlers are taking swimming lessons and attending play programs and exercise sessions at places like Gymboree. Here they practice their developing physical skills on a wide variety of equipment

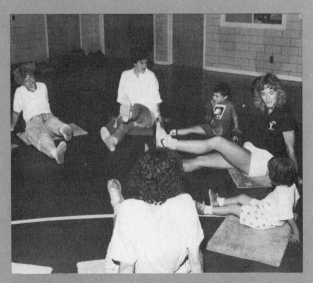

FIGURE 7-13 There are many programs sponsored by companies and agencies designed to provide parents and their children with an environment and materials for play and interaction with other children.

designed to help them develop confidence in their developing physical abilities. In addition, they get to socialize with other children while their parents network with each other and learn parenting skills.

The idea of early learning appeals to many parents. Indeed, it is music to the ears of parents who want their children to learn music as part of their total education. For these parents, Shinichi Suzuki has an answer. Parents play classical music to their infants and toddlers, and then at about age three, children begin to play music on a child-size violin, first by ear and later by sight. Anyone who has seen the young virtuosity of "Suzuki children" cannot help but be impressed.

But early learning is not without its critics and detractors. David Elkind (1987) in particular believes that many early learning activities and programs for young children are inappropriate. Elkind maintains that it's not skills that are important, but the environment provided for children.

*I*N THE SPOTLIGHT

PLAYTIME WITH A PURPOSE

Twenty-month-old Craig loves to climb but doesn't get much of a chance to do it at home. Today, he climbs as much as he wants on a wooden climber and a Versagym. Marianna, fifteen months, spent the last ten minutes on the Choo-Choo Balance Beam. Two-year-old Joel can't seem to make up his mind about which piece of equipment he wants to use. He darts from the Nautilus to the Tunnel of Fun to the Aluminum Gym. No problem. He can take as much time as he wants to discover what interests him. Jennifer, who is three but looks more like two, can't make up her mind if she wants to do anything. She looks from her mother to the thirty, happy, noisy children as they each do their own thing. Jennifer's shy behavior is no problem, either. There is no pressure to learn here, just a stimulating environment and an understanding staff who knows that when Jennifer is ready, she will play in her own way.

It's playtime all over America—play with a purpose and a twist. Twisting, tumbling, and touching are some of the activities that stimulate the sensorimotor systems of young children. Parents and their young children, from three months to four years, are enrolling in record numbers in franchised programs such as Gymboree and Play-o-rena, programs designed to enhance the natural learning process of children through creative play. Such programs are capitalizing on what parents and early childhood educators have known for years: learning occurs through play. These programs satisfy parents' need to have their children play with other children in a safe environment, while satisfying children's natural inclinations to play.

What Would You Do?

Robin Martinez, a thirty-two-year-old attorney, is on a leave of absence from her law firm so she can be a full-time mother to her son, Joel. "I've read a great deal about babies being able to learn more at earlier ages," says Robin. "During my pregnancy, I literally devoured every book I could find on raising a smarter baby. I want Joel to be whatever he wants to be, so I have to start early. I want to do the right things to give him the edge he needs in life to succeed. If I start now, I know he will have an edge over other kids.

"I'm very organized, so I spend a lot of time organizing his time. When he does something, I want it to count. I don't think he needs a lot of unstructured time, so I want him to have a program of learning. When he grows up I don't want to feel guilty that I didn't do all I could do for him. I want him to get admitted to one of the best law schools without any trouble."

Robin has come to you for advice about what "programs for early learning" would be best for Joel. What are you going to tell her?

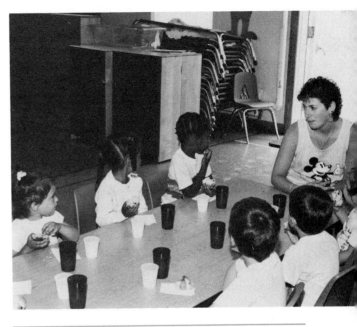

FIGURE 7-14 Today, more toddlers are spending eight and more hours a day in child care programs. Every effort should be made to assure that these programs are quality ones. Indicators of quality include the nature of the environment, the staff and their ability to interact with children, the staff-child ratio and the number of children in each group.

TODDLER CHILD CARE

With increasing numbers of parents in the labor force, the need for toddler care, like the need for all child care, continues to increase. There are primarily three sources of child care available for parents: at-home care in which a care-giver, often a relative, comes to the child's home; family child care in a care-giver's home; and center-based care. The majority of child care is provided by relatives and other individuals in family child care. However, center care is increasing in popularity and availability. Corporate executives in particular are realizing the benefits to their companies and employees of providing accessible, quality child care at or near the workplace. Child care by others—alternative care—is now a permanent, accepted part of child-rearing in American culture.

When making decisions regarding the care of their children, parents should take into consideration four essential factors that determine quality child care for toddlers: environment, the care-givers, the nature of the care, and the curriculum.

The Environment

The physical environment should be clean, bright, and aesthetically pleasing. As a general rule of thumb, parents should not leave their children in a setting in which *they* would not want to spend eight or more hours a day.

The physical environment should be toddler centered. That is, designed and arranged to meet toddler needs, appeal to their interests, and provide for their developmental characteristics.

Health Health guidelines in all programs should provide for the healthy care of toddlers and should focus on the management of infectious diseases. As a minimum, the following policy guidelines are recommended for child care programs that are responsive to the health needs of children and their parents (Aronson & Osterholm, 1986).

1. Notification of public health officials when a possible outbreak of infectious disease is detected or suspected.
2. Frequent hand washing, especially before food handling, after diaper changing or toileting, and after handling of any clothing or other objects contaminated with body secretion or excrement.
3. Cleaning and sanitizing of surfaces used for diapering and food preparation and objects mouthed by toddlers. The sanitizing agent can be household bleach in a concentration of two ounces to a gallon of water. This solution should be made fresh daily.
4. Frequent washing of personal use items, such as stuffed animals and bedding.
5. Enrollment procedures that require that staff and children provide evidence of immunization.
6. Procedures for the exclusion of ill children. (Some programs are providing care for mildly ill children.)

Safety The physical environment provides for the toddlers' safety. Because toddlers are explorers, the environment can be arranged so they can explore in safety. For example, a low barrier around the toddler play area provides for the toddlers' need to explore yet sets a limit on unrestricted exploration. All materials that are potentially hazardous to the toddlers' health and well-being should be stored in areas inaccessible to them.

Learning Materials The learning environment should be rich in a variety of learning materials. These materials should appeal to toddlers and should promote their growing abilities.

Group Size When toddlers are cared for in center settings, group sizes and care-giver–toddler ratios should not exceed those recommended in Table 7–6.

TABLE 7–6

STAFF-CHILD RATIOS AND GROUP SIZE IN TODDLER CHILD CARE										
	Group Size									
Age of Children	6	8	10	12	14	16	18	20	22	24
12–24 months	1.3	1.4	1.5	1.4						
24–36 months		1.4	1.5	1.6						

Note. From *Accreditation Criteria and Procedures of the National Academy of Early Childhood Programs* (p. 24), 1984, Washington, DC: National Association for the Education of Young Children.

Curriculum

The curriculum for toddler child care, whether in a home or center setting, should be *developmentally appropriate* for them. This means it should be consistent with and suitable to the developmental characteristics of toddlers. The National Association for the Education of Young Children (1986) has outlined what such developmentally appropriate practices include:

1. Developmentally appropriate curriculum provides for all areas of a child's development: physical, emotional, social, and cognitive, through an integrated approach.
2. Appropriate curriculum planning is based on teachers' observations and recordings of each

child's special interests and developmental progress.

3. Curriculum planning emphasizes learning as an interactive process. Teachers prepare the environment for children to learn through active exploration and interaction with adults, other children, and materials.

4. Learning activities and materials should be concrete, real, and relevant to the lives of young children.

5. Programs provide for a wider range of developmental interests and abilities than the chronological age range of the group would suggest.

6. Teachers provide a variety of activities and materials; teachers increase the difficulty, complexity, and challenge of an activity as children are involved with it and as children develop understanding and skills.

7. Adults provide opportunities for children to choose from among a variety of activities, materials, and equipment; and time to explore through active involvement. Adults facilitate children's engagement with materials and activities and extend the child's learning by asking questions or making suggestions that stimulate children's thinking.

8. Multicultural and nonsexist experiences, materials, and equipment should be provided for children of all ages.

9. Adults provide a balance of rest and active movement for children throughout the program day.

10. Outdoor experiences should be provided for children of all ages.

Care-givers

Care-givers are the key element of quality child care for any age child. Of course, care-givers must possess those qualities that are critical for working with young children. These qualities include: love of children, caring about children, warmth, kindness, patience, good physical and mental health, compassion, courtesy, dedication, empathy, enthusiasm, honesty, and intelligence.

In addition, care-givers should also demonstrate other characteristics and abilities. As a minimum, they should have:

1. A knowledge of child growth and development of the kind and nature you are reading about in this text.

2. A sensitivity to the needs of children and the ability to respond to these needs in ways that make sense based on the ages, developmental levels, and individual characteristics of the children entrusted to their care.

3. A willingness to learn more about the children they care for and the profession of child care. Children, their parents, and child care programs cannot afford care-givers who know and care little about learning more.

Child Care and Social Policy

As more women enter the work force and as the number of children under five also continues to increase, issues regarding the availability and quality of child care and pay for care-givers have caused federal and state legislators to consider legislation to address these problems. Striking evidence of this is seen in the Alliance for Better Child Care, initiated by the Children's Defense Fund (CDF). The Children's Defense Fund, founded in 1969, provides a voice for the children of America who cannot vote, lobby, or speak for themselves. Based in Washington, DC, CDF has state and local offices throughout the country. The agency gathers and disseminates information on key issues affecting children, and monitors the development and implementation of public policies. It provides information, technical assistance, and support to a network of state and local child advocates. CDF also pursues an annual legislative agenda in the United States Congress and litigates selected cases of major importance. CDF is a private organization supported by foundations, corporate grants, and individual donations.

The Alliance for Better Child Care, which consists of over eighty organizations including the Society for Research in Child Development, has proposed legislation, the Act for Better Child Care, in the U.S. Congress. The purpose of ABC is "to help provide child care for low and moderate income families and to provide incentives for states to improve the quality of all types of child care (center care, family day care, after school care, child care for handicapped children) for all families" (Weintraub & Furman, 1987).

Summary

- The toddler years are characterized by autonomy. Two developmental milestones that contribute to this are independent walking and rapid language development.

- Physical development in toddlerhood is "slow and steady." The average height gain is about eight inches and the average weight gain is about ten pounds. Toddlers, like all children, are individuals, so averages are only that. Toddlers show a wide range of differences in height, weight, and physical appearance. Toddlers are not miniature adults, as close observation of their body proportions reveals. Toddlers at age two are about half their adult height. Toddlers are also "slimming down," which enables them to be actively involved in the physical activity of the toddler years.

- By thirty months, toddlers have their full set of primary teeth. Good dental health begins with the first tooth. This includes dental hygiene and proper nutrition to prevent dental caries.

- Motor development plays a significant role in toddler development. It influences physical, social, and intellectual processes. The average toddler walks at twelve months with a characteristically wide stance, and first attempts at walking are characterized by falling due to body proportions and the learning of a new skill. Toddlers are not able to run well due to imbalance and their inability to start and stop quickly. Since movement is an essential part of the toddler years, parents and other care-givers must support physical activities.

- Fine motor development and fine motor skills enable toddlers to engage in many artistic and self-help activities. Children's artistic expression through age four progresses through four stages: placement, shape, design and pictoral.

- Handedness, or the preference to use one hand over the other, is familial. Most children—90 percent—are right handed.

- Parents influence toddlers' nutritional habits through precept and example. Toddlers develop and demonstrate strong food preferences and want to help themselves during eating. Parents should encourage them to do so.

- Toilet training is largely dependent on physical and neurological maturation and is best accomplished beginning at about the age of two. Parents need to work cooperatively with other care-givers in determining how and when to best train their children. Parents also need to positively support their children during the process of toilet learning.

- Stage V, Experimentation, which occurs between one year and eighteen months, involves *tertiary circular reactions*, in which toddlers repeat actions and modify behaviors over and over to see what will happen. During this stage, children are known as "little experimenters." Object permanence, or the ability to comprehend that an object does not cease to exist simply because it is not visible, continues to develop during Stage V.

■ Stage VI, Representational Intelligence, develops between eighteen and twenty-four months. Representational intelligence begins when toddlers can visualize events internally. During this stage, true object permanence develops. Once they have achieved object permanence, toddlers understand the rudiments of property *identity*, that is, that objects have an identity of their own and exist when the toddler is not present. Representational thought also enables toddlers to engage in one of their favorite activities—pretend play.

■ Children in Stage VI of preoperational intelligence are no longer dominated and controlled by reflexive actions as are infants. The Stage VI child is capable of symbolic thought and is ready to manipulate the environment by the use of symbols through language. The toddler is ready to enter the world of preoperational intelligence.

■ Attention, praise, and compliance with children's requests are examples of how parents use socially mediated reinforcement to help children's language development. Also, children adopt the language usage patterns of their parents by learning the names for things as their parents know them.

■ Children speak their first word at about one year of age. These first words are just that, words relating to the people and things identified and labeled by their parents. Children's one-word utterances are *holophrasic*, meaning they do the work of a whole sentence. Toddlers also use *telegraphic speech*, in which they use two-word sentences to stand for a whole sentence.

■ Mothers use a distinctive method of communicating with their young children called "motherese."

■ "No," one of the toddler's favorite words, progresses through a series of meanings. These levels of meaning include nonexistence, rejection, and denial.

■ The LASS, or language support system, is the means whereby parents and others support children's language development. The ways they do this are through learning basic formats and rules; modeling vocabulary and phrases; involvement in routines and pretend activities; and naming and requesting.

■ Language games provide parents and children an ideal way to interactively engage in the process of language development.

■ Stage One of psychosocial development begins at birth and ends at eighteen months to two years. The primary psychosocial conflict during this stage is the development of trust or mistrust as a result of interactions with parents and other care-givers.

■ Stage Two of psychosocial development begins at eighteen to twenty-four months and continues until age three. During this stage, toddlers develop feelings of autonomy or shame. Toddlers develop autonomy in part through the control of their physical behavior.

■ Toddlers are active and parents must facilitate this activity in a safe and stimulating environment. Parents need to provide toddlers with love and affection; help them become independent; assist in their efforts to do things for themselves; and, allow them to make choices.

■ When selecting child care for their toddlers, parents should take into consideration four essential factors that determine quality child care: environment, the care-givers, the nature of the care, and the nature of the curriculum. The physical environment should be safe and healthy. Staff-child ratios for toddler care should be in accordance with guidelines established by the National Association for the Education of Young Children. The curriculum should be developmentally appropriate. Care-givers should have a knowledge of child development and demonstrate a sensitivity to the needs of children.

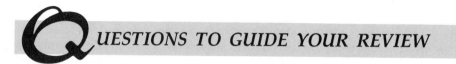

QUESTIONS TO GUIDE YOUR REVIEW

1. What important milestones occur in the toddler period?
2. What are the highlights of toddler physical development?
3. How does toddler dental development differ from infant dental development?
4. What role do motor abilities play in toddler development?
5. What form does artistic expression take in the toddler years?
6. In what ways do toddlers' eating habits influence parenting interactions?
7. What important developmental guidelines should parents follow in supporting children's toilet learning?
8. What are tertiary circular reactions and how do they influence intellectual development?
9. How do Stage V and Stage VI of intellectual development differ?
10. What is object permanence?
11. What is symbolic play and what role does it have in children's development?
12. What is the sequence of language development from one year through three years?
13. What role does socially mediated reinforcement play in language development?
14. What is "motherese" and what roles does it serve in children's language development?
15. How does the LASS support language development?
16. How do games contribute to children's language development?
17. What are the major psychosocial "conflicts" children must reconcile during Stage one and Stage two?
18. What are three major developmental milestones of the toddler years? What transactional influences are there between them and psychological development?
19. In what ways can parents appropriately respond to toddlers' activity, need for love and affection, and their growing independence?
20. What can parents do to "childproof" the toddler environment?
21. What are critical factors care-givers should consider when providing child-care for toddlers?
22. What are important health guidelines that should be followed when providing child care for toddlers?

23. What are the recommended group sizes and toddler–care-giver ratios in a good child care program?
24. What developmentally appropriate practices should be used when caring for and working with toddlers?
25. What qualities should toddler care-givers possess?

ACTIVITIES FOR FURTHER INVOLVEMENT

1. Two important developmental milestones of the toddler period are unassisted walking and rapid language development.
   a. Tell what parents and other care-givers can do to promote these two developmental processes in toddlers.
   b. How can the environment and inappropriate parental practices interfere in the development of language?
2. Toilet training is one of the developmental tasks that causes both parents and children social and emotional distress.
   a. Make a list of the physical and psychosocial factors that children should possess before they are able to appropriately participate in the task of toilet training.
   b. Interview parents of different cultures to determine how and when they toilet trained their children. Summarize your findings.
   c. Comment on the following: "During toilet training, the child is confronted with the conflict of the pleasure of involuntarily letting go and letting go when the mother wills."
3. The style of language a mother uses with her child can influence the child's style of language expression.
   a. Observe different parents across the socioeconomic spectrum to determine the different styles of language used with their toddlers.
   b. Based on your observations, what do you think influences language development in the home?
4. A great deal of emphasis is currently placed on parenting styles.
   a. Why is the authoritative parenting style considered more appropriate than permissive parenting?
   b. What parenting styles or combinations of parenting styles did your parent use with you? What do you believe to be the best parenting techniques they used? Did they do anything as a parent that you will not do as a parent? What?
5. One of the areas of conflict between parents and toddlers is toddlers' quest for autonomy and independence.
   a. Observe parents to determine the positive and negative ways they respond to toddlers' developing independence. Pay particular attention to how the parents react to toddlers when they say "No."
   b. Tell how parental interactions influence toddlers' developing autonomy.
   c. What environmental factors influence the development of autonomy in the toddler years?

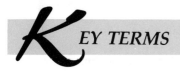

KEY TERMS

Aspiration Inhaling of food or small objects.

Developmentally appropriate Characteristic of curricula, care, and an environment that is consistent with and suitable to the developmental characteristics of individual children and groups of children.

Dominance The preference of one side of the body over another.

Fine motor skills Skills dependent on fine motor activities such as writing and buttoning.

Motherese The distinctive manner in which mothers talk with their young children.

Object permanence The understanding that objects occupy space, have an existence of their own, and continue to exist even when not seen.

Socially mediated reinforcement Reinforcement in the form of such behaviors as attention, praise, and compliance with requests.

Symbolic play Play that utilizes representation, in which something stands for something else.

Tertiary circular reactions Displayed when toddlers repeat actions and modify behaviors over and over to see what will happen. This repetition helps develop an understanding of cause-and-effect relationships and leads to the discovery of new relationships through exploration and experimentation.

Toddlerhood The period from twelve to thirty-six months.

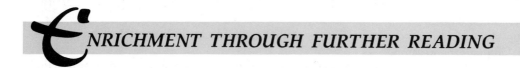

ENRICHMENT THROUGH FURTHER READING

Maynard, Fredelle. (1986). *The Child Care Crisis: The Thinking Parent's Guide to Day Care.* Ontario: Penguin Books.

    Examines all the forms of day care and offers advice about how to evaluate them. Also includes a chapter on what to do if the parent decides to stay home with their young child.

ANSWER TO "WHAT WOULD YOU DO?"

There is a definite dichotomy in the world of young children between those parents who are goal oriented in their efforts to rear the "best and the brightest" and early childhood professionals who view with alarm and apprehension the increasing emphasis on early education. This dichotomy also produces a considerable amount of tension and media attention. More and more early educators are raising their voices to express their concern about what they see as an overzealousness on the part of parents to push and hurry their children toward success. One educator (Buckner, 1988) expresses it this way:

> Clearly, achieving advanced academics at an early age is the goal of many people, but is this race *our* goal for a quality early education? Has our vision as early childhood educators changed? What happened to good old nursery school where children came for the joy of feeding rabbits, building in the block corner, and watching butterflies hatch from cocoons? Are these enriching, time-honored, age appropriate experiences considered "just" play and given a lower status because they do not appear on assessments instruments? Is faster always better? Remember the Aesop fable of the tortoise and the hare (p. 5).

There are many fables that could be cited to explain what is happening in early childhood education today. Some parents and early educators would use the fable of Chicken Little to characterize those critics who are screaming that the sky of early academics is about to fall on all those who advocate it.

Clearly there is a middle ground that provides opportunities both for early academics *and* the "time-honored" practices held dear by many. There are two caveats in all of this. First, times have changed and times are changing. Children who are four today will graduate from high school in the twenty-first century. As society changes, so must educational practices. Many of the things in which young children are involved today, such as computers and interactive learning programs, were not available years ago when "time-honored" practices were developed. Second, any program of activities that unduly stresses children is not in children's best interests.

So, what advice do you give Robin?

*B*IBLIOGRAPHY

Accreditation criteria and procedures of the National Academy of Early Childhood Programs. (1984). Washington, DC: National Association for the Education of Young Children.

Aronson, S., & Osterholm, M.T. (1986). Infectious diseases in child day care: Management and prevention summary of the symposium recommendations. *Reviews of Infectious Diseases, 8,* 672–679.

Bloom, L. (1970). *Language development: Form and function in emerging grammars.* Cambridge, MA: MIT Press.

Brown, R. (1973). *A first language.* Cambridge, MA: Harvard University Press.

Bruner, J. (1983). *Child's talk: Learning to use language.* New York: W. W. Norton.

Buckner, L. M. (1988) On the fast track to. . . .? Is it early childhood education or early adult education? *Young Children, 43,* 5.

Capute, A. J., & Accardo, P. J. (1978, November). Linguistic and auditory milestones during the first two years of life: A language inventory for the practitioner. *Clinical Pediatrics, 17,* 847–853.

Clark, E. V. (1983). Meanings and concepts. In J. H. Flavell & E. M. Markman (Eds.) *Cognitive development: vol. 3 of Handbook of child psychology,* (4th ed.). New York: John Wiley, 787–840.

Dale, P. S., (1976). *Language development* (2nd ed.). New York: Holt, Rinehart & Winston.

de Villiers, P. A., & de Villiers, J. G. (1979). *Early language.* Cambridge, MA: Harvard University Press and William Collins.

Elkind, D. (1987) *Miseducation: Preschoolers at risk.* New York: Alfred A. Knopf.

Espenschade, A. S., & Eckert, H. M. (1980). *Motor development* (2nd ed.). Columbus, OH: Merrill.

Ginsburg, H. & Opper, S. (1979). *Piaget's theory of intellectual development.* Englewood Cliffs, NJ: Prentice-Hall.

Henig, R. M. (1988, May 22). Should baby read? *The New York Times Magazine,* pp. 37–38.

Kellog, R. (1970). Understanding children's art. In P. Cramer (Ed.), *Readings in developmental psychology today.* (pp. 31–39) Delmar, CA: CRM Books.

Longstreth, L. G. (1980). Human handedness: More evidence for genetic involvement. *The Journal of Genetic Psychology, 137,* 275–283.

Macnamara, J. (1982). *Names for things.* Cambridge, MA: MIT Press.

Michel, G. F., Ovrut, M. A., & Harkins, D. A. (1985). Hand-use preference for reaching and object manipulation in 6- through 13-month-old infants. *Genetic, Social, and General Psychology Monographs, 111,* 422.

National Association for the Education of Young Children. (1986, September). Position statement on developmentally appropriate practice in early childhood programs serving children from birth through age eight. *Young Children, 41,* 4–29.

Newport, E. L., Gleitman, H., & Gleitman, L. (1977). Mother, I'd rather do it myself: Some effects and non-effects of maternal speech style, in C. E. Snow & C. A. Ferguson (Eds.), *Talking to children: Language input and acquisition* (pp. 112–129). Cambridge, England: Cambridge University Press.

Piaget, J. (1952). *The origins of intelligence in children.* (M. Cook, Trans.). New York: International Universities Press.

Traub, J. (1986). Goodbye, Dr. Spock: Vignettes from the brave new world of the better baby. *Harper's Magazine, 272,* 57–64.

Weintraub, K. S., & Furman, L. N. (1987, December). Child care: Quality, regulation, and research. *Social Policy Report, Society for Research in Child Development, 2* (4), 1.

Whaley, L. F., & Wong, D. L. (1983). *Nursing care of infants and children (2nd ed.).* St. Louis: C. V. Mosby.

Whitehurst, G. J., & Valdez-Menchaca, M. C. (1988). What is the role of reinforcement in early language acquisition? *Child Development, 59,* 430–440.

CHAPTER EIGHT

The preschool years

◆

VIGNETTE
INTRODUCTION
PHYSICAL DEVELOPMENT
Dental Development
MOTOR DEVELOPMENT
Walking
Running
Climbing
Throwing
Fine Motor Development
Implications of Motor Skills for
    Intellectual Development
Implications of Motor Skills for
    Psychosocial Development
INTELLECTUAL DEVELOPMENT
Preoperational Intelligence
Egocentrism
Implications for Parents and
    Teachers
LANGUAGE DEVELOPMENT
The Importance of Language
    Development
An Interactionist View of

Language Development
From Simple to Complex
Private Speech—"What Piece
    Comes Next?"
What Would You Do?
PSYCHOSOCIAL DEVELOPMENT
Implications for Parents and
    Teachers
GENDER DEVELOPMENT
All I Want for Christmas Is A
    Sex-typed Toy
DEVELOPMENT OF
    AGGRESSION
Biological Factors
Environmental/Social Factors
Sex Differences in Aggression
Implications for Parents
WHY DO CHILDREN PLAY?
Play from a Freudian Perspective
What Is Play?
CLASSIFICATIONS OF PLAY
Social Play
Piaget and Symbolic Play

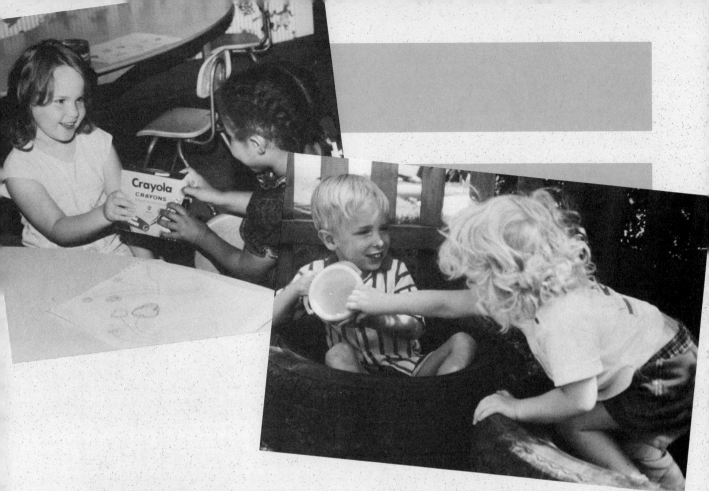

THE COMPETENCIES OF PLAY
PRESCHOOL PLAY
  ENVIRONMENTS
In the Spotlight: Preschool Fitness
ACCIDENTS: CAUSES AND
  PREVENTION
TANTRUMS
WHAT KIND OF PARENT
  SHOULD I BE?
Is There One Best Way to Parent?
A Matrix of Parenting Styles
In the Spotlight: Homeless
  Children
CHILDREN WITH AIDS
What is AIDS?
AIDS Incidence

Children at Risk for AIDS
Implications for Parents and Care-
  givers
Public Policy Implications of AIDS
  for Children and Society
SUMMARY
QUESTIONS TO GUIDE YOUR
  REVIEW
ACTIVITIES FOR FURTHER
  INVOLVEMENT
KEY TERMS
ENRICHMENT THROUGH
  FURTHER READING
ANSWER TO "WHAT WOULD
  YOU DO?"
BIBLIOGRAPHY

⟲IGNETTE

Dawn has just broken across the eastern sky as four-year-old Roberto Sandoval, eager for the day's events, hurries up the dusty street toward the Homestead Migrant Preschool Program. Roberto is accompanied by his thirteen-year-old sister, Anna, who for all intents and purposes is his surrogate mother. In fact, when he really needs comforting and soothing, it is Anna to whom Roberto turns. The other children in the tightly-knit family group include nine-year-old Lorena and two-year-old Miguel. One of the sisters' responsibilities is to escort their younger brothers to the preschool each morning. They then proceed up the winding road to the place where they will catch the school bus for the junior high school.

Roberto's parents, Amelia and Jose, are already at work in the fields of the vast, flat sprawling farmlands of southeast Florida. Since 5:30 AM they have been picking bucket after bucket of tomatoes destined for the tables of families in the Northeast. In some ways, the Sandoval family is more advantaged than their constantly moving counterparts. They are a resident migrant family, and live year round in the Homestead Migrant Camp. However, they will, during the hot summer, travel to Mexico for a two-week vacation with family and friends.

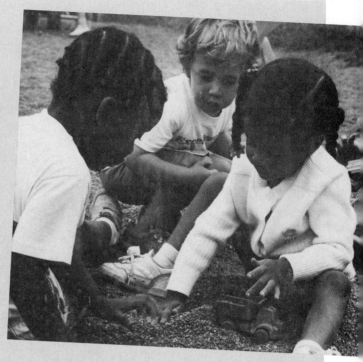

The family of six lives in the migrant camp in a small, square concrete block house consisting of a small kitchen, a small bathroom, and a larger room that is used as a living and sleeping area. They feel they are lucky to have such accommodations.

The Homestead Migrant Program offers the Sandovals and other migrant families much-needed resources as well as referrals to other agencies. These include workshops on alcohol abuse and AIDS prevention, family counseling, free dental services for the children, and, when needed, canned goods, food certificates, and clothing.

The parent involvement component of the Migrant Child Care Program is a vital cornerstone of this organization. These families are in great need of extended services provided by this organization in order to "make it" with their children and meet the many responsibilities that come with having a large family and helping young children get the right start.

The parent involvement component at the Migrant Child Care Program includes an initial interview at the time of registration, daily contacts during the child's (or children's) first week at the program with the teacher, then monthly home visits as support groups, and monthly meetings and workshops to introduce parents to the educational component of the program.

Parents are also encouraged to participate as volunteers, visitors and guests during the daily operation of the child care program.

One of the small group activities that recently occurred and included parents as guests was when one of the mothers brought in fresh fish. She cleaned and skinned it as the children observed. Then they helped to season the fish, cooked it,

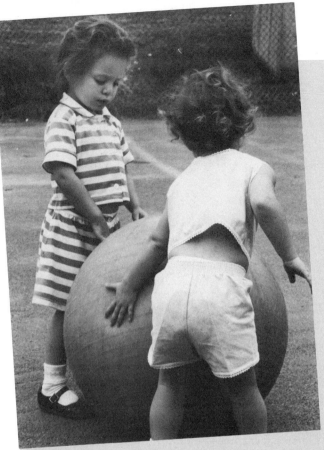

beans, beef, a lettuce and tomato salad, and milk, and concludes with cooked apples for dessert. The two adults, Silvia (the teacher) and Consuelo (the teacher's aide), eat lunch with the children. Prior to their lunch, the children join the teachers in saying grace:

"God is great, God is good,
And we thank Him for our food
By Your hands we all are fed
Give us Lord our daily bread. Amen."

After lunch, Roberto and his other classmates brush their teeth again. Dental hygiene is a very important part of the program, because many of the children enter the preschool program with many cavities.

Following lunch, Roberto takes a nap for an hour and a half. He helps put up and take down his and other children's cots. After his nap, Roberto participates in small group activities such as cooking, which is used to introduce the children to new foods such as celery sticks and peanut butter. Roberto also participates in learning center activities such as seriation, and his teacher asks him to explain how his rows are similar and different. Recently the staff and children transformed the dramatic play area into a flower shop—named "Lupita." Roberto played the role of cashier. He and his other friends made paper flower arrangements to sell for Mother's Day.

Following the learning center activity, Roberto plays on the playground until his sisters arrive. Together with Miguel they will go home to prepare dinner for the family.

and had it for lunch with the rest of the balanced menu planned by the nutritionist. But, to return to Roberto, and his day at the preschool.

By eight o'clock Roberto has had a breakfast consisting of oatmeal, orange juice, and milk. He brushes his teeth and then participates in a circle-time activity. Roberto is involved in a curriculum based in part on the theory of Jean Piaget, which is designed to help him develop language and problem-solving skills. Roberto also participates in outside playground activities including free and structured play. He then cleans up and prepares for lunch, which consists of a flour tortilla, refried

This chapter is about the *preschool years*, the period when children are between thirty-six and sixty months of age, or between the ages of three and five years. While the term *preschool years* is used to describe the years before children enter school, this designation is rapidly becoming obsolete. Today, it is common for many children to be in a school of some kind beginning as early as age two and three. And child care at six weeks is rapidly becoming *de regular* for children of working parents. Likewise, kindergarten as a part of public schooling is now virtually universal for children between the ages of five and six. Whether we like it or not, or agree with it or not, kindergarten is no longer an upward extension of the preschool, and involves much more than cookies and milk as we will see. For this reason, kindergarten-aged children are discussed in Chapter Ten, Middle Childhood: Development during the Elementary School Years. Additionally, with states such as Texas, Florida, California, New York, and North Carolina developing preschool programs for four-year-old children, the term preschool hardly applies to threes and fours anymore.

Some educators and writers utilize the term *early childhood* when referring to the preschool years, but this is out of keeping with the profession's definition of early childhood, the years from birth to age eight. Because of the public's general familiarity with and acceptance of the term *preschool*, we will continue to use it in our discussion of three- and four-year-old children.

PHYSICAL DEVELOPMENT

For preschoolers, height and weight gain is a slow and steady process. Average height gain is about three inches per year, while weight gain averages about four to five pounds a year. (See Tables 8–1 through 8–4.) Although boys tend to be a little taller and heavier than girls, in outward appearances the sexes are similar to each other.

TABLE 8–1

AVERAGE (FIFTIETH PERCENTILE) HEIGHT NORMS FOR PRESCHOOL CHILDREN

Age (Years)	Males		Females	
	Inches	Centimeters	Inches	Centimeters
3	37	95	37	94.1
3.5	39	99.1	38.5	97.9
4	40.5	103	40	101.6
4.5	42	106.6	41.3	105
5	43.2	109.9	42.7	108.4

Note. From "Physical Growth: National Center for Health Statistics Percentiles" by P.V.V. Hamill, T.A. Drizd, R.B. Reed, C.L. Johnson, A.F. Roche, & W.M. Moore, 1979, *The American Journal of Clinical Nutrition, 32*, pp. 607–629.

TABLE 8–2

AVERAGE (FIFTIETH PERCENTILE) WEIGHT NORMS FOR PRESCHOOL CHILDREN

Age (Years)	Males		Females	
	Kilograms	Pounds	Kilograms	Pounds
3	14.69	32.39	13.93	30.71
3.5	15.68	34.57	15.07	33.22
4	16.69	36.80	15.96	35.19
4.5	17.69	39.00	16.81	36.98
5	18.67	41.16	17.66	38.94

Note. From "Physical Growth: National Center for Health Statistics Percentiles" by P.V.V. Hamill, T.A. Drizd, R.B. Reed, C.L. Johnson, A.F. Roche, & W.M. Moore, 1979, *The American Journal of Clinical Nutrition, 32*, pp. 607–629.

Growth spurts in children do not usually occur until the middle school years. The weight gain in preschool children is primarily muscle development, which helps explain why boys are a little heavier than girls.

One thing that is noticeable about preschoolers is that they are starting to look more like adults. One reason for this is that their body proportions are developing more in relation to what they will

TABLE 8-3

AVERAGE WEIGHT AND HEIGHT FOR PRESCHOOL CHILDREN

Age (Years)	Weight (Pounds)		Height (Inches)	
	Males	Females	Males	Females
3	32.4	30.7	37.0	37.0
4	36.8	35.2	40.5	40.0
5	41.2	38.9	43.2	42.7

Note. From "Physical Growth: National Center for Health Statistics Percentiles" by P.V.V. Hamill, T.A. Drizd, R.B. Reed, C.L. Johnson, A.F. Roche, & W.M. Moore, 1979, *The American Journal of Clinical Nutrition, 32,* pp. 607–629.

TABLE 8-4

AVERAGE WEIGHT AND HEIGHT GAIN FOR PRESCHOOL CHILDREN

Age (Years)	Males		Females	
	Weight (Pounds)	Height (Inches)	Weight (Pounds)	Height (Inches)
2–3	4.6	3.5	4.5	3.5
3–4	4.4	2.5	4.5	2.4
4–5	4.4	2.8	3.7	2.7

Note. From "Physical Growth: National Center for Health Statistics Percentiles" by P.V.V. Hamill, T.A. Drizd, R.B. Reed, C.L. Johnson, A.F. Roche, & W.M. Moore, 1979, *The American Journal of Clinical Nutrition, 32,* pp. 607–629.

be as adults. The face grows longer, the waist becomes smaller, the trunk increases in length and by age five, the preschoolers legs are, like adults, about one-half of their body length.

Dental Development

By age three, most preschoolers have their full complement of twenty deciduous or baby teeth. The foundation for good dental health begins in infancy with the emergence of the first tooth, so by the preschool years, brushing and flossing should be regular features of a child's health and self-care routine. Some parents may feel that dental care, including regular visits to a dentist, is unnecessary since the child "is only going to lose his teeth anyway." But for some children, dental caries (tooth decay) are a serious health problem. Proper nutrition also contributes to good dental health, so parents should limit sweet, between-meal snacks as a way of limiting tooth decay.

MOTOR DEVELOPMENT

Motor development plays a prominent role in the lives of preschool children. Preschool children are whirlwinds of energy as they practice and perfect their emerging large muscle physical skills. In addition, fine motor skills play an increasingly significant role in children's cognitive development and academic activities.

Walking

As young children mature from toddlers to preschoolers, they increase their length of stride, develop a consistent step rate, and are able to transfer their weight from heel to toe. By the time they are three, walking is an automatic process. Three-year-old children also begin to demonstrate individuality in their walk and have a personalized way of carrying themselves. By age four, preschool children have achieved an adult manner of walking, characterized by a swinging, rhythmical stride with the ability to walk in a straight line. The preschooler has finally conquered gravity and is now able to coordinate her balance so that walking is a perfected and graceful motor accomplishment (Espenschade & Eckert, 1980, pp. 137–138).

Running

Running requires more strength and coordination than walking. Running is not a fully co-ordinated activity for children between ages two and three because they lack the ability to stop and turn quickly. By age four and five, children have developed control over starting, stopping, and turning.

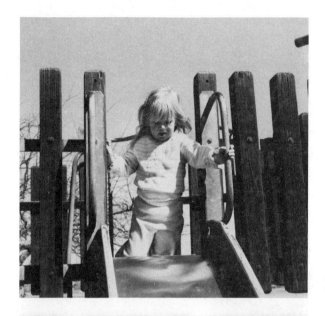
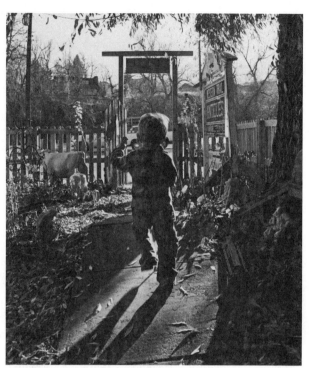
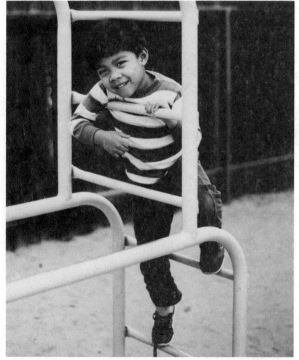
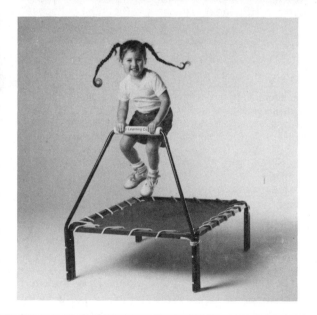

FIGURE 8-1   The preschool years are a time of increased motor activity for preschoolers; motor skills improve dramatically as they physically develop and engage in play activities. Walking, running, jumping, climbing, and throwing and catching are all important preschool activities.

Climbing

Children's ability to climb stairs follows a definite developmental progression (Espenschade & Eckert, 1980):

1. Ascending skill is achieved prior to descending abilities at the same level of accomplishment.
2. A child accomplishes an activity (climbing) of a given level with help before he is able to perform the same activity alone.
3. At each level of achievement, a child is able to negotiate a shorter flight of stairs before he is able to do so with a longer flight.
4. Stairs with low risers can be mastered at each level of achievement prior to stairs of adult height (p. 142).

The height of the step is an important consideration in the child's ability and willingness to use climbing skills. Children who are proficient climbers on low stairs revert to less advanced techniques with higher stairs.

Throwing

As with stair climbing, there are four stages involved in throwing (Espenschade & Eckert, 1980). Each stage progresses toward what is considered a mature level of throwing.

1. During the entire throw, both feet remain firmly in place and the body faces toward the direction of the throw. This is typical of ages two and three.
2. The feet remain horizontal but the body rotates to the right in preparation for the throw and then to the left as the ball is thrown. This is typical in three-and-one-half to five-year-old children.
3. The third stage involves a step forward with the right foot as the ball is thrown. This is accomplished between the fifth and sixth years.
4. The fourth stage involves the transfer of weight to the right foot in preparation for

throwing, and transferring weight to the left foot during the throwing phase. This is usually accomplished at six-and-one-half years and older (p. 152).

Fine Motor Development

Fine motor activities involve the hands and fingers for such actions as holding and manipulating things, and are frequently referred to as *manual skills* and *manipulative skills*. In fact, many preschool activities, such as cutting, pasting, drawing, coloring, and solving puzzles, involve the use of fine motor activities. Preschool teachers frequently identify such tasks as involving *eye-hand coordination*, because the eyes and hands are used in unison to accomplish these activities. As such, much of preschool success is measured by activities involving fine motor skills.

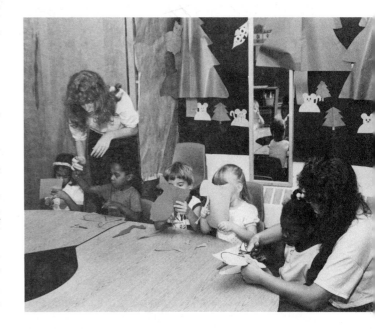

FIGURE 8-2 The ability to manipulate and use the hands for fine-motor activities improves during the preschool years. Many preschool activities involving the use and coordination of hands and fingers such as drawing, tracing, copying, cutting, folding, lacing, and tying form the basis of many school-related activities.

Implications of Motor Skills for Intellectual Development

The importance of motor skills in the development of cognitive abilities cannot and should not be underestimated. First, physical skills contribute to representational thought by enabling children to act on and experiment with their environment. In the process they learn names for things, begin to understand how things work, and are simultaneously practicing their emerging language skills.

Second, children learn as they act on their environments and objects in that environment. For example, as children walk, run, climb, and throw, they learn about space, time, and cause-and-effect relationships, all of which are important concepts in intellectual development.

Third, as children play and interact with others they learn others' points of view and are involved in learning the rules that govern the games they play as well as the game of life.

Fourth, as children develop fine motor skills, they can be involved in many forms of representation *in addition to* language. Some of these are drawing and painting, modeling with clay, cutting and pasting, and construction activities involving wood, styrofoam, and cardboard.

Implications of Motor Skills for Psychosocial Development

During the toddler and early preschool years, children are in the psychosocial stage of Autonomy vs. Shame. They develop a sense of autonomy by controlling their behavior. One way they do this is through the exploration of their environments. And certainly, mastery of physical skills promotes a sense of autonomy.

During the third stage of psychosocial development, Initiative vs. Guilt, preschoolers want to do things for themselves. In fact, a good description for preschoolers is that they are "I-can-do-it-for-myself" persons. This is a desirable attitude and should be encouraged. By using, practicing, and developing their motor skills, children are able to do things for themselves. This leads to initiative and feelings of competence and self-worth. In this sense, the contributions of motor skills to initiative is an interactive cyclical process. The more initiative one has, the better one feels about oneself, which encourages ever higher achievement.

INTELLECTUAL DEVELOPMENT

Preoperational Intelligence

Preoperational thought as designated by Piaget is typical of children two to six years old. The most significant feature of this period is the use of symbols—language—to represent the environment. While the preoperational child can rearrange experiences without actually physically manipulating the environment, she is not yet capable of *operational* thought. An *operation* is reversible mental action whereby an object or experience that is transformed can be returned to its original form. An example of a mental operation is $1 + 2 = 3$ and $3 - 2 = 1$. The process of addition is reversible through subtraction. You know this, but the preoperational child does not.

Preoperational thinking has certain other characteristics. Preoperational children cannot *conserve*; that is, they cannot mentally understand that amount (mass), quantity, and volume stay the same even though appearance (shape, size, and dimensions) changes. In a test of conservation of number, for example, a child is presented with a row of objects, like buttons (Row A). She is then asked to make a second row to exactly match the first. This she can do, as in Row B. When the spacing is changed between the first row and the second (transformation by expanding) as in Rows C and D, so that the endpoints of the rows are not the same, and then the child is asked which row (C or D) has more buttons, the preoperational child will answer, "The second row" (Row D). When asked why the second row (Row D) has more buttons, the child will respond, "Because it is bigger" (or longer). The child really believes that there are more buttons in the second row (Row D) because she confuses length with number. Likewise, when asked which row, E or F, has fewer buttons, she thinks the F (or collapsed) row does. This reflects the inability to conserve.

Egocentrism

The preoperational child is still egocentric, but in different ways than the sensorimotor child. This egocentrism is illustrated by the fact that preoperational children are unable to assume a perspective other than their own. Their view of the world is the only view they take and is the only one that matters to them.

This egocentrism is further illustrated by Piaget's three mountain experiment. A model of three mountains is placed on a table. The child is then shown drawings of views that other children would see if they sat at the other positions around the table. The preoperational child is unable to choose the mountain scene that other children would see if they sat at other places around the table. From this, Piaget concluded that preoperational children do not yet have the cognitive ability to understand that others can see things from a perspective other than theirs. The preoperational child thinks others see what she sees. This egocentrism is demonstrated in other ways in many everyday incidents— what looks big to them they think looks big to teachers; things that they think taste good they want you to eat because they must taste good to you, too; and they think you know exactly what they are talking about even if you join a conversation after it starts.

And speaking of conversation, the preoperational child uses language in a literal sense. The child talks *at* others as opposed to talking *with* them. This is termed *egocentric speech.*

Preoperational children are egocentric in the application of rules as well. They are not afraid to make up rules as they go along, and to them, their rules are all that matter. They are not aware of and therefore are unconcerned with and unaffected by external rules.

The basic egocentrism of the preoperational child then constitutes a barrier to the use of logical thinking. And it is only after maturation and mental development that he will be capable of more logical thought processes.

Other characteristics of preoperational thinking are evidenced by centration and the focusing on states rather than transformations. *Centration* is characterized by focusing on one characteristic of an object, color, for example, while ignoring other attributes such as length and size. Also, children in the preoperational stage focus on the *states* or specific events of a process rather than on the process itself. They focus on the individual steps in baking cookies and have difficulty seeing how all the steps fit together in contributing to the baked cookie. It is as though they are focusing on each frame of a movie rather than seeing the movie as a whole.

Implications for Parents and Teachers

Piaget believed that an active child is a developing child. Or to put it another way, the developing child is active. This inherent capacity for action is reflected both physically and mentally. The child wants to be active in the environment, and in so doing is mentally active in striving for equilibrium. Children need parents and teachers who will enable them to be active in an environment that provides many activities and opportunities to experience new things. Action contributes to intellectual development.

Symbolic representations can be encouraged in a number of ways. First, since children are in a period of rapid language development, the use of language can be supported and encouraged. For most children, language is the major form of representation.

Second, artwork of various kinds can also be used to help children represent their internal thoughts and ideas. Drawing and painting pictures, modeling with clay, cutting and pasting, and construction activities with wood and styrofoam are all meaningful ways to promote and encourage representation. These activities are also meaningful in that they provide children with experiences at a concrete level.

Third, the Language Experience Approach (LEA) helps children express their ideas and allows them to see their thoughts transformed into words and sentences. In the LEA, children tell about their experiences in their own words, and the care-giver or teacher uses pictures, words, and sentences to record their thoughts. This is an excellent way to promote symbolic representation and the writing and reading processes.

Teachers and care-givers should note that preoperational children benefit most from non-abstract experiences because they are still perceptually bound. Their experiences, therefore, should be concrete and have concrete referents, as the suggestions in the previous two paragraphs indicate.

Many kinds of social interactions are necessary to help children *decenter*, or develop out of their egocentrism. Preschoolers, and all children for that matter, need many experiences with a wide range of people, including other children and adults. In this way they learn that others have opinions and thoughts different from their own.

LANGUAGE DEVELOPMENT

The Importance of Language Development

Language development in the preschool years is extremely important because much of children's school success is and will be determined by how well they achieve in school. Much of this achievement is related to how well they know and use language. Learning the language system, then, is important to school and life success. Children who know the names of things, can express themselves well, can talk to the teacher, and understand the language of schooling have a decided advantage in the schooling process.

An Interactionist View of Language Development

We know and take for granted that while children develop physically, all children don't develop physically in the same way. So, too, all children learn language, but all children don't learn language in the same way but results in part from interaction with the environment (Bates, Bretherton, & Snyder, 1988, p. 3).

Interactionism applied is summarized as follows:

> Language is an interactive system that depends crucially on processes and representations from a variety of cognitive domains. The acquisition of language will be shaped and timed by the emergence and development of these requisite cognitive systems (Bates et al., 1988. p. 11).

From Simple to Complex

One of the hallmarks of children's language development in the early years is the progression from the use of simple to more complex sentences. Samples of children's preschool speech patterns show this increase in complexity, with about 25 percent of their sentences being complex (Garrard, 1987). Beginning at age three, children's use of simple sentences such as, "That balloon is big!" and "I ate all my dinner," progresses to the use of more complex sentences, such as the comparative, "My book is bigger than your book." Examples of the type of complex sentences that preschool children use are shown in Table 8–5.

Private Speech—"What Piece Comes Next?"

Jennifer, a four-year-old preschooler, is busily engrossed in putting a puzzle together. As she searches for a piece, she asks herself out loud, "Which piece comes next?" I'm sure you have heard children talk to themselves. More than likely you have talked to yourself. Such conversations with oneself can constitute 20 to 60 percent of the

TABLE 8–5

PRESCHOOL CHILDREN'S COMPLEX SENTENCES

Nature of Complexity	Example
Coordination with and, so, but, or	"Those boys wanted gum, but their mother said 'no.'"
Relatives on the object noun	"That picture is about some birds that got all smeared up."
Relatives on the subject noun	"The boy who lives next door is my friend."
Infinitives	"She wants to put it on to make her shoulders more fresh."
Adverbals with because, since, until, if, before, after	"He can't swim in the pool because there is no water in it."
Indirect complements	"I think that's a picture of George Washington."
Comparatives	"This boy is running faster than that one."

Note. From "Teaching Complex Sentences" by D.L. Tyack, 1981, Language, Speech, and Hearing Services in Schools, 17, pp. 160–174.

language of preschool and elementary school children (Berk, 1986).

Of what value is this private speech? Does it serve any useful purpose? Researcher Berk believes the answer is a resounding "yes." Intrigued by children's private speech, she and a colleague wanted to determine which of two contradictory views of language development, those of Jean Piaget and Lev Vygotsky, was correct. Piaget's view of personal speech—what he termed egocentric speech—is that it serves little useful social purpose. From this point of view, egocentric speech is an indication of children's basic egocentrism and demonstrates that they think other children and adults understand what they are talking about even though they don't. Vygotsky, on the other hand, maintained that private speech helps integrate language and thought. What begins as personal speech gradually becomes, as children grow older, internal thought.

The type of personal speech that children use most often is called "self-guiding" (Berk & Garvin, 1984). This guiding function takes the form of self-answered questions—"Because this is where it is supposed to go"—and self-guiding comments—"Don't put too much glue on it." Private speech also increases when children are confronted with demanding academic tasks (Berk, 1985). So, based on Vygotsky's theory and guided by her research, Berk (1985) provides a number of suggestions regarding preschool classroom practice:

1. Play in social contexts is especially important. Early private speech originates in settings rich in peer social opportunities. Play opportunities should bring together children of different ages, skills, and abilities.
2. In problem-solving situations, children often must rely on guidance and direction from adults before they can function independently. When adults provide the assistance necessary to carry out a new task, then children can structure their own efforts in the same way. They thus have the framework within which to guide—at times with the assistance of private speech—their own efforts.
3. The assistance the adult provides must be of a nature that can eventually be applied by children themselves. By being attentive to children's private speech, teachers can ask children the same kinds of questions to help them solve their own problems.
4. Adults are of most help when their guidance occurs in tasks at the edge of the child's ability and experience, and when their assistance is coordinated with the child's current level of development. In other words, don't make a task too easy or too difficult for a child.
5. Children need learning environments that permit them to be verbally active while solving problems and completing tasks. It is unrealistic, therefore, for teachers to expect a

quiet classroom, especially when children are using self-directed speech to help them learn. Given the opportunity, children's private speech will become internalized (pp. 50–51).

What Would You Do?

The other evening at the local playground, you were conducting observations of young children's play for your course in child development. Your neighbors, Bob and Cynthia Winter, were there and asked your advice about sending their four-year-old daughter, Beth, to a half-day neighborhood nursery school program operated by Alicia Carposa, a certified preschool teacher. Alicia is famous in the area for her program of early learning with and emphasis on early literacy skills. Many parents in the community are sending their children to Alicia's program. Cynthia and Bob, however, have their doubts about what they believe to be the negative effects of early learning on young children's later learning. Lately they have been hearing a lot about the dangers of parents pushing their children.

In your conversation Bob says, "We have made a lot of sacrifices so Cynthia can stay home with Beth. We want Beth to have a normal childhood and enjoy life while she has a chance. Childhood is the most precious period of life— we want her to have time to smell the roses. We don't want a burned-out, psychotic six-year-old because we pushed her into reading and writing at an early age."

You tend to agree with the Winters and want to tell them about how you think too many parents are pushing their young children too much, too soon. Your first reaction is to tell them, "I think you should keep Beth at home until she is ready to begin kindergarten. Let her enjoy life while she has a chance. Once school begins, it seems as though childhood is over." However, you decide to think things over for a day or two.

PSYCHOSOCIAL DEVELOPMENT

We pick up the psychosocial development of the preschool child where we left off in our discussion of the toddler, again utilizing Erikson's theory.

Stage Three—Locomotor-Genital (Initiative vs. Guilt)   This stage is marked by an increasing desire for independence and control over behavior. If given the opportunity, preschoolers will move further away from care-givers in terms of both distance and the nature of the activities in which they are involved. They continually strive to meet their own needs and are characterized by an "I-want-to-do-it-for-myself" attitude.

Children's attempts to develop autonomy and initiative often meet with punishment. Punishment, especially when it is harsh and unreasonable, results in feeling of guilt. The child feels that what was attempted should not have been tried and tends to reduce further attempts at initiative. Furthermore, persistent and harsh punishment encourages the development of aggressive behavior.

Implications for Parents and Teachers

First, working with other care-givers, parents need to develop plans and arrangements for providing continuity, consistency, and sameness in child-rearing patterns. Parents who give their children over to the care of others need to communicate their child rearing goals to assure that there is a match between what they want and what others are able and willing to do. On the other hand, surrogate care-givers may need to help parents articulate what they believe constitute appropriate child-rearing practices. In any event, a high degree of continuity in beliefs and practices needs to exist between parents and others to assure the continuity and consistency that will promote basic trust.

More parents must be willing to seek out acceptable sources of child care that are congruent with their parenting styles, rather than leaving their children in homes and centers where there is a mismatch between what they believe constitutes quality child care and what is being offered. Understandably, this is easier said than done. Also at issue is the unavailability of quality child care to those parents who must work. At stake, however, is the issue of how best to provide for the needs of children.

Second, Erikson's beliefs about developing basic trust, autonomy, and initiative make a great deal of sense. Erikson's ideas are positive in nature and stress the good things that occur as a result of the relationships and interactions between caregivers and children. Building basic trust, autonomy, and initiative in others is a marvelous way to help individual children and affect future generations as well. When viewed in this way, care-giving is seen as an honorable profession, a task to be enjoyed rather than a sentence to be endured.

Third, parents need to balance their desires for perfection and obedience with toddlers' and preschoolers' needs for independence and individual creativity. Adults should compliment children for their efforts rather than criticize them if the end product is not completely finished or is done without the precision the adults would like. Preschoolers are interested in initiating and accomplishing. During this stage of their lives, they are not ready to have their accomplishments judged by adult standards. Doing the task brings success. Success leads to self-confidence, which leads to initiative. These are the ingredients that will enable children as adolescents and adults to achieve well by adult standards.

Fourth, toddlers and preschoolers need opportunities to explore, achieve, go places, and meet people. Overprotection and undue restriction lead to shame and uncertainty. A lesson all care-givers have to learn, albeit a difficult one, is how to let go of their children while they simultaneously provide support and protection.

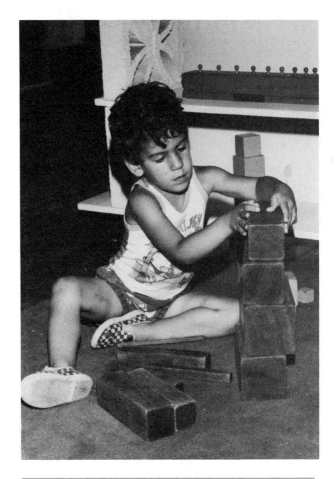

FIGURE 8-3 During the preschool years children's mental schemes develop through activity and involvement. Preschoolers work their way through physical and mental problems through concrete, i.e., physical involvements.

Fifth, care-givers should do nothing for toddlers and preschoolers that they can do for themselves. As Maria Montessori (1967) said, "This is our mission: to cast a ray of light and pass on" (p. 117). Efforts at helping children should be directed toward teaching them the skills they need to be independent of adults. Helping the very young become independent also includes helping

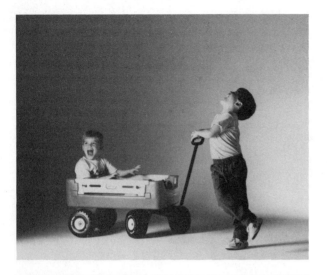

FIGURE 8-4 Preschoolers are in the initiative vs. guilt stage of psychosocial development. They are less dependent on adults and want to do things for themselves. They should be allowed to experiment and explore as a means of developing initiative.

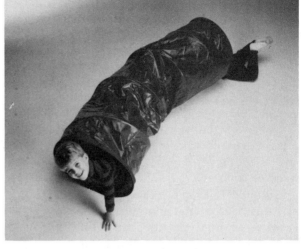

FIGURE 8-5 Psychosocial development is enhanced through exploration. Preschoolers are very curious. They want to know about everything and be involved in everything.

them set and accomplish achievable goals. Appropriate expectations for the age and the maturity of particular children help assure that what they are asked to do is reasonable for them.

Sixth, how much and for what to punish are problems faced by all care-givers. Excessive or punitive punishment stifles attempts at initiative. Guidance and participation in activities with the very young offer a reasonable solution to the punishment dilemma.

Developing routines with children helps them learn what to expect and what behavioral standards are associated with the routine. The toddler's natural desire to do everything, for example, can be channeled into the routine of helping prepare for snack time and clean-up. The care-giver establishes the routine expectation that children, not other care-givers, will put out napkins and cups, pour the beverage, and serve the snack. He or she makes snack time a routine by always having children be the main participants—for example, by making sure cups and pitchers are child size. Such opportunities for involvement not only control behavior, but also provide for feelings of accomplishment, autonomy, and self-worth.

GENDER DEVELOPMENT

Many of your parents had to wait until you were born in order to know if you were a boy or a girl. Today, however, the trend for most parents seems to be that because of increased use of prenatal technology (see Chapter Four), parents know the sex of their children months before they are born. With the first exclamation "It's a girl!" or "It's a boy!", the process of sex role development begins. Through socialization and parenting practices, children learn to identify with one gender or the other. It is during the period from about one and one-half to three years of age that children begin to show pronounced sex-typing of play activities and interests (Huston, 1983). *Sex-typing* is the demonstration of behavior that is typical of a child's sex rather than behavior typical of the opposite sex.

Sex role development consists not only of demonstrating behaviors of a particular sex, it also includes the concept of *gender constancy*, or children's understanding that they are permanently a boy or girl because of genital differences. Development of gender constancy occurs between the ages of three and seven. Also during this time, a child identifies with the parent of the same sex, resulting in a resolution of the Oedipal conflict as described by Freud (see Chapter Two).

All I Want for Christmas is a Sex-typed Toy

Many sex-typed activities involve the use of sex-typed toys, which play a role in sex role development. Children themselves play a considerable role in the selection of their toys, and parents report that one-half of the toys they give their children for Christmas are specifically requested by their children. Furthermore, by the time they reach school age, children are quite sex-typed in their toy preferences (Robinson & Morris, 1986).

DEVELOPMENT OF AGGRESSION

Breathes there an adult who doesn't have childhood memories of the playground bully? Or your memories of childhood may evoke lesser images of aggression, but nonetheless there are images of childhood aggression in all our memories. So the question arises, how do children develop aggressive behavior? Let's begin with a definition of *aggression*, which is "behavior that is aimed at harming or injuring another person or persons" (Parke & Slaby, 1983, p. 550). This behavior is both physical and verbal. When Billy screams at Barbie, "I hate you. I'm going to give you a karate kick," Billy is demonstrating aggressive behavior.

Biological Factors

When you think of aggressive behavior, you probably also think of raging hormones, especially testosterone in males, which cause persons to be aggressive toward another. While such a relationship may exist during adolescence, the general opinion is that "there is no tyrannical control of aggressive behavior by hormones; instead, hormones should be viewed as a part of a multivariate set of determinants rather than as a sufficient cause of aggression" (Parke & Slaby, 1983, p. 562).

Other biological factors that may contribute to aggressiveness include temperament, the basic nature of a child, sex (boys are larger and stronger than girls), and physical characteristics (negative views toward unattractive children may result in aggression) (Parke & Slaby, 1983).

Environmental/Social Factors

According to *social learning theory*, children learn to be aggressive by the imitation of models such as parents, siblings, and peers, and by feed-

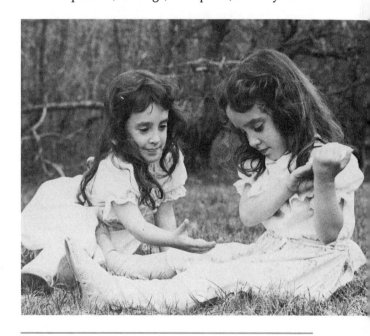

FIGURE 8-6 Signs of anger and aggression are common in the preschool years; preschoolers often display these emotions when they don't get their own way. Parents and care-givers can help children manage their aggression by providing alternative means for them to achieve their goals.

back from people and the environment. In the case of modeling, it is a case of "monkey see, monkey do." The leading proponent of the social learning theory is Albert Bandura (1977), who has done a significant amount of work relating to the role of modeling in the development of aggression.

Sex Differences in Aggression

Are boys more aggressive than girls? Yes. There are clear sex differences in aggression, with boys displaying more aggression than girls (Parke & Slaby, 1983). Part of the reason for this difference in aggressive behavior can be attributed to the fact that parents treat boys differently than they do girls; parents encourage boys to participate in sex-typed activities, for example, play with guns; and boys have different opportunities to acquire aggressive behavior, such as participation in sports and physical activities (Parke & Slaby, 1983).

*I*MPLICATIONS FOR PARENTS

What is the best way for parents to deal with an aggressive child? First, parents should try their best to avoid developing aggressive behavior in their children. For example, they can avoid, in so far as possible, the use of physical punishment, since children who are physically punished tend to demonstrate more aggressive behavior than their counterparts. Parents should model for children the resolution of conflict situations so that children will be able to do the same.

Second, parents can be judicious in the kinds of toys they provide for their children. Parents can reduce the numbers of guns, war toys, and action figures they give their children while at the same time monitoring how they play with such toys.

Third, parents can provide nonaggressive environments and programs for their children. For example, parents can select child care programs with uncrowded and humane environments that have care-givers who are sensitive to parents' desires for nonaggressive activities. Child care programs for their part can utilize curricula that help children develop prosocial behaviors, in other words, helping and getting along with others. Such curricula will help children develop skills for the peaceful resolution of differences as alternatives to aggressive acts.

WHY DO CHILDREN PLAY?

A number of theories have been advanced for why children play. One of the most persistent reasons given is the surplus energy theory (Spencer, 1878). This view is consistent with Victorian views of children, namely that they are little savages and that play serves the purpose of draining their surplus energy. Is this theory sufficient to account for children's play in the twentieth century? Not entirely. While the release of surplus energy is therapeutic and does provide relief from stress and tension, there is more to children's play than their emptying themselves of surplus energy. The surplus energy theory of play, however, is a consistently popular one and is reinforced when teachers and parents observe young children energetically engaged in playground activities.

Play from a Freudian Perspective

Sigmund Freud believed that play is important to children's emotional development. Primarily, play enables children to rid themselves of negative emotions resulting from unpleasant and/or traumatic experiences. Within the context of Freudian theory, play is a *cathartic* or cleansing function enabling children to empty themselves of feelings such as anger, aggression, and hurt. For example, while playing in the doll corner, Brian, who was punished at home before school, may pick up a doll and give it a smack or two and aggressively exclaim, "Shut your mouth, you naughty boy." In this way, Brian rids himself of hostile feelings through his actions and by reversing roles and transferring his negative feelings to the doll. This is one reason advocates of play in children's programs believe that children need settings and opportunities to engage in pretend play free from intrusive care-giver interference.

What Is Play?

A number of definitions have been advanced to address the persistent questions regarding play. Morrison (1988) defines play as a self-motivated activity through which learning occurs. Children do not have to be told to play and, as such, play is a self-initiated activity. Frequently, professionals try to distinguish between work and play and end up with the observation that play is child's work. For children, however, play is what they decide to do, work is what others direct or tell them to do, even though the activity may have play-like qualities about it.

Play enables the child to engage in many activities that contribute to mental and physical activity, and consequently results in the construction of intelligence and the acquisition of knowledge.

Johnson, Christie, and Yawkey (1987) believe that play must possess five characteristics in order to be properly classified as play.

1. It must be separated from everyday experience, so that the actions are performed differently than in nonplay settings.
2. The motivation for the play comes from within the individual rather that externally.
3. Attention is focused on the activity rather than the goal of the activity.
4. Free choice is involved as opposed to an activity assigned by the teacher.
5. Pleasure and enjoyment are involved (pp. 11–12).

Am (1986) views play, especially pretend play, as a process of communication. As such, play consists of two parts, what children say ("Ummmm, this food tastes good"), and the context of the play, which also communicates (for example, Marty pretends to eat the "food" on her plate while Sherri stands by ready to give her another serving).

CLASSIFICATIONS OF PLAY

Social Play

Mildred Parten (1932) observed children at play in social settings and classified their play into six developmental stages. This classic description of play is widely used as a basis for understanding children's play behavior. Parten's developmental stages of social play are shown in Table 8–6. Through observing children at play we can determine a great deal about their cognitive and social developments, as well as their play and play material interests.

Piaget and Symbolic Play

Piaget (1962) describes four stages of play through which children progress as they develop: functional play, symbolic play, play involving games with rules, and constructive play. (See also Chapter Ten.)

Functional Play   *Functional play* is the play of the sensorimotor period and occurs in response to muscular activities and the need to be active. Functional play is characterized by repetitions, manipulations, and self-imitation. Piaget (1962) described

TABLE 8-6

MILDRED PARTEN'S DEVELOPMENTAL STAGES OF SOCIAL PLAY		
Stage	Age (years)	Characteristics of Play
Unoccupied behavior	0–2	Children are not playing, but are engaged in "unoccupied behavior," e.g., looking around the room and following adults.
Onlooker behavior	2 and older	Children spend their time watching others play. They may verbally interact with others but do not engage in play with them.
Solitary play	2½ and older	Child engages in play by himself. He plays with his toys or materials on his own. His play is not dependent on or involved with the play of others.
Parallel play	2½–3½ and older	Child plays near other children. Child may choose a toy, material or activity that brings him alongside others or others alongside him. He is still involved in his own play, however.
Associative play	3½–4½ and older	The child plays with others in a group. Children may exchange materials. Although children are playing together, there is no intended purpose of the play. Children are involved in interpersonal relations during play. Children at a water table frequently exhibit this kind of play.
Cooperative play	4½ and older	The child plays in and with a group that has some intended purpose or goal, e.g., building a fort, making a sand sculpture, playing a game, or dramatizing (such as playing house).

Note. From "Social Play Among Preschool Children" by M. Parten, 1932, *Journal of Abnormal and Social Psychology, 27,* pp. 243–269.

functional play—which he also called *practice play* and *exercise play*—this way:

> The child sooner or later (often even during the learning period) grasps for the pleasure of grasping, swings [a suspended object] for the sake of swinging, etc. In a word, he repeats his behavior not in any further effort to learn or to investigate, but for the mere joy of mastering it and of showing off to himself his own power of subduing reality (p. 162).

Symbolic Play   This second stage of play, *symbolic play*, is the play of the preoperational period.

Piaget also refers to this stage of play as the "let's pretend" stage of play. During this stage, preschoolers freely display their creative and physical abilities and social awareness in a variety of ways.

THE COMPETENCIES OF PLAY

In the continuing debate about what preschool curriculum should be, many people respond that play is the most appropriate curriculum. However, to say that is to say that play is the nutrient or fertilizer of young children. Play is the *process* by which the curriculum is implemented. To say play is the curriculum begs the issue of what children are to learn. It is true that children learn *through* play. This means then that early educators must plan for what they want that learning to be!

What good preschool programs do—in fact what any good educational program does—is to take each child at whatever point she is in her development and provide a set of guided experiences that enables her to go as far as possible *without* pushing, hurrying, bullying, belittling, or overstressing. But the essence of early education becomes the set of guided experiences—both cognitive and affective. Without them there is really no program. Unfortunately, some early educators have responded to the issues of pushing and hurrying by either doing nothing or by saying that the solution is play. Play is not the solution. The set of guided experiences is the solution. And it is entirely possible and appropriate that these guided experiences can be conducted *in part* through play activities.

PRESCHOOL PLAY ENVIRONMENTS

Play enables children to develop new skills, to practice already existing skills, and to learn more about themselves and others. Play, especially outdoor play, also provides opportunities for risk-taking. Jambor (1986) believes play environments must provide children opportunities to participate at their own levels of abilities and should encourage children to advance in levels of participation after each has developed feelings of competence, confidence and security. These conditions are met in an environmental playground that combines the natural environmental features of trees, bushes, and dirt mounds with vertical and horizontal ropes, and walks and tire swings. Such an environment enables children to play at levels suited to their abilities and needs. Furthermore, children are able to "challenge and test their limitations, contemplate risk factors and set their own standards for safety based on their own experiences and levels of competence and security" (Jambor, 1986, p. 25).

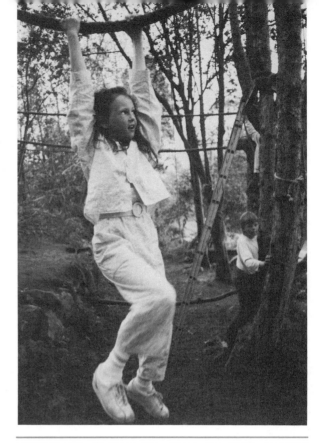

FIGURE 8-7 Outdoor play areas should be designed to help children develop physical skills and feelings of confidence and accomplishment.

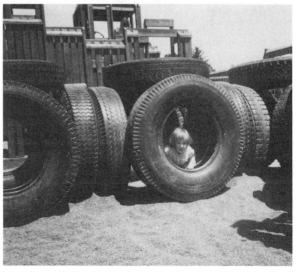

FIGURE 8-8 Outdoor play areas and playgrounds provide children numerous opportunities to develop many of the physical, social, intellectual and interpersonal skills they need as they grow and develop.

*I*N THE SPOTLIGHT

PRESCHOOL FITNESS

The fitness craze is no longer limited to Father jogging or Mother participating in aerobics classes. A healthy lifestyle is "in," and many of America's preschoolers are included. Today, preschoolers participate in a wide variety of activities designed especially for them such as swimming, exercise classes, and massage sessions. Many resorts' package vacations are designed to specifically involve the preschooler. No longer must the family forgo a vacation of skiing or water sports. It is as common to see three- and four-year-old children at ski resorts as it is to see them at shopping malls. Local Y's have been quick to

capitalize on the fitness craze and now their swimming pools are full of infants, toddlers, and preschoolers participating in "Mommie and Me" swimming classes. In fact, many preschoolers may have been introduced to the fitness lifestyle in utero, since more mothers are participating in exercise programs while they are pregnant.

Of course, in keeping with the current trend to dress the part regardless of the activity, preschool fashions include special designer exercise outfits. Many preschoolers are as fashion conscious as their older siblings and parents.

ACCIDENTS: CAUSES AND PREVENTION

Accidents, not illnesses, are the major causes of death and injuries in young children. Boys are twice as likely as girls to be injured, and of both sexes, automobile accidents and falls account for 38 percent of all injuries. Also, about one-third of the children who survive injuries have long-term disabilities.

America's fascination with cars and its dependency on the automobile as a means of transportation affects the lives of preschoolers. Preschoolers can spend considerable amounts of time in automobiles, accompanying their parents and being transported to child care, preschool, and the many functions in which preschoolers are now involved. Automobile injuries could be greatly reduced through the regular use of safety seats and seatbelts. Although all fifty states have some kind of mandatory child restraint law, it is still the

responsibility of the parents and other care-givers to properly use car seats and seat belts.

The most common cause of childhood facial injury is a fall from a bicycle. Falls from stairs are the second most common cause of facial injuries ("All Fall Down," 1986).

TANTRUMS

Undoubtedly you have seen and heard a tantrum, for there is no mistaking it. In fact, you may have thrown one or two of your own. It very often happens in the aisles of a toy store, at a checkout counter, or in front of an audience of some kind. A child sits hopelessly and forlornly on the floor screaming her head off, all because she can't have her own way. If you can't remember if you ever threw a tantrum, ask your parents. Their memory is pretty accurate in matters such as this. However, the chances are pretty good that you didn't throw one, for only about ten percent of children do,

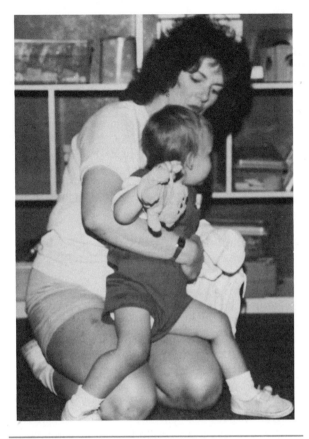

FIGURE 8-9 Many parents try to cope with children's tantrums by giving in to them. However, the best way to eliminate tantrums is to ignore them. Also, when parents set limits as to what is acceptable behavior, then children have a basis by which to control their behavior.

with three-year-old children throwing the most (Bax, 1985).

Tantrums usually occur when children can't get their own way and progress through three stages (Bax, 1985). First, the child becomes cranky or begins crying intermittently while trying to get her own way. Then when her repeated demands are denied, she begins full-blown screaming, which lasts three to five minutes, or longer. If the child is left alone, the crying decreases and becomes an intermittent sobbing. This phase lasts about five minutes. Attempts to comfort the child usually trigger off another bout of loud crying. So, it is best to wait until the crying and sobbing end before trying to console her.

What is the best way to handle a tantrum? Ignore it. But this is easier said than done, depending on where the child is when he throws the tantrum. A tantrum in a supermarket, a doctor's office, or in the presence of friends and relatives is pretty hard to ignore. One way to deal with it when others are present is to take the child to another room and just let him cry.

Keep in mind that the psychosocial period of initiative vs. guilt is a time in which children want to demonstrate independence and have control over their behavior. Tantrums are one way, albeit a not very pleasant or acceptable way, of getting and maintaining this control. How best to deal with tantrums is only part of the many tasks involved in parenting and leads us to raise the question most parents have asked at one time or another.

WHAT KIND OF PARENT SHOULD I BE?

For many parents, parenting the preschooler does not seem to be the leisurely and effortless task that they thought it would be. Given the fact that life and life-styles have changed dramatically over the last several decades, it is only natural that parenting would also change. Today, many women with young children routinely return to work shortly after childbirth, requiring that arrangements be made for proper child care. Then, too, there are many other things for children to be involved in today that their parents were not involved in when they were preschoolers. There seems to be a constant round of activities, from pee-wee baseball, football, and soccer to karate lessons (for Mom, too!) to music lessons.

Many frazzled parents ask the question, "What kind of parent should I be?" The trite and easy answer to this question is, "A good one." Some purveyors of parenting books make pronouncements about how their product can produce perfect parents. Wiser counsel advises a compromise. The result is "a good enough parent," and this is precisely what Bruno Bettleheim (1987) suggests. But what is involved in being a good enough parent? Bettleheim, like Spock, believes that good parents trust their judgment, or what he calls their "inner experiences."

> All of us must struggle to understand ourselves better, not the least because our efforts to achieve greater clarity about ourselves make it possible for us to achieve clarity in our relation to our child, with a consequent enrichment to our life. Such understanding of ourselves around some issue of child-rearing cannot be handed to us by someone else, no matter how great their expertise may be; it can be achieved only by ourselves, as we struggle to remove whatever has obscured this understanding from our conscience (p. 32).

Bettleheim advocates that rather than create the kind of children they want, parents should help their children fully develop in their own way and in their own time, so that they will become the kind of persons they wish to become. When parents do this, then:

> Their struggles [to find solutions to child-rearing problems] will make them good enough parents, to their own and their children's benefit. The good enough parent will always be aware that conceiving and bearing a child and bringing it into this world are the most wondrous events in the life of a child. The more they can enjoy together, each in their own ways, what follows from it—the parents raising the child, the child being raised by his parents—the happier their lives will be (p. 377).

Is There One Best Way to Parent?

Parenting style leads us to another question about parents. Is there only one best way to be a good parent? Two people who have spent a lot of time researching this question, Stella Chess and Alexander Thomas (1987), believe the answer is "no," and that "there is no single style of parenthood that is best for all children." Rather, they recommend what they call "goodness of fit." They describe it this way:

> Goodness of fit exists when the demands and expectations of the parents and other people important to the child's life are compatible with the child's temperament, abilities and other characteristics. With such fit, healthy development for the child can be expected. . . . Poorness of fit, on the other hand, exists when the demands and expectations are excessive and not compatible with the child's temperament (p. 56).

For example, (and it is one provided by Chess and Thomas), some parents can attend to their children's crying at night without too much effort. This effort involves a minimal loss of sleep and they still wake refreshed in the morning. They have easily attained a "goodness of fit" with their children. On the other hand, some parents respond differently to the same nighttime demands. They are slow to wake up, are groggy and irritable while they attend to their children's needs, have trouble going back to sleep, and are exhausted the next day. One way for such parents to attempt to achieve their "goodness of fit" would be to take turns with their partner dealing with such nighttime interruptions, while encouraging the child to sleep through the night. The point is that parents must seek to develop this fit between themselves and their children. This process involves *both* parents and children making efforts to adjust to each other.

A Matrix of Parenting Styles

Two developmental psychologists, Eleanor Maccoby and John Martin, (1983) reviewed the literature relating to parenting styles and developed a matrix of parental characteristics (see Table 8–7). Four characteristic parenting styles—authoritative, authoritarian, permissive, and indifferent—are demonstrated by parents in their day-to-day interactions with their children. While it may be easy to spot one parent's style as fitting easily into one of these categories, another parent's may have a style that reflects two or more of the categories. Then, too, some parents may change their styles from time to time, exhibiting some or all of the listed characteristics. What is important for children's development is the consistent style used by parents across developmental time.

Authoritative Parenting Being an authoritative parent means being involved in the right way. Baumrind (1971) provides us with a comprehensive portrait of authoritative parents. They expect mature behavior from children, set clear standards, enforce rules, encourage children to be independent and to express themselves as individuals, communicate well with their children, encourage children to express their points of view, and recognize their parental rights and the rights of their children.

What kind of children does authoritative parenting produce? According to Baumrind, such children are more competent, independent, self-reliant, self-controlled, content, friendly, and cooperative. This array of positive attributes makes the children of authoritative parents sound almost too good to be true. They are the type of children most parents want. As with many things, being an authoritative parent is easier said than done. Many parents lack the knowledge and skills necessary to be authoritative. Therefore, they will need help to gain the necessary parenting skills.

TABLE 8–7

		CLASSIFICATION OF PARENTING PATTERNS	
		Acceptingness	
		Parent is accepting, responsive; relationship is child-centered.	Parent is rejecting, unresponsive; relationship is parent-centered.
Demandingness	Parent is demanding and controlling.	1. *Authoritative* Characterized by reciprocal relations; high in bidirectional communication.	2. *Authoritarian* Characterized by emphasis on parent's assertion of authority over child.
Demandingness	Parent is undemanding, makes few attempts to control.	3. *Permissive* Characterized by parental indulgence of child's desires.	4. *Indifferent* Characterized by parental neglect of child; parent tends to neglect child and avoid involvement.

Note. Adapted from "Socialization in the Context of the Family; Parent-Child interaction" by E.E. Maccoby & J.A. Martin, in *Socialization, Personality, and Social Development*, Ed. E.M. Hetherington, vol. 4 of *Handbook of Child Psychology* (4th ed.), Ed. P.H. Mussen, 1983, (New York: John Wiley) p. 39.

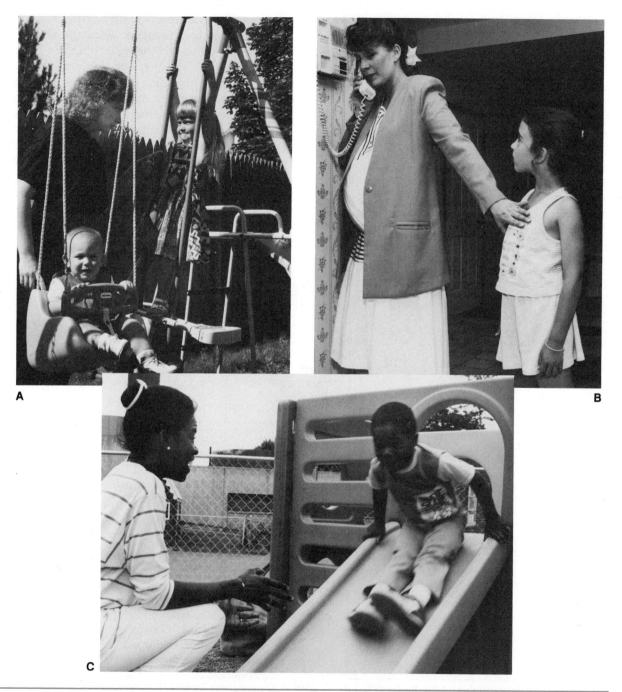

FIGURE 8-10 Different parenting styles have differing consequences on children. Children of (A) authoritarian parents tend to lack social competence; children of (B) indifferent parents tend to be immature; children of (C) authoritative parents tend to be more self-confidence and self-controlled.

Authoritarian Parenting Maccoby and Martin describe the authoritarian style of parenting this way:

> In the authoritarian pattern, parents' demands on their children are not balanced by their acceptance of demands from their children. Although it is understood that children have needs that parents are obligated to fulfill, power-assertive parents place strict limits on allowable expression of these needs by children. Children are expected to inhibit their begging and demanding, and in extreme cases they may not even speak before being spoken to. Parents' demands take the form of edicts. Rules are not discussed in advance or arrived at by any consensus or bargaining process. Parents attach strong value to the maintenance of their authority, and suppress any efforts their children make to challenge it. When children deviate from parent requirements, fairly severe punishment (often physical) is likely to be employed (p. 39).

The important issue in a discussion of parenting styles is the ultimate effect they have on children and psychosocial development. Maccoby and Martin summarize the relation of authoritarian parenting styles to children's personality characteristics this way:

> Children of authoritarian parents tend to lack social competence with peers: They tend to withdraw, not to take social initiative, to lack spontaneity. Although they do not behave differently from children on contrived measures of resistance to temptation, on projective tests and parents' reports, they do show lesser evidence of "conscience" and are more likely to have an external, rather than internal, moral orientation in discussing what is "right" behavior in situations of moral conflict. In boys, there is evidence that motivation for intellectual performance is low. Several studies link authoritarian parenting with low self-esteem and external locus of control (pp. 43–44).

Many parents believe reality is the opposite of what research data depict as reality. The folklore of childhoods remembered is full of accounts of parents (as children) being "taken out behind the woodshed." Many parents believe that controlling children with a "firm hand" lays the foundation for right behavior. Parents believe that "to spare the rod is to spoil the child." In the case of child-rearing practices, however, a heavy hand and parents' insisting on their way appear to be undesirable approaches and not in the best interests of children.

Permissive (Indulgent) Parenting Maccoby and Martin say that permissive parenting consists of a cluster of behaviors, including:

1. The ideological belief that it is "right" for children to display their feelings and emotions. This belief, however, can lead to frustration with children's behavior and result in harsh punishment.
2. Inattention.
3. Indifference.
4. Nonintervention in children's affairs because of tiredness, depression, or preoccupation.

What are the consequences of permissive parenting? Diana Baumrind (1967) provides us with a picture of the consequences of failing to be actively involved in parental responsibilities. She found that children of permissive parents are immature, and their behavior is characterized by a *lack* of impulse control, self-reliance, independence, and social responsibility (1971).

Indifferent-uninvolved Parenting Maccoby and Martin (1983) characterize uninvolved parents as wanting to keep their children at a distance. Such parents "orient their behavior primarily toward the avoidance of inconvenience. Thus they will respond to immediate demands from the children in such a way as to terminate them" (pp. 43–44). The extreme result of uninvolved parenting is psychological detachment from children and disinterest in them. Another consequence is neglect, which is a component of abuse. On the other hand, involvement is an elusive characteristic. How much involvement is too much or too little? The amount of involvement parents have in children's lives is a function of where they are in their growth and development as parents. The author, for example, is constantly involved in his children's lives, but there are times when he exerts more or less guidance, depending on the needs of each child. The point is that involvement in children's lives is essential, but too much involvement may be just as bad as too little.

*I*N THE SPOTLIGHT

HOMELESS CHILDREN

You have no doubt heard and read a great deal about the homeless. Perhaps your image of a homeless person is a slouching, gray-haired, elderly man with two weeks of stubble on his chin, sleeping on a heating grate in front of a wealthy cooperative condominium. Or perhaps you think of a toothless bag lady pushing her shopping cart, purloined from the local supermarket and laden with all her worldly possessions (other people's castoffs), up the skyscraper canyons of a major urban city. But what about homeless children? What is your image of them? Maybe you don't have one, because homeless children are easily left out of discussions relating to one of America's most visible and pressing social problems. Children are often the unknown and neglected in the world of the homeless. Yet they represent a significant portion of the homeless population. Over 25 percent of the homeless are homeless families, many with preschool children (Bassuk & Rubin, 1987). Most of these families consist of single mothers with preschool children.

From a social and public policy point of view, the fact that single mothers and their children are an increasing part of the homeless population should not be surprising to you. This frightening social trend is part of the feminization of poverty in which many women, as a result of divorce, unemployment and underemployment, are sinking deeper and deeper into poverty. The sad reality is that many young children born to, or living with, single mothers will spend much of their developmental years in poverty. The chances are pretty good, too, that they may also spend their adult years in poverty and have children who will do likewise, thus making both poverty and homelessness an intergenerational phenomena.

From a developmental perspective, homeless children do not fare very well at all. In one sample of homeless children five years of age or younger, 47 percent had one developmental delay and 30 percent had two or more. Also, when compared to emotionally disturbed children, data revealed that they were equal to or had higher scores in the following areas: sleep problems, shyness, withdrawal, and aggression (Bassuk & Rubin, 1987).

Clearly, there is a need for schools, social service agencies, and other groups to intervene in the lives of these children and their families. The alternative is a group of children who will fail to reach their full potential, and who are considered not their nation's greatest wealth, but rather as their nation's discards.

As a social policy report of the Society for Research in Child Development states:

The experience of the homeless has profound long-term consequences for children. For younger children homeless with their families, it may result in irreversible disruption in their education. The developmental delays associated with homelessness and social instability may never be overcome (Solarez, 1988, p. 11).

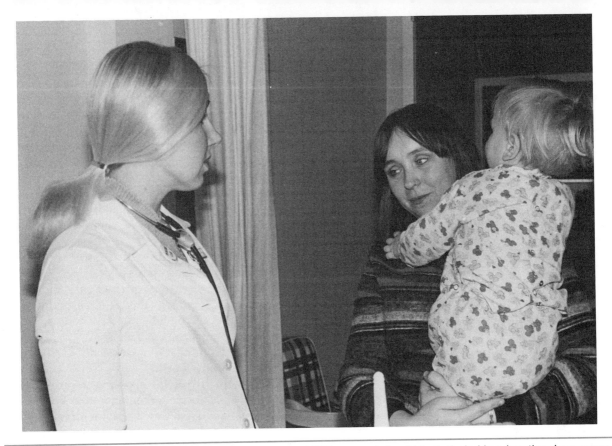

FIGURE 8-11 Children with medical problems such as AIDS can and should be included in educational programs. Preschool officials should work within Federal, State and agency laws and guidelines to provide appropriate educational services to preschoolers with special needs. (From Lesner/PEDIATRIC NURSING, copyright 1983 by Delmar Publishers Inc.)

CHILDREN WITH AIDS

What is AIDS?

AIDS, or *Acquired Immune Deficiency Syndrome*, is a relatively new disease that was described in 1981 and named in 1982. AIDS is caused by the Human Immunodeficiency Virus (HIV). HIV weakens or destroys the immune system, thus allowing diseases and infections to develop. Children and adults with HIV may not get AIDS; they can develop symptoms not normally associated with AIDS but which are referred to as AIDS Related Complex (ARC); while others develop AIDS symptoms. The manifestation of AIDS in children is different from adults. For example, Kaposi's Sarcoma, a form of cancer, is found in about 25 percent of adult AIDS cases, but seldom in children.

More commonly, children with AIDS develop infections such as pneumonia and central nervous system disorders. Also, some children with the AIDS virus are born with facial and cranial abnormalities.

AIDS Incidence

The number of children with AIDS is growing. As of July 1989, the Center for Disease Control in Atlanta (1988) estimated that 1,613 children below age thirteen have developed AIDS. At least 75 percent of these cases have been transmitted from an infected mother to her fetus or infant during the perinatal period.

A woman infected with AIDS always passes the AIDS antibodies to her fetus. However, the actual virus is passed only about 40 percent of the time through mixing of blood at birth or through the presence of the AIDS virus on the cervix. It is not until children are about fifteen months old that they start making their own antibodies if they have the virus. The reason for this is that children's immune systems do not fully function until that time and therefore they cannot produce AIDS antibodies. This explains why the HIV virus cannot be determined in babies under fifteen months.

Researchers and medical practitioners are now contemplating the treatment of babies with AIDS virus before they become ill. They believe that AZT (azidothymidine, an AIDS drug) may suppress or eliminate the virus if given early. There is even discussion of treating the fetuses of infected mothers (Kolata, 1988).

Children at Risk for AIDS

A question that everyone asks about AIDS is, "How do you get it?" Children can become infected with AIDS in the same ways adults become infected. However, one method of infection over which children have no control is being born to an infected mother. Following are the ways children can acquire or are at risk for AIDS:
- Born to an infected mother
- Victim of sexual abuse
- Being the recipient of a blood transfusion
- Being a hemophiliac
- Engaging in homosexual practices
- Engaging in IV drug use
- Being breast-fed by an HIV-infected person (Raper & Aldridge, 1988)

Implications for Parents and Care-givers

Everyone, not just parents and care-givers, needs to know what AIDS is and is not. In 1986, then Surgeon General of the United States, C. Everett Koop, advocated teaching young children about AIDS "at the lowest grade possible."

Child care centers and preschool programs must develop an AIDS policy. This AIDS policy is not a "stand alone" policy, but part of a larger infection and disease control policy. This AIDS policy also has to include such things as how to handle children with the AIDS virus when they are biters, have bloody diarrhea, bloody noses, or other bloody discharges. Although at the present time there is no evidence that HIV is transmitted through saliva, parents and care-providers need to have available a policy that addresses the biting by HIV-infected children of those who are not infected.

The Center for Disease Control in Atlanta, Georgia recommends that children with HIV be allowed to attend their own child care and school programs. Exceptions to this general guideline include but are not limited to HIV children who:
- Have open sores on their skin
- Have uncontrollable nosebleeds
- Have bloody diarrhea
- Are at high risk for exposing a care-giver or other child to blood-contaminated body fluids
- Have habitual biting behavior or are neurologically impaired and don't have control of their body fluids (Merahn, Shelov, & Mc-Cracken, 1988).

Every program must develop a plan for disease and infection control. This plan should include procedures for diaper changing, food preparation, and handwashing. All care-givers should wash their hands before and after each diaper change and whenever they come into contact with any body fluids of any kind. These procedures should be part of the infection control and health management program of any child care and school program.

Guidelines for infection control include the following (Merahan, Shelov, & McCracken, 1988):

1. Wash hands. Hand washing, by both children and adults, is the primary method to stop the spread of all illnesses.
2. Maintain supplies such as running water, liquid soap, paper towels, disposable latex gloves, and a disinfectant such as household bleach.
3. Use latex gloves for handling blood. As a

general rule, anytime a care-giver is dealing with blood (such as from a bloody nose or stool), he should wear rubber or latex gloves.

4. Maintain a clean and healthy environment.
5. Seek help from the local health department.

The HIV virus is very fragile outside the body and is killed with soap, detergents, peroxide, alcohol, and chlorine. A solution of ten parts water to one part household bleach makes an ideal disinfectant for use in a child care center. The solution must be made fresh each day.

Also, all blood or body-fluid-soaked items should be placed in a leak-proof bag for washing or disposal.

Public Policy Implications of AIDS For Children and Society

A number of serious problems and issues are posed by AIDS. These must be addressed in a forthright manner, with the best interests of children and their families as the primary consideration.

Children's rights are at the heart of many AIDS deliberations. Issues of mandatory testing, access to child care and public schooling, and the right to medical care are topics being actively pur-

sued by legal experts and child advocates. In addition, efforts to exclude and quarantine AIDS children are being hotly contested by children's rights advocates.

Basic human care and protection is also an issue. Some AIDS children are "throw-away children," who are not wanted by parents or relatives. Others are orphaned when their parents die of AIDS. For them, foster care in a loving home is not easy to find, and many spend their lives in clinics and other public facilities as "hospital boarder children" without the benefits of a normal home life. This isolation leads to psychological scarring and developmental delays because of the lack of consistent nurturing and care.

Some child advocates fear that society may be too willing to "write off" AIDS children because they are dying. They maintain that AIDS children have as much a right to a full life as do other children.

The implications for society and its health care and education systems are great and far reaching. Issues relating to this area include how to pay for the cost of medication, hospitalization, and basic care. In addition, controversies over how much and at what age to teach children about AIDS are far from settled.

*S*UMMARY

- The preschool years cover the period when preschool children are between thirty-six and sixty months of age. More three- and four-year-old children are entering preschool, child care, and other educational programs than ever before.
- Physical development of preschool children is characterized as slow and steady. Preschoolers are starting to look more like adults as their body proportions change. Preschool children gain an average of four pounds in weight and three inches in height each year. By age three, most preschoolers have their full complement of twenty teeth. The preschool years are an ideal time to begin a personal program of dental hygiene.
- By the age of three, walking is an automatic process, and by four years is a perfected and graceful motor accomplishment. Preschool children's abilities to climb stairs and throw objects follow predictable developmental sequences that enable them to master these motor tasks during the preschool and early elementary years.
- The development and use of physical skills play important roles in preschool children's cognitive, psychosocial and language development. In addition, they also have an influence on children's school success. Their importance should not be overlooked or underestimated by parents, teachers, and care-givers.
- Preschool children are in the preoperational stage of cognitive development. They are not capable of *operational* thought. An *operation* is a reversible mental action whereby an object or experience that is transformed can be returned to its original form. Preoperational children cannot *conserve;* that is, they cannot mentally understand that amount (mass, quantity, and volume) stays the same even though appearance (shape, size, and dimensions) changes. Preschool children are also egocentric in thought and speech.
- Language plays an important role in children's school achievement. One of the hallmarks of children's language development in the preschool years is the progression from the use of simple to more complex sentences. Preschoolers also engage in "private speech," which helps them integrate language and thought. Private speech also serves a "self-guiding" function for children and helps them solve problems.
- Preschool children are in the locomotor-genital (initiative vs. guilt) stage of psychosocial development. This stage is marked by an increasing desire for independence and control over behavior.
- During the period from about one and one-half to three years of age children begin to show pronounced *sex-typing* of play activities and interests, which is the demonstration of behavior that is typical of a child's sex rather than behavior typical of the opposite sex. Sex role development also consists of *gender constancy*, or children's understanding that they are permanently a boy or girl. Development of gender constancy occurs between the ages of three and seven. The development of *aggression*, or behavior that is aimed at harming or injuring another person, is attributed to biological and social factors.

■ Many reasons are given for why children play. One reason is that it enables children to expend surplus energy. Freud believed that play enabled children to expend emotional energy, and play, therefore, served a cathartic function.

■ Play is defined as self-motivated activity through which learning occurs. Parten identified six developmental stages of children's social play: unoccupied, onlooker, solitary, parallel, associative, and cooperative. Piaget classified children's play into four stages: functional play, symbolic play, play involving games with rules, and constructive play.

■ Outdoor playgrounds and play environments enable children to develop new skills, practice already existing skills, and to learn more about themselves and others.

■ Parenting the preschooler today is a much more demanding and involved process than it was in previous decades. Parents must do all they can to protect children from automobile accidents and falls, which account for 38 percent of all children's accidents.

■ Bruno Bettleheim advocates that parents try to be "good enough" parents, which involves helping their children fully develop, in their own way, and in their own time. Alexander Thomas and Stella Chess advocate that parents work to develop a "goodness of fit" with their children, which involves matching parental demands and expectations to children's temperament and abilities. Eleanor Maccoby and John Martin believe that of four parenting styles—authoritative, authoritarian, permissive, and indifferent—that the authoritative works best.

■ All who work with young children must be knowledgeable about AIDS, or *Acquired Immune Deficiency Syndrome*. AIDS is caused by the Human Immunodeficiency Virus (HIV), which weakens or destroys the immune system and allows diseases and infections to develop.

■ Children are at risk for AIDS who are born to an infected mother, the victims of sexual abuse, the recipients of a blood transfusion, hemophiliacs, engaging in homosexual practices, engaging in IV drug use, or are being breast-fed by an HIV-infected person. Every child care and preschool program must develop a plan for disease and infection control. Such plans should include procedures for diaper changing, food preparation, and handwashing.

■ A number of important public policy issues involve AIDS and young children. These include the rights of children, basic child care and protection, and the cost of AIDS care.

*Q*UESTIONS TO GUIDE YOUR REVIEW

1. What years are included in the preschool period?
2. How is parenting a preschooler today different from when you were a preschooler?
3. Why is the physical development of preschool children often characterized as "slow and steady?"

4. What are the main hallmarks of preschool children's motor development?
5. What is the developmental progression of children's stair-climbing ability?
6. What are the four stages involved in learning to throw?
7. What are some implications children's motor development has for intellectual development?
8. What is preoperational thought?
9. What are the characteristics of children's preoperational thought?
10. In what ways are preoperational children egocentric?
11. What can parents, teachers and care-givers do to enhance the intellectual development of preschool children?
12. Why is it important that young children learn language and learn it well?
13. How do children's sentences develop from simple to complex?
14. What is private speech? What roles does it play in learning? How can teachers and others enhance children's private speech?
15. What are the characteristics of psychosocial development during the locomotor-genital stage?
16. What implications does the locomotor-genital stage of psychosocial development have for teachers and parents?
17. How does gender development occur in young children? How are sex-typing and gender constancy alike and different?
18. What is aggression and how does it develop? Are there sex differences in aggression?
19. What is play?
20. What are Parten's classifications of social play?
21. What are Piaget's four stages of play?
22. What are some essential characteristics of children's preschool play environments?
23. What are the most frequent causes of accidents in the preschool years?
24. What are the essentials of being a "good enough parent" and "goodness of fit?"
25. Why is the authoritative parenting style considered better than other parenting styles?
26. What is AIDS? What causes AIDS?
27. In what ways are children at risk for AIDS?
28. Under what conditions might children with AIDS not be allowed to attend preschool and other programs?
29. What can teachers and care-givers do to control the spread of AIDS and other diseases in preschool programs?
30. What are the public policy implications of AIDS?

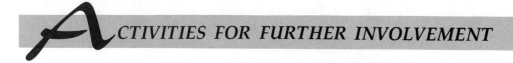

ACTIVITIES FOR FURTHER INVOLVEMENT

1. Piaget believed that one of the cognitive characteristics of preschool children is that they are egocentric, meaning that they have difficulty differentiating their perspectives from other's points of view.

a. Observe preschoolers to determine how and in what ways they are egocentric.

b. How does language contribute to the lessening of egocentric thought and actions? What can parents and others do to promote communication between preschoolers as a means of facilitating exchanges of views?

2. Cognitive development in the preschool years is different from cognitive development in infancy.

   a. Develop a chart that shows the differences in the cognitive development of infants, toddlers, and preschoolers.

   b. Tell how preschoolers' abilities to represent contribute to their cognitive development.

3. Preschool children are in the stage of initiative and guilt.

   a. Identify what parents can do in the home and community to help their children develop initiative rather than guilt.

   b. What role does risk-taking play in the development of initiative? What role should parents play in helping their children learn to take risks? What parental behaviors discourage children from being risk-takers?

   c. Observe preschoolers to find instances of guilt in their psychosocial development. What do you think contributed to such guilt?

4. You have been invited to address the Preschool Parents Club.

   a. Tell how parents must adjust their behavior and parenting styles in the preschool years to foster favorable development.

   b. Describe the negative outcomes that come from ridicule and punishment.

   c. Provide five guidelines for positive parenting during the preschool years.

5. Biology, environment, and experiences influence child development.

   a. Tell how individual differences in children, such as curiosity, can be accounted for by one of the above factors.

   b. Make a list of experiences that you think would be most beneficial for all children to have. Tell why.

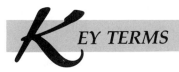

KEY TERMS

Aggression Behavior that is aimed at harming or injuring another person or persons.

Centration Characterized by children focusing on one characteristic of an object. For example, focusing on color while ignoring other attributes, such as length and size.

Conserve The cognitive ability of children to mentally understand that amount (mass, quantity, and volume) stays the same even though appearance (shape, size, and dimensions) changes.

Decenter To develop out of egocentrism.

Early childhood The years from birth to age eight. Also defined as the years from conception to age eight.

Egocentric speech The speech used by children in the preoperational stage of cognitive development. Children use language in a literal sense, whereby they talk *at* others as opposed to talking *with* them.

Eye-hand coordination Coordination of sight with manual dexterity. In the preschool years this usually involves such activities as cutting, pasting, etc. (See *Manual skills.*)

Functional play The play of the sensorimotor period and occurs in response to muscular activities and the need to be active. Functional play is characterized by repetitions, manipulations, and self-imitation.

Gender constancy Children's understanding that they are permanently a boy or girl because of genital differences.

Manual or manipulative skills Fine motor activities involving the hands and fingers, such as holding and manipulating things. Activities such as cutting, pasting, drawing, coloring, and solving puzzles involve the use of fine motor activities.

Operation A reversible mental action whereby an object or experience that is transformed can be returned to its original form. An example of a mental operation is $1 + 2 = 3$ and $3 - 2 = 1$.

Preschool years Period when children are between thirty-six and sixty months of age, or between the ages of three and five years.

Sex-typing The demonstration of behavior that is typical of a child's sex rather than behavior typical of the opposite sex.

Symbolic play The play of the preoperational period. Piaget also refers to this stage of play as the "let's pretend" stage of play.

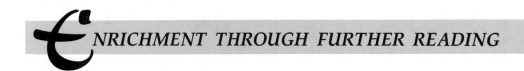

ENRICHMENT THROUGH FURTHER READING

Bettleheim, B. (1987). *A good enough parent.* New York: Alfred A. Knopf.
   Bettleheim encourages parents to trust their own judgments in order to gain their own insights into child rearing. He views child rearing as a creative act. Informative and enjoyable reading.

Chess, S. & Thomas, A. (1987). *Know your child.* New York: Basic Books.
   The authors advocate a "goodness of fit" between children's basic temperaments and parents' expectations and attitudes. The authors provide much sensible and important information.

Masters, W., Johnson, V., & Kolodny, R. (1988). *Crisis: Heterosexual behavior in the age of AIDS.* New York: Grove Press.
   The first couple of sexology have created another storm with their new book. They make many controversial statements including the claim that AIDS is transmitted through casual contact.

Shiff, Eileen (Ed.). (1987). *Experts advise parents.* New York: Delacorte.
   Leading parenting authorities from Benjamin Spock to Burton White provide parents with useful advice regarding many common child-rearing problems.

Tobin, J.J., Wu, D.Y.H. and Davidson, D.H. (1989). *Preschool in three cultures.* New Haven: Yale University Press.

This is an interesting and challenging book about what administrators, teachers and parents in three cultures—Japan, China and America—believe are the purposes of good preschools. The challenge comes from two sources. The reader is forced to confront cultural preconceptions about early schooling. Second, the book is difficult to read—but worth the effort.

ANSWER TO "WHAT WOULD YOU DO?"

Your first reaction was to advise the parents to forget the early learning; to relax and enjoy parenting and to avoid pushing their child. On second thought, though, such advice may be a little hasty and only half right. Increasingly, researchers and early childhood educators are suggesting that literacy begins to emerge in the cradle. Writer Melanie Wells (1988) says that this view "suggests that children may be ready to learn the elements of literacy in infancy. Indeed, those who support the new view believe that literacy skills will almost inevitably develop if the child is placed in a literate environment and given some encouragement" (p. 21). So, while your advice to parents not to push their children is sound, you can also encourage them to involve their children in literacy activities such as reading and being read to, letting them help "write" letters to grandparents and others, and drawing and scribbling.

Keep in mind that what makes "sense" isn't always true, and that just because many people are railing against early learning doesn't necessarily make it bad for children. As with most things, there often is a middle ground that offers the best choice. Pressuring, stressing, and overstimulating children in order to promote early learning is not good for parents or their children. Yet, on the other hand, providing an environment for literacy development from the day of birth makes sense if you want—and most parents probably do—a literate child.

BIBLIOGRAPHY

All fall down. (1986, July–August). *American Health*, p. 29.

Am, E. (1986). Play in the preschool: Some aspects of the role of the adult. *The International Journal of Early Childhood, 18*(2), 90–97.

Bandura, A. (1977). *Social learning theory.* Englewood Cliffs, NJ: Prentice-Hall.

Bassuk, E., & Rubin, L. (1987). Homeless children: A neglected population. *American Journal of Orthopsychiatry, 57,* 279–286.

Bates, E., Bretherton, Snyder, L. (1988). *From first words to grammar.* Cambridge, England: Cambridge University Press.

Baumrind, D. (1967). Child care practices anteceding 3 patterns of preschool behavior. *Genetic Psychology Monographs, 43–88.*

Bax, M. (1985). Crying: A clinical overview. In B. Lester & C. F. Z. Boukydis (Eds.), *Infant Crying* (pp. 341–348). New York: Plenum Press.

Berk, L. E. (1985). Why children talk to themselves. *Young Children, 40,* 46–52.

Berk, L. E. (1986). Private speech: learning out loud. *Psychology Today, 20,* 35–42.

Berk, L. E., & Garvin, R. A. (1984). Development of private speech among low-income Appalachian children. *Developmental Psychology, 20,* 271–286.

Bettleheim, B. (1987). *A good enough parent.* New York: Alfred A. Knopf.

Centers for Disease Control. (1989, July). *HIV-AIDS Surveillance Report.*

Chess, S., & Thomas, A. (1987). *Know your child.* New York: Basic Books.

Espenschade, A. S., & Eckert, H. M. (1980). *Motor development.* Columbus, OH: Merrill.

Fong, B. C., and Resnick, M. R. (1986). *The child: Development through adolescence* (2nd ed.). Palo Alto, CA: Mayfield.

Garrard, K. R. (1986). Helping young children develop mature speech patterns. *Young Children, 42,* 16–21.

Hamill, P. V. V., Drizd, T. A., Reed, R. B., Johnson, C. L., Roche, A. F., & Moore, W. M. (1979). Physical growth: National Center for Health Statistics Percentiles. *The American Journal of Clinical Nutrition, 32,* 607–629.

Huston, A. C. (1983). Sex-typing. In E. M. Hetherington, *Socialization, personality and social development:* Vol. 4 of P. H. Mussen (Ed.), *Handbook of child psychology* (4th ed.). New York: John Wiley. (pp. 387–467).

Jambor, T. (1986). Risk-taking needs in children: An accommodating play environment. *Children's Environment Quarterly, 3,* 22–25.

Johnson, J. E., Christie, J. F., & Yawkey, T. B. (1987). *Play and early childhood development.* Glenview, IL: Scott, Foresman.

Kolata, G. (1988, May 24). Children and AIDS: Drug tests raise hope and ethical concerns. *The New York Times,* p. 23.

Maccoby, E. E., & Martin, J. A. (1983). Socialization in the context of the family: Parent-child interaction. In E. M. Hetherington (Ed.), *Socialization, personality and social development:* Vol. 4 of P. H. Mussen (Ed.), *Handbook of child psychology* (4th ed.). (pp. 1–101). New York: John Wiley.

Merahn, S., Shelov, S., & McCracken, G. (1988, March). AIDS: What teachers, directors and parents want to know. *Scholastic Pre-K Today,* pp. A3–6.

Montessori, M. (1967). *The discovery of the child.* Notre Dame, IN: Fides.

Morrison, G. S. (1988). *Education and development of infants, toddlers and preschoolers.* Glenview, IL: Scott, Foresman.

Parke, R. D., & Slaby, R. G. (1983). The development of aggression. In E. M. Hetherington (Ed.), *Socialization, personality and social development:* Vol. 4 of P. H. Mussen (Ed.), *Handbook of child psychology* (4th ed.) New York: John Wiley (pp. 547–641).

Parten, M. (1932). Social play among preschool children. *Journal of Abnormal and Social Psychology, 27,* 243–269.

Piaget, J. (1962). *Play, dreams and imitation in childhood.* New York: W.W. Norton.

Raper, J., & Aldridge, J. (1988, February). What every teacher should know about AIDS. *Childhood Education,* pp. 146–149.

Robinson, C. C., & Morris, J. T. (1986). The gender-stereotyped nature of Christmas toys received by 36-, 48-, and 60-month-old children: A comparison between requested and nonrequested toys. *Journal of Sex Roles, 15,* 21–32.

Solarz, A. L. (1988, Winter). Homelessness: Implications for children and youth. *Social Policy Report: Society for Research in Child Development, 3* 1–18.

Spencer, H. (1878). *The principles of psychology.* London: Appleton.

Tyack, D. L. (1981). Teaching complex sentences. *Language, Speech, and Hearing Services in Schools, 17,* 160–174.

Wells, M. (1988). The roots of literacy. *Psychology Today, 22,* 20–22.

CHAPTER NINE

Learning and education in the preschool years

◆

VIGNETTES
INTRODUCTION
PRESCHOOL ENROLLMENT
REASONS FOR THE
  POPULARITY OF PRESCHOOLS
Disadvantaged Children
Working Parents
Divorce Rate
Importance of the Early Years
VISIONS OF YOUNG CHILDREN
Miniature Adults
Growing Plants
The Competent Child
Future Investments
PRESCHOOL PROGRAMS
Academic Orientation
Preschools as Preventative
  Programs
Multiplicity of Programs
NURSERY SCHOOLS
Nursery School Activities

HEAD START
THE MONTESSORI PROGRAM
Basic Features
THE BANK STREET PROGRAM:
  A DEVELOPMENTAL-
  INTERACTIONIST APPROACH
THE HIGH/SCOPE CURRICULUM
TRANSITIONS
PREDICTING PRESCHOOL
  SUCCESS
Implications of Preschool
  Screening
DO PRESCHOOL PROGRAMS
  MAKE A DIFFERENCE?
FACILITATING PRESCHOOLERS'
  LANGUAGE DEVELOPMENT
FACILITATING PRESCHOOLERS'
  LITERACY DEVELOPMENT
When Does Writing Begin?
COMMUNICATION IN THE
  PRESCHOOL YEARS

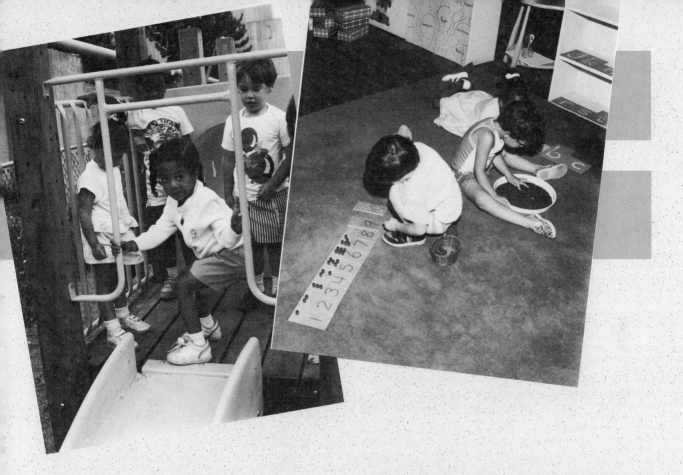

Implications for Teachers and
   Parents
In the Spotlight: Preschool Peer
   Interaction
SPECIAL NEEDS
   PRESCHOOLERS
Public Law 94-142
Public Law 99-457
Mainstreaming
Matching Children's Needs to
   Setting Resources: The Match-up
   Matrix
Gifted Preschoolers
PRESCHOOL ISSUES
The Developmentally Appropriate
   Curriculum
"At Least Have Them on the Old
   Side"

Who Should Attend?
Who Should Teach Preschoolers?
Unrealistic Expectations
What Would You Do?
In the Spotlight: Crisis and Stress
   in Children's Lives
SUMMARY
QUESTIONS TO GUIDE YOUR
   REVIEW
ACTIVITIES FOR FURTHER
   INVOLVEMENT
KEY TERMS
Enrichment through Further
   Reading
ANSWER TO "WHAT WOULD
   YOU DO?"
BIBLIOGRAPHY

VIGNETTES

"Before be five be four"—*Pogo* (Walt Kelly)

"What I know of children I have learned from them. There have been moments when I have felt like Columbus discovering America."—*Caroline Pratt*

Four-year-old Robyn Decker has attended school for three years. Her parents enrolled her in the Midtown Early Learning Center when she was one, and then at age three, she entered the Kiddie Kampus Nursery School, because according to Robyn's mother, Linda, "It has a reputation for stressing the academics."

Robyn has learned a lot of "academics" in school and her parents are proud of her accomplishments. Her teachers regard her as "very bright and smart." Robyn can name all the letters of the alphabet, both upper and lower case, and she has a sight reading vocabulary of 35 words. Robyn is highly motivated and enjoys learning. After school recently she informed her mother, "I want to learn to read all the color words just like Jennifer and Mandy," two of her older friends in the kindergarten program.

In addition to all of her schooling activities, Robyn attends ballet classes two days a week and a ceramics class once a week. Both she and her sister, Karen, attend summer camp for six weeks where they swim, ride on horseback, and work with computer learning programs.

Linda and Byron Decker want their children to do well in school. As Linda explains it, "I want Robyn and Karen to grow up to have good jobs so they can support themselves at an above average level. I know that by giving them an early start they will do better throughout life."

Every day, Mary Fernandez drops off her son, Michael, at KIDCO Preschool. She feels she doesn't have a choice. Mary is a CPA and has a large clientele at a "Big Eight" accounting firm where

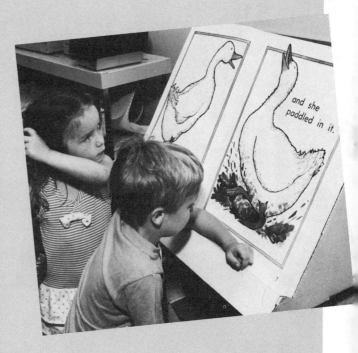

she is a junior partner. Besides, Mary has to work. She and her husband were divorced when she was four months pregnant with Michael. Michael has never seen his father, who now lives in Venezuela.

Michael's teachers say he is "average" and that he doesn't seem to be a happy child. He is shy, withdrawn, and frequently comes to school in clothes that are either too big or too small. As Phyllis Margolis, the lead teacher of the four-year-old program explains, "There doesn't seem to be a loving relationship between Michael and his mother. She is a real cool person. The other day we had parent-teacher meetings after school, and when she came in she didn't even greet Michael; she acted as though he didn't exist."

Mary has high hopes though for her son. "I want him to be a doctor and make lots of money. He's a good kid, he really is. I just think his teachers could get him interested in more things."

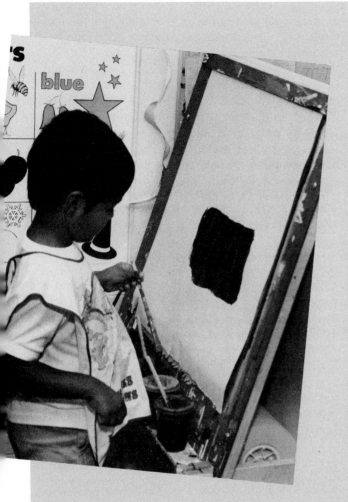

while his mother was raped; saw his fourteen-year-old cousin, Calvin, shot in the arm in a gang war, and watches from his second floor window as the police routinely sweep through the neighborhood looking for drugs and confiscating weapons.

Raynaud seems small for his age. His mother says he was born a month too soon. His actions are skitterish and he is easily startled by loud noises. When he hears what sounds like gunshots, which frequently happens during the late afternoons and evenings, he hides behind a chair or under the bed. Violence has obviously had an influence on Raynaud, but its extent will not be known for years. According to Gayle Kron, a psychiatric social worker assigned to work with school counselors in the housing project school attendance area, "The climate of steady violence that many children such as Raynaud experience in their lives is bound to leave emotional scars. It can be very psychologically crippling to children. We have to figure out ways to help these children while we find ways to end the violence."

Two years ago, the city school administration opened a preschool for children in the housing project. It is funded by special state early intervention program monies and a grant from a local charitable foundation. The best available records indicate that there are 200 three- and four-year-old children in the sprawling housing project. School administrators planned a program for fifty children, but only twenty-two are enrolled and many of those attend only occasionally. Raynaud is one of the occasional attenders, coming one or two days a week. His mother can't give a good reason for not sending Raynaud to school except to say that "He likes to stay home and watch television. I think he is scared to go out."

Three-year-old Raynaud lives with his teenage mother in one of the city's worst housing projects, known for its crime, violence, and crack dens. During his young life, Raynaud has been witness to many events that most people will not experience in a lifetime. He watched from the kitchen

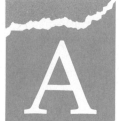

A s these vignettes indicate, preschool children have changed remarkably from what you were like as a three- or four-year-old and from what others might think today's average preschooler is like. Many children are "old for their age" in the sense that they have done and seen things that were not probable or possible for preschoolers decades ago. For children like Raynaud, these experiences are not life's best and they undoubtedly will have negative effects. On the other hand, for children such as Robyn, early experiences have had a beneficial influence.

Many preschool children have spent years in child care and/or preschool programs, some having been enrolled as early as six weeks of age. Many preschoolers have traveled widely, watched thousands of hours of television, have experienced the trauma of child abuse, and have lived in families that have undergone the stress and tensions of divorce. Collectively and individually, preschool children today are vastly different from their counterparts in the era of "Leave it to Beaver."

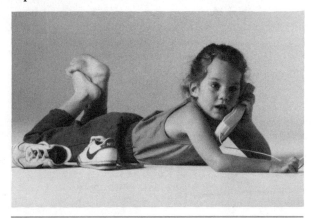

FIGURE 9-1 Many preschoolers have already gone places and done things that would have been impossible for their counterparts of a decade ago. Some think that as a result, children are growing up too fast, too soon. But as society changes, so do the opportunities available to its children.

While there has always been an acceptance of preschool programs for the very young, and while some children have always attended preschool programs, recent societal changes have altered our thinking about preschool programs and who should attend them. The entry of more women into the workplace as a result of the economic restructuring of the American economy and the women's movement have created an almost insatiable need for child care. The public schools have responded in part by opening their doors to four-year-old children. First, it was to disadvantaged children, and now it is to all children.

PRESCHOOL ENROLLMENT

The number of children enrolled in preschool programs is at an all-time high. In 1986, 2.6 million children ages three and over were attending a preschool (U.S. Bureau of the Census, 1988). These enrollments will increase, and projections through 1993 place preschool enrollment at 3.7 million children in both private and public settings "(The Statistical Trends," 1985). No longer are children staying at home with their parents, engaging in blissful play. Rather they have joined the ranks of older children and are spending eight and more hours engaged in the business of learning.

REASONS FOR THE POPULARITY OF PRESCHOOLS
Disadvantaged Children

The nation's poor children have long been the focus of public concern. Child advocates maintain that this concern is often too little and inadequately translated into programs and services that will help poor children and their families. Many children, because they share Raynaud's social and economic status, will not have access to the opportunities nor realize the dreams envisioned for them in this land of promise. Nine million children do not have access to basic health care and eighteen million have never been to a dentist (Save the Children Federation, 1985, p. 67). Over 40 percent of New

York's children live below the poverty line and in 1986, the city had 11,000 homeless children, known as *boarder babies*, living in municipal shelters (Stein, 1987). The Head Start program, initiated in 1965, is one noteworthy attempt to meet the needs of disadvantaged preschool children. Unfortunately, only 20 percent or one-fifth of the nation's eligible children are enrolled in a Head Start program.

Working Parents

One of the realities of the 1990s is that more mothers are employed, out of economic necessity and/or because they want to be, than at any other time in our nation's history. (See Table 9–1.) Maternal employment has created a tremendous demand for child care. The fact is that there is not enough quality child care to satisfy the needs of parents. The public schools have responded in part by providing before- and after-school care for school-age children and this is helpful. However, the tremendous need for child care for children prior to kindergarten and first grade remains like turbulent floodwaters behind a bursting dam. This pent-up child care demand creates pressure on the public schools to add at least a year of schooling to the K–12 grades. Many states are responding by providing special allocations to begin public preschool programs for three- and four-year-old children. We are fast becoming a nation with a Pre-K–12 system of public schooling consisting of fourteen grades.

TABLE 9–1

WOMEN IN THE LABOR FORCE WITH CHILDREN

Ages of Children	Number of Women	Percentage of all Mothers with Children in Age Category
Under 6	9 Million	56.7
3–5	4 Million	62.4
Under 3	5.6 Million	52.9

Note. Bureau of Labor Statistics, U.S. Department of Labor, 1988.

Divorce Rate

The high divorce rate is one reason many women with young children must work. In 1985, the divorce rate was 21.7 percent per 1,000 married women. Over half (53 percent) of these divorces involved children (National Center for Health Statistics, 1988). Single women with children are the most needy when it comes to child care. Consequently, preschool programs, especially those operated by the public schools at public expense, appeal to them.

Importance of the Early Years

People who advocate schooling for preschool children do so on the basis that the early years are educationally important in a number of ways. First, many parents and professional educators consider the preschool years as a time when children get "ready" for school. Viewed from this perspective, what a four-year-old does or does not learn influences how successful she will be in future school grades. Preschools, then, are considered the foundation for future school and life-long learning.

Second, advocates of early schooling see the early years as a way to combat some of the persistent problems of later schooling, such as school failure and attrition. In addition, these early education advocates are quick to cite the economic advantages to taxpayers and to individuals themselves that result from high school education. Thus, *early intervention*, or the process of addressing root causes of later school and life problems as early as possible is used as a persuasive argument for preschool education. Prevention, not remediation, is the rallying cry of those who see the schools as an effective instrument of social policy.

VISIONS OF YOUNG CHILDREN

Adults and the general public have certain ways of looking at—viewing—children. And how people view children helps determine how children are treated, reared, educated and the priority they have in the hearts and minds of those who control the nation's purse strings. Some historical, traditional, and contemporary ways of viewing children follow.

Miniature Adults

In earlier times, children were viewed as little more than miniature adults. This perspective is seen in the famous painting of children's games by Brughel the Elder, where children, although they are participating in children's games, still look like adults. They all have the same proportions as adults, they are simply scaled down, much like today's miniaturists scale down houses and trains in exact detail and proportion. This view of children as adults remains a powerful and pervasive image, whereby children model adult products, where children's fashions copy those of adults, and where children on television are often wiser, smarter, and more sophisticated than their parents and care-givers. When teachers and care-givers view children, who are chronologically and developmentally three and four years old, as adults, then they are likely to teach children as they would an adult, interact with them in adult ways, and have adult expectations for them.

Growing Plants

Frieddrich Froebel (1782–1852), the founder of the kindergarten (garden of children), popularized the view that children are similar to growing plants. A child is a seed or tender plant that needs the care and nurture of the gardener—the parent or teacher. As such, children grow and learn by a process of *unfolding*. The parent's and teacher's role is to observe, respect, and provide activities— mainly through play—for children to learn what they are able to learn when they are ready.

Many modern day kindergartens and preschool practices are based on ideas that have their roots in this view of children. For example, if children are not learning it is because they are not "ready" and therefore need more time to mature

or unfold. This view then supports grade retention, in other words, failing, and holding children out of kindergarten or first grade until they are ready. This later practice is euphemistically referred to as giving a child "the gift of time." For people who believe in unfolding, time cures all things. Also, other educational and social policies are based on the concept of unfolding, such as proposals and legislation to increase the age requirements for enrollment in preschool and kindergarten programs.

The Competent Child

The competent child is a more contemporary view and one promoted by the emphasis on the intellectual importance of the early years, a concept fashionable since the late 70's. According to Elkind (1986) the competent child concept is in keeping with life in the last decade of the twentieth century. Essentially, the competent child can cope with early separation from parents, early child care and high-pressure academic programs. Parents justify all their efforts on behalf of the child as necessary for his own good in order that he can and will keep up with his equally pressured and competent peers. Educationally then, parents are willing to seek out the best programs for their children at the earliest ages possible in order to capitalize on their competence and in efforts to make them more competent.

Future Investments

A continually persistent view since the 1960s and a contemporarily popular view of children is that they represent the future wealth or economic potential for parents and the nation. Thus, the education and care of young children is seen as an economically sound and cost-effective investment in the future. Many social policies and state and federal programs are based on this premise. Programs such as Head Start and child welfare programs, for example, are built on the underlying assumption that preventing problems in childhood results in a more productive adulthood, which in turn means that the nation will benefit from having employed citizens who will pay their share of the taxes. Furthermore, and perhaps more importantly, it means these productive citizens will not be consumers of expensive assistance, remedial, or rehabilitative programs. It is not uncommon, therefore, to hear social planners talk in terms of "human capital," "investment strategies," and "cost effectiveness" when justifying the funding of preschool programs, especially those for the disadvantaged.

The implications that preceding and other views of young children have for educational practice are several. First, how we as individuals and collectively as a society view children determines how we care for, treat, and educate them. Second, views of children provide a focus for discussion and public interest, which in turn helps direct economic allocations. A nation and its citizens are willing to support those programs that are congruent with their views of the world of children.

PRESCHOOL PROGRAMS
Academic Orientation

One of the significant changes in preschool programs over the last several decades is that educators have deemphasized the social adjustment and socialization orientations that were traditional preschool objectives and have replaced them with an academic orientation. The emphasis in preschools on an academic focus coincided with the back-to-basics movement in the public schools, a movement which began in the 1970s as a reaction against public perception that children were not learning how to read or write.

Traditionally, play has always been viewed as a major activity through which preschool children learn. In this sense, play is viewed as children's work, and children work at their job of learning *through* play. When children play house, for example, they are really working in preparation for adulthood. Today, however, there is more emphasis on having preschool children sit and engage in activities designed to either "get them ready for

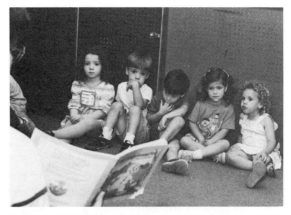

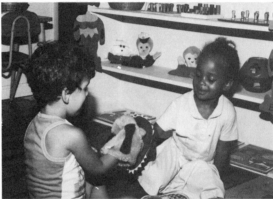

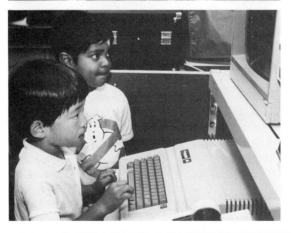

FIGURE 9-2 More states are funding preschool programs for three- and four-year-old children, especially those who are at risk for developmental delays and possible school failure. Also, quality preschools are viewed as one means of helping address societal problems.

school" or meet parents' expectations that early learning contributes to later life success. Preschool children, like all children, are always being prepared for the next step, phase, or program, where real learning will occur and where their previous learning will be put to good use.

Preschools as Preventative Programs

Education is very much a "top down" process in which ever greater demands are made of teachers and children in the early years as a means of assuring later learning and as an antidote for the problems of the middle and adolescent years. Consequently, educators and public policy developers see the early years as the beginning of such major schooling problems as the high drop-out rate and societal problems as drug usage. Viewed from this perspective, the responses are predictable—prevent the problems before they begin. Thus, preschools and early learning are seen as ideal ways to intervene in the lives of children—often disadvantaged children and their families. When preschools

and accompanying programs are perceived as a primary way to attack societal ills, then they are more likely to receive public support and legislative funding.

Multiplicity of Programs

In addition, there are now many more different kinds of preschool programs than there were in the past, depending on the funding sources, the philosophies of the directors, the desires of parents, and the needs of children. The tremendous range of these programs is shown in Table 9–2. A major problem that will likely continue to confront preschool professionals, parents, and children is the lack of quality, assessable preschool programs.

NURSERY SCHOOLS

The nursery school is one of the earliest and most traditional types of preschool programs. Nursery schools provide for a full range of services and emphasize educational experiences. Although many people think that early schooling for young children is a recent innovation of the last two

TABLE 9–2

TYPES OF PRESCHOOL PROGRAMS		
Program	Purpose	Age
Early childhood	*Multipurpose*	*Birth to third grade*
Child care	Play/socialization; babysitting; physical care; provide parents opportunities to work; cognitive development	Birth to 6 years
Employer child care	Different settings for meeting child care needs of working parents	Variable; usually as early as 6 weeks to the beginning of school
Corporate child care	Same as employer child care	Same as employer child care
Industrial child care	Same as employer child care	Same as employer child care

Proprietary care	Provide care and/or education to children; designed to make a profit	6 weeks to entrance into first grade
Nursery (public or private)	Play/socialization; cognitive development	2–4 years
Preschool (public or private)	Play/socialization; cognitive development	2½–5 years
Parent cooperative preschool	Play/socialization; preparation for kindergarten and first grade; babysitting; cognitive development	2–5 years
Babysitting cooperatives (Co-op)	Provide parents with reliable babysitting; parents sit for others' children in return for reciprocal services	All ages
Prekindergarten	Play/socialization; cognitive development; preparation for kindergarten	3½–5 years
Junior kindergarten	A prekindergarten program	Primarily 4-year-olds
Head Start	Play/socialization; academic learning; comprehensive social and health services; prepare children for first grade	2–6 years
Home Start	Provide Head Start service in the home setting	Birth–6 or 7 years
Laboratory school	Provide demonstration programs for preservice teachers; conduct research	Variable; from birth through senior high
Child and Family Resource Program	Deliver Head Start services to families	Birth–8 years
Montessori School (preschool and grade school)	Provide programs that use the philosophy, procedures, and materials developed by Maria Montessori	1–8 years
Open education	Child-centered learning in an environment characterized by freedom and learning through activities based on children's interests	2–8 years
British primary school	Implement the practices and procedures of open education	2–8 years

Note. From *Education and Development of Infants, Toddlers and Preschoolers* (p. 178) by George S. Morrison, 1988, Glenview, IL: Scott, Foresman.

decades, this is not the case. In fact, nursery schools have a long and illustrious history. Nursery school pioneers were innovators of practices today's teachers use daily and customarily take for granted. In 1916, Harriet Johnson started the Nursery School of the Bureau of Educational Experiments, which is today known as the Bank Street College of Education. She enrolled children between the ages of fourteen months and three years. Her curricula consisted of active experimentation based on play. Caroline Pratt, another educational pioneer, is famous as a developer of nursery school practices, unit blocks, and a leader in the child study movement.

Most nursery schools conduct programs that provide for the *whole child* and place an emphasis on learning through play. Many nursery schools that operated previously for only half a day are now responding to parents' needs and conduct full day programs.

Also, many preschool teachers, when asked what kind of a program they operate, say they have an eclectic one whereby they take the best from each program and use it to help children learn in the best way possible. Many have developed a *gestalt*, or integration of ideas from several programs, to help them best meet the needs of their children. They use whatever teaching/learning strategies work best for each child or group of children.

Nursery School Activities

Many nursery school activities are designed to help young children develop their motor skills. Toys that children can push and pull are favorites. Wagons, tricycles and riding toys are also favorites with children and, at the same time, give them opportunities to exercise and use the large muscles in their arms and legs. Play activities, the traditional curriculum of many nursery schools, are motor based.

Activities and tasks requiring fine motor skills play a larger role in the lives of preschoolers than they do in the lives of infants and toddlers. The reason for this is simply a matter of development—gross motor skills develop before fine motor skills. With the increased development of the hands and fingers, children are able to participate in self-help activities such as buttoning, zipping, and tying. They are also able to engage in many activities that are considered preschool and readiness activities because parents and educators view them as ingredients of school success. These include solving puzzles together, stringing beads, coloring, painting, drawing and "writing."

HEAD START

In 1964, a social and educational revolution began in America. In this year, Congress passed the Economic Opportunity Act, which among other things, funded the Head Start program for preschool children. Later, in 1967, Congress also funded the Follow Through program, which extends the services of Head Start and provides services for primary age children considered at educational risk.

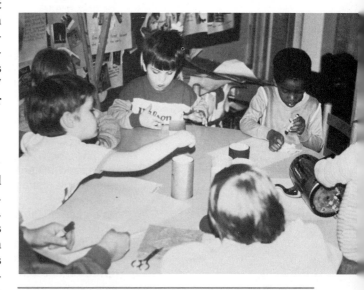

FIGURE 9-3 Head Start provides a comprehensive education and social service program for disadvantaged children and their families. Head Start is very popular with the constituency it serves and with the public at large. Unfortunately, Head Start serves only about one fifth of the eligible children.

The national Head Start program annually serves about one-half million children in 1,305 programs throughout the United States. Eighty-three percent of the children served are between the ages of three and four.

Head Start is designed to provide a comprehensive developmental program for preschool children from low-income families. The overall goal is to promote social competence by providing children with opportunities to achieve their potential in cognitive, language, socioemotional, and physical development. To achieve this goal, Head Start has the following program components: education, parent involvement, health services (including psychological services, nutrition, and mental health),

social services, and career development of staff, parents, and administration.

The educational program of Head Start has the following objectives (U.S. Department of Health & Human Services, 1984):

1. Provide children with a learning environment and the varied experiences that will help them develop socially, intellectually, physically, and emotionally in a manner appropriate to their age and state of development toward the overall goal of social competence.
2. Integrate the educational aspects of the various Head Start components in the daily program of activities.

TABLE 9–3

NINTH DISTRICT (BANKS COUNTY, GEORGIA) HEAD START DAILY SCHEDULE 1988–89	
7:30–8:00 AM	Greet children as they arrive at the Center. Encourage peer conversation during bus arrivals.
8:00–8:45 AM	Breakfast is served. Discuss foods that are eaten and why they are important. Encourage conversation throughout mealtime. Clean up and return to Head Start Center.
9:00–9:30 AM	Brush teeth. Visit bathroom. As children finish, they select their activity for learning centers.
9:30–10:15 AM	Large group activity (unit study, story, finger play, music).
10:15–11:15 AM	Small group activities (math, language, fine motor, science, art).
11:20–11:50 AM	Outdoor play (activities and games inside if weather doesn't permit outdoor play).
11:50 AM–12:00 PM	Visit bathroom and wash hands.
12:00–12:50 PM	Lunch. Children serve themselves with milk and tray. Use mealtime as a time for conversation and for children to verbalize.
12:50–1:00 PM	Brush teeth and visit bathroom.
1:00–2:30 PM	Quiet time and rest time with soft music. The children that wake early will select an activity of their choice.
2:30–2:45 PM	Group discussion (review day's activities).
2:50–3:00 PM	Load bus to go to high school to transfer children to their buses. At a convenient time to the children, staff works individually with children who have special needs.

3. Involve parents in the educational activities of the program to enhance their role as the principal influence on the child's education and development.
4. Assist parents to increase knowledge, understanding, skills, and experience in child growth and development.
5. Identify and reinforce experiences that occur in the home that parents can utilize as educational activities for their children (pp 8–9).

These educational objectives guide local Head Start agencies in developing their own educational programs that are unique and responsive to the children, families, and communities they serve. Consequently, and contrary to popular opinion, there is really no national Head Start curriculum. Many Head Start programs stress activities generally typical of nursery school and kindergarten programs, and include activities designed to promote children's success in school.

Table 9-3 shows the daily schedule of the Ninth District (Banks County) Head Start program, which serves over 1,000 children in Gainesville, Georgia.

THE MONTESSORI PROGRAM

Maria Montessori (1870–1952) developed one of the better-known and more influential preschool programs. Almost every town in the United States has a school bearing the name of the woman who devoted her life to developing an educational program. Montessori's ideas have greatly influenced early childhood materials, curriculum, and teaching methods.

Montessori began her career as the first woman physician in Italy, after which she turned her attention to finding an educational solution for mental retardation. While working with mentally handicapped children, she developed materials and activities that enabled many of them to read and write, accomplishments that were unheard of at the time. The opportunity to perfect her methods and apply them to normal children came in 1906, when she was invited to organize educational pro-

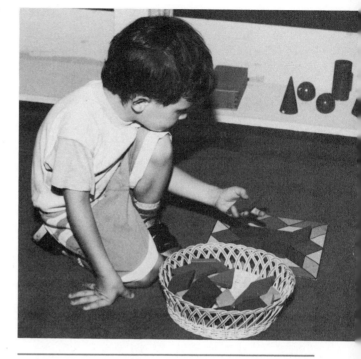

FIGURE 9-4 Montessori programs have always been popular with parents who want to give their children early learning experiences. In a Montessori classroom, multi-age children use sensory materials and engage in practical life activities to learn concepts and skills related to school success.

grams for the Roman Association of Good Building to benefit children living in tenement housing. Her first school was called the *Casa dei Bambini*, or *"Children's House,"* a name still used by many Montessori programs.

Basic Features

A number of features form the foundation for the Montessori program and help make it unique among all the others.

Sensory Materials Montessori believed children learn through their senses. Accordingly, she developed a set of materials designed to train the senses and, at the same time, to help children learn basic concepts important in school success. Montessori sensory materials are identified and described in Table 9-4.

TABLE 9-4

MONTESSORI SENSORY MATERIALS

1. Pink tower—(visual discrimination of dimension). Ten wood cubes of the same shape and texture, all pink, the largest of which is ten centimeters cubed. Each succeeding block is one centimeter smaller. The child builds a tower beginning with the largest block.
2. Brown stairs—(visual discrimination of width and height). Ten blocks of wood, all brown, differing in height and width. The child arranges the blocks next to each other from thickest to thinnest so the blocks resemble a staircase.
3. Red rods—(visual discrimination of length). Ten rod-shaped pieces of wood, all red, of identical size but differing in lengths from ten centimeters to one meter. The child arranges the rods next to each other from largest to smallest.
4. Cylinder blocks—(visual discrimination of size). Four individual wood blocks, which have holes of various sizes. One block deals with height, one with diameter, and two with the relationship of both variables. The child removes the cylinders in random order, then matches each cylinder to the correct hole.
5. Smelling jars—(discrimination involving the olfactory sense). Two identical sets of white, opaque glass jars with removable tops through which the child cannot see but through which odors can pass. The teacher places various substances, such as herbs, in the jars, and the child matches the jars according to the smell of the substance in the jars.
6. Basic tablets—(discrimination of weight). Sets of rectangular pieces of wood which vary according to weight. There are three sets, light, medium, and heavy in weight, which the child matches according to the weight of the tablets.
7. Color tablets—(discrimination of color and education of the chromatic sense). Two identical sets of small, rectangular pieces of wood are used for matching color or shading.
8. Sound boxes—(auditory discrimination). Two identical sets of cylinders are filled with various materials such as salt and rice. The child matches the cylinders according to the sound the materials make.
9. Tonal bells—(sound and pitch). Two sets of eight bells, which are alike in shape and size but differ in color. One set is white, the other brown. The child matches the bells according to the tone they make.
10. Cloth swatches—(sense of touch). The child identifies two identical swatches of cloth according to touch. This activity is performed first without a blindfold, but is later accomplished using a blindfold.
11. Temperature jugs or thermic bottles—(thermic sense and the ability to distinguish between temperatures). Small metal jugs are filled with water of varying temperatures. The child matches jugs of the same temperature.

Note. George S. Morrison, *Early Childhood Education Today*, 4th ed. (Columbus, Ohio: Charles E. Merrill, 1988).

Respect for Children Montessori believed that respect for children is an essential foundation of all education. She emphasized that children should be treated with dignity, and this belief permeates all Montessori practice. According to Montessori, children's essential natures are good, not bad. This respect for children is operationalized in practice in a number of ways. Children are made the focus of learning, they are provided with individualized programs, they are not treated as miniature adults, and they are treated in mannerly and humane ways.

Sensitive Periods Montessori believed there are genetically programmed *sensitive periods* during which children are more capable learning certain things. She felt this was particularly true of language development. The teacher's role, in part, is to determine, through observation when these sensitive periods occur, and when they do, to provide an environment and activities that support learning.

Autoeducation Montessori believed in the capacity of all children to educate themselves. The key to self-education is a prepared environment where children can do things for themselves, be independent, and become independent of adults.

The Prepared Environment One of the key tasks of a Montessori teacher is to prepare an environment in which children can learn for themselves. Preparing the environment means having ready and available materials and activities that are developmentally appropriate and that match children's sensitive periods and learning backgrounds.

THE BANK STREET PROGRAM: A DEVELOPMENTAL-INTERACTIONIST APPROACH

In 1919, Harriet Johnson started the Nursery School of the Bureau of Educational Experiments in New York, devoted to the study of children and educational practice. The Bureau later became the Bank Street College of Education, which sponsors the Bank Street School for Children. The Bank Street early childhood program is based on a developmental-interactionist point of view. This approach to education has its roots in the philosophy of John Dewey, the preeminent American educator who did much to influence what is often called *progressive education,* which basically is a theory of schooling emphasizing children and their interests rather than subject matter. Because of this attention to children, the terms *child-centered, child-centered schools,* and *child-centered curriculum* are frequently used to denote early childhood programs designed with the needs and interests of children in mind. This is the way Dewey described the child-centered approach.

All of the schools . . . as compared with traditional schools . . . [exhibit] a common emphasis upon respect for individuality and for increased freedom; a common disposition to build upon the nature and experience of the boys and girls that come to them, instead of imposing from without external subject matter standards. They all display a certain atmosphere of informality, because experience has

proved that formalization is hostile to genuine mental activity and to sincere emotional expression and growth (Archambault, 1964; pp. 170–171).

TABLE 9–5

A BANK STREET DAY (INTERAGE GROUP—4–5 YEARS OF AGE)	
Time	Activity
8:30–9:00 AM	Children arrive. Parent-child interaction. Teacher observation of interactions (children and parents interact with materials). Free choice of activities.
*9:00–10:15 AM	Outside play—large muscle activities
	OR
	Inside work period. Use of blocks, paints, etc., and dramatic play
*10:15–11:15 AM	Outside Activities
	OR
	Inside Work Period
AM Activity.	Music/Movement (once a week the children are provided music/movement activities by a special teacher)
11:45–12:15 PM	Lunch
12:15–1:15 PM	Rest/Quiet time
1:15–1:45 PM	Circle time/Story discussion
1:45–2:45 PM	Work time (similar to morning activity)
2:45–3:00 PM	Clean up
3:00–3:15 PM	Wraps/Pick up

*Note. Generally, while one half of a group are playing outside, the other half is inside and vise-versa

In a child-centered approach, learning initiatives come *primarily* from the children. The teacher's role is that of facilitating and providing an environment in which children can follow their

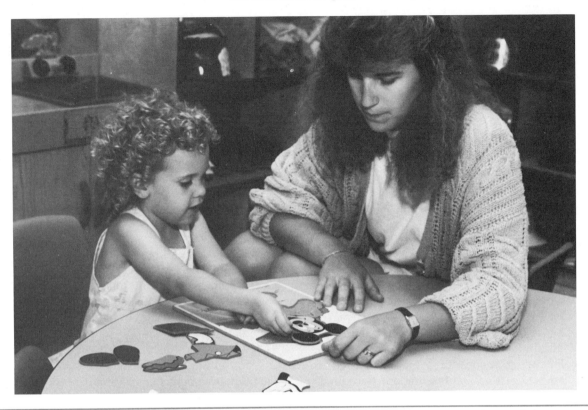

FIGURE 9-5 In a child-centered program, children and their needs and interests are the focus of the program. Contrary to popular opinion however, children's interests are not the basis for determining the curriculum. However, the interests of children within the preschool curriculum do determine specific activities and involvement.

interests and learn within the context of the activities resulting from these interests. Play is the primary context within which children discover, extend, and develop their interests. Thus, a predetermined curriculum is not imposed from the outside, rather the natural development of the child is the key.

The Bank Street program represents this "child-centered" approach to learning and education, and constitutes the "middle ground" or "center" of American preschool educational thought and practice. This child-centered focus maintains that children's development, needs, and natures, not adults' or society's, should determine the goals, objectives, and teaching practices of early childhood programs.

The developmental-interactionist model has the following four general goals (DeVries, 1987):

1. To enhance competence. This goal includes the use of knowledge, self-esteem, self-confidence, resourcefulness, resilience, and a feeling of competence.

2. To promote individuality or identity. This goal includes identifying self-qualities and roles occupied, for example, worker, learner, member of group, etc.

3. To promote socialization. Two primary abilities are necessary to achieve this goal: first, sensitivity to others' points of view and the ability to engage in cooperative relations in play, work, talk, and argument; and second, the ability to communicate in a variety of ways.

4. To develop integration of functions and the ability to be open to a wide range of phenomena (pp. 303–304).

Barbara Biber (1903–), long a proponent of the whole child approach and a leading spokesperson for the developmental-interactionist point of view, suggests the following eight developmental-educational goals and accompanying preschool activities (Biber, 1984):

1. To serve the child's need to make an impact on the environment through direct physical contact and maneuver.
   - Exploring the physical world: for example, equipment, space, and physical protection.
   - Constructive, manipulative activities with things (presymbolic): for example, a variety of materials—blocks, clay, sand, and wood.
2. To promote the potential for ordering experience through cognitive strategies.
   - Extending receptiveness and responsiveness: for example, variety of sensorimotor-perceptual experiences, focus on observation and discrimination.
   - Extending modes of symbolizing: for example, gestural representation; two-dimensional representation with pencil, crayons, paints; and three-dimensional representation with clay, blocks, and wood.
   - Developing facility with language; for example, word meanings and usage, scope of vocabulary, mastery of syntax, playful and communicative verbal expression.
   - Stimulating verbal-conceptual organization of experience and information: for example, verbal formulation; integration of present and nonpresent; accent on classification, ordering, relationship, and transformation concepts in varied experiential contexts.
3. To advance the child's functioning knowledge of his environment.
   - Observation of functions within school: for example, heating systems, water pipes, kitchen, and elevator.
   - Story-reading: for example, stories about nature, work processes, people's roles and functions.
   - Observation of functioning environment outside the school: for example, to observe work forces, natural processes—buildings, construction, traffic regulation; to visit police, fire fighters, farm and dairy.
   - Discussion of contemporary events that children hear about: for example, war, demonstrations, strikes, space activities, street violence, explorations, and earthquakes.
4. To support the play mode of incorporating experience.
   - Nourishing and setting the stage for dramatic play activity: for example, experiences, materials, and props.
   - Freedom to go beyond the restraints of reality in rehearsing and representing.
5. To help the child internalize impulse control.
   - Communicating a clear set of nonthreatening controls: for example, limits, rules, and regulations.
   - Creating a functional adult authority role: for example, understandable restraints, alternative behavior patterns, and nonpunitive sanctions.
6. To meet the child's need to cope with conflicts intrinsic to this stage of development.
   - Dealing with conflict over possession displaced from the family scene: for example, fostering special relation of child to a single adult, guidance in learning to share things as well as people.
   - Alleviating conflict over separation related to loss of familiar context of place and people: for example, visits from people to school, interchange of home and school objects, and school trips to school neighborhoods.
   - Accepting ambivalence about dependence and independence: for example, selection of areas of curriculum most suited to independent exploration and acceptance of regressive dependent behavior under stress.
7. To facilitate the development of an image of self as a unique and competent person.
   - Increasing knowledge of self: for example,

identity, family, and ethnic membership, and awareness of skills.
- ■ Clarifying sense of self: for example, as initiator, learner, and autonomous individual.
- ■ Advancing integration of self: for example, self-realization through reexpression in symbolic play, latitude for individual mix of fantasy with knowledge of objective reality.

8. To help the child establish mutually supporting patterns of interaction.
- ■ Building informal communication channels, verbal and nonverbal: for example, adult-child, child-child.
- ■ Cooperative and collective child-group relations: for example, discussion periods, joint work projects.
- ■ Creating supportive adult roles: for example, source of comfort, troubleshooter, solver of unknowns, investor in child's learning. (pp. 245–254).

Classroom practice is really what defines a child-centered approach. Consequently, the teacher in a Bank Street program has two fundamental roles. One is to act as a mediator between the world of the family and the world of the peer group and larger society. The second role is to foster the child's ego development and mental health (DeVries, 1987, p. 310). These roles are accomplished by developing a sense of trust between the teacher and child. Above all, the teacher needs to be a trusting person. As a result of this trust bond, the teacher can promote the child's initiative in interacting with the world outside the family.

It is fair to say that traditional education approaches generally value conformity, whereas the Bank Street program does not. In addition, from the Bank Street perspective, cognitive education does not by itself solve all children's problems or account for all their development. Having children learn only cognitive skills will not help them in today's demanding and complex world. So, the challenge in the Bank Street program is how to integrate the cognitive and affective domains while keeping the child at the center of the program. This is done in part by:

1. Nurturing individuality
2. Valuing creative expression
3. Encouraging children to express themselves—their feelings and ideas
4. Stimulating children to take initiative, make choices, and to have and assume responsibility
5. Sponsoring and encouraging free and spontaneous play
6. Educating for values by balancing individual fulfillment with the values of society
7. Developing a curriculum in response to children's needs and development

THE HIGH/SCOPE CURRICULUM

The High/Scope curriculum has its roots in Piaget's theory of cognitive development and, as such, is based on the principle of *constructivism*. Simply stated, the constructivist approach maintains that children literally construct their knowledge of the world and their level of cognitive functioning. "The more advanced forms of cognition are constructed anew by each individual through a process of 'self-directed' or 'self-regulated activity' " (Kuhn, 1981, p. 353). Constructivism then means that "knowledge is built by an active child from the inside rather than being transmitted from the outside through the senses" (Kamii, 1981, p. 234). The child as knower and doer constructs knowledge. Constructivism then stands in direct opposition to the behaviorists, who see stimuli acting on passive children, who then react in response to that stimuli. Constructivists, on the other hand, see an active child operating on the environment and creating a reaction because of his active involvement.

How does the constructivist view then get translated into educational practice? The High/Scope curriculum:

> . . . .is based upon the assumption that children are natural inquirers, who need assistance and direction in the pursuit of knowledge at their level of development. The acquisition of knowledge is viewed as an active, exploratory process, whose primary aims are questioning–problem solving contexts and forming tentative hypotheses based upon the child's experience and interests. Knowledge thereby becomes realistic and useful, and is essentially for the sake of practical activities (Weikart & Tompkins, 1988, p. 3).

The teacher's role in the High/Scope curriculum is to assist children in the natural process of inquiry, to arrange the classroom to promote active learning, to make plans and review activities with children, to interact with individual children, and to lead small- and large-group sessions. Whereas in a child-centered approach, activities are initiated by the child, and in a teacher-centered approach, learning activities are initiated by the teacher, the High/Scope approach is a mutually cooperative process.

Two processes constitute the central core of the High/Scope program, the plan-do-review sequence, and key experiences. In the three-stage plan-do-review process, children—in cooperation with the teacher—plan for an activity they will undertake. This can include an oral plan—telling the teacher what she will do—and later a "written" plan. The child then completes the activity she planned, for example, sorting objects according to color and shape. The child and the teacher then review what the child did, how she did it, and learning outcomes, for example, "Tell me why you put the round shapes in this box." Key experiences are the second essential part of the High/Scope curriculum. Key experiences in the area of active learning for children between the ages of four and six are:

- Exploring actively the attributes and functions of materials with all the senses.

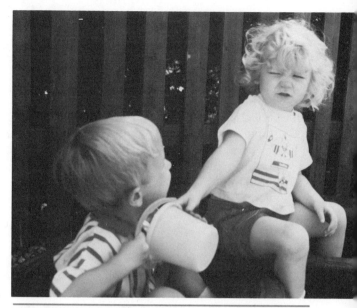

FIGURE 9-6 Preschool programs should provide opportunities for children to be actively involved with the environment, materials and with peers. Children during the preschool years are in the stage of initiative vs. guilt and need to express their ambition and purpose through activities and projects.

- Discovering relations through direct experience.
- Manipulating, transforming, and combining materials.
- Acquiring skills with tools and equipment.
- Using small and large muscles.
- Taking care of one's own needs.
- Predicting problems and devising ways of solving them (D. McClelland, personal communications, 1988).

Whereas in a child-centered approach, the social-emotional development of children is a primary and central theme, in the High/Scope program, such development is dealt with indirectly. The rationale is clear:

> It is easier and more productive to focus directly on, say children's planning than on group dynam-

ics, on classifying objects and events than on interpreting fantasies—the one is concrete and intellectual, the other abstract and esoteric (Homann, Banet, & Weikart, 1979, p. 1).

TABLE 9–6

A SCHEDULE FROM HIGH/SCOPE	
9:00 AM	Arrival
9:10 AM	Bathroom (washing hands)
9:20 AM	Breakfast/Snack
9:30 AM	Planning Time
9:40 AM	Work Time
10:30 AM	Clean Up Time
10:40 AM	Recall Time
10:55 AM	Growth Motor Time
11:15 AM	Small Group Time/Teacher Directed Activity
11:40 AM	Large Group Time (music, songs, stories)
11:55 AM	Bathroom
12:00 PM	Lunch
12:30 PM	Dismissal

(Courtesy of the authors and High/Scope Press)

TRANSITIONS

Preschool children face many transitions in their lives as they are left with baby-sitters, enter child care programs, attend preschool, and prepare to enter kindergarten and first grade. Depending on how adults help children make these transitions, they can be unsettling and traumatic or joyful and rewarding. The transition from home to preschool and from preschool to kindergarten can influence positively or negatively children's attitudes toward schooling. Also, a transition is just that—a transition from one learning setting to another. Under no circumstances should the transition from preschool to kindergarten or first grade be viewed as

the beginning of "real learning." Following are some things parents, care-givers, and professionals can do to help children make transitions easily and confidently:

- Educate and prepare children ahead of time for any new situation. For example, children and preschool teachers can visit the kindergarten or first grade program the children will attend. Also, toward the end of the preschool year, or as time to enter the kindergarten approaches, children can practice doing certain routines the way they will encounter them in their new school setting.
- Work with parents to alert them to new and different standards, expectations regarding curriculum, achievement standards, dress, behavior, and parent/teacher interactions. Preschool teachers in cooperation with the kindergarten teachers should share curriculum materials with parents so they can be familiar with what their children will learn.
- Provide parents of special needs children and bilingual parents with additional help and support during the transition process.
- All professionals should visit the programs their children will attend in the future. This is essential in order to better understand the physical, curricular, and affective climates of the receiving programs. As a result, professionals will be better able to incorporate into their own curricula methods that will help children adjust to new settings.
- Work cooperatively with the staff of any program the children will attend in order to work out a "transitional plan." Continuity between programs is important for social, emotional, and educational reasons. Children should see their new setting as an exciting place where they will be happy and successful.

PREDICTING PRESCHOOL SUCCESS

School entrance, whether preschool, kindergarten, or first grade, is a critical developmental and life event. The events of schooling frequently determine how successful a child will be in school and life. School success affects children's life success and also the school success of their children. Given, then, the importance of school success, educators, social workers, and health personnel are increasingly interested in identifying those children who are at risk for school success in order to focus resources prior to and at the time of school entrance. There are a number of ways to determine children's risk for school failure.

One way is to identify those children who are "poor." This is how Head Start selects children for participation in its program. Being poor by the federal definition means that you and your family do not have an income sufficient to purchase adequate health care, food, housing, clothing, and educational services. The federal government annually publishes family income guidelines. In 1985, the poverty level for a family unit of four was $11,000.

A second way is to conduct *developmental screening*, using a *developmental screening test*. Such tests are designed to alert professionals of the possibility of developmental delays. When children are identified as having a delay, then professionals can conduct diagnostic testing to determine the exact cause and extent of the delay and propose appropriate intervention strategies. A list of some tests used to screen children follows. Keep in mind that there are many assessment and diagnostic instruments available. A good way to become more familiar with such tests is by looking through publishers' catalogs and professional journals.

- *Denver Developmental Screening Test (DDST)* (Frankenburg, Sciarillo, & Burgess, 1981)—Evaluates four aspects of child development—gross motor skills, fine motor adaptive skills, language skills, and personal-social skills—in children two months to six and one-half years.
- *Developmental Indicators for the Assessment of Learning–Revised (DIAL-R)* (Mardell-Czudnowski & Goldenberg, 1983)—Evaluates three areas—motor skills, concepts (naming colors, identifying body parts, naming letters and sorting chips), and language—in children two to six years of age.

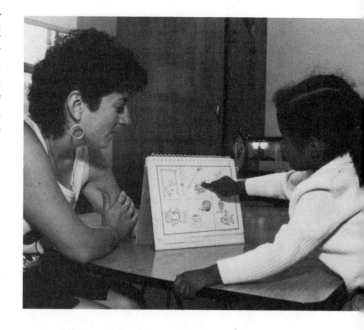

FIGURE 9-7 Today, preschool screening tests are assuming greater importance in the determination of whether or not children are ready for schooling experience. They also identify those children who may benefit from special programs and services designed to remediate developmental delays and other risk factors.

- *Diagnostic Inventory for Screening Children (DISC)* (Amdur, Mainland, & Parker, 1984)—Identifies delays in eight developmental areas: fine motor skills, gross motor skills, receptive language, expressive language, visual attention and memory, auditory attention and memory, self-help skills, and social skills. Can be used with children between birth and five years.

A third way to determine those children who are at risk for grade failure is to determine social and environmental factors related to school success and failure, and to assess children in relation to them. One such method is the RISC (Risk Index of School Capability) Scale (Fowler & Cross, 1986). The scale is shown in Table 9–7.

TABLE 9–7

RISC SCALE	
Maternal education	0–3
Family history of learning problems	0–2
Age/gender	0–2
Attention span	0–4
Total score	0–11

For example, a child at highest risk for grade failure would be one:

1. Whose mother has a ninth grade education or less (0 points);
2. Who is a male and is within three months of the cut-off age for school entrance (0 points);
3. Whose family has a history of learning difficulties (0 points); and
4. Who is very distractible (0 points).

Children with scores of seven or above have a 98 percent positive predictive value for successful grade completion; a score of four, five, or six carries an intermediate risk for grade failure (a score of five has a 39 percent positive predictive value for grade success), and a score of three or less has a positive predictive value for grade failure.

Implications of Preschool Screening

Parents and professionals should not view the results of screening instruments and predictive scales in a deterministic way. No child should be "written off" at any stage in their progress through the educational system. Rather, such scales are of value in two regards. First, they are enlightening to professionals and parents in that they show what contributes to success and failure. For example, in the sense that maternal education is a factor in children's school success, current efforts at reducing the number of school dropouts and programs designed to encourage teenage parents to complete their high school education will benefit future generations of children.

Second, when children are identified as being at risk for learning and grade failure, then teachers and others can design programs to help children and their parents in order to *prevent* grade failure. The whole point of early screening and diagnosis is to provide the services necessary to help assure success for children.

DO PRESCHOOL PROGRAMS MAKE A DIFFERENCE?

The preschool movement has generated a great deal of controversy over the last several decades. Part of the controversy revolves around whether or not preschool programs are effective. When the public and preschool critics question the success of preschool programs, they usually do so in two ways: on the basis of students' academic achievement and on future economic return. Student achievement is generally measured by test scores and economic effectiveness by future employability.

In 1962, the Perry Preschool Program was initiated in Ypsilanti, Michigan to assess the impact of a preschool program on low-income minority children. Each year for five successive years, two matched groups of preschool children were selected and one group was randomly assigned to attend preschool. A total of fifty-eight children attended preschool and sixty-five served as controls. The children participating in the program had IQ's of between sixty and ninety, almost half came from single-parent homes, and fewer than twenty percent of the parents had graduated from high school. The preschool children participated in a high-quality educational program two and one-half hours per day from October to May. The adult-child ratio was approximately 1:5, and teachers visited the homes of the children for about ninety minutes a week. All study participants were followed through to age nineteen. The results of this longitudinal study indicate that children who participated in the preschool program:

1. Had higher academic achievement and higher achievement motivation;
2. Were placed less often in special education classes;
3. Experienced fewer months of unemployment, with 50 percent of the preschool group employed at age nineteen versus 28 percent for the control group;
4. Had fewer incidents of delinquency—by age nineteen, 22 percent of the preschool group had been arrested one or more times as compared to 38 percent for the control group; and
5. Experienced less teenage pregnancy—the twenty-five women in the preschool group had seventeen births by age nineteen as compared to the twenty-four women in the control group, who had 28 births.

All these results are statistically significant except for the fertility comparison.

What may be even more significant from a public policy point of view is the cost-benefit ratio of the Perry Preschool Program. This is important since in the public's eye, economic cost-effectiveness is frequently the basis for judging the worthiness of a program. When all the costs of the preschool program are deducted from the monies that were *not* spent on welfare payments and costs of special education; and when additional taxes paid by the preschool participants through increased employment are considered, the estimated gain to the public is $2,290 per preschool participant through age nineteen (Berrueta-Clement, Schweinhart, Barnett, Epstein, & Weikart, 1984).

FACILITATING PRESCHOOLERS' LANGUAGE DEVELOPMENT

Since language usage is so important to school success, teachers and parents must provide an environment in which children's language can flourish and in which they can, in the constructivist sense, develop language. This flourishing can occur with the assistance of appropriate instructional strategies, with teacher modeling, and with opportunities for children to be involved in language.

Some things teachers and parents can do are:

- Provide children with opportunities for learning to use elaborated/complex sentences. These opportunities can include providing role models—teachers, parents, adults, and other children—as a means of enabling children to hear complex language and to have the opportunity to practice language skills.
- Provide instructional activities that cause children to practice the use of complex language, for example, children describe pictures and relate experiences.
- Provide children the opportunity to use language in social contexts with others who have the desired language skills. Playing with children who are good communicators enables children who are not to have the opportunity to learn from their peers. Also, children become good communicators in part by having opportunities to practice language. It is extremely important for children to have opportunities to exchange opinions and viewpoints with other children, not only because such encounters facilitate language development, but because they also promote cognitive development.
- Provide a language-rich environment that includes reading to children, utilization of the language experience approach, dramatic play opportunities, role playing, show and tell, and the general encouragement of children's use of language. A preschool classroom should be one in which language usage is prized and valued rather than one in which silence is the criterion by which children's behavior is assessed.

FACILITATING PRESCHOOLERS' LITERACY DEVELOPMENT

In order to fully understand children's *total* language development in the preschool years, you need to be familiar with a number of terms used with increasing frequency in early childhood and preschool settings. First is the term *literacy*. Formerly, many teachers and parents tended to think of reading, writing, and speech as separate processes and, as a result, taught them as separate and often highly isolated subjects and skills. Now, however, the term *literacy*, the ability to read and write, is used to more adequately reflect contemporary thinking that reading and writing are both part of the process of becoming literate.

A second important term is *emerging literacy*. There is a strong tendency to think of reading and writing as beginning when children go to school. Thus we talk about children *learning* to read and write as a result of being *taught* in school. The term *emerging literacy*, on the other hand, indicates that children begin the process of being literate at birth. Viewed in this way, children are always in the process of developing literacy skills.

Third is the term *whole language*. The term *whole language* is used to convey the concept that language development, reading, writing, and speech are not separate and unrelated processes. Rather, they are and should be treated as an integrated whole. "Students learn about reading and writing while listening; they learn about writing from reading and gain insights about reading from writing" (Newman, 1985, p. 5).

When Does Writing Begin?

The process of writing begins almost as soon as children are able to hold a writing instrument, as evidenced by the scribbling of fifteen-month-old Andrew (see Figure 9–8). The examples of children's writing in Figures 9–9 and 9–10 show how their writing develops in the preschool years. Andrew at fifteen months does not relate writing

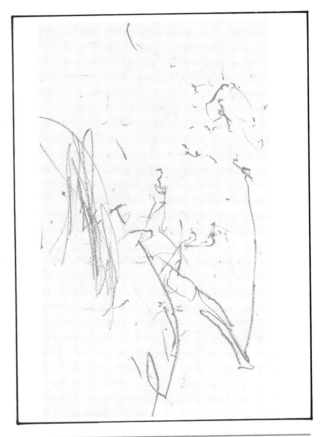

FIGURE 9-8 Andrew's scribble. Toddlers such as 15-month-old Andrew like to "write." Today, the emphasis is on literacy development, which is viewed as beginning at birth.

with speech or communication. Rather he is interested in the product of "writing."

Next, children use shapes to correspond to objects. These shapes (circles, squares, and triangles) form a basis for writing, in which children combine shapes to create forms. This process leads to recognition of objects in the environment and the use of shapes to represent objects in the environment. Children are still more interested in the process than the product, as shown in Michael's and Emily's "writings" (see Figures 9–9A and 9–9B).

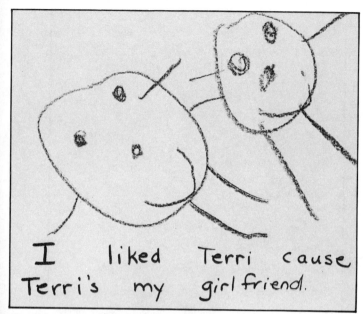

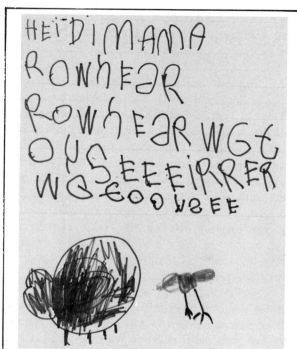

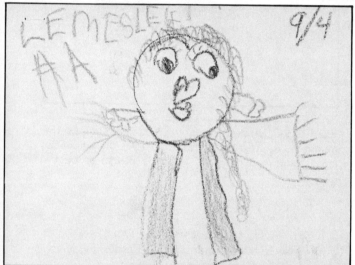

FIGURE 9-9 Michael's (top) and Emily's (bottom) "writing" use shapes to represent objects in the environment. They are still more interested in the process rather than the product.

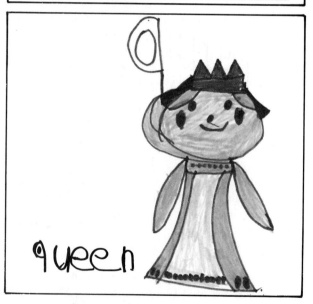

FIGURE 9-10 Heidi's (top) and Jamie's (bottom) writing. The progression of their writing is from shapes for objects, to figures in the environment, to having letters and words be the symbols which stand for objects and ideas.

On the other hand, four-year-old Heidi shows by her product that she is aware of figures in the environment and her shapes are more controlled. Five-year-old Jamie combines lettering with drawing to show an understanding of the relationship of letters to objects and words (see Figures 9–10A and 9–10B).

Today, preschool teachers recognize that oral and written language are integrated with each other. Therefore, there is more of an effort to promote language development as an integrated whole rather than as separate and distinct processes.

COMMUNICATION IN THE PRESCHOOL YEARS

The ability to communicate with others develops rapidly during the preschool years. Some of these communicative abilities include (Shatz, 1983):

- The adoption and use of parental conversational styles and responses. For example, when a child says, *"By the way,* I'm going to the movies with my mom," she has probably adopted that particular way of opening a sentence from the parent.
- Development of a sense of responsibility regarding conversational rules. Children make attempts to respond appropriately in situations calling for a particular response.
- Giving appropriate specific answers to specific requests (by age three).
- Making specific requests (by age four).
- Using ellipsis, which involves eliminating from conversations elements of a grammatical sentence that is understood in context, thereby eliminating redundancies. For example, when the care-giver asks a child, "What do you want?" and the child responds, "A drink," he considers "I want" an unnecessary part of the conversation.
- The use and understanding of appropriate linguistic reference, which is an indication of something existing in the environment. For example, when a child's mother says, "See the doggies. Which one do you like?", the child understands the referent "which" and responds, "The brown one." Also, referential

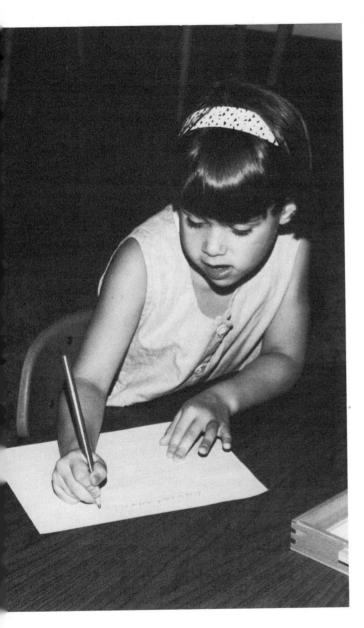

FIGURE 9-11 Literacy development is viewed as an integrated whole which consists of writing, reading and spelling. Teachers provide preschoolers with opportunities to become immediately involved in literacy development through writing. This process is often referred to as the language experience approach.

skill involves understanding the role gestures play in language. Thus, while saying that he prefers the brown dog, the child also points to it.

■ Learning language appropriate to scripts, routines, and rituals. There are certain routine situations that call for certain language, such as saying "Hi" when greeting someone and saying "Goodbye" when leaving. Certain rituals also call for certain kinds of language. A social interaction ritual, for example, involves asking someone how they are. A script is a conceptual framework that describes a sequence of events in a particular situation. For example, in a Montessori classroom, the understanding by children of how they will use materials and engage in a particular learning activity constitutes a script. This script is shared by all children. Conversation with other children and the teacher is therefore easier because a child knows the script—the events, sequence of activities, and dos and don'ts of using materials.

Implications for Teachers and Parents

As teachers, care-givers, and parents involve children in language development, there are a number of things they can keep in mind:

1. Children's involvement in and use of language grows out of their experiences. The point is that as children have rich, varied, and meaningful experiences, they have a framework within which to express themselves. Also, experiences help provide the extrinsic motivation and help develop the intrinsic motivation for language use. Children who are involved in *doing* things, *going* places and *interacting* with people have experiences about which to talk, write, and read.

2. From the time they are born, children are surrounded with speech and print. Teachers and parents can and should use the context of daily living to help children learn language. The environment provides many natural ways for language learning, and, at the same time, children learn that speaking, writing, and reading are embedded in and essential to daily living.

3. The roots of literacy begin early in the mother-infant attachment process. The atmosphere surrounding the interaction of securely attached dyads is more positive than that of anxiously attached dyads. In securely attached dyads, there is less need to discipline and the children are less distracted than in anxiously attached dyads. Therefore, mothers of securely attached infants can demand more of their children because the children have developed more trust. The quality of attachment has implications for emerging literacy. Securely attached dyads pay more attention to the formal aspects of maternal reading instruction, in other words, the mother naming letters, trying to make the child recognize sounds, and connecting letters to well-known words (Bus & van Ijzendoorn, 1988). Thus, competence in emerging literacy can be enhanced by working with new parents and parents-to-be to provide them with the rationale and skills for developing secure attachment relationships with their young children.

*I*N THE SPOTLIGHT

PRESCHOOL PEER INTERACTION

When parents respond to the question "Why do you want your child to go to preschool?", they frequently say, "So they can make friends and to learn how to get along with others." For parents, socialization is a primary goal for any kind of preschool or child care experience. But what is the socialization reality for children? What are peer interactions like in the early years?

During the preschool period, children's ability to use language more effectively to communicate also enables them to play with a wider range of children. For example they are able to name activities—"Ride bikes"—and to specify the conditions of play—"You're the mommy and I'm the baby." As a result, preschoolers play with a wider range of playmates than do toddlers (Howes, 1988, p. 4).

Also during the preschool years, children begin to differentiate between friends and playmates, and they play with children they do not consider friends. Preschoolers use temporary friendship status to gain entry into play and play groups—"I'll be your friend if I can play" (Howes, 1988).

Social classifications (for example, rejected) play an important role in peer social development. Children with rejected social classifications are more likely to be rebuffed by their peers, and are described by their teachers as having more difficulty with their peers. Socially inactive children (for example, withdrawn) engage in less complex play interactions. And children with no mutual friends have a harder time entering play groups, engage in less skillful interaction, and receive lower teacher ratings (Howes, 1988, p. 51).

Young preschool children develop many of their social interactions on the basis of sex. Mutual friends are almost always of the same sex, the amount of time children spend with same-sex children is greater than with opposite-sex children, and boys tend to have a larger friendship network than do girls (Hartup, Laursen, Stewart, & Eastenson, 1988).

Friendships play a major role in the social conflicts that occur between preschoolers. As you might expect, because preschoolers play with their friends more often, they also have more conflicts with their friends. But there is a difference in how these conflicts are handled and resolved. Mutual friends manage their conflicts differently. Their conflicts are less "heated," they use disengagement more often with friends than with nonfriends, and equality is more evident between friends than nonfriends so that there are fewer "winner-loser" outcomes of the conflicts. Furthermore, following conflict, mutual friends are more likely than nonfriends to stay in physical proximity with each other and continue their social interactions (Hartup et al., 1988).

A question frequently raised about early child care is its effects on children's social development. There is not universal agreement on the nature and extent of the influence. Carollee Howes (1988), for example, maintains that child care, particularly for those children in stable peer groups, is beneficial for social development. She puts it this way: "Children who enter child care earlier appear to have an easier time with peers as preschoolers" (p. 69). On the other hand, Belsky and Rovine (1988) assert that for infants, twenty or more hours of nonparental child care results in insecure infant-attachment relationships. This early insecure attachment implies that such children may be at risk for later social development.

Implications So what are the implications of preschoolers' social interactions for parents and teachers? First, awareness is a key. Teachers, through observation, can be perceptive to and aware of peer interactions. Rather than merely accepting children's social classifications or friendship patterns for what they are, and rather than reinforcing children's social skills, (withdrawal, for example), teachers can recognize that they can and should help children in their social development and peer interactions.

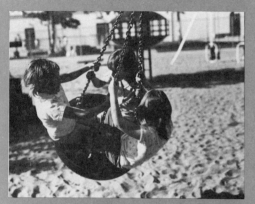

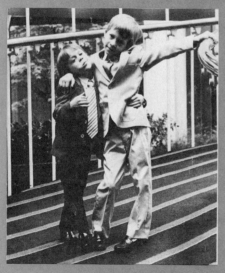

FIGURE 9-12 Preschoolers have many opportunities to learn many things in peer group situations. They make new friends; learn how to get along with others; learn new ideas and exchange different points of view; and, as a result, become less egocentric.

Second, preschool teachers can help children make friends. This can occur in part by arranging opportunities for children to work on projects and school activities together. Also, teachers can teach children skills for making friends. Children can learn many skills that will assist them in social interactions. For example, watch how socially adept preschoolers interact with others. They introduce themselves: "I'm Craig—what's your name?" They also make invitations to others: "Do you want to play?" These and others are the skills children can learn to help them socially.

Third, teachers, parents, and care-givers can model social skills for children. Their interactions with both adults and children set the tone for social interactions in preschools and child care centers.

Fourth, professionals can provide children with contexts within which it is possible to have positive social contacts and to make friends. When children are in small groups, they have a better chance of making friends than when they are constantly in large-group settings. This is why some parents and professionals are critical of large, impersonal child care programs. Adult-child ratios that encourage and foster children's social interactions are also important.

Furthermore, peer interaction fosters cognitive development by allowing children to acquire new skills and restructure their ideas through discussion. Collaboration in preschoolers can lead to greater learning than independent work. It would appear then that two heads are indeed better than one (Azmitia, 1988). The point is, however, that children have to have the opportunity to collaboratively work with each other, and they have to have preschool teachers who recognize the importance of such collaborative involvements.

Finally, with all the emphasis on conflict resolution and curriculum designed to teach preschool children conflict resolution strategies, it would seem that one of the best things parents, teachers, and care-givers can do for children is to teach them how to make friends. In the final analysis, teaching children how to make friends and how to be a friend may be one of the best things that can come from preschool programs.

SPECIAL NEEDS PRESCHOOLERS

All young children don't fit the description of the "normal" preschooler. Some children have physical and mental conditions that require special services and provisions for their education and care. These "special needs" children include the handicapped, those "at risk," the gifted, and those with multicultural heritages. All involved in the education and care of young children are interested in providing them with services that are appropriate to their physical, mental, social, and emotional abilities. In particular, professionals are interested in early intervention in order that children's development will not be delayed, to reduce family stress, and to lessen the likelihood of costly services later in life.

To provide for and facilitate services to handicapped children and their families, the federal government has passed two landmark pieces of legislation, Public Laws 94-142 and 99-457.

Public Law 94-142

Public Law 94-142, known as the Education for all Handicapped Children Act of 1975, has these important provisions:

- Provides for a *free* and *appropriate* education for all children between the ages of five and twenty-one, regardless of the nature and severity of their handicaps.
- Provides for an *individualized* and appropriate educational program that matches services to meet each child's unique educational need. The basis for this program is the IEP (Individualized Educational Plan). The IEP describes the child's current status, specifies educational goals and objectives, describes the special educational services that will be provided, and specifies evaluation criteria for determining if the objectives have been met.
- Provides that the child will be placed in the *least restrictive environment*, in other words, the one in which the child will benefit the most.
- Provides due process for children and their families. For example, parents have a right to question and challenge decisions made about their children, and parents may be represented by legal council.
- Provides for parent involvement in the development of educational policy and in developing and implementing children's IEPs.

Public Law 99-457

In 1986, Congress passed Public Law 99-457, the Education of the Handicapped Act Amendments. Two provisions of P.L. 99-457 are important in our discussion of preschool children.

First, the law establishes a preschool grant program that extends the rights of P.L. 94-142 to children between the ages of three and five. By the 1990–1991 school year, states applying for P.L. 94-142 funds will have to show that they are providing services to the three to five-year-old age group.

The second significant provision of P.L. 99-457 is the Handicapped Infants and Toddlers Program. This provision provides for services to handicapped and at-risk children from birth to age three *and* their families. Eligible children under this pro-

388 ■ CHAPTER NINE Learning and education in the preschool years

vision include (1) those experiencing developmental delays in one or more of the following areas: cognitive, physical, language and speech, psychosocial, or self-help skills, (2) those who have a physical or mental condition that has a high probability of resulting in a developmental delay (for example, Down syndrome and cerebral palsy) and (3) those at risk medically or environmentally for developmental delays. For example, environmental risk can include such things as poverty, child abuse, and parents who are themselves handicapped in some way.

In order to provide services to children, a multidisciplinary assessment is developed by a multidisciplinary team of professionals, who, with the parents, make recommendations regarding the child and family. Services to children can include special education, speech and language pathology and audiology, occupational therapy, physical therapy, psychological services, parent and family training and counseling services, transition services from one program or programs to another, diagnostic services, and health services.

Also, the infant and toddler provision of P.L. 99-457 provides that families may receive services as needed to facilitate in the development of their children. The Individualized Family Services Plan (IFSP) must contain the following:

1. A statement of the child's present levels of development (cognitive, speech/language, psychosocial, motor, self-help)
2. A statement of the families strengths and needs relating to enhancing the child's development
3. A statement of major outcomes expected to be achieved for the child and family
4. The criteria and procedures, and timeliness for determining progress
5. The specific early intervention services necessary to meet the unique needs of the child and family, including the method, frequency, and intensity of services
6. The projected dates for the initiation of services and their expected duration
7. Procedures for the transition from early intervention into preschool programs

Mainstreaming

The concept of the least restrictive environment means that handicapped children, regardless of their handicap, will be placed in a program that is most appropriate for them and in which they will benefit the most. The process of *mainstreaming* means then that special needs children will be placed in the least restrictive environment, where they will be educated and cared for in as normal a manner as possible. Figure 9–13 shows a continuum of settings from the least to the most restrictive.

1. Regular programs, with or without supportive services.
2. Regular programs plus supplementary instruction and support.
3. Part-time regular program and part-time special program.
4. Full-time special program placement.
5. Home-bound with home services.
6. Hospital, residential, or total care settings.

FIGURE 9-13 Services and programs for children with special needs are designed to occur in a least restrictive environment. The least restrictive environment is the regular program, whatever that may be. The most restrictive setting, on the other hand, is an institutional setting.

Matching Children's Needs to Setting Resources: The Match-up Matrix

A primary goal of all professionals who work with special needs children is to mainstream them into the least restrictive environment. Consequently, more special needs preschool children are being placed in regular program settings. However, a successful placement depends on many factors and this is how a match-up matrix is helpful.

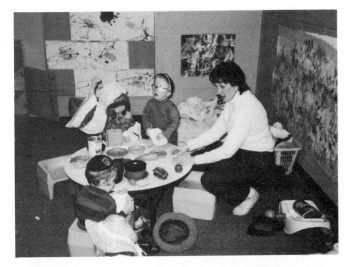

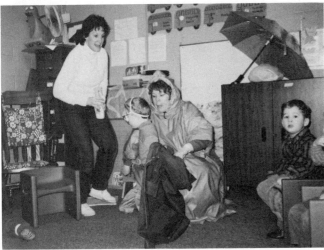

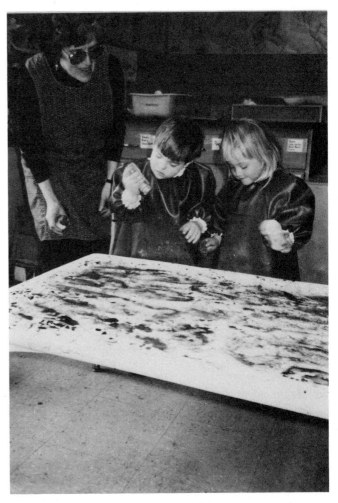

FIGURE 9-14 More attention than ever before is being given to children with special needs. These special-needs children are being mainstreamed into regular programs to the benefit of themselves and other children.

Following is a description of how a match-up matrix works in a real-life setting, as developed by Mary Ann Wilson, Director of The Early Childhood Program at Sullivan County (New York) Community College, and Barry H. Pehrsson, Administrator of the Southwinds Center, Middletown, New York.

Given the mandate to increase services for children with special needs, decisions will need to be made regarding the best program to serve a child's and a family's needs. How do parents decide which program is best for their child? How do programs decide if their services are appropriate for a specific child's needs? How do teachers and therapists decide when they should refer a child to another program? In short, how does one transition a child from early intervention services to early childhood education programs?

The match-up matrix allows parents, educators, therapists, and administrators to make these

TABLE 9–8

MATCH-UP MATRIX FOR ADAM AT SUNSHINE PRESCHOOL

Child Needs/ Setting Resources	Training	Specialists	Equipment and Materials	Appropriate Peers	Aide/ Helper	Action
Motor	− Traffic patterns; seating mobility	+ Therapist from hospital	+ Walker from home	− Not independent; some limits	N.A.	1
Language	+	N.A.	N.A.	+	N.A.	
Cognitive	+	N.A.	N.A.	+	N.A.	
Social	− Sharing independent play	N.A.	N.A.	+	N.A.	3
Self-help	− Independent dressing, toileting	N.A.	− Traffic patterns	+	N.A.	2
Behavior	+	N.A.	N.A.	+	N.A.	
Medical	− Information on seizures	N.A. Family doctor/ neurologist	N.A.	N.A.	N.A.	4
Home	− Teenage brother, parent demands	N.A.	N.A.	− No young siblings; no playmates	N.A.	

Note. A + indicates a child's needs can be met with current setting resources; a − indicates a setting resource need followed by action resource need. The numbers in the action column indicate priority: #1 is what staff will do first. N.A. is not applicable.

decisions based upon information rather than emotion, prejudice, assumptions, and/or false expectations. Quite simply, the setting resources are listed as they relate to an individual child's needs. The specific areas of need are also listed for the individual child. The team who is attempting to make a placement decision examines each need as compared with the setting resources to determine if there is a match in each category. Actions to meet any unmet needs are identified and assigned a priority. With this strategy, a decision can be made with concrete information regarding the program's abilities to meet the child's needs. An example follows.

Two-and-a-half year old Adam has been diagnosed with diplegic cerebral palsy (involvement of the lower extremities) with an accompanying seizure disorder resulting from a head injury he received in a car accident at eighteen months of age. Shortly after the accident, Adam received physical therapy through the hospital's outpatient services. On the recommendation of his therapist who continues to work with him regularly, Adam's parents are seeking to enroll him in a preschool.

Adam uses a walker to move around his environment. Though he is able to do many things easily, he often asks for help. His language and cognitive skills have been assessed at or above age-level; however, self-help skills have been affected by his gross motor delays. Though seizures occurred frequently after the accident, with daily medication there has been no recurrence except with a high fever. Adam relates well to adults, though he sometimes appears unnecessarily dependent upon them. Adam has limited opportunities to interact with children his own age. He has a teenage brother who seems to cater to him, both parents work, and a housekeeper/baby-sitter watches Adam in his home. Both parents are concerned about Adam's care and want him to be happy.

In the match-up matrix of Adam's needs and the preschool's resources, we see a match in many areas; nevertheless, a few actions are needed before the team can recommend that Adam enroll in the Sunshine Preschool (see Table 9–8). The greatest area of concern involves motor, with self-help as a close second. The use of a walker in a busy classroom is possible but the staff must organize the space differently for the ease of traffic patterns.

Adam's seating must be situated for easy use of the walker and planning is needed to make sure that Adam will be able to maneuver easily around the classroom, especially in small spaces such as the bathroom. The physical therapist has offered to come to the preschool to share suggestions for Adam's independence. As with many young children who have not attended school, Adam will need help to learn independent play skills and social skills with his peers. Though the parents have been assured that the seizure disorder is under control, the staff have requested specific information from the physician and neurologist to know what to expect and what to do if such an episode should occur.

As a result of the match-up matrix, the team has decided to take the actions identified in the order of priority. Once completed, the team agrees to recommend that Adam be enrolled in the Sunshine Preschool. A team conference is planned to review progress at the end of two months.

When Adam's parents visit the program for the meeting, they are amazed by how much Adam can do for himself. They are sending their teenage son to visit on his next school holiday and they are beginning to demand more independence in daily routines at home. Adam's physical therapist reports an increase in his progress in their weekly sessions, particularly in Adam's motivation, compliance, and pride in his achievements.

It is possible that the match-up matrix would show many areas where a match does not easily occur between a program's resources and the child's needs. In this case, it can be clearly seen why the specific team is not recommending enrollment for the child. Furthermore, the matrix can help the team identify programs or services that would be appropriate, as the child's needs have already been outlined. The match-up matrix also provides a clear definition of what skills or what setting resources are needed to make the most appropriate placement decision. Thus, if an individual child or program do not "match" at a particular time, it is possible to define under what conditions the placement might be considered. If the child or the program isn't "ready," the team can look forward to the time when the child is indeed "ready" for the program, and the program can prepare the most appropriate services for the child, within their resources.

Gifted Preschoolers

Gifted preschoolers may be the most neglected group of preschool special needs children. In order to provide programs for gifted preschoolers, they first must be identified. There are a cluster of personal and environmental characteristics that help identify young children who have the potential for being gifted. These are (Lewis & Michalson, 1985):

1. Cognitive abilities—curiosity, attention, and superior memory.
2. Language abilities—early use of sounds, first words, and speech.
3. Affective characteristics—pleasure in learning, positive self-concept, persistence, and task orientation.
4. Social knowledge and relationships—development of social knowledge (knowledge of others and their behaviors) and good socioemotional adjustment. (Young children who show signs of giftedness may have behavior problems, however.)
5. Family interaction and environment—Parental responses that provide experiences, support, and encouragement for learning and independence.
6. Demographic variables—birth order may be a factor in giftedness, since mothers give first-born children more attention and stimulation.

There are certain indicators of giftedness; the earliest sign is rapid development. Many gifted children do things earlier than their normal counterparts; they are very alert and interested in almost everything. Other indications of giftedness are:

1. Early learning of any kind.
2. Above-average curiosity.
3. Enhanced linguistic abilities, including an advanced vocabulary and a high frequency of questions.
4. Good memory skills.
5. Above average physical development and health.
6. Ability to concentrate for long periods of time.
7. Independence.

Teachers can encourage children who may be gifted in the following ways:

1. Provide opportunities for children to develop more advanced skills. In preschool programs, the curriculum enrichment approach is the preferred method of providing for the gifted. In this way, the gifted remain with their age peers and learn and develop appropriate social skills.
2. Enrichment provides opportunities for gifted children to have broader, kinds of experiences in areas related to a particular talent or ability.
3. Help gifted children in the areas in which they are not gifted.
4. Provide an environment in which gifted children can use their talents and abilities. The primary factor in helping children develop their potential for giftedness is an interactive environment that supports the development of their abilities.

PRESCHOOL ISSUES
The Developmentally Appropriate Curriculum

The development of public school programs for four-year-old children has created a number of issues. First is the issue of what to teach. Many critics of early schooling maintain the four-year-old children are not ready for academics, and that preschool programs should not be kindergarten programs redesigned for four-year-olds. Critics are worried about rushing young children into early academics.

The solution that has been most often suggested for this perceived danger is the *developmentally appropriate curriculum*, in which the needs and learning styles of children are the determiners of the instructional process. This means that in theory at least, there is no *predetermined* and set curriculum that *all* four-year-olds, regardless of ability or development level, must receive. In other words, "Pedagogy should not bow to chronology. Age does not define learning needs" (Futrell, 1987, p. 252).

"At Least Have Them on the Old Side"

Yet age is precisely the criteria that some opponents of early schooling would use as a determiner of whether or not children are ready for school. At issue here are two ways of determining age: chronological age and developmental age. *Chronological age* is the age of a child since birth, her age in years. *Developmental age*, also referred to as *behavior age*, indicates the behavior level that is average for a child's age.

The contemporary followers of Arnold Gesell (1928), such as Louise Bates Ames (1980), maintain that school placement should take place on the basis of developmental or behavior age rather than on the basis of chronological age. Developmental age for the purposes of school placement is generally determined through the use of a preschool readiness test, such as the *School Readiness Test* published by the Gesell Institute of Child Development (1978). The results of this and/or other tests and other data such as parents' and other teachers' observations are used to make decisions regarding children's entry into preschool, kindergarten, and first grade. Where such developmental evaluation does not occur, then Ames offers the following advice: "We encourage parents to allow their children to be among the oldest in their classes rather than the youngest" (Ames, 1987, p. 139). For those who advocate developmental placement, *development over time* is the factor that contributes to children's school readiness and for children who are not "ready" for schooling, time is the remedy.

Who Should Attend?

The issue of the age of children attending preschool is really part of the larger issue of *who* should attend preschools. Preschool programs for low-income and disadvantaged children seem to be a generally accepted proposition. However, the thought of universal, compulsory preschools for all four-year-olds meets general resistance. So social and class issues, as well as economic issues, are at work in any determination of public preschool programs accessible to all children.

Who Should Teach Preschoolers?

Child care and early childhood professionals see public school personnel as being unequipped, lacking in training, and not understanding of the issues involved in preschool education. There is a tremendous difference between three- and four-year-old, kindergarten, and first grade children. Younger children are more dependent on care-givers, and critics of the public schools maintain that the way public school teachers teach kindergarten children is inappropriate for preschool children.

Of course, there are many social and economic issues that underlie the main issue of who can best teach young children. As the public schools increasingly move into the education of four-year-old children, this means that some care-givers and aides will be displaced by higher paid and certified personnel.

Control is also an issue. As public schools take over the responsibility for preschools, they also control who teaches in them and how they will be operated.

Unrealistic Expectations

With the increase in the numbers of preschools, there may be the tendency for the public to expect too much of and from them. For example, given the economic benefits of preschools reported from the Perry Preschool Program, advocates may want preschools to be even more effective instruments of public policy. Thus, faced with too many and/or unrealistic expectations, preschools are at risk for failure.

What Would You Do?

Nancy Overholt considers herself a modern parent. She tries to keep abreast of all the latest child development information by reading books and magazines. Nancy recently enrolled in a course at the local junior college called "Helping Your Children Learn Through Toys and Games." After several classes, Nancy developed some serious concerns about toys and violence. In her last class, the professor concluded her lecture by saying, "A parent with any sense wouldn't let her children play with toy guns or any kind of war toys. We have got to teach our kids peace, not how to murder each other!" Nancy has tried to read as much as she can about the effects of toy guns and war toys on children, but she's confused by what seems to be conflicting evidence. Furthermore, one of her classmates, Gloria Yotraw, keeps cornering her during class breaks and wants her to join a local campus group called Students and Mothers United to End Violence.

Nancy's son, Daryl, will celebrate his fourth birthday in a month. Nancy is thinking about sending out birthday invitations with a note that says, "Since I believe that toy guns and war toys promote violence, please don't buy Daryl these kinds of presents." However, before Nancy sends out the invitations, she wants to talk with you in order to get your ideas and opinions. What are you going to say to Nancy?

*I*N THE SPOTLIGHT

CRISIS AND STRESS IN CHILDREN'S LIVES

Children are subjected to many personal crises and social stressors as they grow and develop. One way of conceptualizing the crises children face is to examine them in the context of Bronfenbrenner's (1979) model, which depicts children as influenced by personal, community, and national influences. (See also Chapter One.) Examples of stress and crisis at the personal level include illness, injury, rejection, abuse, and divorce. At the community level, gang violence, shoot-outs with drug dealers, moving, changing nursery schools, and community opposition to admitting children with AIDS to school are just a few of the many sources of stress and crisis. At the national level, stress and crises come from economic depression resulting in an altered standard of living, natural disasters, and wars and threats of wars (especially nuclear disasters).

Dimidjian (1986) suggests that adults have to assist children in developing adaptive behavior resulting in responsible and autonomous actions. In doing so, she outlines the following adult roles:

1. *Mediator*—The adult clarifies communication, provides correct information, and assists in the expression and understanding of affect.

2. *Information-provider*—The adult extends emotional support and straightforward, developmentally appropriate information that assists the child's intellectual understanding and psychological integration of feelings generated by the crisis.

3. *Buffer*—The stable adult acts as a buffer for stress, helping children recognize and understand feelings.

4. *Provider of coping strategies*—Adults can describe alternative actions as well as prepare and reassure children as they deal with crisis and stress.

5. *Referral source and facilitator*—Adults help parents and their children find professional help and services as necessary.

6. *Role model*—Adults provide for the observing child a model of proactive advocacy for and on behalf of children and their parents.

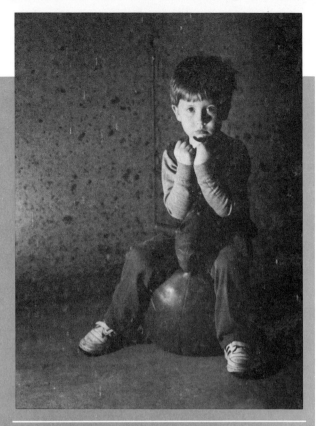

FIGURE 9-15 Today, children are experiencing more stress in their lives than ever before. Parents and teachers can help children deal with stress by reducing, as much as possible, the stressful situations children have to cope with and by teaching children specific stress reducing techniques.

SUMMARY

- Preschool enrollment is at an all-time high. In 1986, 2.6 million children ages three and over were attending a preschool. These enrollments will increase and projections through 1993 place preschool enrollment at 3.7 million children.
- Reasons for the increase in the popularity of preschools and preschool enrollments include disadvantaged children, working parents, and the high divorce rate. Also, the early years are considered by many to be important years for a number of reasons. They are the foundation of later school learning and are considered as years in which to address later school problems, such as failure and "dropping out."
- Our views of children help shape and determine how we care for and teach them. Likewise, how a nation views its children determines what kind of programs it is willing to provide and to what extent it is willing to support those programs. Some view children as: miniature adults, growing plants, competent, and future investments.
- A significant change in preschools in the past decade is the shift from a social-emotional-play orientation to an academic orientation. This reorientation results in part from the back-to-basics movement and parents' desires for their children to begin to learn early in life. Also, preschools and early learning are seen as ideal ways to intervene in the lives of children—often disadvantaged children and their families—as a means of preventing many of society's problems, such as crime, drugs, and the problem of school dropouts.
- Today, there are now many more kinds of preschool programs than there were in the past. This is because of the interest in preschool programs and the many agencies conducting and funding early childhood programs.
- Nursery schools provide for a full range of services and emphasize educational experiences. Most nursery schools conduct programs that provide for the *whole child* and place an emphasis on learning through play.
- Head Start is designed to provide a comprehensive developmental program for preschool children from low-income families. The overall goal is to promote social competence by providing children with opportunities to achieve their potential in cognitive, language, socioemotional, and physical development.
- Maria Montessori (1870–1952) developed one of the better-known and more influential preschool programs. Montessori programs are characterized by their use of sensory materials, their respect for children, helping children educate themselves, and a prepared environment in which children can learn for themselves.
- The Bank Street program of preschool education is a "child-centered" approach to learning and education. This developmental-interactionist program maintains that children's development, needs, and natures, should determine the goals, objectives, and teaching practices of early childhood programs.
- The High/Scope curriculum has its roots in Piaget's theory of cognitive development, and is based on the constructivist approach, which maintains that children literally construct their knowledge of the world and their level of cognitive functioning. The

teacher's role is to assist children in the natural process of inquiry, to arrange the classroom to promote active learning, to make plans and review activities with children, to interact with individual children, and to lead small- and large-group sessions. Two processes constitute the central core of the High/Scope program—the plan-do-review sequence and key experiences.

■ Increasingly, preschool professionals are using screening tests to help place children for instructional purposes and for identifying developmental delays. These tests include the Denver Developmental Screening Test (DDST), the Developmental Indicators for the Assessment of Learning–Revised (DIAL-R), and the Diagnostic Inventory for Screening Children (DISC). Parents and professionals should avoid being deterministic about screening results. Such results are, however, enlightening to professionals and parents in that they show what contributes to success and failure, and enable professionals to design programs to help children and their parents.

■ When preschool children participate in a high-quality program, research results indicate that they have higher academic achievement and higher achievement motivation, are placed less often in special education classes, experience fewer months of unemployment, have fewer incidents of delinquency, and experience less teenage pregnancy.

■ Language usage and development are critical for preschool and later life success. Today, the emphasis is on children's literacy development, and this process is viewed as beginning at birth. Also, the term *whole language* conveys the concept that language development, reading, writing, and speech are integrated, not separate processes.

■ The ability to communicate develops rapidly during the preschool years and involves the use of parental conversational styles, more attention to conversational rules, making specific requests, the use of ellipses, the use of appropriate linguistic reference, and learning language appropriate to routines, scripts, and rituals.

■ Some children have physical and mental conditions that require special services and provisions for their education and care. These special needs children include the handicapped, the "at risk," the gifted, and those with multicultural heritages. To provide for and facilitate services to handicapped children and their families, the Federal government has passed two landmark pieces of legislation, P.L. 94-142 and 99-457.

■ One way professionals attempt to meet the needs of special needs children is through *mainstreaming* or placing special needs children in the least restrictive environment, where they will be educated and cared for in as normal a manner as possible. Also, providing for special needs children includes matching their needs to the setting resources. This is accomplished in part through a match-up matrix.

■ Gifted preschoolers may be one of the most neglected groups of special needs children. More efforts are being made to identify and provide for gifted preschoolers. Teachers and others need to be alert to the characteristics of giftedness in children.

■ There are a number of current and controversial issues involved in preschool education. These include how to design and implement curricula and activities that are developmentally appropriate; who should attend preschools; who should teach preschoolers; and the appropriate expectations for preschool programs.

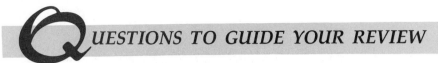

QUESTIONS TO GUIDE YOUR REVIEW

1. Preschool children have changed in a number of ways over the last several decades. Review these changes and tell what implications they have for how children are cared for and reared.
2. What are the reasons for increases in preschool enrollments and the popularity of preschools?
3. What are some current popular views that adults have of children? How do these views influence how adults rear and educate children?
4. What are the reasons why many preschools have adopted an academic orientation to their curricula and activities?
5. What are the primary features of a nursery school program? How is a good nursery school program different from other preschool programs?
6. What is the primary purpose of Head Start? How are the educational objectives of Head Start different from the objectives of other programs?
7. What are the distinguishing features of a Montessori program? What are the purposes of the sensory materials in a Montessori program?
8. How and why is the Bank Street program child-centered? In what ways is the Bank Street Program similar to and different from other programs?
9. What forms the basis of the High/Scope curriculum? What are the key features of this program?
10. What are transitions and why are they important in children's lives?
11. What are the purposes of developmental screening?
12. What are some frequently used developmental screening tests?
13. In what ways do quality preschools make a difference in children's later lives?
14. What can parents and teachers do to enhance preschoolers' language development?
15. Why are preschool teachers emphasizing literacy development and the whole language approach to literacy?
16. How can parents and teachers facilitate children's social development?
17. What are the major provisions of P.L. 92-142 and 99-457?
18. What should teachers and parents look for as identifying characteristics of the gifted?
19. How can parents and others facilitate the development of gifted children?
20. What can parents and teachers do to help children deal with stress?

ACTIVITIES FOR FURTHER INVOLVEMENT

1. Increasingly, preschools are playing larger roles in the lives of children and their parents.

   a. Based on research and the recommendations of professional organizations, develop goals for a preschool program. Make sure that you account for all of the developmental areas: cognitive, language, physical, and psychosocial.

   b. Interview parents of preschool children. Identify what they think are desirable qualities and characteristics of preschool programs. How do these compare with standards set by early childhood educators?

2. There are many different program models for educating preschoolers.

   a. Observe in preschool programs that use the Montessori system, a play-oriented approach, and a cognitively-oriented curriculum. Tell which you think is best and why.

   b. Why are "models" of preschool education so popular?

3. *Developmentally appropriate* is a term used with increasing frequency in early childhood programs.

   a. Explain what *developmentally appropriate* means and provide examples for its application in the classroom and home.

   b. Observe in preschools and child care centers in order to identify developmentally appropriate and inappropriate practice. Give specific answers.

4. The topic of early learning is a controversial issue.

   a. What are the major issues involved in the topic of early learning?

   b. Interview parents and develop position statements for and against early learning.

   c. How does the trend toward early academics play a role in the early learning controversy?

5. One of the hallowed and accepted traditions of early childhood education is that learning occurs through play.

   a. Observe in preschool settings and identify specific instances in which children did and did not learn through play.

   b. Identify what parents and preschool teachers can do to promote learning through play.

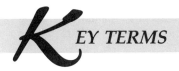

*K*EY TERMS

Boarder babies Young, homeless children living in municipal shelters.

Early intervention The process of addressing root causes of later school and life problems as early as possible.

Emerging literacy The idea that the foundations of literacy begin in early childhood and that becoming literate is a continual process begun early in life.

Literacy The ability to read, write, and speak.

Whole language The concept that language development, reading, writing and speech are not separate and unrelated processes, and should be treated as an integrated whole.

ENRICHMENT THROUGH FURTHER READING

Morrison, G. S. (1988). *Early childhood education today* (4th ed.). Columbus, OH: Merrill.
A comprehensive overview of early childhood education philosophy, theory, and curriculum. Particularly useful are chapters on Montessori, Piaget, child care, and preschool programs. An excellent book as an introduction to the field of early childhood education.

Morrison, G. S. (1988). *Education and development of infants, toddlers, and preschoolers.* Glenview, IL: Scott, Foresman/Little, Brown.
An interesting and informative explanation of how developmental theory relates to classroom and program practice. Contains many interesting program vignettes as well as practical suggestions for parents, teachers, and care-givers.

Warger, C. (Ed.). (1988). *A resource guide to public school early childhood programs.* Alexandria, VA: Association for Supervision and Curriculum development.
This informative book enables the reader to learn about the issues and various points of view associated with increasing demands for preschool programs. Also has a section which describes preschool programs around the United States.

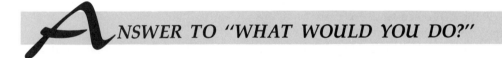

ANSWER TO "WHAT WOULD YOU DO?"

First, you have an obligation to tell Nancy some of the issues and information involved:

Research suggests that guns increase the chances of doing serious injury, and also heighten some people's instigation of aggression (Turner, Simons, Berkowitz, & Frodi, 1977).

The ready availability of handguns in the home and their accessibility to children are two contributing factors in the unintentional firearm deaths of young children by young children (Wintemute, Teret, Kraus, Wright, & Bradfield, 1987).

Look-alike toy guns are a special problem for parents and law enforcement agencies. In some cases, children think all guns are alike because many toy guns look like the real thing. In some instances, police have shot children because the guns they were playing with looked real. As a result, many cities have banned the sale of toy gun look-alikes. Furthermore, some national retailers of children's toys are phasing out their sale of toy gun look-alikes (*Discount Store News*, 1988).

Children do need to learn how to solve problems in nonaggressive ways. However, this means that they have to be taught prosocial and conflict resolution skills that will enable them to solve their differences in nonviolent ways. Some ways that parents and professionals can teach and model nonviolent conflict resolution skills are by encouraging positive social relationships in interactions with adults and children; providing opportunities for children to share, take turns, form friendships, and be cooperative; promoting the use of language to express feelings (instead of hitting) as a means of resolving conflicts; teaching the use of language to express positive as well as negative feelings; and encouraging children to learn how to say "I'm sorry."

Your best advice to Nancy is that how parents feel about guns, their purpose, and use is a matter of individual values and beliefs. Therefore, Nancy is justified in her views and is certainly justified in sending out the invitations requesting no toy guns or war toys. Since Nancy believes that toy guns can cause violence in children's lives, she should also examine the roll and place of guns in her family setting. You can advise Nancy about the risks to children associated with keeping guns in her home. Since Nancy is concerned about the use of guns, you can assume that this would mean that she should also be concerned about the risks of handgun ownership.

Additionally, you can encourage Nancy to critically examine other forms of violent influences in Daryl's life. The violent content of television and movies can teach children the wrong lessons about how to deal with life's problems. Consequently, Nancy may also want to monitor her son's television viewing.

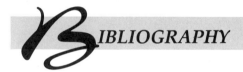

BIBLIOGRAPHY

Amdur, J. M., Mainland, M. C., & Parker, K. C. H. (1984). *Diagnostic inventory for screening children.* San Antonio, TX: The Psychological Corporation.

Ames, L. B. (1987). Respect for readiness. In Eileen Shiff (Ed.), *Experts advise parents.* New York: Delacorte, pp. 123–145.

Ames, L. B., & Chase, J. A. (1980). *Don't push your preschooler.* New York: Harper & Row.

Archambault, R. D. (Ed.). (1964). *John Dewey on education—Selected writings.* New York: Random House.

Azmitia, M. (1988). Peer interaction and problem solving: When are two heads better than one? *Child Development, 59,* 87–96.

Belsky, J., & Rovine, M. J. (1988). Nonmaternal care in the first year of life and the security of infant-parent attachment. *Child Development, 59,* 157–167.

Berrueta-Clement, J. R., Schweinhart, L. J., Barnett, W. S., Epstein, A. S., & Weikart, D. P. *Changed lives: The effects of the Perry preschool program on youths through age 19.* Ypsilanti, MI: The High/Scope Press.

Biber, B. (1984). *Early education and psychological development.* New Haven: Yale University Press.

Bronfenbrenner, U. (1979). *The ecology of human development: Experiments by nature and design.* Cambridge, MA: Harvard University Press.

Bureau of Labor Statistics, U.S. Department of Labor. (1988). Telephone interview with Howard Hayghe, June 2, 1988.

Bus, A. G., & van Ijzendoorn, M. H. (1988). Mother-child interactions, attachment, and emergent literacy: A cross-sectional study. *Child Development, 59*, 1262–1272.

DeVries, R. (1987). *Programs of early education: The constructivist view.* New York: Longman.

Dimidjian, V. J. (1986). Helping children in times of trouble and crisis. *Journal of children in contemporary society, 17*, 113–128.

Discount Store News. (1988, May 9). p. 85.

Elkind, D. (1986). Formal education and early education: An essential difference. *Phi Delta Kappan, 67*, 634.

Fowler, M. G., & Cross, A. W. (1986). Preschool risk factors as predictors of early school performance. *Developmental and Behavioral Pediatrics, 7*, 237–241.

Frankenburg, W. K., Sciarillo, W., & Burgess, D. (1981). The newly abbreviated and revised Denver developmental screening test. *The Journal of Pediatrics, 99*, 995–999.

Futrell, M. H. (1987). Public schools and four-year-olds. *American Psychologist, 42*, 251–253.

Gesell, A. (1928). *Infancy and human growth.* New Haven, CT: Gesell Institute of Human Development.

Gesell Institute of Human Development. (1978). *Preschool readiness test.* New Haven, CT: Author.

Hartup, W. W., Laursen, B., Stewart, M. I., & Eastenson, A. (1988). Conflict and the friendship relations of young children. *Child Development, 59*, 1590–1600.

Homann, M., Banet, B., & Weikart, D. P. (1979). *Young children in action.* Ypsilanti, MI: The High/Scope Press.

Howes, C. (1988). *Peer interaction of young children. Monographs of the Society for Research in Child Development, 53* (1, Serial No. 217).

Kamii, C. (1981). Application of Piaget's theory to education: The preoperational level. In I. Sigel, D. M. Brodzinsky, & R. M. Golinkoff (Eds.), *New directions in Piagetian theory and practice.* Hillsdale, NJ: Lawrence Erlbaum.

Kuhn, D. (1981). The role of self-directed activity in cognitive development. In I. Sigel, D. M. Brodzinsky, & R. M. Golinkoff (Eds.), *New directions in Piagetian theory and practice.* Hillsdale, NJ: Lawrence Erlbaum, 353–363.

Lewis, M., & Michalson, L. (1985). The gifted infant. In J. Freeman (Ed.), *The psychology of gifted children.* New York: John Wiley.

Mardell-Czudnowski, C., & Goldenberg, D. (1983). *DIAL-R: Developmental indicators for the assessment of learning—revised.* Edison, NJ: Childcraft.

Morrison, G. (1988). *Early childhood education today,* (4th ed.). Columbus, OH: Charles E. Merrill.

Morrison, G. S. (1988). *Education and development of infants, toddlers and preschoolers.* Glenview, IL: Scott, Foresman.

National Center for Health Statistics. (1988). *Advanced report of final divorce statistics, 1985* (Monthly Vital Statistics Report, Vol. 36, No. 8 Supplement, DHHS Publication No. (PHS) 88-1120). Hyattesville, MD: Author.

Newman, J. M. (1985). *Whole language: Theory in use.* Portsmouth, NH: Heinemann.

Save the Children Federation. (1985). *Hard choices: Portraits of poverty and hunger in America.* Westport, CT: Author.

Schatz, M. (1983). Communication. In J. H., Flavell & E. M. Markman (Eds.), *Cognitive development: Vol. 3 of Handbook of child psychology.* (4th ed.), New York: John Wiley, pp. 858–871.

The statistical trends. (1985, May). *The Principal, 64,* 16.

Stein, A. (1987, January 17). New York's poor children: A tinderbox. *New York Times,* p. 27.

Turner, C. W., Simons, L. S., Berkowitz, L., and Frodi, A. (1977). The stimulating and inhibiting effects of weapons on aggressive behavior. *Aggressive Behavior, 3,* 355–378.

U.S. Bureau of the Census. (1988). Telephone interview with Paul Siegel, June 2, 1988, regarding the Current Population Survey, October, 1986.

U.S. Department of Health and Human Services. (1984, November). *Head Start performance standards* (45-CFR 1304) Washington, DC: U.S. Government Printing Office.

Weikart, D., & Tompkins, M. (1988, February). Introduction to the High/Scope curriculum. A paper distributed at the Florida Leadership Conference, Tampa, Florida.

Wintemute, G. J., Teret, S. P., Kraus, J., Wright, M. A., & Bradfield, G. (1987). When children shoot children. *Journal of the American Medical Association, 257,* 3107–3109.

CHAPTER TEN

Middle childhood: development during the elementary school years

VIGNETTES
INTRODUCTION
PHYSICAL DEVELOPMENT
Physical Appearances—Obesity
Weight Reduction
Implications for Parents
NUTRITION DURING THE
  MIDDLE YEARS
Good Nutrition
MOTOR DEVELOPMENT
Large Muscle Development
In the Spotlight: Little League
  Baseball
Fine Motor Development
COGNITIVE DEVELOPMENT
Concrete Operational Skills
Family Influences on Cognitive
  and Affective Development

LANGUAGE DEVELOPMENT
Vocabulary Development
Phonological Development
Use of Sentences
Implications for Parents and
  Teachers
PSYCHOSOCIAL DEVELOPMENT
Implications for Parents and Care-
  Givers
AGGRESSION
What Would You Do?
PEER RELATIONSHIPS
Friendships
Shyness
PSYCHOSEXUAL DEVELOPMENT
Differences Between the Sexes
In the Spotlight: Why Do Boys Do
  Better in Math than Girls?

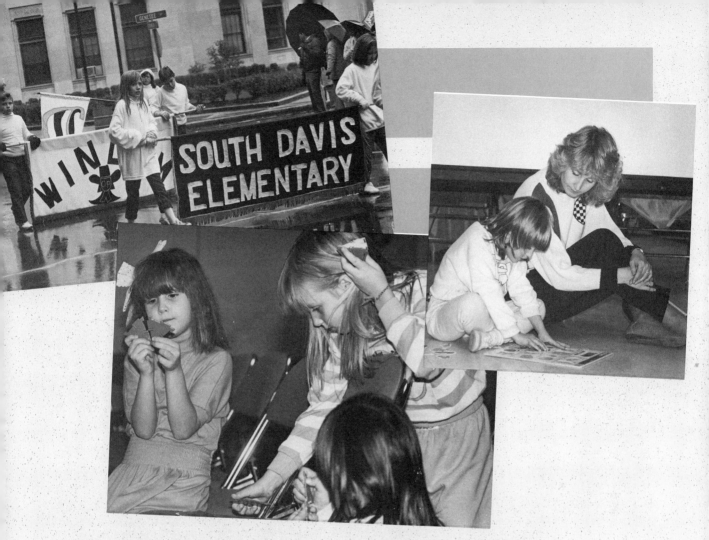

Could Mind Sex Be the Answer?
In the Spotlight: Is Biology
   Destiny or Can We Have
   Androgyny, Too?
MORAL DEVELOPMENT
Piaget's Stages of Moral Thinking
Kohlberg's Levels of Moral Growth
Implications for Teachers
In a Different Voice: The Voice of
   Carol Gilligan
GIFTED CHILDREN
Public Policy and State Definitions
   of Giftedness
Eligibility Criteria
In the Spotlight: Understanding

Measurement Terms
System of Multicultural Pluralistic
   Assessment (SOMPA)
Programs for the Gifted
SUMMARY
QUESTIONS TO GUIDE YOUR
   REVIEW
ACTIVITIES FOR FURTHER
   INVOLVEMENT
KEY TERMS
ENRICHMENT THROUGH
   FURTHER READING
ANSWER TO "WHAT WOULD
   YOU DO?"
BIBLIOGRAPHY

VIGNETTES

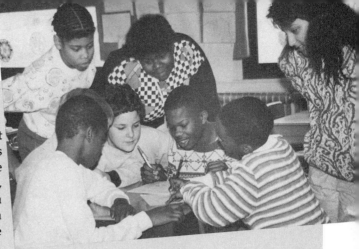

Ten-year-old Aram attends the fifth grade at Calaway Elementary School. Aram likes school, is an average student, and his favorite subjects are math and art. Aram's art teacher, Mrs. Rodriguez, says, "Aram has a talent for art." Aram spends a lot of time drawing, especially football players in action, and whenever he goes to a movie, he usually sketches several of the actors from memory. Aram is also very interested in sports. He took judo lessons for three years and earned an orange belt. He stopped taking judo lessons because it was inconvenient for his parents to get him there. As his mother says, "With all the things the two other children are involved in, it was just too much of a hassle, what with me working and all."

Six months ago Aram started playing baseball. He plays shortstop for the Tigers, a team in a local Optimist league. At this age, Aram is very attached to his father, Hector. They are both involved in sports, and Hector makes a point of practicing with his son at least two times a week. Aram wants to be a football player when he grows up—or he may be a policeman. Hector's cousin is a policeman and Aram is impressed by his manner and uniform. But for now, Aram is mainly interested in playing the latest computer games, going to baseball practice, and drawing pictures of athletes.

Twelve-year-old Buster Raines and his ten-year-old cousin, Lester, walk across the dusty, barren, litter-strewn patch of land that separates two housing projects in a low-income, inner-city residential complex. Suddenly, the duo hears what sounds like gunfire and they duck their heads and run for cover. Such flights for cover are a normal part of Buster's life. In fact, he seems to have grown accustomed to violence and the threats it brings. Buster brags, "Shootin' don't scare me man—if I had a gun, I'd shoot back!"

Instead of ducking bullets, Buster should be in the sixth grade at P.S. 215 two blocks up the street, but he doesn't have much time for school.

Buster has started standing security for the Blackrock Warriors, the gang that controls the drug traffic in the two housing projects. It is doubtful that Buster will attend much school, for his world is now focused on earning money and living life within the code of conduct that governs gang life.

Buster's mother doesn't want him to be involved in the gangs, but she's apathetically resigned to it. She complains, "I keep telling Buster, 'Don't you get mixed up with those people,' but I know it don't do no good to tell him nothing, he's gonna do it anyhow."

Eight-year-old Craig Orvieto weighs sixty-four pounds, is forty-six inches tall and is a head shorter than all the other members of his second grade class. Craig is often described as a "miniature fullback." Craig attends Elmhurst Elementary School and is an above average student. Craig is in the top reading and math groups of his class. His teacher, Mrs. Evans, says, "I just love Craig because he is eager to learn and he does a lot of things to help around the classroom. He is a such a good sport, too. Last month he lost the class election for president, but he congratulated the boy that won and has just gone on about his business. Craig also really knows right from wrong."

Craig enjoys going to school and says, "I like school because the teachers are nice and I have a lot of good friends. The sports teachers teach us sports that I've never played before, like four-way soccer. I also like math because the teacher teaches us math that I've never learned before. I learn more things in math than in any other subject."

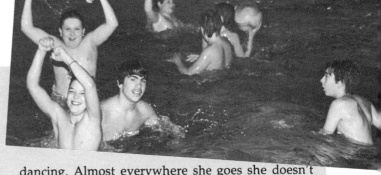

Craig's favorite activity and pastime is baseball. He memorizes baseball facts from books, loves to watch baseball on television, and will talk baseball to anyone willing to listen. For his eighth birthday, Craig's parents sent him to a week-long baseball camp sponsored by the local university. Craig is so involved in baseball that when he grows up, he wants to sell baseball cards and play baseball. Craig also collects baseball cards and has a complete 1988 Tops collection. Craig also has a Jose Canseco rookie card. "This card is the best in my collection," brags Craig. "It's worth about $100.00. I know because my dad helped me look it up in a baseball card book."

The thing that people notice first about Abigail Morris is her red hair. It immediately makes her special in peoples' eyes, and her tresses set her apart from other children. Abigail is used to people talking to her about her gorgeous hair and how beautiful it makes her look. Although Abigail sometimes feels self-conscious about the constant attention, she does enjoy being noticed, and, if the truth were known, she would miss not getting the compliments.

Abigail is ten years old, four feet eight inches tall, and weighs seventy-five pounds. She is in the fourth grade at Wesley Elementary School, which is her "home base school." Two days a week she attends Sunnydale School, a program for gifted children operated by the school district. Abigail fits the typical profile of a gifted child. She has a high intelligence; her parents won't say how high, just that it is "very high." Abigail is articulate, curious, highly motivated, sensitive, one or more grade levels above the average in all her school subjects, and very comfortable in the gifted program. Abigail says, "The gifted program gives me the freedom to do my own thing. I'm accepted for who I am. Also, I like the less structured environment here at Sunnydale. I get to pick the subjects I want to take and I get to set my own schedule. It's a lot of fun!"

Abigail swims, takes art classes, plays the violin, and dabbles in cartooning—she has created a cartoon dog. Most of all, though, Abigail enjoys dancing. Almost everywhere she goes she doesn't walk or run—she dances. When people ask her what she wants to be when she grows up, she responds without hesitation, "A professional dancer."

According to her parents, if Abigail has a major fault it is that she is interested in *everything*. She gets interested in something for a while and then loses interest. But this is something the Morris' are able and willing to overlook, for Abigail, an only child, fits their ideal. As her mother, Karen, says, "I always wanted to be the mother of a girl. I realize now Abigail is everything I wanted in a daughter. She is bright, talented, and sensitive. I couldn't ask for more."

At six years of age, Jonathan Greenberg is well on his way to his ultimate goal of earning a black belt in karate. Jonathan started taking karate lessons because other kids were picking on him in kindergarten. Today, instead of picking on Jonathan, the kids in his first grade class seek him out as a leader and someone with whom they want to be. Although Jonathan knows that "karate is just for self defense," his parents nonetheless are quick to extol the benefits it has had in Jonathan's life. "It has improved his self-confidence to the point where Jonathan now believes there is nothing he can't do," says his father, Sam. His mother, Sarah, is quick to add, "We never pushed Jonathan into karate; it was something he wanted to do so he could defend himself from the other kids. Karate has had a real positive impact on his life. His self-esteem is better and he's much more popular at school." Jonathan's teacher agrees. "He's one of the best students—if not the best student—I have. There is nothing he won't do or attempt to do. He is a very bright child. He's going to go far. If karate is what has done it, then I recommend it to other parents."

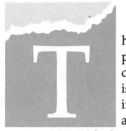

The middle years are the years between preschool and adolescence when children are five to twelve years old. This is the time period when children are in kindergarten through sixth grade and attend elementary school. However, with the growing popularity of middle schools (see Chapter Eleven), more children in grades five and six are going to school with seventh and eighth graders. Kindergarten children, five- and six-year-olds are discussed in this chapter, and kindergarten programs in Chapter Eleven, because of the increasing inclusion of compulsory kindergarten as part of public schooling. With most five- and six-year-old children enrolled in a public school kindergarten of some kind, it is no longer appropriate to classify kindergarten as a preschool program.

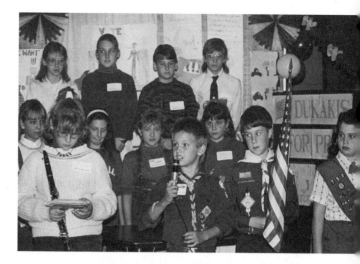

FIGURE 10-1   **During the early part of the middle childhood years boys are a little taller and heavier than girls. However, beginning at about ages 9 and 10, girls begin the early phase of their growth spurt and out gain boys in both height and weight.**

PHYSICAL DEVELOPMENT

A number of interesting physical developments are recognizable in middle childhood children. (See Table 10–1.) From ages five to seven, children's weight and height approximate each other. For example, at age six, boys weigh forty-six pounds and are forty-six inches tall, while girls weigh forty-three pounds and are forty-five inches tall. Up to age nine, the weight of boys and girls tends to be the same. However, beginning at age nine, girls start to pull ahead of boys in both height and weight. This is normal in the sense that girls begin their growth spurt a year or two ahead of boys, so that by the end of the elementary grades, girls are generally taller and heavier than boys.

By the end of the middle years, children's physical appearances tend to resemble more the characteristics of adults. However, because some parts of the body may grow faster than others, they may look out of proportion and gangly. This unevenness in physical development is known as *asynchrony.*

TABLE 10–1

AVERAGE (FIFTIETH PERCENTILE) WEIGHT AND HEIGHT NORMS FOR MIDDLE CHILDHOOD CHILDREN				
	Males		Females	
Years	Weight (Pounds)	Height (Inches)	Weight (Pounds)	Height (Inches)
5.0	41	43	39	43
5.5	43	45	41	44
6.0	46	46	43	45
6.5	48	47	45	46
7.0	50	48	48	48
7.5	53	49	51	49
8.0	56	50	55	50
8.5	59	51	58	50
9.0	62	52	63	52
9.5	65	53	67	53
10.0	69	54	71	54
10.5	73	55	76	56
11.0	78	56	81	57
11.5	82	58	86	58
12.0	88	58	91	60

TABLE 10-2

	Girls: Percentiles			Boys: Percentiles		
PERCENTILE WEIGHTS (IN POUNDS) FOR OBESE GIRLS AND BOYS						
Age in years	75th	90th	95th	75th	90th	95th
6.0	47.25	52.75	56.75	49.50	53.50	58.00
7.0	53.25	60.50	65.50	55.00	60.25	66.50
8.0	61.50	70.75	76.50	61.50	68.50	76.00
9.0	71.50	83.00	89.50	69.25	78.50	87.75
10.0	82.75	96.25	104.00	78.50	90.00	99.75
11.0	94.50	110.25	119.00	89.00	102.75	113.50
12.0	106.00	123.50	134.00	101.00	116.25	128.00
13.0	116.75	135.50	148.25	114.25	130.25	143.25
14.0	125.75	145.50	161.00	128.50	144.50	159.00
15.0	133.00	153.25	171.50	142.75	158.50	174.50
16.0	137.25	158.00	178.50	155.00	172.00	188.75
17.0	138.75	159.50	181.75	163.50	184.25	201.25
18.0	138.50	159.25	181.75	167.75	195.00	211.00

Note. From *Nelson Textbook of Pediatrics* (12th ed., pp. 30–31) by R.E. Behrman and V.C. Vaughan, III, 1983, Philadelphia, PA: W.B. Saunders. Copyright 1983 by W.B. Saunders. Adapted by permission.

Physical Appearances—Obesity

How many times have you heard a child being teased because he is overweight? You undoubtedly felt sorry for the teased child and wished that there was something you could do. What is obesity, what causes it, and what can parents and others do to help those who are obese? *Obesity* is defined by body weight, normed for height, age, and sex, which exceeds the ninetieth percentile (Johnson & Corrigan, 1987). (See Table 10–2.)

Obesity is a problem facing as many as 10 to 20 percent of school-age children (Anspaugh, Ezell, & Goodmann, 1987, p. 13). It is difficult to set one absolute standard for obesity since children have different builds and body shapes, but it is generally evident in the eye of the beholder.

Have you ever asked yourself why children are fat? Many reasons are given for obesity; some of these include psychological, cultural, physiological, and genetic influences. Family eating patterns and physical activity also play a role in obesity. (Anspaugh et al., pp. 12–13). A child

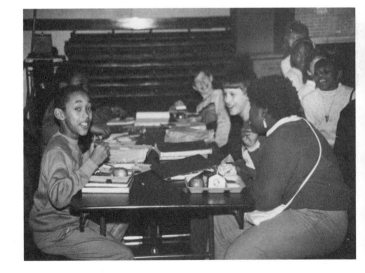

FIGURE 10-2 In years past, a fat baby was thought to be a healthy baby. No more. Today, with over 10% of school-age children in the obese category, there is an emphasis on helping all children learn and practice habits relating to good nutrition and exercise that will enable them to lead a healthy life.

reared in a family in which overeating and snacking are routine will have a harder time maintaining her ideal weight than will a child living in a family where such habits are not the norm. Also, you have no doubt heard a great deal about "couch potatoes," children and adults who snack while they sit in front of the television for long periods of time. These people are more prone to being overweight.

There are basically two schools of thought regarding the causes of obesity. One maintains that obese people are the way they are because of overeating. According to this point of view, then, the solution to obesity is to provide people the help they need so that they don't overeat.

A second opinion regarding the cause of obesity maintains that its roots are physiological and hereditary. There is a strong correlation between the obesity of parents and the obesity of their children. By age seventeen, the children of obese parents have three times the chance of being obese as the children of lean parents (Woolston, 1987). The metabolic theory of obesity is gaining more acceptance as new studies (Kolata, 1988) show that obese people have low metabolic rates. *Metabolism* is the rate at which the body transforms food into energy. This metabolism view also suggests that obesity has a physiological basis and tends to run in families.

TABLE 10–3

WEIGHT REDUCTION PROGRAM FOR CHILDREN AND ADOLESCENTS

Lesson 1: Should you lose weight?
- Thin-crazy and fat facts
- How much overweight are you?
- Why are you overweight?
- Can you lose weight safely and permanently?

Lesson 2: Measuring current eating and exercise habits
- An objective look at your eating and exercise
- Developing a positive attitude

Lesson 3: Beginning to change
- Decreasing eating situations
- Scheduling meals
- Limiting snacking
- Focusing on hunger feelings
- Exercising regularly

Lesson 4: Food, nutrition, and weight
- How to eat a balanced diet
- Keeping track of calories
- Making eating a pure experience
- Eating only in eating places
- Increasing exercise

Lesson 5: Calorie reductions
- Estimating daily energy requirements
- Eating deliberately
- Rewarding yourself for changes in eating and exercise

Lesson 6: Useful thoughts and images
- Making eating areas distinctive
- Using aversive imagery to reduce snacking
- Developing positive thoughts

Lesson 7: Becoming an assertive eater
- Appreciating your food
- Eating in social situations

Lesson 8: Coping with stress
- Using relaxation to cope with stress and curb emotional eating

Lesson 9: Goals and problem solving
- Effective problem solving

Note. From "The Behavioral Treatment of Child and Adolescent Obesity" by W.G. Johnson and S.A. Corrigan, 1987, *Journal for Child and Adolescent Psychotherapy, 4,* p. 97.

The relation of obesity to heredity is one that has intrigued researchers for a long time. Now they may have come up with another piece to the obesity puzzle. Researchers think that abnormally low levels of a protein, *adipsin*, may be the culprit, by affecting appetite and metabolism (Kolata, 1989). Researchers have found that animals that are obese for genetic or metabolic reasons have low levels of adipsin. While this relationship is proven to exist only in animals at the present time, the discovery of such a link further strengthens the belief that obesity is inherited. Such a discovery could mean that people with obesity could be treated with adipsin.

Weight Reduction

Of course, the problem of how to lose weight is one that confronts all who are overweight. Table 10–3 outlines a weight reduction program for children and adolescents.

IMPLICATIONS FOR PARENTS

Parents cannot abandon their parental responsibilities when it comes to helping their children lose weight *and* practice good nutrition. Following are some things parents can do to help their children in their efforts to lose and control their weight (Rubin, 1988). Parents should:

- Examine their own eating habits. Parents can be a good role model for their children as far as food and eating habits are concerned. For example, parents should not help themselves to fattening desserts while admonishing their children for not being able to resist desserts.

- Seek professional advice about the diets their children should follow.
- Clear most of the sweets and fattening foods out of the house so children will not be tempted while they are dieting.
- Restrict the amount of time children watch television and establish limits on what children can eat while watching television.
- Be an ally with children in their battle to lose weight.
- Remember that the success or failure of children to lose weight hinges on inner motivation.

NUTRITION DURING THE MIDDLE YEARS

I'm sure you have heard the saying, "Breakfast is the best meal of the day." But what does this mean? Does it mean that it is the best-tasting meal of the day, or does it mean that it makes more difference than the other two meals of the day? This saying has been interpreted by many teachers to mean that children who eat breakfast do better in school. But is this interpretation an accurate one? As of now, we have to say that we are not sure. One study found that there is no difference in the *test* performance of breakfast eaters and non–breakfast eaters (Dickie & Bender, 1982). On the other hand, in another study children's performance on a continuous performance test was measured at 9:50 AM, 11:00 AM, and 12:10 PM. The results indicated that as the morning progressed, both the breakfast eaters and the non–breakfast eaters made more errors, and their performances were more variable. However, the

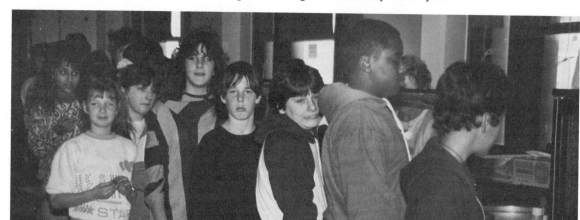

FIGURE 10-3   Good eating habits begin at birth and must continue through the school years. Many elementary schools have programs designed to teach good nutritional habits. Many school cafeterias are reexamining their menus and food service practices to emphasize better eating habits.

children who ate breakfast (milk, cereal with sugar, egg, juice, and toast) made fewer errors and were less variable than those children who did not eat breakfast (Connors & Blouin, 1983). So, *when* a teacher teaches something to her students may be as important as *what* her students did or didn't have for breakfast.

What implications does this information have for professional practice? There are several. First, a breakfast as part of a program of services for all children whose economic background and family life-style demand it is a legitimate programmatic effort to enhance their health and nutritional status. Second, what children eat and when they eat it are important nutritional and educational concerns. Perhaps for some children, a mid-morning snack, as practiced in many preschool programs, would be also beneficial to children in the elementary grades. Third, just as we stress the need to be aware of children's cognitive and affective needs,

so also must we be aware of their nutritional needs. For some children, going without breakfast may not interfere with their morning's activities. For other children, going without breakfast may prevent them from doing the best they can.

Good Nutrition

Parents and care-givers need to help children develop good nutritional habits early in life. This can be accomplished in part by helping children learn what constitutes good nutrition and by helping them monitor their eating habits. Table 10-4 shows a food guide for children ages four to ten. Frequently children and their parents forget how many calories are in certain foods and the sodium and sugar content of those foods. These are often greater than we realize. Table 10-5 shows the sugar content of selected foods.

TABLE 10–4

Food Group	Recommended Number of Servings	Average Serving Size
BASIC FOUR FOOD GUIDE FOR CHILDREN: PRESCHOOL-AGED CHILDREN, 4–10 YEARS		
Milk (or equivalent)	4	
Milk, preferably low fat or skim		¾–1 cup
Powdered milk		3–4 tbsp.
Cheese		¾–1½ oz.
Cottage cheese		¾–1 cup
Yogurt		¾–1 cup
Meat, fish, poultry (or equivalent)	2 or more	2–3 oz.
Eggs		1 whole
Peanut butter		2–3 tbsp.
Cooked dried peas or beans		½–¾ cup
Luncheon meat		2 slices
Vegetables and fruits	4 or more	
Citrus fruits (vitamin C source)	1 or more	
Orange or grapefruit juice		½–1 cup
Strawberries		1 cup
Tomatoes or tomato juice		½–1 cup
Yellow or green vegetable or fruit (vitamin A source)	1 or more	
Broccoli		¼ cup
Spinach		¼ cup
Carrots		¼ cup
Squash		¼ cup
Cantaloupe		¼–½ fruit
Apricots		5–8 halves
Other fruits and vegetables	2 or more	
Fresh, frozen, canned fruits and vegetables		½ cup
Potato, turnip, most whole vegetables		½–1 veg.
Apple, banana, most whole fruits		½–1 fruit
Breads and cereals (whole grain or enriched)	4 or more	
Bread		1–2 slices
Dry cereal (unsweetened)		1 cup
Cooked cereal, rice, pasta		½ cup
Others (to meet calorie needs)	as needed	
Butter, margarine, mayonnaise, oil		1–2 tbsp.
Desserts		
Pudding		½ cup
Ice cream or ice milk		1 cup
Cookies		2–3 medium
Cake		1 oz.
Pie		1½ oz.
Sugar, honey, molasses, jelly, jam		2 tbsp.

Note. From *Parents' Guide to Nutrition* (pp. 123–124) by the Boston Children's Hospital, 1986, Reading, MA: Addison-Wesley.

TABLE 10–5

		Sugar	Sugar
Food	Serving Size	(gm)	(tsp.)
Beverages			
Cola-type soft drinks	12 fl. oz.	40.7	10.2
Ginger ale	12 fl. oz.	29.0	7.25
Orange soda	12 fl. oz.	45.8	11.5
Kool-aid	8 fl. oz.	24.2	6.1
Lemonade, canned, frozen, mix	8 fl. oz.	22.5	5.6
Tang, orange	3 tsp. in 6 fl. oz. water	21.7	5.4
Candy and Candy Bars			
Chocolate chips	1 oz.	17.0	4.25
Chocolate-flavored chips	1 oz.	7.6	1.9
Milk chocolate	1.07 oz. bar	17.0	4.25
Milk chocolate, almonds	1 oz.	14.0	3.5
Peanut butter cups	1.6 oz	21.0	5.25
Jelly beans	10	26.4	6.6
Lifesavers	1 each	2.4	0.6
Chewing gum	1 stick	2.4	0.6
Salt-water taffy	1 piece	2.4	0.6
Bubble gum	1 piece	4.0	1.0
Marshmallows	4 large	21.2	5.3
Cereals (all cup sizes are 1 ounce of cereal)			
Boo Berry	1 cup	13.0	3.25
40% Bran	¾ cup	5.0	1.25
Cheerios, regular	1¼ cup	1.0	0.25
Honey Nut	¾ cup	10.0	2.5
Cocoa Krispies	¾ cup	12.0	3.0
Corn Flakes	1 cup	2.0	0.5
Crazy Cow, chocolate/strawberry	1 cup	12.0	3.0
Frankenberry	1 cup	13.0	3.3
Froot Loops	1 cup	13.0	3.3
Kaboom	1 cup	6.0	1.5
Puffed Rice or Wheat	1 cup	0.0	0.0
Raisin Bran	¾ cup	12.0	3.0
Rice Krispies	1 cup	3.0	0.75
Shredded Wheat	1 biscuit	0.0	0.0
Sugar Smacks	¾ cup	16.0	4.0
Total	1 cup	3.0	0.75
Trix	1 cup	12.0	3.0
Wheaties	1 cup	3.0	0.75
Desserts			
Pudding, instant, chocolate, lemon, vanilla	½ cup	26.5	6.6
Pudding pops, average for all flavors	1 pop	14.4	3.6
Toaster pastry	1 each	15.0	3.8
Twinkies	1 each	19.2	4.8

Fruits and Fruit Juices			
Apple	3½ oz.	9.9	2.5
Banana	3½ oz.	14.0	3.5
Blueberries	3½ oz.	5.8	1.45
Cantaloupe/honeydew	3½ oz.	11.1	2.78
Grapes	3½ oz.	13.6	3.4
Grapefruit	3½ oz.	6.8	1.7
Orange	3½ oz.	8.2	2.1
Peach	3½ oz.	6.7	1.68
Strawberries	3½ oz.	5.2	1.3

Note. Adapted from *Bowes and Church's Food Values and Portions Commonly Used* (14th ed.) by J.A.T. Pennington and H.N. Church, 1985, Philadelphia: J.B. Lippincott.

MOTOR DEVELOPMENT
Large Muscle Development

Running   Between the ages of five and six, children have reasonably mastered the process of running and are able to use these skills in play and recreational activities.

Climbing   By the time children are six years of age, 90 percent are classified as reasonably proficient climbers. Keep in mind, however, that there are wide variations in the abilities of children to perform all motor tasks (Espenchade & Eckert, 1980, p. 143).

Throwing   As indicated in Chapter Eight, it is during the school years that children master the last two stages of throwing. Between the ages of five and seven, children are able to transfer their weight to their right foot in preparation for throwing (stage 3) and are able to transfer their weight to their left foot during the act of throwing.

As children develop during the middle years, the above-mentioned skills that rely on skill and strength continue to improve. Thus as a child becomes stronger and taller, she becomes more capable of improved performances in these areas. However, dramatic improvements in physical skills are observed in tasks involving timing and coordination. These increased skills enable children in the elementary grades to participate in many athletic activities involving throwing, catching, hitting, and kicking. During these years, children are noticeably more proficient in being able to time the swing of a bat and to judge distances that balls are hit or thrown, making it much easier for them to succeed in sports activities. This increased physical ability accounts in part for the popularity of athletics with this age group. With increased physical ability comes competence, achievement, and recognition.

It is not only children's physical development that enables them to participate in athletic activities. Their cognitive development enables them to take part in and make sense of rules with games. In fact, children's abilities to understand game rules makes athletic involvement such as soccer and baseball more enjoyable and interesting for them.

*I*N THE SPOTLIGHT

LITTLE LEAGUE BASEBALL

Most towns and cities have organized programs enabling children to participate in the nation's pastime—baseball. Little League baseball is "one form of preadolescent play that is directed by adults ostensibly for the benefit of preadolescents" (Fine, 1987, p. 39).

Certainly Little League has critics who maintain that it is an adult-dominated sport that makes too heavy a demand on children. However, the popularity of Little League can hardly be denied by the large number of boys—and, increasingly, girls—who play on the diamond. Fine (1987) has this to say about Little League:

The arguments of the critics of the program, although valid in individual cases, appear invalid generally. Similarly we must view with caution claims made by the proponents of the program that Little League has major benefits. While the conclusion may not be glamorous, Little League does not seem to have the dramatic effects its proponents hope or its critics fear. Basically, Little League is fun for those preadolescents who participate, and while we should never stop trying to curtail its flaws, we should be satisfied that it brings a little joy to the lives of children (p. 221).

Furthermore, Piaget (1932) maintains that by playing rule-bound games, children learn respect for rules. Such process as learning rules and reconciling conflicts and disputes are contributory to children's moral development.

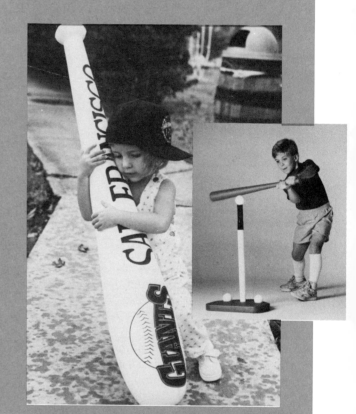

FIGURE 10-4 Children in middle childhood develop the ability to play games with rules and many of these are adult sponsored. While organized sports have positive benefits such as learning cooperation and achievement motivation, some of the negative factors include risk of injuries and overemphasis on winning.

Fine Motor Development

There are sex-related differences in the performance of fine motor tasks in the early years and these continue into the middle years. You may have heard that girls are better in school-related tasks than boys. This is true, and has a basis in the ability to complete fine motor tasks. For example, while both first grade boys and girls perform equally well on a task of dotting the circle, boys perform significantly worse on symbol copying (Judd, Siders, Siders, & Atkins, 1986).

COGNITIVE DEVELOPMENT

As you will recall from Chapter Two, Piaget's *concrete operations* stage of intellectual development covers the entire middle childhood period. This stage is called *concrete* because children's thought is restricted to what they encounter through direct experience (Bybee & Sund, 1982, p. 97). During the years from age seven through age eleven, children's thinking is more internalized and they are capable of engaging in problem solving. But, as we discussed in Chapter Two, they can only do this concretely, meaning that they think about problems involving identifiable objects and their properties.

In the earliest stages of concrete operations, when a child is given a problem to solve, for example, "If Jose has four checkers and Silvia has three checkers, how many checkers are there?", being able to physically see and manipulate the checkers contributes to his ability to solve the problem. A child in the later stages of concrete operations is able to solve the problem by mentally visualizing the checkers. However, a difficulty that children have in the concrete operational stage is that they are unable to conceptualize all of the relevant components of a problem.

Concrete Operational Skills

In their development through concrete operations toward the formal operations stage, children undergo a number of transitions in the conceptual

TABLE 10–6

AGES AT WHICH MIDDLE CHILDHOOD CHILDREN ATTAIN CONSERVATION

Type of Conservation	Age	Characteristic Response of Child
Substance	6–7	Realizes amount of substance doesn't change by dividing it.
Length	6–7	Realizes bending a wire doesn't change its length.
Number	6½–7	Realizes rearranging objects doesn't change their number.
Continuous Quantity	6–7	Realizes pouring liquid from one container to another doesn't change the quantity.
Area	7	Realizes the area of a paper split in half covers just as much area as if it were whole.
Weight	9–12	Realizes a mashed piece of clay weighs the same as when it was a sphere.
Volume	11–12 and beyond	Realizes that a mashed piece of clay immersed in a liquid will occupy as much volume as when it was a sphere.

Note. From *Piaget for Educators* (p. 102) by R.W. Bybee and R.B. Sund, 1982, Columbus, OH: Merrill.

structures that are necessary in order to think logically, as is required in formal operations.

Conservation One of the hallmarks of the concrete operational stage is the appearance of *conservation*, the ability to understand that properties of an object remain the same in spite of changes in its appearance. Yet, the middle school child

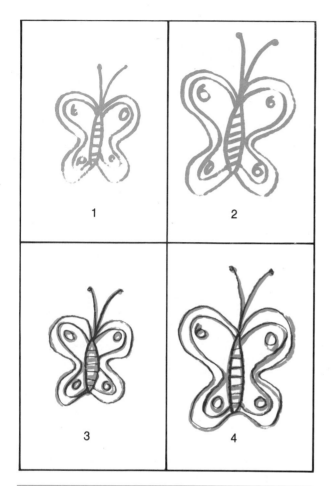

FIGURE 10-5 In multiple seriation, children are able to use two properties to order objects as shown with these butterflies of different size and color.

There are three types of seriation that are important from a Piagetian perspective: simple seriation, multiple seriation, and transitive inference. In *simple seriation*, children are asked to order five to ten objects according to some property, such as length. The Montessori red rods and brown stairs are examples of such seriation tasks (see Chapter Nine). In *multiple seriation*, children must use two properties to order objects. For example, children are asked to establish the order between *size* and *color*, such as with (1) a small butterfly that is light blue, (2) a large butterfly that is light blue, (3) a small butterfly that is dark blue, and (4) a large butterfly that is dark blue. Solving this seriation task requires a 2 by 2 matrix, as shown in Figure 10–5. The third type of seriation, *transitive inference*, requires that children order objects without direct comparison of all the objects. This mode of deductivity is known as *transitivity*. For example, $A < B$ and $B < C$, therefore $A < C$. The cognitive ability involved is to draw a conclusion without all the elements being included, in other words, comparing B to C in order to know that $A < C$. Transitivity is an important logical reasoning operation, and enables the concrete operational child to solve this problem, a problem that would be impossible for a preoperational child. Jane is taller than Mary and Mary is taller than Sally. Therefore Jane is taller than Sally.

Classification   *Classification* is the ability to identify relationships among objects, persons, and events. There are three types of classification: simple, multiple, and class inclusion. In *simple classification*, there are two developmental levels. In the first, the child groups objects according to one characteristic—she puts all the blue blocks in one pile. In the second, the child can mentally represent the classification task—putting the blue blocks in one pile and the green blocks in another pile. Thus, if the child is given a set of blue and green blocks and is asked to classify them, she can classify according to how things go together. In this case, the blue blocks belong in one group and the green blocks belong in another group.

does not suddenly function equally well in all areas of conservation. For example, the ability to conserve substance and length occurs before the ability to conserve weight and volume. Table 10–6 shows the approximate age levels at which conservation is attained.

Seriation   Seriation is the ability to order a group of objects using a property common to all objects.

Multiple classification involves classifying objects using two mutually exclusive attributes, for example, classifying objects according to color and shape. When given red triangles, red squares, blue triangles, and blue squares, the child can classify in more than one way—the red triangle with the blue triangle and the red square with the blue square. Things can go together by color and shape.

In *class inclusion*, children understand that one or more classes can exist within another class. A child who has a bouquet of ten red silk roses and ten yellow silk roses can classify the roses into two groups—red and yellow. If the roses are then made into a bouquet and the child is asked, "Are there more red roses or flowers?" and the child responds "Flowers," then she recognizes that red roses are a member of the flowers class and understands class inclusion.

In their attainment of the concrete operations stage, children are capable of a number of important operational processes. One of these is the ability to *decenter*, which is the ability to take many aspects of a situation into consideration rather than focusing on only one particular one, as is the case with preoperational children. The ability to decenter enables elementary children to solve class inclusion problems.

Concrete operational children are also capable of *reversibility*, or the ability to mentally go back to the beginning of a problem and think about what happened.

Number Many teachers and parents think that counting represents children's total understanding of numbers. It is not. Understanding of numbers is based on more than just rote counting. Other concepts are also included, such as *equivalence*, the concept that one of anything is equivalent to one of anything else. For example, one apple is equivalent to one orange, as far as number is concerned.

Understanding number also includes an understanding of *ordinal* and *cardinal* number. *Ordinal* number means the order of objects in an ordered sequence. Again, using as our example the Montessori materials—red rods in a sequenced row according to length—there is a first, second, third, and fourth rod. *Cardinal* number refers to how many objects are contained in a set, for example, five blocks, four dolls, three spoons.

Recall in Chapter Eight, when we talked about preoperational children's ability to conserve, we said that when given two equivalent rows of checkers, children base their numerical judgment on the length of the rows. They do not have the ability to *conserve number*. In the concrete operations period, children come to understand that the number in a group remains equivalent regardless of how the items are arranged.

Space Spatial relations during the concrete operations stage deal with the position of objects in space. A common task for understanding spatial relations involves the ability to identify the horizontal position of colored water in a closed container, such as a jar. To determine a child's understanding of spatial relations, the child is then shown a picture (see Figure 10–6) of the container

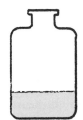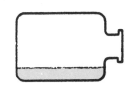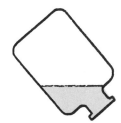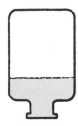

FIGURE 10-6 Children in the concrete operations stage develop the cognitive ability to understand horizontal and vertical as shown in this test, which Piaget used to test children's spatial understanding. Children who do not understand the horizontal and vertical will draw the liquid the same way the container is tipped.

in different positions and is asked to indicate, by drawing a line, how ne water would look. In the preoperational stage, the child cannot show how water will appear in the various positions. Children in the concrete operational stage, on the other hand, can show how the water remains in the horizontal position regardless of the position of the container (right side up, on its side, upside down, etc.).

Time Understanding of time involves three basic kinds of mental operations. These are seriation of experiences, (teeth are brushed after lunch); time between events (how long is it until lunch?); and calculation of how much time something will take (if a car travels fifteen feet a minute, how long will it take to go two feet?). During the concrete operational period, children are able to reason correctly about time.

Family Influences on Cognitive and Affective Development

Families and Television Viewing Families and family environments play important and powerful roles in children's lives by influencing the nature and direction of cognitive and affective development. There are a number of family patterns that are important to children's acquisition of cognitive skills, development of motor restraint, reduced aggression, and better school behavior. These patterns are demonstrated by parents who (1) value imagination and resourcefulness or responsibility and stability, (2) do not emphasize power-assertive discipline and physical punishment, (3) actively mediate the outside world for children through explanation and discussion rather than preemptory discipline or judgmental assertions, and (4) watch less television themselves and who hold a less mean and scary view of their environment (Singer & Singer, 1986).

Aspects of family environment and parents' child-rearing attitudes and skills are associated with how much television children watch, their viewing patterns, and viewing preferences (Tangney, 1988).

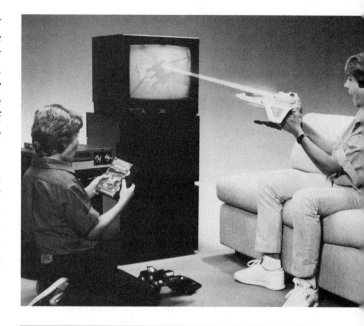

FIGURE 10-7 The influences of television viewing on children extend beyond the contents of a particular show. Other viewing influences include who the child views television with; what is done while viewing, e.g., eating; and the purpose of watching the program.

Also, in families where parents lack empathy, sensitivity, and adaptive role expectations, children view television programs with violent and fantasy-oriented content more often. There are a number of explanations for how parents with the traits mentioned influence their children's television viewing habits. First, if a child has experienced a history of unrealistic expectations, then the child selects fantasy–escapist-oriented programs. It is as though the child "takes a break" from the demanding aspects of his home environment. Second, children of parents with dysfunctional child-rearing patterns avoid relationship-oriented and family situation comedies. Apparently for these children, there is little in their home life that is light-hearted and humorous. Third, parents with authoritarian and nonempathetic attitudes may themselves prefer the kind of programs their children are watching, and therefore they are both acting as a model for their children as well as selecting the programs that they and their children watch. What is also important for children with dysfunctional parents is that these children spend more time than their peers—more than twenty-five hours per week—watching television. What is significant is that these children are watching the programs that are least likely to provide them with the role models they need, and which are least likely to contribute to their cognitive growth.

LANGUAGE DEVELOPMENT
Vocabulary Development

Generally, when people think of language development in the early years, they think of vocabulary development. Indeed the number of words a child adds to her vocabulary in these years is truly impressive and astounding. From the first year, when first words begin, how many words a day does a child add to her vocabulary? Make a guess. Estimates range from nine a day (Carey, 1978) to thirteen a day (Miller & Gilda, 1987). Certainly a child doesn't add this number of words every day, but when you realize that the average high school graduate at seventeen years of age has a vocabulary of 80,000 words (Miller & Gilda, 1987), then the average child has to learn at the rate of 5,000 words per year or about thirteen words a day!

So how do children accomplish this? Preschoolers employ a number of techniques. First, they associate sound with meaning. However, many repetitions of a word may be necessary before the sound of a new word becomes familiar.

Second, children's understanding of words grows in two stages—fast and slow. In the fast stage, children quickly notice new words and assign them to broad categories. For example, a three-year-old, after hearing the word *chromium*, assigned it to the category of color names. In the slow stage, on the other hand, children still have to work out differences and relations between words, for example, the difference between the words for different colors of reds.

Third, children learn words by *overextension.* They apply the attributes associated with one word—apple—to something else—a tomato.

When children enter the elementary grades, one way they learn words is through reading. However, they are expected to learn many more words than it is possible to learn merely by reading. Children can also learn new words through conversation and by asking others what new words mean. But classroom teachers seldom have time for this kind of individual interaction. This is one reason that many teachers provide children with dictionaries. However, dictionary use requires many skills and the student must still pay attention to the reading task. For these reasons, many students lose interest in using the dictionary. One frequently recommended method compatible with modern technology is the use of an interactive video display to mobilize the natural ability of children to learn words from context (Miller & Gilda, 1987).

Phonological Development

All children develop a phonological or sound system for the language they use—in our case, English. They also learn the phonetic system—the rules—by which this sound system is governed. This mastery is usually attained by age four or five, but it is not uncommon to hear school-age children of seven and eight saying *cwack* for crack, birthday may be pronounced as *birfday*, and toothbrush as *toofbrush*, and that is pronounced *dat* and them is *dem* (DeStefano, 1978, p. 52). Children's phonological development has a number of implications for teachers. First, children's ability to produce phonemes should be viewed as developmental; second, phonological differences in children may be due to social and geographic differences; and third, students may not perceive differences in the way they use words and how adults use them. (DeStefano, 1978, pp. 52–53).

Use of Sentences

During the middle years, children use a greater variety of sentences and their sentences become more complex. Also, older children learn to *embed*, as a means of combining ideas (Hoskisson & Tompkins, 1987, p. 22). For example, a preschool child will say, "My dog named Checkers ran away and got lost and won't come home and we can't find him." An older child will say, "My dog, Checkers, ran away from home and is lost." Also, older children will use such connectors as *because*, *if*, *unless* and *meanwhile*.

Implications for Parents and Teachers

During this stage of language development, children need opportunities to read a wide variety of literature as a means of learning about different syntactic forms and styles. In addition, by being involved in writing activities, children learn how to use syntax in written expression.

It is also during the middle years that children's ability to understand the meanings of words increases. This understanding includes knowing the different meanings for words—the word *home* has twenty-two meanings (The American Heritage Dictionary, 1982, p. 618), synonyms—*happy* and *glad*, antonyms—*happy* and *sad*, and homonyms—*sew* and *so*. Children must also learn idiomatic expressions, such as, "She flew off the handle."

As previously indicated, elementary school children need activities and experiences for learning words other than looking them up in dictionaries. Some of these activities should include reading literature, participating in dramas, and conversations with a wide variety of individuals.

PSYCHOSOCIAL DEVELOPMENT

As you will recall from our discussion of developmental theories in Chapter Two, children in the middle school years are in Erikson's *industry vs. inferiority* stage of psychosocial development and in Freud's *latency* period of development. (See Table 10–7.) According to Freud, children's sexual and aggressive energies are latent, and their phys-

TABLE 10–7

STAGES OF PSYCHOSOCIAL DEVELOPMENT ACCORDING TO FREUD AND ERIKSON	
Freud	Erickson
Stage 1—Oral (Birth to one year)	*Stage 1*—Oral-Sensory: Basic Trust vs. Mistrust (Birth to eighteen months)
Stage 2—Anal (Two to three years)	*Stage 2*—Muscular-Anal: Autonomy vs. Shame and Doubt (Eighteen months to three years)
Stage 3—Phallic or Oedipal (Three to four years)	*Stage 3*—Locomotor-Genital: Initiative vs. Guilt (Three to five years)
Stage 4—Latency (Five to thirteen years)	*Stage 4*—Latency: Industry vs. Inferiority (Five to eleven years)
Stage 5—Mature Genital (Twelve/thirteen to eighteen years)	*Stage 5*—Puberty and Adolescence: Identity vs. Role Confusion

ical and psychic energies are directed toward physical and intellectual achievements. The reason for this latency is because children have *repressed*, or pushed from their consciousness, feelings for intimacy with one parent or the other. During this period they are bringing a resolution to the Oedipal and Electra complexes of the earlier phallic stage. Freud believed the reason for the industriousness of this period was to enable the child to develop competence as a *defense*, an unconscious protective behavior, against the sexual desire for the parent. Thus, accomplishments and achievement unconsciously help the child to resolve feelings of not being able to be intimate with the parent of the opposite sex. Thus, for both Freud and Erikson, psychosocial development during the middle school years is achievement oriented.

Children in the middle years are involved in developing feelings of self-worth and industry, and in this regard, the middle years are important for the development of competence. Children are involved in developing self-confidence and they also have a desire to achieve to the best of their ability. Self-confidence and achievement are key contributors to competent behavior.

The other side of the industry coin is inferiority. Children develop a sense of inferiority when they are not able to achieve or when they are belittled by others. When children develop a sense of inferiority, they are not able to acquire the necessary feelings of industry that are so important for this developmental stage. The implication for teachers and parents in this regard is clear—helping children develop a sense of industry and achievement is much easier and developmentally healthy than trying to counteract inferiority once it has developed.

Implications for Parents and Care-givers

There are a number of implications children's psychosocial development has for parents and care-givers. First, middle school children are literally the sum of their achievements, and are influenced by what others say about them and their achievements. Parents and teachers should avoid being negative and overly critical of children's achievements. Rather they should support children's efforts to achieve and should help them develop standards by which their work and other's work are judged.

Second, achievement motivation plays a major role in children's learning and their self-view. *Achievement motivation* is the desire to achieve as well as one behaviorally and cognitively can. A child becomes involved in an activity and wants to do the best that she can. Individuals with an inner sense of achievement motivation strive for a high level of excellence in any activity, especially those in which it is reasonable for them to think they should do well. Thus, a child who possesses a strong sense of achievement motivation strives to do better without underachieving—doing less than what she is capable of doing—or overachiev-

ing—constantly striving to do more than what she is capable of doing. Teachers and parents can and should instill in children a sense of achievement motivation.

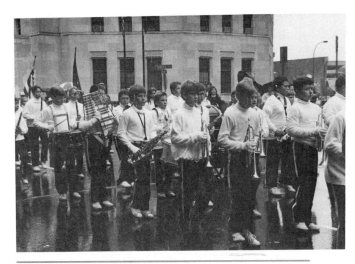

FIGURE 10-8 Children in the middle childhood years are in Erickson's psychosocial stage of industry vs. inferiority. Children need opportunities to achieve and be good at what they are involved in. Parents and teachers can help to develop achievement motivation in children.

AGGRESSION

Do you remember the classroom bully of your grade school days? We all remember such persons and occasionally we wonder what they are doing to themselves and others. Children in the middle years demonstrate their aggressiveness in a number of ways. They get into fights, belittle others, and are hostile to teachers, schoolmates, and family members. Chances are such children as adolescents will continue to be aggressive and will have trouble getting along with their schoolmates and families. It seems as though aggression in the middle years creates problems for children in the adolescent years (Goleman, 1988). There are particular traits that underlie children's aggressiveness: (1) during the heat of anger, they cannot think of other ways to react other than to strike out at someone, and (2) they are prone to perceive slights where none were intended (Goleman, 1988).

What Would You Do?

Eight-year-old Albert Boardner is in the second grade at Logpile Elementary School. His teacher, Mrs. Thatcher, is very concerned about little Al's behavior. He is demonstrating a cluster of behaviors that Mrs. Thatcher feels will lead to later delinquency. Specifically, Al takes pleasure in teasing and tormenting his classmates, rushes through his school work and works sloppily, delights in telling exaggerated stories, and frequently interrupts Mrs. Thatcher when she is talking.

Mrs. Thatcher sent a note home to Mr. and Mrs. Boardner requesting a parent-teacher conference to discuss Al's behavior. Since you are conducting observational activities at Logpile as part of the requirements for a child development class you are taking at the university, Mrs. Thatcher thinks you could benefit by sitting in on the conference.

During the conference, the Boardner's seem unconcerned about Mrs. Thatcher's description of Al's behavior. Mr. Boardner in particular feels Mrs. Thatcher is making too much of small things, and repeatedly stresses how he and Al engage in a lot of rough-and-tumble play at home. "A little teasing never hurt anybody," says Mr. Boardner. "I want Al to be able to dish it out as well as take it." In addition, Mr. Boardner commented, "Al's all boy. I like him the way he is. He's really a chip off the old block. This is how I acted when I was a kid. He'll grow out of this stage. All he needs is more control, which he'll get in the upper grades when he starts to have male teachers."

When the conference was over, Mrs. Thatcher felt frustrated and unsure about what she should do. "Maybe I am making too much of all this," she offers. "Perhaps Mr. Boardner is right, and Al is just going through a stage and he'll outgrow his negative behaviors. Maybe if I just ignore Al everything will work out in the long run." Turning to you for support, Mrs. Thatcher asks, "What do you think?"

PEER RELATIONSHIPS
Friendships

The development of friendship relationships is stage related. Friendship development occurs in five stages of overlapping ages (Selman & Selman, 1979). These stages are:

- Stage zero: momentary playmates (ages three to seven)

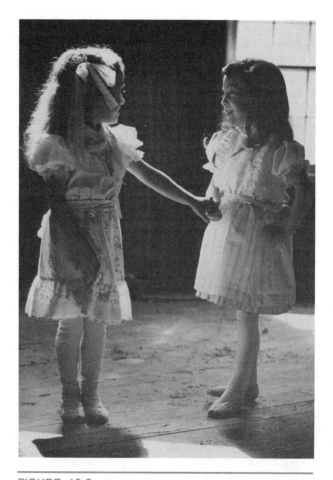

FIGURE 10-9 Friendships serve many useful functions. In some ways friends act as surrogate parents, providing emotional support and affection. Likewise, children can learn many useful skills and habits from friends. Of course, the opposite is also true.

- Stage one: one-way assistance (ages four to nine)
- Stage two: two-way, fair weather cooperation (ages six to twelve)
- Stage three: intimate, mutually-shared relationships (ages nine to twelve)
- Stage four: mature friendships (ages twelve and older)

There are a number of specific things teachers can do to promote children's friendship development (Kotselink, Stein, Whiren, & Soderman, 1988, pp. 356–362):

1. Provide opportunities for children to be with their friends informally—to talk, to play, and to enjoy one another's company.
2. Plan ways to pair children in order to facilitate interactions.
3. Pair a shy child with a younger playmate who is less sophisticated socially.
4. Take children's friendships seriously.
5. Carry out group discussions that focus on children's self-discovered similarities.
6. Help children learn each other's names.
7. Give children on-the-spot information to help them recognize the friendly overtures of others.
8. Help children recognize how their behavior affects their ability to make friends.
9. Get children involved at the beginning of a play episode so they will not be viewed as interlopers.
10. Help children endure the sorrows of friendship.

Shyness

You have all seen them and perhaps you are one yourself. They stand apart from others. It is hard for them to interact with and make conversations with others. They often play alone and like to be alone. The unfamiliar is a source of fear, and they avoid novel and new situations. They are shy children. How do they get that way? Are they born that way or did something happen to make them shy and introverted? The answer to both questions is "yes," with our best explanation being a combination of the two. Shyness seems to be a combination of both inherited temperament and chronic environmental stress (Kagan, Reznick, & Snidman, 1988). Shy children show more activity in certain biological systems, such as increases in heart rate, dilation of the pupils, and muscle tension when confronted with novel situations than do children not rated as shy, indicating an inborn biological basis for shyness. On the other hand, "the actualization of shy, quiet and timid behavior at two years of age, requires some form of chronic environmental stress acting upon the original disposition present at birth. Some possible stressors include prolonged hospitalization, death of a parent, marital quarrelling or mental illness in a family member" (Kagan, et al, 1988, p. 171).

PSYCHOSEXUAL DEVELOPMENT

Normal heterosexual development involves the adoption of standard measures of masculine and feminine behavior. This includes the attraction to and preference for members of the opposite sex. For some children, this normal development does not occur and in childhood they demonstrate patterns of cross-gender behavior. Extreme patterns of such behavior are associated with postpubertal homosexuality (Zucker, 1987). A comprehensive discussion of homosexuality is found in Chapter Twelve.

Differences Between the Sexes

There are a number of well-established differences between the sexes (Maccoby & Jacklin, 1974). These are:

- Girls have greater verbal ability than boys. During the preschool and elementary levels, boys' and girls' verbal abilities are about the same. However, beginning at about age eleven, female verbal superiority increases and continues through high school and possibly beyond.

- Boys excel in visual-spatial ability. This ability is found in adolescence and adulthood, but not in childhood.
- Boys excel in mathematical ability. The two sexes are similar in childhood, but beginning at about twelve or thirteen, boys' mathematical

aptitudes increase faster than girls.

- Boys are more aggressive than girls. This difference is found as early as two to two and a half years, and while the aggressiveness declines with age, boys and men remain more aggressive (pp. 351–352).

*I*N THE SPOTLIGHT

WHY DO BOYS DO BETTER IN MATH THAN GIRLS? COULD MIND SEX BE THE ANSWER?

Why is it that boys do better in mathematics than girls? While many ideas, from biology to testing bias, have been offered, the primary reason may be sexual bias. Simply put, boys may get all the attention in the classroom while girls get short-changed. Field researchers in over a hundred fourth, sixth, and eighth grade classes found that boys dominated classroom communication (Sadker & Sadker, 1985). The Sadkers' research is contradicting many traditional notions of what goes on in America's classrooms. Not only do boys dominate communication, they also are more assertive in the classroom. And, despite what is commonly thought, that girls get more attention in reading and that boys get more attention in math, the fact is that boys get more attention in all subject areas, period! Part of this is due to what the Sadkers call "mind sex." *Mind sex* is the tendency of teachers to keep calling on students of the same sex after they have called on a boy or girl. When a teacher calls on a boy, she keeps thinking of that sex. Since boys are more assertive and dominate classroom communication, they are more in the teacher's attention and will therefore get more than their fair share of attention.

Also, the Sadkers found that in half the classrooms they surveyed, children are segregated by sex into rows or sides of the room.

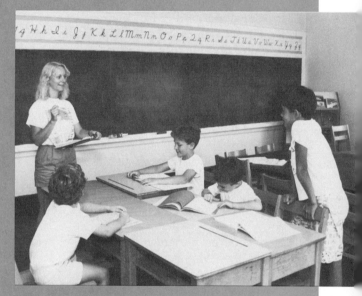

FIGURE 10-10   One of the reasons that boys may do better than girls in math is that they tend to receive more attention from their teachers. When teachers are aware of such bias, they can change their teaching methods to equalize, as much as possible, their attention to both sexes.

Sometimes teachers do the segregation, sometimes the children themselves do. Thus, when a teacher focuses on one row or side of the room, she tends to interact with that section longer, especially the boys.

Furthermore, children who are given accurate and precise feedback about their work and behavior tend to achieve better academically. And—you guessed it—teachers tend to do just that, give boys more accurate and precise feedback about their schoolwork and behavior.

So what are classroom teachers to do if they hope to correct their bias? There are a number of things, which the Sadkers call "equity principle" (Sutton, 1986). First, they can recognize their own sex biases. This may mean that they have a principal or faculty colleague observe them to see how they interact with the children in their classrooms. Second, they can make a concerted effort to call on all the children in their classroom, especially the girls. Third, they can increase their "wait time," the amount of time they give a student to answer a question, in order that those who hesitate or are not used to responding have an opportunity to do so.

*I*N THE SPOTLIGHT

IS BIOLOGY DESTINY OR CAN WE HAVE ANDROGYNY, TOO?

I'll bet you have heard the argument that people are who they are, and that it is foolish to try to change what biology has destined. Such arguments about the role of biology on the sexual development of boys and girls are frequently heard and have implications for parenting and teaching. There is increasing interest in the concept of *androgyny*, the realization that beneficial male and female characteristics can and should exist in the same person. Rather than possessing sharply polarized male or female characteristics, the androgynous person blends characteristics. Whether male or female, such a person can be both assertive and nurturing when considered within the framework of traditional gender roles. As Maccoby and Jacklin (1974) so eloquently advocate:

We suggest that societies have the option of minimizing, rather than maximizing, sex differences through their socialization practices. A society could, for example, devote its energies more toward moderating male aggression than toward preparing women to submit to male aggression, or toward encouraging rather than discouraging male nurturance activities. In our view, social institutions and social practices are not merely reflections of the biologically inevitable. A variety of social institutions are viable within the framework set by biology. It is up to human beings to select those that foster the life styles they most value (p. 374).

However, the socialization practices of a population are hard to change, and efforts to promote androgynous personalities meet resistance from those who hold stereotypical views of sex roles. For example, men still hold very traditional sex-role expectations for themselves and their sons (Emihovich, Gaier, & Cronin, 1984). In addition, in single-parent families headed by women, over 90 percent of the time mothers give their children either sex neutral or toys traditionally associated with their children's gender. The same pattern holds true for household chores. Boys are more likely to do "male" chores and girls are more likely to do "female" chores (Richmond-Abbott, 1984).

MORAL DEVELOPMENT
Piaget's Stages of Moral Thinking

The leading proponents of a developmental concept of children's moral growth are Jean Piaget and Lawrence Kohlberg. Piaget identified the two stages of moral thinking typical of children in the elementary grades as the stage of *heteronomy*—being governed by others regarding right and wrong—and the stage of *autonomy*—being governed by oneself regarding right and wrong.

> The analysis of the child's moral judgments has led us perforce to the discussion of the great problem of the relations of social life to the rational consciousness. The conclusion we came to was that the morality prescribed for the individual by society is not homogenous because society itself is not just one thing. Society is the sum of social relations, and among these relations we can distinguish two extreme types: relations of constraint, whose characteristic is to impose upon the individual from outside a system of rules with obligatory content, and relations of cooperation, whose characteristic is to create within people's minds the consciousness of ideal norms at the back of all rules. Arising from the ties of authority and unilateral respect, the relations of constraint therefore characterize most of the features of society as it exists, and in particular the relations of the child to its adult surrounding. Defined by equality and mutual respect, the relations of cooperations, on the contrary, constitute an equiliberal limit rather than a static system (Piaget, 1965, p. 395).

The stage of heteronomy is characterized by "relations of constraint." In this stage, the child's concept of good and bad and right and wrong is determined by the judgments pronounced by adults. An act is "wrong" because one's parents or teacher say it is wrong. The child's understanding of morality is based upon the authority of adults and those which "constrain" her.

Gradually, as the child matures and has opportunities for experiences with peers and adults, moral thinking may change to "relations of co-operation." This stage of personal morality is characterized by exchange of viewpoints between children and between children and adults as to what is right, wrong, good, or bad. This level of moral development is not achieved by authority, but rather by social experiences within which one has opportunities to try out different ideas and discuss moral situations. Autonomous behavior does not mean that children agree with other children or adults, but autonomous people exchange opinions and try to negotiate solutions.

The relations of constraint stage is characteristic of children up through first and second grades, while the relationships of cooperation stage is characteristic of children in the middle and upper elementary grades. The real criterion for determining which developmental stage a child is operating in, however, is how she is thinking, not how old she is.

Kohlberg's Levels of Moral Growth

Lawrence Kohlberg, a follower of Piaget, also believes children's moral thinking occurs in developmental levels. The levels and substages of moral growth as conceptualized by Kohlberg (1973) are preconventional, conventional, and postconventional.

Level I—Preconventional Level (Ages Four to Ten) Morality is basically a matter of good or bad, based on a system of punishments and rewards as administered by adults in authority positions. In Stage 1, the punishment-and-obedience orientation, the child operates within and responds to physical consequences of behavior. Good and bad are based upon the rewards they bring, and the child bases judgment on whether an action will bring pleasure. In Stage 2, the instrumental-relativist orientation, the child's actions are motivated by satisfaction of needs. Consequently, interpersonal relations have their basis in arrangements of mutual convenience based on need satisfaction ("You scratch my back; I'll scratch yours").

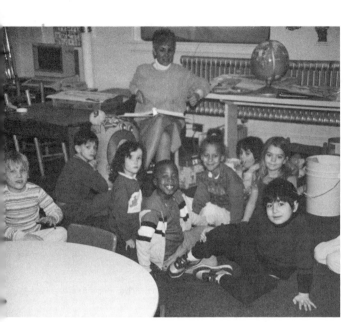

FIGURE 10-11 Classrooms are excellent environments in which to help children with issues, values and questions of moral behavior. While many teachers may think that promoting moral development is not part of their responsibility, the failure to do so may deny children the opportunity to develop to their fullest moral potential.

Level II—Conventional Level (Ages Ten to Thirteen) Morality is doing what is socially accepted, desired, and approved. The child conforms to, supports, and justifies the order of society. Stage 3 is the interpersonal concordance or "good boy-nice girl" orientation. Emphasis is on what a "good boy" or "nice girl" would do. The child conforms to images of what good behavior is. In Stage 4, the "law-and-order" orientation, emphasis is on respect for authority and doing one's duty under the law.

Level III—Postconventional Level (Ages Thirteen and Beyond) Morality consists of principles beyond particular group or authority structure. The individual develops a moral system that reflects universal considerations and rights.

Stage 5 is the social-contract legalistic orientation. Right action is guided by individual rights agreed upon by all society. In addition to democratic and constitutional considerations, what is right is relative to personal values. At Stage 6, the universal-ethical-principle orientation, what is right is determined by universal principles of justice, reciprocity, and equality. The actions of the individual are based on a combination of conscience and these ethical principles.

Just as Piaget's cognitive stages are fixed and invariant for all children, so, too, are Kohlberg's moral levels. All individuals move through the process of moral development, beginning at Level I, and progress through each level. No level can be skipped, nor does an individual necessarily achieve every level. Just as intellectual development may become fixed at a particular level of development, so may an individual become fixed at any one of the moral levels.

Implications for Teachers

What implications do the theories of Piaget and Kohlberg and programs for promoting affective education have for classroom practice?

- The teacher must like and respect children.
- The classroom climate must be accepting of individual values. Respect for children means respect for and acceptance of the value system the child brings to school. It is easy to accept an individual with a value system similar to one's own; it takes more self-discipline and maturity to accept an individual with a different value system.
- Teachers and schools must be willing to deal with issues, morals, and value systems other than those they promote for convenience, such as obedience and docility.
- Kohlberg maintains that a sense of justice must prevail in the schools, instead of the injustice that arises from imposing arbitrary institutional values.
- Children must have opportunities to interact with peers, children of different age groups,

and adults to enable them to move to the higher levels of moral functioning.

- Students must have opportunities to make decisions and discuss the results of decision making. The development of a value system cannot occur through listening to others or through a solitary opportunity at decision making.

In a Different Voice: The Voice of Carol Gilligan

Not everyone agrees that the way Freud, Piaget and Kohlberg describe moral development is the way that moral development really occurs for all children, especially females. One of those with a dissenting view—and an increasingly popular dissenting view—is Carol Gilligan. Gilligan believes that moral thinking among women is different from moral thinking among men. Women's moral thinking, Gilligan maintains, is based on consideration and preservation of human relationships. Here is what she has to say (Gilligan, 1982):

> The subject of moral development not only provides the final illustration of the reiterative pattern in the observation and assessment of sex differences in the literature on human development, but also indicates more particularly why the nature and significance of women's development has been for so long obscured and shrouded in mystery.
>
> The criticism that Freud makes of women's sense of justice, seeing it as compromised in its refusal of blind impartiality, reappears not only in the work of Piaget but also in that of Kohlberg. While in Piaget's account of moral judgment of the child, girls are an aside, a curiosity to whom he devotes four brief entries in an index that omits "boys" altogether because "the child" is assumed to be male, in the research from which Kohlberg's derives his theory, females simply do not exist. Kohlberg's six stages that describe the development of moral judgement from childhood to adulthood are based empirically on a study of eighty-four boys whose development Kohlberg has followed for a period of over twenty years. Although Kohlberg claims universality for his stage sequence, those groups not included in his original sample rarely reach his higher stages. Prominent among those who thus appear to be deficient in moral development when measured by Kohlberg's scale are women, whose judgement seem to exemplify the third stage of his six-stage sequence. At this stage morality is conceived in interpersonal terms and goodness is equated with helping and pleasing others. This conception of goodness is considered by Kohlberg and Kramer [a coauthor] to be functional in the lives of mature women insofar as their lives take place in the home. Kohlberg and Kramer imply that only if women enter the traditional arena of male activities will they recognize the inadequacy of this moral perspective and progress like men toward higher stages where relationships are subordinate to rules (stage four) and rules to universal principles of justice (stages five and six).
>
> Yet herein lies a paradox, for the very traits that traditionally have defined the "goodness" of women, their care for and sensitivity to the needs of others, are those that mark them as deficient in moral development. In this version of moral development, however, the conception of maturity is derived from the study of men's lives and reflects the importance of individuation in their development (pp. 17–18).

> When one begins with the study of women and derives developmental constructs from their lives, the outline of a moral conception different from that described by Freud, Piaget or Kohlberg begins to emerge and informs a different description of development. In this conception, the moral problem arises from conflicting responsibilities rather than from competing rights, and requires for its resolution a mode of thinking that is contextual and narrative rather than formal and abstract (p. 19).
>
> The moral imperative that emerges repeatedly in interviews with women is an injunction to care, a responsibility to discern and alleviate the "real and recognizable trouble" of this world. For men, the moral imperative appears rather as an injunction to respect the rights of others and thus to protect from interference the rights to life and self-fulfillment (p. 100).

> As Freud and Piaget call our attention to the differences in children's feelings and thought, en-

abling us to respond to children with greater care and respect, so a recognition of the differences in women's experience and understanding expands our vision of maturity and points to the contextual nature of developmental truths. Through this expansion in perspective, we can begin to envision how a marriage between adult development as it is currently portrayed and women's development as it begins to be seen could lead to a changed understanding of human development and a more generative view of human life (p. 174).

GIFTED CHILDREN

At the beginning of this chapter, you read about Abigail, who is gifted. Who are gifted children? All of us have met children whom we thought were gifted in one way or another, but were they gifted? One way to determine who is gifted is to consider the federal definition of giftedness. A generally accepted definition of giftedness comes from P.L. 97-35, the Education Consolidation and

Improvement Act, which defines giftedness this way:

> Gifted and talented children are now referred to as "children who give evidence of high performance capability in areas such as intellectual, creative, artistic, leadership capacity, or specific academic fields, and who require services or activities not ordinarily provided by the school in order to fully develop such capabilities (Sec. 582).

Notice in the definition that the concept of gifted has been broadened to include the talented. While the public may tend to think of the gifted as only those children with high intelligence, a child who has average intelligence may have exceptional abilities in dance. In such a case, then, she would be considered talented and appropriate activities and services would be in order.

Public Policy and State Definitions of Giftedness

Over the last decade, federal policy has focused in part on states' rights. The implication of this policy is that federal monies for special programs such as those for special needs children have been given to the states rather than distributed directly by federal agencies. The effect of this policy is that all of the fifty states have developed definitions of giftedness and guidelines for the delivery of services. While these definitions have common similarities, you must be familiar with the definitions of giftedness in your state and the procedures for the delivery of services.

For example, in the State of Florida, the definition of giftedness is: "One who has superior intellectual development and is capable of high performance. The mental development of a gifted child is two (2) standard deviations or more above the norm."

Eligibility Criteria

Based on the definition of giftedness, the School District of Dade County, Florida, the nation's fourth

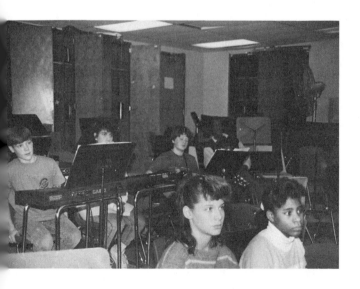

FIGURE 10-12 Gifted and talented children are receiving more attention and school districts are developing more programs to provide appropriate services and activities for them.

largest school district, has the following eligibility criteria:

1. Superior intellectual development—an intelligence quotient of two (2) standard deviations or more above the mean on an individually administered standardized test of intelligence.

The standard error of measurement may be considered on individual cases.

2. A majority of characteristics of gifted children according to a standard scale or checklist.
3. Need for a special program.
4. Age of student—meaning that eligible students between kindergarten and graduation may participate.

IN THE SPOTLIGHT

UNDERSTANDING MEASUREMENT TERMS

In our discussion of the eligibility requirements for gifted programs in the school district of Dade County, there are several terms with which you may not be familiar, *standard deviation* and *standard error of measurement*.

Standard Deviation The standard deviation, usually abbreviated as SD, is the most frequently used index of variability or how spread out test scores are from the mean. The more spread out the scores, the more the variability. For example, let's say you gave a math test to a group of first grade children. Their scores are 17, 17, 17, 17, 19, 19, 19, and 19. The *mean,* or average, of this set of scores is 18. The scores are very close to the mean. The next day, you give another math test to another group of children and their scores are 12, 14, 15, 15, 19, 21, 23, and 25. The mean of this set of scores is also 18, but the variance from the mean is much larger. It would be accurate and correct for you to say that for both groups, the mean score was 18, but you would not be providing the whole picture. The children in the first group performed closer to the mean than did the children of the second group. In order for us to know how spread out the scores are, we need a measure of variability. This is what the SD tells us. The SD is calculated by (1) subtracting the mean from each score, (2) squaring the difference, (3) adding the squares, (4) dividing by the number of scores, and (5) finding the square root.

Mean

a) 17, 17, 17, 17, 19, 19, 19, 19 $n = 8$
    $\Sigma x = x/n$ $= 144/8$

b) 12, 14, 15, 15, 19, 21, 23, 25 $n = 8$
    $\Sigma x = x/n$ $= 114/8$

Standard Deviation $SD = \sqrt{(x - x)^2 / n}$

a) *Step 1:* $17-18 = -1$, $17-18 = -1$, $17-18 = -1$, $17-18 = -1$, $19-18 = 1$, $19-18 = 1$, $19-18 = 1$, $19-18 = 1$

    Step 2: $(-1)^2 = 1$, $(-1)^2 = 1$, $(-1)^2 = 1$, $(-1)^2 = 1$, $(1)^2 = 1$, $(1)^2 = 1$, $(1)^2 = 1$, $(1)^2 = 1$

    Step 3: $1 + 1 + 1 + 1 + 1 + 1 + 1 + 1 = 8$

    Step 4: $8/8 = 1$

    Step 5: $\sqrt{1} = 1$

b) *Step 1:* $12-18 = -6$, $14-18 = -4$, $15-18 = -3$, $15-18 = -3$, $19-18 = 1$, $21-18 = 3$, $23-18 = 5$, $25-18 = 7$

    Step 2: $(-6)^2 = 36$, $(-4)^2 = 16$, $(-3)^2 = 9$, $(-3)^2 = 9$, $(1)^2 = 1$, $(3)^2 = 9$, $(5)^2 = 25$, $(7)^2 = 49$

    Step 3: $36 + 16 + 9 + 9 + 1 + 9 + 25 + 49 = 154$

    Step 4: $154/8 = 19.25$

    Step 5: $\sqrt{19.25} = 4.3875$

FIGURE 10-13 Standard deviation.

Standard Error of Measurement The standard error of measurement is an indicator of *reliability* or how consistently a test measures what it is supposed to measure. A small standard of error measurement indicates high reliability and a high standard error of measurement indicates low reliability. No test is absolutely reliable in that if a test is administered to a group of children twice, the individual scores from one testing to the other will vary. The less they vary, the more reliable the test is. This is why the standard error of measure of the WISC-R, which is 3, is added to the score of each child and explains why a child can score 127 and meet the 130 eligibility requirement.

The School District of Dade County uses the Wechsler Intelligence Scale for Children—Revised (WISC-R), which has a mean of 100 and a standard deviation of 15. This means that in order to qualify as gifted, the child would have to have an I.Q. of 130. The standard error of measurement is 3, so a student could have a measured intelligence on the WISC-R of 127, and be eligible for the gifted program.

Note also that the characteristics of gifted children specified by the School District of Dade County include four areas: learning, motivation, creativity, and leadership.

System of Multicultural Pluralistic Assessment (SOMPA)

Any standardized test is normed on a particular population. This means that for some children, cultural bias may exist in the test. In order to overcome this bias, additional tests may be used to identify minority gifted students. For example, in the School District of Dade County, when a minority student has an IQ of 118 or above, then school psychologists administer to parents the sociocultural scales of the SOMPA. These scales are designed to determine a student's Estimated Learning Potential (ELP). If the child's IQ is 118 with an ELP of 130, then he is admitted to the gifted program. The sociocultural scales gather data relating to family size, family structure, socioeconomic status, and urban acculturation.

Programs for the Gifted

As school districts pay more attention to the gifted, the gifted are provided more and different kinds of services. There are a number of kinds of programs for the gifted. These include:

- A self-contained program, which a classroom teacher provides for any gifted children she might have in her classroom.
- A pull-out program in which a child is taken out of his classroom for a portion of the day and instructed in a special program, usually by a teacher trained to provide activities for the gifted.
- A home-based program in which programs for the gifted are provided in the school the child attends. The home-based program could be a pull-out program. If the school population is large enough and if there are enough gifted children, then other home-based options are possible. For example, in the 1550-pupil Kendale Lakes Elementary School in the School District of Dade County, the gifted program

for the 160 gifted children is conducted through a "school within a school" program. In this program, the children attended a gifted school within the elementary school.

■ A full-time gifted program. The pupils in the "school within a school" at the Kendale Lakes Elementary School are in a full-time program.

■ A gifted program by grade level, where the gifted children from a grade level are together.

■ A multi-age program in which gifted elementary children are, regardless of their age or grade level, grouped for instructional purposes. For example, in the Kendale Lakes Elementary Gifted Program, children in grades three to six are grouped part of the day based on projects of their interests. Thus a third grader and a sixth grader might be involved in a project relating to inventors and inventions.

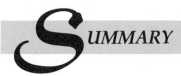 UMMARY

■ The middle years are the years between preschool and adolescence when children are five to twelve years old. This is the time period when children are in elementary school, from kindergarten through sixth grade. However, increasing numbers of children in grades five and six are also enrolled in middle schools.

■ In the early middle years, boys' and girls' heights and weights approximate each other. Beginning at about age nine, girls start to pull away from boys in height and weight. Such development is normal since girls begin their growth spurt earlier than boys. By the end of the middle childhood years, then, girls are taller and heavier than boys.

■ Obesity, or weight that exceeds the ninetieth percentile, may affect as many as 10 to 20 percent of the nation's children. Obesity is attributed to a number of factors including psychological, cultural, physiological, and genetic influences. Two major theories for the cause of obesity are overeating and lowered metabolism. New research indicates that low levels of a protein called adipsin may be a reason for lowered metabolism, which in turn gives rise to obesity. Such findings lend increased credibility to the heredity theory.

■ Breakfast per se may not be the best meal of the day. Much depends on what children eat and when they eat it. Teachers must be sensitive to the impact of food and eating schedules on children's classroom performances.

■ Parents and care-givers need to help children develop good nutritional habits early in life. This can be accomplished in part by helping children learn what constitutes good nutrition and by helping them monitor their eating habits.

■ Large muscle development in children's middle years is largely a matter of continuing development. Most children are reasonably proficient at running, climbing, and throwing. Improvement in coordination and timing enables children to engage in athletic activities.

■ During the period of middle childhood, children from ages seven to eleven are in the concrete stage of cognitive development. In their development through concrete operations toward the formal operations stage, children undergo a number of necessary transitions in conceptual structures that enable them to think logically as required in formal operations. These include: conservation, the ability to understand that properties of an object remain the same in spite of changes in its appearance; seriation, the ability to order a group of objects using a property common to all objects; and classification, the ability to identify relationships among objects, persons, and events.

■ Children during the middle years are able to decenter, which is the ability to take many aspects of a situation into consideration rather than focusing on only one particular one. In addition, they are able to engage in reversibility, the ability to mentally go back to the beginning of a problem and think about what happened.

■ Children's understanding of number includes the concept of equivalence, the idea that one of something is equivalent to one of something else. Also, children learn the properties of cardinal and ordinal numbers. Understanding of spatial relations and time concepts enables children to use concrete operations.

■ Families and family environments play important and powerful roles in children's lives by influencing the nature and direction of cognitive and affective development. Family patterns and child-rearing practices influence how much television children watch, their viewing patterns, and their viewing preferences. Children's television-viewing habits in turn influence their cognitive development.

■ One of the hallmarks of children's language development during the middle years is a tremendous growth in vocabulary development. Teachers can facilitate vocabulary development through the use of computer programs in which children have the opportunity to understand meanings of new words.

■ Phonological development continues during the middle years and children learn to use increasingly complex and sophisticated sentences.

■ Children in the middle school years are in Erikson's *industry vs. inferiority* stage of psychosocial development and in Freud's *latency* period of development. Achievement is a big factor in children's psychosocial development, and parents and teachers should facilitate opportunities for children to develop feelings of accomplishment.

■ Shyness seems to be a combination of both inherited temperament and chronic environmental stress.

■ There are a number of differences between the sexes. Girls have greater verbal ability than boys, and boys excel in visual-spatial and mathematical ability. Also, boys are more aggressive than girls. However, parents and teachers should minimize sex differences and should encourage the development of the best characteristics of both sexes in all children.

■ Sexual bias may be one reason boys' academic achievement exceeds that of girls. A cause of this may be teachers' preferential attention to boys. Some ways teachers can avoid bias and preferential treatment is to be aware of their own biases, pay as much attention to girls as they do to boys, and give all children in their classrooms the opportunity to participate.

■ According to Piaget and Kohlberg, moral development occurs in predictable and identifiable stages. Critics of Piaget's and Kohlberg's theories of moral development, such as Carol Gilligan, maintain that these theories are limited to males and fail to include research that indicates women's moral thinking is different from men's.

■ The needs of gifted children, those with high intellectual and performance ability, are being provided for through appropriate programs and services to meet their special needs. These programs and services are offered in home-based, gifted center and classroom settings.

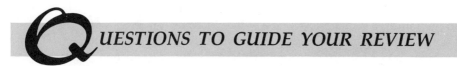

QUESTIONS TO GUIDE YOUR REVIEW

1. What are the middle years, and why are these years developmentally important?
2. How are boys and girls physically different during the middle years?
3. What are the causes of obesity? How can teachers and parents help children deal with obesity?
4. What constitutes good nutrition during the middle years?
5. What are the highlights of children's motor development during the middle years?
6. What is conservation, and what role does it play in cognitive development?
7. What are the differences between simple and multiple seriation?
8. What role does transitivity play in cognitive development?
9. What are the different kinds of classification that children use during the middle years?
10. How do number, space, and time contribute to cognitive development?
11. What are the characteristics of children's language development during the middle years?
12. What role does industry and inferiority play in children's psychosocial development?
13. What can teachers do to promote friendships between and among children during the middle years?
14. What are the hallmarks of boys' and girls' moral development during the middle years?
15. What are the differences in children's moral development in levels I, II, and III?
16. According to Carol Gilligan, how does women's moral thinking differ from men's?
17. What is giftedness, and how can teachers and parents provide for gifted children?
18. What is SOMPA, and what role does it play in the determination of a child's giftedness?

CTIVITIES FOR FURTHER INVOLVEMENT

1. Topics relating to children's nutrition and health habits in the middle years receive frequent attention in the news media.
   a. Why are nutrition and obesity given so much press and attention?
   b. What accounts for increasing numbers of children during the middle years being involved with diets and dieting?
   c. As a parent, what would you do to assure that your children learn good nutritional practices?
   d. Make a survey of children's snacking habits. What does this data tell you?
2. Although increasing numbers of critics decry the involvement of children in organized sports, nonetheless, the number of children involved in such activities increases.
   a. What factors account for the increase in children's organized sports?
   b. What benefits accrue to children through involvement in organized sports?
   c. Develop guidelines that you think should be used to govern children's involvement in organized sports.
3. Television exerts a powerful influence on the lives of children and families.
   a. In what specific ways does television affect children positively and negatively?
   b. Give examples of how children can learn through television.
   c. Why is television called an "electronic baby-sitter?
4. Children's interactions with others are an important part of growing up.
   a. What can parents, teachers, and others do to reduce aggression in children's interpersonal relationships?
   b. What can parents and teachers do to help children overcome their shyness?
   c. Why do parents place such a heavy emphasis on having their children learn to get along with others?
5. Gifted children are sometimes referred to as the "most neglected of special needs children."
   a. Why are gifted children frequently neglected?
   b. Why is there an increase in the number of programs for the gifted?
   c. Visit programs for the gifted in your area. Are they meeting the needs of gifted children? What would you do to improve these programs?

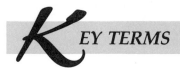

KEY TERMS

Adipsin A protein. Low levels of adipsin may cause lowered metabolic rates leading to obesity.

Asynchrony Characteristic of physical development when some parts of the body may grow faster than others, causing children to look out of proportion and gangly. Unevenness in physical development.

Concrete operations The stage of cognitive development in which children's thought is restricted to what they encounter through direct experience.

Conservation The ability to understand that properties of an object remain the same in spite of changes in its appearance.

Metabolism The rate at which the body transforms food into energy.

"Mind sex" The tendency of teachers to keep calling on students of the same sex after they have called on a boy or girl.

Multiple seriation The ability to use two properties to order objects.

Obesity Defined by body weight, normed for height, age, and sex, which exceeds the ninetieth percentile.

Seriation The ability to order a group of objects using a property common to all objects.

Simple seriation The ability to seriate objects according to some property, such as length.

Transitive inference The ability to order objects without direct comparison of all the objects.

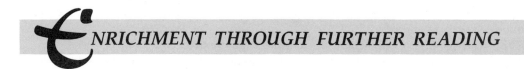

ENRICHMENT THROUGH FURTHER READING

Fine, G. A. (1987). *With the boys: Little League baseball and preadolescent culture.* Chicago: The University of Chicago Press.

    An interesting and readable description of Little League baseball. Provides many useful and fascinating insights into preadolescent behavior and culture.

Hale-Benson, J. E. (1986). *Black children: Their roots, culture and learning styles.* Baltimore: The Johns Hopkins University Press.

    Provides valuable information about black children's learning and expressive styles. There are many implications for how to accommodate the natural learning styles of black children with the teaching/learning styles encountered in the process of schooling.

ANSWER TO "WHAT WOULD YOU DO?"

As we have discussed before, many people feel that time cures all things, from a broken heart to student misbehavior. As we also know, maturation does play a large role in development, learning, and behavior. However, in this case, the chances are pretty good that little Al, the classroom bully and terror of today, may grow up to be big Al, the juvenile delinquent of tomorrow.

Al's behavior pattern is a high-risk one for later misconduct in school and the community (Spivack, Marcus, & Swift, 1986). In their research, Spivack and his associates found that high-risk behavior patterns related to later conflict with adult authority are:

(a) The tendency to become involved in poking and annoying social behavior, as well as in excessive talking and noisemaking in the classroom; (b) impatience, reflected in the tendency to rush into things before listening or judging what is best to do and in an apparent need to move ahead constantly without looking back or reflecting upon the past; (c) negative and defiant behavior with the teacher; and (d) self-centered verbal responsiveness characterized by interruption of others with remarks irrelevant to what is said in the context of ongoing conversation and by blurting out personal thoughts with insufficient prior self-examination (p. 128).

The researchers go on to state that:

Given the cluster of elements, it is easy to see how such a child might easily come into early conflict with adult authority, especially in settings that demand self-restraint and accommodation to numerous social and task demands, such as the classroom. Although such behaviors may not have their origins in hostile intent, it is easy to imagine such children quickly becoming involved in negative peer interchanges and angry adult reactions, all of which would quickly snowball, with increasing age, into the kinds of behavior we label as antisocial (p. 128).

So there is reason for Mrs. Thatcher to be concerned. She should not and cannot ignore Al's behavior. She should work with school personnel, such as a counsellor and a psychologist, to develop an intervention program that will enable Al to develop socially acceptable inter-personal skills. Furthermore, she and school personnel must also work with Al's parents so that they can have the child development knowledge and parenting skills necessary to remedy Al's at-risk behaviors. If Mrs. Thatcher and school personnel consciously ignore Al's symptoms, then it may well be that they will pay for Al's progress through the juvenile justice system.

*B*IBLIOGRAPHY

The American Heritage Dictionary. (1982). Boston, MA: Houghton-Mifflin.

Anspaugh, D., Ezell, G., & Goodman, K. N. (1987). *Teaching today's health.* Columbus, OH: Merrill.

Boston Children's Hospital. (1986). *Parents' guide to nutrition.* Reading, MA: Addison-Wesley.

Bybee, R. W. & Sund, R. B. (1982). *Piaget for educators* (2nd ed.). Columbus, OH: Merrill.

Carey, S. (1978). The child as word learner. In M. Halle, J. Bresnan, & G. A. Miller (Eds.), *Linguistic theory and psychological reality* (pp. 263–293). Cambridge, MA: MIT Press.

Conners, K. C. & Blouin, A. G. (1983). Nutritional effects on behavior of children. *Journal of Psychiatric Research, 17,* 193–201.

DeStefano, J. (1978). *Language, the learner and the school.* New York: John Wiley.

Dickie, N. H. & Bender, A. E. (1982) Breakfast and performance in schoolchildren. *British Journal of Nutrition, 48,* 482–496.

Emihovich, C. , Gaier E. L., Cronin, M. C. (1984). Sex role expectation changes by fathers for their sons. *Sex roles, 11,* 861–868.

Espenchade, A. S. & Eckert, H. M. (1980). *Motor development.* Columbus, OH: Merrill.

Fine, G. A. (1987). *With the boys: Little League baseball and preadolescent culture.* Chicago: The University of Chicago Press.

Gilligan, C. (1987, Fall). Adolescent Development reconsidered. In C. E. Irwin, Jr. (Ed.) *Adolescent social behavior and health.* (New Directions for Child Development, No. 37). San Francisco: Josey-Bass.

Goleman, D. (1988, October 6). Aggression in children can mean problems later. *New York Times,* p. 22.

Hoskisson, K. & Tompkins, G. E. *Language arts: Content and teaching strategies.* Columbus, OH: Merrill.

Johnson, W. G., & Corrigan, S. A. (1987). The behavioral treatment of child and adolescent obesity. *Journal of Child and Adolescent Psychotherapy, 4,* 91–100.

Judd, D. M., Siders, J. A., Siders, J. Z., & Atkins, K. R. (1986). Sex-related differences on fine-motor tasks at grade one. *Perceptual and Motor Skills, 62,* 307–312.

Kagan, J. J., Reznick, S. & Snidman, N. (1988). Biological bases of childhood shyness. *Science, 240,* 167–171.

Kohlberg, L. (1973, October 25). The claim to moral adequacy of a highest stage of moral judgment. *The Journal of Philosophy, 70,* (18), 630–646.

Kolata, G. (1989, January 3). Fat-cell protein is implicated in obesity. *The New York Times,* pp. 15, 19.

Kolata, G. (1988, February 15). New obesity studies indicate metabolism is often to blame. *The New York Times,* pp. 1, 17.

Kostelink, M. J., Stein, L. C., Whiren, A. P., & Soderman, A. K. (1988) *Guiding children's social development.* Cincinnati, OH: South-Western Publishing Co., pp. 359–362.

Maccoby, E., & Jacklin, C. (1974). *The psychology of sex differences.* Stanford, CA: Stanford University Press.

Miller, G. A., and Gilda, P. M. (1987, September). How children learn words. *Scientific American, 257,* 94–99.

Piaget, J. (1932). *The moral judgment of the child* (M. Gabin, Trans.). New York: The Free Press.

Richmond-Abbott, M. (1984). Sex role attitudes and children in divorced, single parent families. *Journal of Divorce, 8,* 61–81.

Rubin, N. (1988, February). Baby fat or just plain fat. *Parents,* p. 103.

Sadker, M., & Sadker, D. (1985, March). Sexism in the school room of the '80s. *Psychology Today,* 54–57.

Selman, R. L., & Selman, A. P. (1979, October). Children's ideas about friendship: a new theory. *Psychology Today, 13,* 71–114.

Singer, J. L., & Singer, D. G. (1986). Television-viewing and faimly communication style as predictors of children's emotional behavior. *Journal of Children in Contemporary Society, 17,* 75–91.

Sutton, C. (1986, November 11). Why do boys score higher? *The Washington Post,* p. 85.

Tangney, J. P. (1988). Aspects of the family and children's television viewing content preferences. *Child Development, 59,* 1070–1079.

Woolston, J. L. (1987). Obesity in infancy and early childhood. *J. amer. acad. child adol. psychiat., 26,* 123–126.

Zucker, Kenneth. (1987). Commentary of Kohlberg, Ricks, and Snarey's (1984): Childhood development as a predictor of adaption in adulthood. *Genetic, Social and General Psychology Monographs, 11,* 127–130.

CHAPTER ELEVEN

Learning and education during the middle years

◆

VIGNETTES

INTRODUCTION—THE NEW
  CURRICULUM

Arrivederci Recess

In the Spotlight: Just Say "No" to
  Guns

Human Growth and
  Development—AKA Sex
  Education

COOPERATIVE LEARNING

Benefits of Cooperative Learning

Pros and Cons of Cooperative
  Learning

Implications of Cooperative
  Learning for Schooling

TEACHING THINKING

THINKING: WHAT IS IT?

Critical Thinking

Teaching Children to Think
  Creatively

Implications for Teachers and
  Parents

INFORMATION PROCESSING
  AND COGNITIVE
  DEVELOPMENT

INFORMATION PROCESSING AT
  WORK

Sensory Processes

Perception

Attention

Memory

Metamemory

Information Processing and
  Implications for Teachers

Metacognition

THE TWO BRAINS

In the Spotlight: The Right Brain
  in Action

Organizing the Curriculum for the
  Right and Left Brains

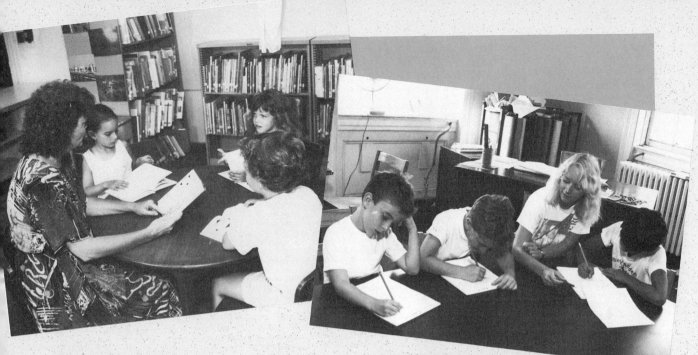

KINDERGARTEN EDUCATION
Who is Kindergarten for?
Universal Kindergarten
In the Spotlight: School
    Readiness—Who Gets Ready for
    Whom?
Promoting Readiness
Basic Skills Orientation
Reading in the Kindergarten
Kindergarten's Future
EMERGING LITERACY
Implications for Teachers and
    Parents
"George He Here Now"—Helping
    Black Children to Write
BILINGUALISM—MAKING
    CHILDREN LITERATE IN TWO
    LANGUAGES
Is There a Critical Period for
    Second Language Learning?
Implications for Teachers and
    Parents
In the Spotlight: A Just Community

What Would You Do?
CHILD CARE FOR SCHOOL-AGE
    CHILDREN
Before- and After-school Child
    Care
Latchkey Children—Caring for
    Themselves
TRANSITIONS
Helping Children Make
    Transitions
In the Spotlight: The Dieting
    Craze
SUMMARY
QUESTIONS TO GUIDE YOUR
    REVIEW
ACTIVITIES FOR FURTHER
    INVOLVEMENT
KEY TERMS
ENRICHMENT THROUGH
    FURTHER READING
ANSWER TO "WHAT WOULD
    YOU DO?"
BIBLIOGRAPHY

⌣IGNETTES

"Like most fifth graders, Amanda Cave spends much of her days on the three R's. But one recent day, she also worked on an architectural drawing, played the trumpet, did improvisational dancing, went on a scavenger hunt in the park and studied Spanish.

"The diversity of Amanda's day was no accident. It reflected the standard curriculum at the Key School, a new public elementary school dedicated to helping children develop a wide range of abilities that is based on the ideas of Howard Gardner, one of a growing number of scholars who are challenging traditional notions about human intelligence" (Fiske, 1988, p. A16).

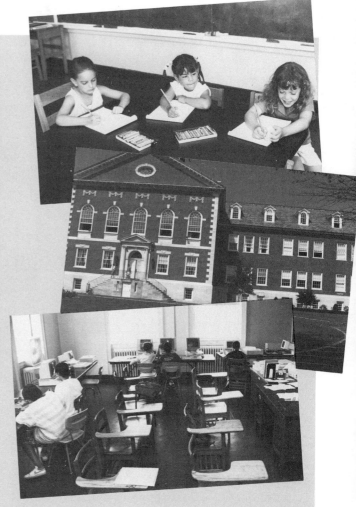

"In an unusual approach to learning history and writing, the children in Milly Sturman's fourth-grade class are spending the entire year writing biographies of the Rev. Dr. Martin Luther King, Jr. The biographies are full of facts and anecdotes and the pristine sense of injustice of 9-year-olds.

" 'One day Martin and his brother, A.D., were coming back from a trip,' goes one passage in Chrissy Della Corte's 40-page biography. 'They went on a train. The air was full of sunshine and happiness until they got down to the South again. Boom! The train conductor pulled the curtain closed so nobody would see them. How sad they felt, not wanted to be seen by the whites!"

"Although pupils have always written book reports and biographical compositions, the project at P.S. 201 in Flushing, Queens, is distinctive because the children have been working on the biographies daily for almost a year, doing much of their work in social studies and writing through the lens of one person's life" (Berger, 1988, p. 24).

"A new concept that advocates the unification of reading, writing and speaking in instructional programs is gaining popularity among teachers nation wide. 'Whole language' as it is called, rejects the skills-driven approach of most basel reading programs in favor of a 'holistic' view that capitalizes on literacy abilities that young students are already developing" (O'Neil, 1989, pp. 2, 6, 7).

"Looking for new ways to improve the education of black children, growing numbers of parents and educators in urban school districts are supporting requirements that teachers include or emphasize the contributions of blacks and other minorities in a wide range of subjects.

"These parents, educators and many psychologists say that one of the biggest obstacles to educational achievement among blacks is low self-esteem. And, they say that while the teaching in most of the nation's schools is seldom overtly racist, the lessons far too often use the accomplishments of whites at the expense of offering positive images of minorities" (Johnson, 1989).

The New Curriculum. When you were in the elementary grades, you probably were taught subjects like reading, language arts, mathematics, social studies, and health, with physical education and recess included to help break the routine. But, just as times have changed, so, too, the curriculum of many elementary schools has also changed as is apparent from the preceding vignettes.

Today, in addition to the basic skills, students are learning such subjects as how to cope with stress and the dangers of drugs and guns. Typical of these new curricula are: Gun Awareness; Coping with Death; Substance Abuse Education; Human Growth and Development; Say "No" to Drugs; Sexual Abuse Prevention; Coping with Stress; and Career Awareness. Many of these new curricula reflect the problems and concerns of contemporary society. The public believes that schools should be places where children learn the basic skills, and in addition, schools and teachers have a responsibility to help solve society's problems. This is why school curricula frequently mirror society's problems and why new curricula emerge as societal problems change.

Arrivederci Recess

As new curricula compete with the basic skills for time in the crowded school day, and as parents demand more from school systems, school officials look for programs to cut. One of the casualties in this curriculum cutting struggle is recess, the favorite subject of every child in school (Kass, 1989). Recess is often muscled out of children's daily schedules because it is easy to eliminate and is not always looked on with favor by educators.

*I*N THE SPOTLIGHT

JUST SAY "NO" TO GUNS

The third graders at Olinda Elementary School, located in the Liberty City area of Dade County, Florida, do more than learn how to read or write. They also participate in a gun awareness program designed to teach children that guns can kill. The school board, concerned about gun-related deaths in children, enlisted the help of a committee representing police departments, the teachers' union, teachers, parents, administrators, and the PTSA to develop a program of gun awareness.

According to Bill Harris, Supervisor for Safety and Driver Education in Dade County, the goal of the program is to reduce or eliminate the number of incidents involving injuries and deaths related to hand guns. "We want to counteract the messages of television that deaths are not real, but that in real life, death is forever." The Gun Awareness Curriculum, which may be the first of its kind in the nation, was initiated with a Gun Awareness Day in all of the district's 243 elementary, middle, and senior high schools.

According to Leorna Smith, principal of Olinda Elementary School, "The children in our community are exposed to guns more than ever before. We've had children bring toy guns to school and they see real guns and are exposed to them in the community. In the gun awareness program, we don't try to glamorize guns or to encourage children to go look for guns, but to remind them that guns kill!"

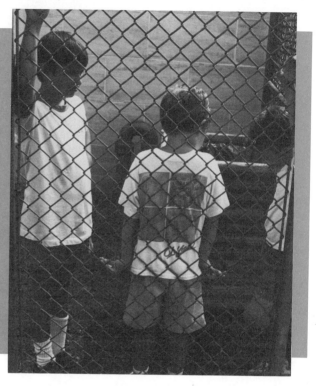

FIGURE 11-1 One of the challenges facing today's schools is to address, through curriculum and activities, early causes of many contemporary social problems such as drug abuse and delinquency. Increasingly, schools are viewed as more than places to teach reading, writing and arithmetic.

Human Growth and Development—AKA Sex Education

William Shakespeare said that a rose by another name would smell just as sweet, and Gertrude Stein said that a rose is a rose is a rose. They were both right. In the world of elementary education, "human growth and development" is the curricular euphemism to describe programs that include heavy doses of sex education. Educators have had to resort to such terminology in order to allay parents' fears that their children are being taught about sex, and to appease those who don't want the schools to teach about sex at all. Many parents and teachers feel that sex education is imperative, especially in these times when sex is used to sell food, toothpaste, and automobiles; countless references to sexual activity are routine ingredients of television programs, music videos, and movies; and the specter of AIDS is hanging over our society. While some seek a solution by yearning for a return to the more pristine era of "Leave It to Beaver" and "Father Knows Best," others maintain that today's children must have the facts about sex and sexuality in order to make sense of the sexual stimulation that bombards and surrounds them. Children need help in developing knowledge about sex and the skills necessary for sexual decision making.

Of course, human growth and development curricula include more than sex education. They also generally include family life topics and developmental information designed to help children and youth better understand themselves and others.

COOPERATIVE LEARNING

Competition is one of the hallmarks of our democratic society. Competition is part of the marketplace, the workplace, and the classroom. You may remember your elementary school days as times in which you competed with other students

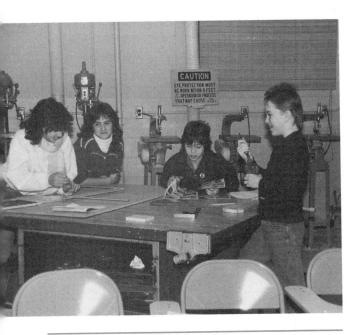

FIGURE 11-2 Peer relationships are an important part of children's development in the middle years. Peers help children learn many things, such as other's points of view and how to give and take. Now schools are involving students in cooperative learning in an effort to help them learn better.

for the top grades. You competed to be the first with the right answer, but in some classrooms today, things are a little different. Now there is a tendency to downplay competition and place more emphasis on cooperation. Cooperative learning is seen as a way of boosting student achievement and enhancing self-esteem. Instead of competition, the emphasis is on cooperation in the form of cooperative learning.

Cooperative learning is an instructional and learning strategy that has captured the attention of many educators. Cooperative learning refers to a set of instructional methods in which students are encouraged or required to work together on academic tasks (Slavin, 1987b). In cooperative learning, teachers employ a set of instructional methods in which students work in small, mixed-ability learning groups (Slavin, 1987a). The co-

operative learning group normally consist of four students who are responsible themselves for learning and for helping their group members learn. In one form of cooperative learning, called "Student Teams—Achievement Division," four mixed-ability students—usually one high achiever, two average students, and one low achiever—participate in a regular cycle of activities (Slavin, 1987a):

- The teacher presents the lesson to the group.
- Students work to master the material using worksheets or other learning materials. Students are encouraged to not only complete their work, but to explain their work and ideas to group members.
- Students take brief quizzes.

In a cooperative learning group, children are assigned certain tasks, for example, there is a group leader, who announces the problem or task; a praiser, who praises group members for their answers and work; and a checker. Group responsibilities rotate as the group engages in different tasks. Children are also encouraged to develop and use interpersonal skills, such as addressing classmates by their first names, saying "Thank you," and explaining to their groupmates why they are proposing an answer.

On the classroom level, there are five basic elements that need to be incorporated into the instructional process in order for cooperative learning to be successful (Brandt, 1987).

- "Positive independence"—The students have to believe they are in the learning process together and that they care about each others' learning.
- Verbal, face-to-face interaction—Students have to explain, argue, elaborate, and tie what they are learning now to what they previously learned.
- Individual accountability—Every member of the group has to realize that they have to learn.
- Social skills—Students must learn—be taught— appropriate leadership, communication, trust-

building, and conflict-resolution skills.
- Group processing—The group has to assess how well they are working together and how they can do better.

Benefits of Cooperative Learning

The benefits of having students engage in cooperative learning are several (Slavin, 1987a):

- It motivates students to do their best.
- It motivates students to help one another.
- It significantly increases student achievement.

Pros and Cons of Cooperative Learning

Supporters of cooperative learning maintain that it enables children to learn how to cooperate, and that children learn from each other. And since schools are such competitive places, it gives them an opportunity to learn cooperative skills, which they will need later in life.

However, not all teachers agree that cooperative learning is a good idea. They maintain that it is time consuming in that a group can take longer than an individual to solve a problem. Other critics charge that time spent on cooperative learning takes away time from learning the basic skills of reading, writing, and arithmetic.

Implications of Cooperative Learning for Schooling

Given the pressure on the public schools for accountability for learning, it makes sense that teachers would want to use a humanistic approach that increases student achievement. Furthermore, school critics say that frequently classrooms are too competitive and that students who are not competitive or high achievers are left behind. Cooperative learning would seem to be one of the better ways to reduce classroom competitiveness and foster "helping" attitudes.

The implications of cooperative learning go beyond the individual classroom. For example, we might assume that if classsroom teachers are involving their children in cooperative learning, then they (the teachers) are also involving themselves in cooperative activities with their colleagues, with the intent of enhancing the schooling process.

TEACHING THINKING

The back-to-basics movement has been a dominant theme in American education for the past two decades. It is likely to continue as a curriculum force to be reckoned with well into the twenty-first century. When we think of the basic skills, we generally think of reading, writing, and arithmetic. Indeed, in many elementary schools, these subjects garner the lion's share of time and teacher emphasis. Yet for some of the critics of education, and for the advocates of basic education, the ultimate basic of sound education is not the basics of the 3 Rs. Rather, the *real* basic of education is *thinking*. The rationale is that if students can think, then they can meaningfully engage in subject matter curriculum and the rigors and demands of the workplace and life. As a result, teachers are including the teaching of thinking in their daily lesson plans.

In classrooms that emphasize thinking, students are encouraged to use their "power of analysis," and teachers are asking higher level questions. Teachers are being encouraged to challenge their children to think about classroom information and learning material, rather than just giving them information for which rote, memorized responses are acceptable. So, rather than merely asking their children to recall information, teachers are asking their children to think critically about information given, solve problems, and reflect on information.

THINKING: WHAT IS IT?

By now you are probably asking yourself what teachers mean when they say they are teaching thinking. Well, since there are a number of different kinds of thinking, we must define each.

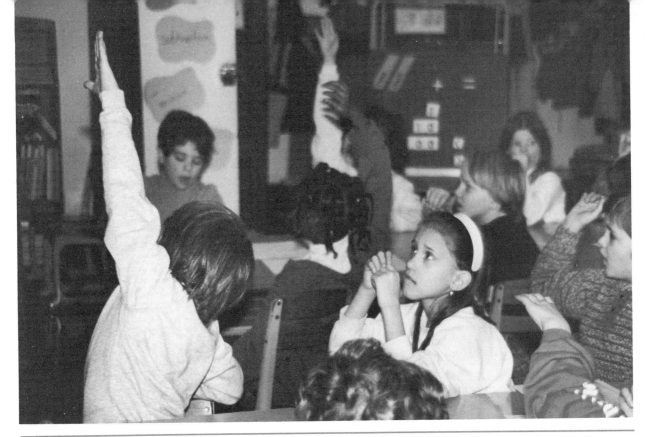

FIGURE 11-3 Teaching thinking is now considered the most basic of the basic skills. Many teachers are incorporating thinking skills into their regular curricula.

Critical Thinking

Critical thinking is reasonable, reflective thinking that is focused on deciding what to believe or do (Ennis, 1987). *Creative thinking*, on the other hand, is *divergent thinking* in which a child generates many different answers, solutions and approaches to a particular problem. Following is a list of critical thinking skills recommended for third graders (McTighe, n.d., p. 5).

1. Clarifying Issues and Terms
    a. Makes careful observations.
    b. Identifies and expresses main idea, problem, or central issues.
    c. Identifies similarities and differences.
    d. Organizes items into defined categories.
    e. Defines categories for unclassified information.
    f. Identifies information relevant to a problem.
    g. Formulates questions.
    h. Recognizes different points of view.
2. Judging and Utilizing Information
    a. Identifies obvious stereotypes.
    b. Distinguishes between fact and opinion.
    c. Identifies and explains sequence and prioritizing.
    d. Identifies evidence that supports (or is related to) a main idea.
    e. Identifies obvious assumptions.
    f. Identifies obvious inconsistency and contradiction.
    g. Identifies cause and effect relationships.
3. Drawing Conclusions
    a. Recognizes the adequacy of data.
    b. Identifies cause-and-effect relationships.
    c. Draws conclusions from evidence.
    d. Puts simple hypotheses into "if, then" sentences.

Most programs designed to teach thinking skills are based on the following basic beliefs and assumptions (Chance, 1986):

1. Thinking is a skill and can be taught.
2. Thinking is best taught by direct and systematic instruction.
3. The emphasis of instruction in thinking should be upon the process of thinking, not the products.
4. Students must use the thinking skills they are to learn.
5. Teachers should reinforce the appropriate use of thinking skills.
6. Teachers should make allowances for individual and developmental differences among students.
7. Thinking should be taught in a relaxed, nonthreatening atmosphere.
8. Thinking must be taught over a period of years.
9. An effort must be made to see that the skills taught in the program carry over to other subjects.
10. The teacher is the single most important determinant of the success of a thinking program (pp. 133–139).

In addition, critical thinking is characterized by certain attributes or criteria that separate it from ordinary thinking. These enable teachers and children to assess children's activities and make judgments about whether or not they are engaging in critical thinking as opposed to ordinary thinking. Table 11–1 compares the characteristics of ordinary thinking with the characteristics of critical thinking.

Teaching Children to Think Creatively

There are four basic concepts involved in promoting children's *creative* thinking (Doutre, 1988). They are:

- Fluency, the ability to think of an abundance of ideas, possibilities, consequences, and objects.
- Originality, the ability to come up with unusual, unique, or clever responses to a lesson or problem.
- Flexibility, the ability to use many different approaches or strategies to solving a problem.
- Elaboration, the ability to expand, develop, and embellish ideas, plans, and stories.

TABLE 11–1

COMPARING ORDINARY THINKING TO CRITICAL THINKING	
Ordinary Thinking	Critical Thinking/Reasoning
Guessing	Estimating
Preferring	Evaluating
Grouping	Classifying
Believing	Assuming
Inferring	Inferring logically
Associating concepts	Grasping principles
Noting relationships	Noting relationships among other relationships
Supposing	Hypothesizing
Offering opinions without reasons	Offering opinions with reasons
Making judgments without criteria	Making judgments with criteria

Note. From "Critical Thinking—What Can It Be?" by M. Lipman, 1988, *Educational Leadership, 46,* p. 40.

Implications for Teachers and Parents

Teachers and parents who want to promote creative thinking in children need to be aware of several things. First, children need the freedom *and* security to be creative thinkers. Many teachers and school programs are focused on helping children learn the *right* answers to a problem. Thus, children soon learn from the process of schooling that there is only one right answer. So, children may be so "right-answer"-oriented that they may be uncomfortable with searching for other answers or think that to do so is a waste of time.

Second, the environment must support children's creative efforts. Teachers must create classroom settings in which children have the time, opportunity, and materials with which to be creative. Letting children think creatively only when all their subjects are completed or scheduling creative thinking for only certain periods of time will not encourage creative thinking to the extent it should be.

Third, creative *and* critical thinking must be *integrated* into the total curriculum, so that children are taught to think critically and creatively across the curriculum, the school day, and throughout their lives.

INFORMATION PROCESSING AND COGNITIVE DEVELOPMENT

While Piaget's theory of cognitive development gets a great deal of attention and is the basis for much of the discussion regarding cognitive development, a growing competitor is information processing. In the *information processing* approach to the study of human cognition:

The human mind is conceived of as a complex cognitive system, analogous in some ways to a digital computer. Like a computer, the system manipulates or processes information coming in from the environment or already stored within the sys-

tem. It processes the information in a variety of ways: encoding, recoding, or decoding it; comparing or combining it with other information; storing it in memory or retrieving it from memory; bringing it into or out of focal attention or conscious awareness and so on (Flavell, 1985, p. 75).

The information that is processed consists of knowledge of word meanings and facts; how to do various things; perceptual distinctive features that help a child recognize letters; meanings of sentences; and higher order units such as schemes, plans, strategies, and rules used in thinking. And, in a single "burst" of information processing, all of these components can be involved (Flavell, 1985).

Some researchers who study the information processing approach to cognition attempt to explain what the mind does when dealing with a problem and the sequences in which problems are solved. The ultimate goal of the study of information processing is, as Flavell (1985) points out, "to achieve a model of cognitive processing in real time that is so precisely specified, explicit and detailed that it can actually be run successfully as a working program on the computer" (p. 76).

The comparisons between cognitive functioning and the computer are intriguing and, in many respects, surprisingly similar. For example, the human brain is the hardware that is "upgraded" through developmental processes and experiences. Just as a computer needs programs, in other words, software, to operate, so does the mind, in the form of information and strategies. Given this model, then, the purpose of teaching children thinking skills, for example, is to provide them with better software.

INFORMATION PROCESSING AT WORK

Let's see how this information processing model works in the life of a child. In order for the system to work, information must get into the system. Three critical processes for "inputting" information into the human system are sensory processes, perception, and attention.

Sensory Processes

One way for children to gather data is through the senses, which are physical. Using the senses, children gain information from the environment through seeing, hearing, touching, tasting, and moving. Many school programs design their curricula to focus on such sensory activities, because teachers and parents realize the importance they play in learning. For example, the Montessori program, you will recall, is devoted in part to training the senses, enabling children to better take in sensory data. Many preschool programs help children learn skills and concepts that have their bases in sensory processes, for example, learning to identify colors and sounds.

Perception

There is more to sensory data than merely taking it into the system. No doubt you have been in a particular situation with other people and your impressions of the situation were different from theirs. How do you account for this? One way is through *perception*, which is the ability of children to recognize, organize, and interpret sensory data and experiences. Perception is the process of making sense of what one sensorially experiences. Throughout the earlier chapters you have read how infants, toddlers, and preschoolers learn about the world through perceptual processes.

Attention

Attention, or the selective focusing of our concentration, plays an important role in children's learning processes because attention determines what and how they learn. In fact, there is the *zero-order theory* that says, "No attention, no learning" (Simon, 1986). Teachers and other professionals plan and organize for learning, but it is the child that must attend to that learning experience and learn from it. Attention consists of three components: *state, resource,* and *process* (Picton, Stuss & Marshall, 1986). As a state of mind, children expect certain information and prepare to perceive and act on that information. As a resource, attention is allocated to particular mental processes. As a process, attention chooses certain information, strategies, etc., for response while ignoring other information.

Watch some television commercials and determine what the creators of these ads did to capture your attention. Generally such things as size, color, sound, and novelty are employed separately and in combination to attract and keep your attention. Also, as many of you have learned from interpersonal relationships, what interests us also attracts us.

Motivation and Attention In teacher training programs, one area that is almost always included in the curriculum is methods and activities for helping teachers learn how to motivate students to attend to the learning process. In designing classroom activities and exercises that students will attend to, teachers must keep in mind that students give their attention to activities that are neither too simple or too complex (Simon, 1986). When a student is presented with a task that is too simple, it is boring, and when it is too complex, it is also boring. Teachers' tasks then become determining what is novel enough *for each child* to motivate them and keep them interested in the learning task. One way that many educators choose to solve this pedagogical problem is to base instructional activities on the interests of children, as first advocated by John Dewey (1975). This approach to classroom practice was and is evident in the instructional practices of the open classroom, and is also somewhat evident in thematic and integrated approaches to teaching and learning.

Now that information has been put into the system, something has to be done to and with it. In computer parlance, it has to be stored—so, too, with the mind. And the way for storing information in both humans and computers is through memory. One of the questions asked about a computer is, "How much memory does it have?" Unlike computers, however, we humans have all the memory we will ever need, barring illness, accident, or senility. Our problem as humans is to use the memory we have.

Memory

Did you ever wonder why phone numbers are seven digits and zip codes are five digits (nine, if you use the expanded version)? The reason is a very practical one. These bits or chunks of information represent the average storage capacity of your short-term memory (STM). The human short-term memory is limited to about seven items of information (Miller, 1956). This is why once you've looked up a telephone number and dialed it, it's forgotten. It also accounts for why you have to look up a number again to redial it because the line was busy! Short-term memory does, indeed, put a limit on our ability to process information.

Information stored in our long-term memory (LTM), on the other hand, stays with us forever, enabling us to recall events years after they have happened. We might not always be able to recall what is in our long-term memory, but it is there nonetheless. (Sometimes you may hear short-term memory referred to as "near" and long-term memory as "far.")

Memories of very early childhood are memories involving visual or emotional responses because of a lack of language skills necessary to store the events. In fact, it is rare for people to remember things that happened to them before they learned how to talk (Stark, 1984). However, memory in the "wide sense," in which past experiences exert an effect on current and future behavior, is probably present from birth. Memory in the "strict sense," a memory for a particular event at a particular time and place, begins to develop at eight to nine months (Restak, 1986, p. 151).

In our discussion of attention, we talked about the zero-order of learning. There is also a *first-order* of learning, which says that if an individual pays attention to a "chunk" of information for about eight seconds, that something is going to be stored in his long-term memory (Simon, 1986).

There are some things all of us can do to enhance our ability to remember, both for the long and the short term.

Rehearsal When you repeat a phone number that you are going to dial, you are conducting maintenance rehearsal for short-term memory. *Elaborative rehearsal*, on the other hand, is designed to commit information to long-term memory. A child who practices memorizing a part for a school play is committing her lines to long-term memory.

Organization Information is remembered more easily when it is organized. One of the organizers of this text is frequent headings that tell what the following paragraphs are about. These organizers make it easier to recall information read.

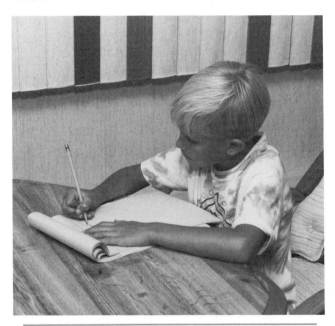

FIGURE 11-4 What children already know influences not only what they can learn but also what they remember and recall. Children with little knowledge or experience in an area have little to recall. Providing children with special experiences and opportunities therefore enhances both learning and memory.

Meaningfulness When information is meaningful, it is easier to remember. Meaningfulness is a function of how what we want to memorize is related to what we already know. If there is no relationship, there is little if any meaning. Interest also plays a role in meaningfulness. When children are interested in what they are learning, it is meaningful to them and it is more easily remembered.

Mnemonic Devices   Everyday, people who want to remember something employ the use of *mnemonics*, a system, strategy or plan to develop or improve the memory. (The word "mnemonic" comes from the Greek *mnemosune*, for "memory." Mnemosyne is the Greek goddess of memory and mother of the Muses.) One mnemonic device is the association of what you want to remember with an image. For example, a reminder to study becomes an image of your notebook and a reminder to call your best friend becomes an image of a telephone.

Keywords are frequently used to help children remember, and are common in many basic phonetic systems. Children are taught certain key words in order to help them remember the sounds of certain letters. For example, in order to recall the sound of the long vowel "a," the key word is "cake." Children are taught to refer to "cake" in order to obtain the sound of the letter "a."

Another mnemonic is one you have probably used to help you remember information for a test. This is the "first-letter" mnemonic. For example, the categories on the APGAR scale are *A*ppearance, *P*ulse, *G*rimace, *A*ctivity, and *R*espiration.

The sentence mnemonic is another useful aid to memory. For example, the sentence, "There is an *A*dvantage *I*nvolved *I*n *I*nitially *I*ntending *G*ood *E*xpectations," can help you remember in order the eight stages of Erikson's psychosocial development (TAIIIIGE).

Mnemonic devices are useful for all kinds of daily memory applications. For example, let's say that you wanted to remember, in the order in which they were created, the United States Cabinet level departments. The following mnemonic sentences would help: "See the dog jump in a circle. Leave her home to entertain educated veterans." (For your information, the departments in order are: State, Treasury, Defense, Justice, Interior, Agriculture, Commerce, Labor, Health and Human Services, Housing and Urban Development, Transportation, Energy, Education, and Veterans Affairs.) (Donovan, 1989)

Metamemory

You have certain notions and understandings about your ability to use memory and your ability to memorize. You know what kind of information is difficult for you to memorize and what kind of data is easy for you to memorize. Such self-knowledge of one's memory is *metamemory*, which is an individual's knowledge or cognition about anything pertaining to memory (Flavell, 1985, p. 209).

Information Processing and Implications for Teachers

One of the first rules of teaching at any level is to, first of all, get the students' attention. As obvious as this basic pedagogic rule may seem, it is surprising how often it is ignored! Second, the particular meaning information or activities have for children plays a powerful role in whether or not they will learn as well as how well they learn. Flavell (1985) puts it this way:

> Inputs that have little meaning for the individual—that do not fit readily into his acquired knowledge structure, that cannot easily be assimilated into his existing cognitive schemes, and so on—tend to be hard to store and retrieve. . . . Thus, what the head knows has an enormous effect on what the head learns and remembers (p. 213).

Consequently, it is important for teachers to help children learn and, in the process, match existing tasks to previous learnings. In this sense then, teaching and learning are reciprocal and accumulative processes—helping children learn increases their potential and presumably their ability to learn even more.

Metacognition

Over the last decade, one of the most influential and popular topics related to middle childhood and adolescent thinking and education deals with metacognition, a key component of information processing. *Metacognition* refers to an individual's knowledge of the factors that affect cognitive and learning activity and the control of these factors. In the reading process, for example, three sets of such factors include: knowledge of oneself as a reader, the demands of the reading task, and the strategies one employs in reading (Palincsar & Ransom, 1988). A child's knowledge of herself as a learner, the requirements of the learning task, and the strategies she uses for the task at hand, determine how she accomplishes the task and how successful she is. Her success in monitoring her learning in these ways in turn will contribute to her success—or failure—in subsequent cognitive activities.

The strategies a child uses in a learning task are important, because strategies differ in their accuracy, the amount of time needed to use them, the amount and kind of memory needed, and the range of problems to which they apply (Siegler, 1988).

While all students monitor their learning and achievement, successful achievers monitor their learning in order to use strategies that bring successful results (Brown, 1978). Some of these successful strategies include:

■ Clarifying and understanding the implicit and explicit requirements of a task.

■ Identifying the important parts of a message.
■ Engaging in self-questioning in order to determine if students are meeting their goals.
■ Taking corrective steps when students realize failures in understanding material.

THE TWO BRAINS

With all our discussion of thinking and memory, it is only natural that these topics should lead us to a consideration of the brain and its role in learning, because memory and thinking are functions of the brain. Today, there is general agreement that the two halves of the brain—the right and left hemispheres—while functioning as an integrated whole, also function differently. This view of the brain was not always the popular one. Previously, researchers thought that the whole brain was involved in every function. Then they thought that the left hemisphere was dominant. Now we know that both brains, with their specialized functions, contribute to learning in important ways.

Physically, the two brains are symmetrical in keeping with the left-right symmetry of the human body. Body movements are evenly controlled between the two brains, with the left hemisphere controlling the right side of the body and right hemisphere controlling the left side of the body. However, this asymmetry of functioning is mis-

TABLE 11–2

PROCESS CHARACTERISTICS OF THE TWO BRAINS	
Left Hemisphere	*Right Hemisphere*
Verbal	Nonverbal, visuo-spatial
Sequential, temporal, digital	Simultaneous, spatial, analogical
Logical, analytical	Gestalt, synthetic
Rational	Intuitive
Western thought	Eastern thought

Note. From *Left Brain, Right Brain* (p. 237) by S.P. Springer and G. Deutsch, 1985, New York: W.H. Freeman.

TABLE 11-3

DICHOTOMIES OF RATIONAL (LEFT BRAIN) AND INTUITIVE (RIGHT BRAIN)	
Left	*Right*
Convergent	Divergent
Intellectual	Intuitive
Deductive	Imaginative
Rational	Metaphorical
Vertical	Horizontal
Discrete	Continuous
Abstract	Concrete
Realistic	Impulsive
Directed	Free
Differential	Existential
Sequential	Multiple
Historical	Timeless
Analytical	Holistic
Explicit	Tacit
Objective	Subjective
Successive	Simultaneous

Note. From *Left Brain, Right Brain* (p. 237) by S.P. Springer and G. Deutsch, 1985, New York: W.H. Freeman.

leading, for you know that one side of your body is dominant. If you are right-handed, you probably kick with your right leg and prefer your right eye for looking. In this sense, the two brains are asymmetrical. Another way in which brain function is asymmetrical is that in most persons, speech is localized in the left hemisphere (Springer & Deutsch, 1985, p. 37).

The left hemisphere is the analytical brain. It engages in rational, linear, and sequential thinking, and is efficient in dealing with verbal information. The right hemisphere is involved in synthesis and recognizing patterns between separate parts. Table 11–2 shows the processes of the two hemispheres, and Table 11–3 shows the differences between the processing styles of the right and the left hemispheres.

*I*N THE SPOTLIGHT

THE RIGHT BRAIN IN ACTION

With all the emphasis on the two brains, we tend to forget that both are necessary for intelligent and creative activities. We think of the sciences as rational and precise, yet the intuitive plays a significant role in many great discoveries. Here is how Richard Rhodes (1986) describes the discovery of the basic idea for the splitting of the atom, a first key step on the road to the making of the first atomic bomb. Leo Szilard, famed scientist who helped in the development of the first atomic bomb, is on one of his daily walks:

"As the light changed to green and I crossed the street," Szilard recalls, "it . . . suddenly occurred to me that if we could find an element which is split by neutrons and which could emit two neutrons when it absorbs one neutron, such an element, if assembled in sufficiently large mass, could sustain a nuclear chain reaction."

"I didn't see at the moment just how one would go about finding such an element, or what experiments would be needed, but the idea never left me. In certain circumstances it might be possible to set up a nuclear chain reaction, liberate energy on an industrial scale, and construct atomic bombs."

Leo Szilard stepped up onto the sidewalk. Behind him the light changed to red (p. 28).

Organizing the Curriculum for the Right and Left Brains

In the curriculum field today, there is a prominent group that argues that the two halves of the brain—the right and the left—carry out two different kinds of thinking. Therefore they argue that the curriculum and instructional practices should be focused toward both sides. Furthermore, children's individual learning styles, right brain or left brain, should be accounted for in daily planning and activities. Some educators maintain that because the preponderance of school time is devoted to reading, writing, and arithmetic, the school curriculum develops primarily the left brain and is therefore biased against the right brain. In this sense, schooling provides an impoverished environment for the development of the right brain. Because of the concern that half of students' brains—the right halves—are being neglected, more educators are advocating curricula specifically designed to develop the right brain. Some activities suggested specifically to promote right brain thinking are (Williams, 1983):

- Visual thinking—Verbal techniques can be balanced with *visual strategies*, such as expressing ideas through pictures, maps, diagrams, and charts.
- Fantasy—Fantasy, or the ability to generate and manipulate mental imagery, can be used to help translate verbal information into images.
- Evocative language—*Objective language* has as its goal precision of meaning. *Evocative language* is rich in associations, highly sensual, and much less precise. "My love is like a red, red, rose," is an example of evocative language.
- Metaphor—Metaphorical or analogical thinking is the process of recognizing a connection between two seemingly unrelated things. The comparison of cognitive functioning to a computer is one example of metaphorical thinking.
- Direct experience—Much of the schooling experience is textually based and the extent of this textually-based learning increases as chil-

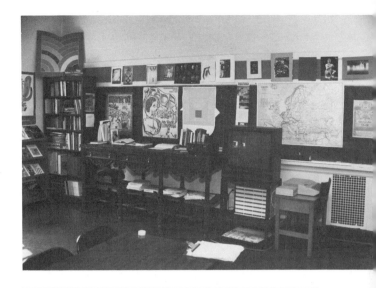

FIGURE 11-5 With so much emphasis on teaching to the two brains, more teachers are structuring classroom activities and environments to provide for both the left and right brains.

dren progress through school. Direct experiences with people, places, and things provide for nonverbal and nontextual interaction. Direct experiences include laboratory experiments, field trips, manipulation of materials, primary sources, real objects, simulation, and role playing.
- Multisensory learning—In addition to the auditory and visual senses, the tactile and kinesthetic (movement) senses also provide opportunities for learning.
- Music—Most listeners use their right hemispheres to process music, and music can be used as a source of instruction (for example, learning about the different kinds of music and music appreciation) and enjoyment (pp. 30–36).

KINDERGARTEN EDUCATION

Friedrick Froebel (1782–1852) is known as the father of the kindergarten ("garden of children"). Froebel's educational concepts and kindergarten program were imported to the United States virtually intact by individuals who believed in his ideas and methods. Especially innovative was Froebel's idea that learning can be based on play and children's interests. In addition, Froebel was the first to advocate a communal education for young children outside the home. Until Froebel, young children were educated in the home, by their mothers.

The kindergarten movement in the United States was not without growing pains. Over a period of time, the kindergarten program, at first ahead of its time, became rigid, and methods became teacher centered rather than child centered. By the turn of the century, many kindergarten leaders thought kindergarten programs and training should be open to experimentation and innovation. The chief defender of the Froebelian status quo was Susan Blow. In the more moderate camp was Patty Smith Hill, who thought that, while the kindergarten should remain faithful to Froebel's ideas, it should nevertheless be open to innovation. She believed that to survive, the kindergarten movement would have to move into the twentieth century. She was able to convince many of her colleagues and, more than anyone else, is responsible for the survival of the kindergarten as we know it today.

Patty Smith Hill's influence is evident in the format of many present-day preschools and kindergartens. Free, creative play, where children can use materials as they wish, was Hill's idea, and represented a sharp break with Froebelian philosophy. She also introduced large blocks and centers where children could engage in housekeeping, sand and water play, and other activities as they wished, rather than as the teacher dictated.

Who Is Kindergarten for?

Froebel's kindergarten was for children three to seven years of age; in the United States, kindergarten age has been considered the year before children enter first grade. Since the age at which children enter first grade varies, however, the ages

at which they enter kindergarten also vary. People tend to think that kindergarten is for five-year-old children rather than four-year-olds, and most teachers tend to support an older rather than a younger entrance age because they think "older" children are more ready for kindergarten and learn better.

There is wide public support for tax-supported public kindergartens and for making kindergarten attendance compulsory. A Gallup (1986) poll showed that 80 percent of the respondents favored "making kindergarten available for all those who wish it as part of the public school system," 71 percent favored compulsory kindergarten attendance, and 70 percent think children should start school at ages four or five (29 percent favored age four and 41 percent favored age five) (pp. 55–56). The question today is not so much whether a child will attend kindergarten, but when.

Universal Kindergarten

Kindergarten has rapidly become universal for the majority of the nation's five-year-olds. Today, kindergarten is either a whole or half-day program and within the reach of most of the nation's children. (See Table 11–4.)

TABLE 11–4

PROJECTED TRENDS IN PRESCHOOL ENROLLMENT BY AGE: 1990 TO 1993 (IN THOUSANDS)				
	Public Schools (Age)		Private Schools (Age)	
Year	5 Years	6 Years	5 Years	6 Years
1990	2,644	314	529	46
1991	2,667	318	533	46
1992	2,683	321	537	46
1993	2,693	323	538	46

Note. From "The Statistical Trends," May 1985, *The Principal,* *16*, p. 16.

*I*N THE SPOTLIGHT

SCHOOL READINESS—WHO GETS READY FOR WHOM?

In discussions of kindergarten programs, few issues generate as much heat as school readiness. Some school districts have raised the entrance ages for admittance to kindergarten and first grade, and require that children be five years old by the first of September to be admitted to kindergarten. This decision is based on the reasoning that many children are "not ready," and teachers, therefore, have difficulty teaching them. There is renewed emphasis on getting children ready for life processes and events such as child care, nursery school, preschool, kindergarten, and first grade. The early childhood education profession is reexamining "readiness," its various interpretations, and the various ways the concept is applied to educational settings.

For most parents and early childhood educators, readiness means the child's ability to participate and succeed in beginning schooling. Readiness includes a child's ability, at a given time, to accomplish activities and engage in processes associated with schooling, whether nursery school, preschool, kindergarten, or first grade. *Readiness* is thus the sum of a child's physical, cognitive, social, and emotional development at a particular time. Readiness does not exist in the abstract; it must relate to something. Increasingly, in today's educational climate, readiness is measured against the process of formal public schooling. By the same token, a child's lack of readiness may be considered a deficit and a deterrent, because it indicates a lack of what is needed for success in kindergarten and first grade.

Promoting Readiness

Some early childhood educators and many parents believe that time cures all things, including a lack of readiness. They believe that as time passes by, a child grows and develops physically and cognitively and, as a result, becomes ready to achieve. This belief is manifested in school admissions policies that keep children out of school for a year if they demonstrate lack of readiness as measured by a readiness test.

The modern popularizer of the concept of unfolding was Arnold Gesell (1880–1961), whose ideas and work continue at the Gesell Institute of Human Development in New Haven, Connecticut. Gesell made fashionable and acceptable the notion of inherent maturation that is predictable, patterned, and orderly. He also developed a series of developmental or behavioral norms that specify in detail children's motor, adaptive, language, and personal-social behavior according to chronological age. Gesell also coined the concept of *developmental age* to distinguish children's developmental growth from chronological age. For example, a child who is five years old may have a developmental age of four because he demonstrates the behavioral characteristics of a four-year-old rather than a five-year-old. Gesell believed that parents make their greatest contribution to readiness by providing a climate in which children can grow without interference according to their innate timetable and blueprint for development. The popularity of this *maturationist view* has led to a persistent sentiment that children are being hurried to grow up too soon.

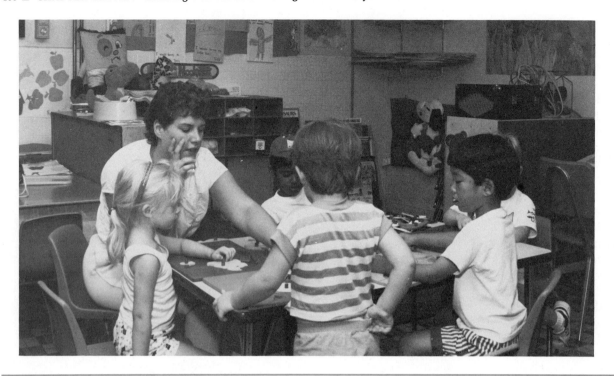

FIGURE 11-6 Kindergartens today are really part of the first year of school and are no longer considered as part of the preschool scene. What was once taught in first grade is now taught in many kindergartens. Kindergarten is no longer just a place for milk and cookies.

For Froebel, play was the energizer, the process that promotes unfolding. Montessori believed the prepared environment, with its wealth of sensory materials specifically designed to meet children's interests, is the principal means to help children educate themselves. For Piaget, the physically and mentally active child in an environment that provides for assimilation and accommodation develops the mental schemes necessary for productive learning.

Providing young children with *quality* preschool programs is another way to promote and assure their readiness. As more and more kindergarten teachers see that children are not ready for basic skills curricula, agencies such as Head Start, child care centers, and public schools have implemented programs for three- and four-year-olds to provide the activities and experiences necessary for kindergarten success.

Basic Skills Orientation

There is a great deal of tension in kindergarten education between those who advocate a readiness-play orientation and those who advocate a basic skill orientation. For example, Florida, the first state to mandate compulsory kindergarten education for all five-year-olds (students must be age five by September 1), has a primary education program that requires screening all children within the first six weeks of school for placement into one of three instructional groups: developmental (normal grade level); enrichment (above grade level), and preventative (below grade level). In Dade County, the kindergarten program operates according to a "balanced curriculum," where basic objectives and minimal instructional times are specified for subject matter areas.

Reading in the Kindergarten

Most elementary schools and many kindergartens focus on readiness and teaching reading. Students and teachers spend much of their time and energy in this process and related activities. Methods of organizing the classroom, such as grouping and scheduling, are frequently based on reading, and social patterns are often established according to membership in reading groups.

Learning to read in the primary grades is not an unreasonable expectation, and children look forward to it. Parents assume that when their children enter school, they will be taught to read. Learning to read is not only a social dictate, it is an academic necessity; how well a child reads often determines how successful he is in school. But with the greater emphasis on early schooling and basic skills, the teaching of reading is being pushed down to the kindergarten. Many parents and early childhood educators question a number of factors associated with early reading: first, its appropriateness and advisability; second, the teaching methods; and third, the pressure on children and the consequent stress this *pressure* can cause.

Developmentally Appropriate Reading Practices The Texas Association for the Education of Young Children has issued a description of a developmentally appropriate kindergarten reading program.

1. Young children learn through experiences that provide for all of the developmental needs—physical, socioemotional, as well as intellectual.
2. Young children learn through self-selected activities while participating in a variety of centers that are interesting and meaningful to them.
3. Young children are encouraged to talk about their experiences with other children and adults in the classroom.
4. Young children are involved in a variety of psychomotor experiences, including music, rhythm, movement, large and small motor manipulatives, and outdoor activities.
5. Young children are provided with many op-portunities to interact in meaningful print contexts: listening to stories, participating in shared book experiences, making language experience stories and books, developing key word vocabularies, reading classroom labels, and using print in the various learning centers.

Kindergarten's Future

The trend in kindergarten education is toward full-day, cognitive-based programs. Kindergartens give public schools an opportunity to provide children with the help they need for later success in school and life. Children come to kindergarten programs knowing more than their counterparts of twenty years ago. Children with different abilities and a society with different needs require that kindergarten programs change accordingly.

EMERGING LITERACY

In Chapter Nine, we began a discussion of emergent literacy regarding children's abilities to learn to speak, read, and write. We continue that discussion here. The concept of literacy as an emerging process has its basis in a number of areas. First, a small number of researchers (Smith, 1982) began to regard reading as a natural process, rather than an artificial process that teachers imposed on children when they came to school. In addition, literacy has come to be defined as a process that involves cognitive as well as social activities. In this sense, literacy is a meaning-based activity. Children want to make sense of what they speak, write, and read (Hall, 1987, p. 5). The current popularizer of the emerging literacy concept is Yetta Goodman, who maintains that "literacy develops naturally in all children" (Goodman, 1980, p. 4).

The emerging literacy concept is based on a number of beliefs about literacy that are different from how much of it was viewed in the past (Hall, 1987, p. 8).

■ Reading and writing are cognitive and social abilities involving a whole range of meaning-

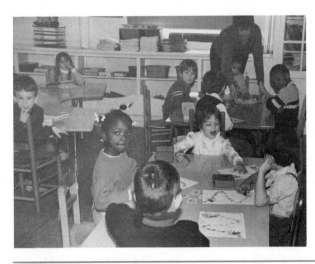 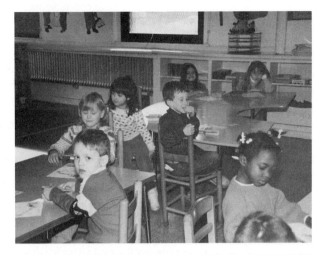

FIGURE 11-7   Learning to write and read are now considered "natural" rather than "artificial" processes, meaning that they should occur as a natural and regular part of children's in- and out-of-school lives. In this sense reading and writing are also seen as social processes.

gaining strategies.

■ Most children begin to read and write long before they arrive at school. They do not wait until they are taught.

■ Literacy emerges not in a systematic, sequential manner, but as a response to the printed language and the social environment experienced by the child.

■ Children control and manipulate their literacy learning in much the same way they control and manipulate all other aspects of their learning about the world.

■ Literacy is a social phenomenon and, as such, is influenced by cultural factors. Therefore, the cultural group in which children grow up will be a significant influence on the emergence of literacy.

Given these points, children are seen as competent individuals who can, on their own, develop knowledge about and abilities for literacy.

Implications for Teachers and Parents

The emerging part of literacy also has several significant implications for parents and teachers.

The term "emergent" implies: (1) that development takes place within a child; (2) that emergence is a gradual process; (3) that for literacy—or anything else—to emerge, there has to be something there in the first place; and (4) that cognitive and language processes and concepts emerge best in the conditions that facilitate such emergence, for example, in contexts that support efforts and involvements, facilitate inquiry, respect performance, and provide for involvement in real literacy acts (Hall, 1987, pp. 9–10).

"George He Here Now"—Helping Black Children Write

Writing, like reading, is one of the basic tasks of schooling. Some children come to school knowing how to write, all children come to school with the expectation and anticipation that they will write. But what does a teacher do with children who use nonstandard English, such as "My momma sick"? The answer is simple—you teach them to write. While some inexperienced and culturally insensitive teachers may believe that black English is a barrier to learning to write, it is not, and it should not be used as an excuse for not empowering young children with the ability to write in standard

English. Becoming proficient in the use of standard English is a goal of schooling. Black English is used by many children and possesses some of the characteristics illustrated in the two sentences above: the use of double subjects and the deletion of some form of the verb "to be."

Lynda Markham (1984) provides some useful suggestions to help young children learn to write:

1. Black English is a problem only if the teacher allows it to be. Being informed about black English and black children and having a positive attitude are important to helping children write.
2. Remember that the basics of writing are racial.
3. Provide children many opportunities for oral language development in order for them to expand their language base as a basis for writing.
4. Reading to children and allowing children opportunities to read provides models of syntax and form as well as expanding their understanding of the world.
5. Provide children something to write about as well as the time, materials, and support for writing.
6. Avoid correcting too frequently or without regard for children's feelings. Yet, at the same time, teachers can help children correct and improve their writing.

BILINGUALISM—MAKING CHILDREN LITERATE IN TWO LANGUAGES

The term *bilingualism* creates different emotions in people. Some see it as an unnecessary and unpatriotic endeavor, while others see it as a humane and culturally sensitive way of introducing children and adults into pluralistic American society and helping them become proficient in English. The emotional tensions are all the more evident when states such as California and Florida hold referendums to declare English as their official state language. Ethnic groups oppose such actions because they believe they are designed to curtail cultural diversity.

The Bilingual Education Act of 1968 was the first official federal recognition of the needs of students with limited English-speaking ability. This act has been extended by Congress over the years and most recently when the 1988 Bilingual Education Act (BEA) was reauthorized for a three-year period under the Hawkins-Stafford Elementary and Secondary School Improvement Act of 1988.

The 1988 BEA authorizes 75 percent of total grant funds under BEA to school districts for *transitional* bilingual education. The other 25 percent of the funding goes to other alternative instructional programs, such as general English as a Second Language (ESOL) programs, which do not use native language in the instructional process (Stewner-Manzanares, 1988, p. 7).

A central issue in the great bilingual education debate is how to best teach English to limited English proficient (LEP) students. There are several ways to accomplish this task. One is through *immersion*, or what is often referred to as the "sink or swim" method. A child is put into a classroom with her English-speaking peers and she learns the language by being surrounded by it all day long. This is the way many immigrants of previous decades learned English, and many maintain that it was good enough for them and therefore should also be good enough for modern-day immigrants.

A second way to teach LEP children English is through a *transitional* program of bilingual education in which children are taught in their native language *while* they are learning English. Officially, *transitional bilingual education programs* are programs that incorporate a native language instructional component into their curriculum and instructional programs. A child is given a transitional program only until he becomes proficient enough to use English to learn, and then no further instruction is provided. According to the BEA, a child may spend no more than three years in a transitional bilingual program. A transitional program also includes the incorporation into the instructional process of the child's cultural heritage and that of other children in American society. Critics

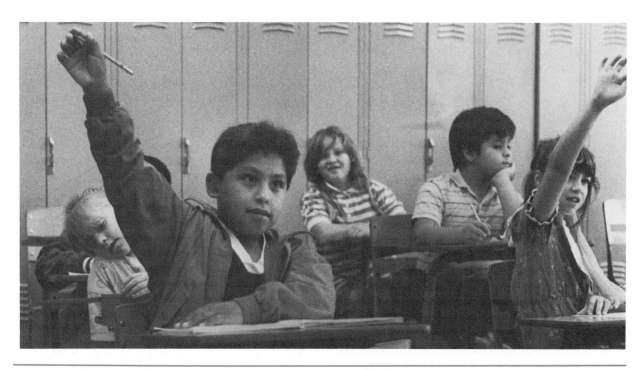

FIGURE 11-8 A great deal of controversy surrounds how to teach English to children who are non-native speakers. A particular problem for many large urban school districts is that many children are illiterate in their native language as well as non-speakers of English.

of such programs maintain that children keep on using their native language and never learn English at all or learn too little to help them make the transition.

A third method of teaching English to LEP or non-English-speaking students is through TESOL (*Teaching English to Speakers of Other Languages*), in which students are taught English without benefit of instruction in their native language. Many adult education programs are taught in this way.

A fourth program of bilingual education is a *maintenance* program in which the child's proficiency in his native language is maintained and improved while he learns English. This is also a program for children who are bilingual, and is an effort to maintain the home language. Critics of maintenance programs say they are unnecessary and costly. These programs are also referred to as *developmental* bilingual programs.

A current problem facing many urban school systems in the United States is that a growing number of immigrant children, particularly those from third world and revolution-torn countries in which the education programs have been disrupted or are nonexistent, are illiterate in their native tongues. Thus, they enter the school systems without being able to communicate well in their own language and not at all in English.

Is There a Critical Period for Second Language Learning?

I'm sure you have heard that the best time to learn a second language is as early as possible. The tales of adults who tried and failed to become fluent in a second language add to the public perception that you either learn a language early or not at all. Second language learning by young children is rhapsodized as relatively effortless and practically automatic. But is such a belief true? Not according to Catherine Snow (1987), who maintains that:

> Second language learning appears, upon more careful examination [of research data] to be slow, effortful, and often less perfectly successful for younger as well as older learners. In fact, speed of second language acquisition seems in general to be positively correlated with age. For most domains of acquisition studied, older learners acquire more in the same amount of time than younger learners.
>
> Of course, it is not the case that age is the only factor of influence in speed of second language learning. It is well documented that such factors as amount of exposure, quality of language exposure, motivation to learn, desire to identify with the second language group, tolerance for the psychological stress associated with functioning in two cultural settings, and language aptitude play important roles as well (pp. 192–193).

Implications for Teachers, Parents and Adults

What implications does such information have for child development and education professionals? There are a number. First, the critical period for second language development probably extends beyond the pubertal stage. Generally, the classical critical period of language development is given as from about age one through puberty. Thus our conception that "older students" cannot learn a second language has to be modified. Second, the life period over which people can reasonably be expected to learn a second language can include the mature adult years.

*I*N THE SPOTLIGHT

A JUST COMMUNITY

In Chapter Ten we discussed moral development during the middle years based on the theory of Lawrence Kohlberg. This theory has many implications for classroom practice such as those that occurred in the development of a "Just Community" at Birch Meadow Elementary School, Reading, Massachusetts (Murphy, 1988). Concerned by students' uncaring attitude toward others and their frequent bickering, teachers decided to use the ideas of Kohlberg to develop a program that would improve the quality of life in the school. According to Kohlberg, in a just community, teachers do not concede authority or leadership to children, but they do listen to children and are willing to adjust procedures, rules, and decisions when there is no good reason *not* to. In the Birch Meadow program, there are two ongoing activities: circle meetings in all classrooms, and two student councils, one for the primary and one for the intermediate grades.

In a circle meeting, there are four basic steps:

1. Chairs are arranged in a circle so that all students can maintain eye contact with each other.
2. The discussion leader—not necessarily the teacher—controls the order in which students speak.
3. Anyone can refrain from speaking by saying "pass."
4. While students are sharing their ideas, no interruptions, comments, or laughter, are permitted.

However, when a meeting is called to solve a particular problem, then four other steps are also employed in addition to those listed. These are:

1. All suggestions are recorded.
2. Suggestions are discussed in order to arrive at consensus.
3. A timetable is set for implementing the solution, necessary tasks are assigned, and the solution is given a trial.
4. The outcomes are discussed at a later circle meeting.

Circle meetings are called to discuss student behaviors, injustices, safety matters, and differences of opinion relating to classroom rules. In addition, classroom circles are used to discuss current events, review subject matter, explore feelings related to tragic events, and discuss any event of importance to teachers and children.

The intermediate grades (grades four to six) hold elections for student council officers and then individual classrooms elect representatives to the council. The vice president of the intermediate council is the chairperson of the primary council, whose members are elected by the students or appointed by the teachers.

Among the many accomplishments of the student councils are a playground cleanup; fund-raisers for UNICEF, the renovation of the Statue of Liberty, and St. Jude's Children's Research Hospital ($3,400 in ten days); getting skim milk, chocolate milk, and ice cream treats added to the cafeteria menu; and the return of paper towels to the restrooms.

The just community at Birch Meadows has enabled the 400 children to develop a sense of ownership in the school and a sense of responsibility for their classmates. They are also learning to care for and share with others. And, perhaps just as importantly, the community grows stronger each year as students become more experienced living in it.

What Would You Do?

Mercedes McCallum is in the third grade at Jefferson Elementary School. In first and second grades, Mercedes was an above average student, she enjoyed going to school, and was happily involved with school-related activities. At the end of the first grading period this year, however, Mercedes grades were all Cs. Also, she is growing more apathetic toward school and there are days when she doesn't care whether or not she attends.

Last week, Mrs. McCallum met with Mercedes' teacher to find out why Mercedes' grades had fallen and what could be done about her emerging negative attitude toward school. During the conference, Mercede's teacher, Muriel Baylish, a new teacher to the district, told Mrs. McCallum that Mercedes' past school performance was highly overrated and that her grades were inflated by about a full letter. "One of my jobs," Mrs. Baylish said, "is to help students see themselves as they really are. It's no favor to parents or children letting them go through life thinking they can do more than they are capable of. It only catches up to them later in life. Mercedes is an average to below-average student, so there is no use my mincing words about it."

Mr. and Mrs. McCallum are stunned by Mrs. Baylish's attitude and what she said about Mercedes. The McCallums know that you, as their next-door-neighbor, are taking courses in child development and education at the university. They have invited you over to discuss what you think they should do. Since you have some time to plan for the visit, what will you tell the McCallums?

CHILD CARE FOR SCHOOL-AGE CHILDREN

With the increase in the number of working mothers, the demand for child care has greatly outstripped its availability. The public has put heavy pressure on the public schools to help meet the need for child care in two ways. One result, which we have already discussed, is the rapid growth of preschool programs for four-year-old children. While the justification for four-year-old programs is most often made on the basis of providing much-needed services for disadvantaged children, we cannot overlook the reality of the present. Public schooling for all four-year-olds is becoming more of an accepted proposition by many states and school districts. The point is that the public schools provide a tremendous baby-sitting service to the nation's children and parents. That service now includes four-year-old children and is called pre-school.

Before- and After-School Child Care

The second way that public schools have responded to the public's need for child care is through before- and after-school care. Typical of this response is that provided by the Kendale Lakes Elementary School in Miami, Florida, which has an enrollment of 1550 children in grades K–6. This before- and after-school program is what is known as a principal-operated program, in that the principal administers the program and the school provides all the services and personnel. Some other schools provide a program of contracted child care services through the YWCA, which administers the programs and provides the personnel and services.

Before-school care at Kendale Lakes Elementary is from 7:00 AM to 8:20 AM, five days a week, and costs $1.20 a day (1989 figures). Enrollment is about eighty children. After-school care begins at 2:00 PM (for kindergarten children) and ends at 6:00 PM and services approximately 275 children. The after-school care costs $3.50 a day. The school also stays open for child care on all spring and winter breaks, and is open from 8:00 AM to 6:00

PM at a cost of $10.00 per day. Following are the before- and after-school care schedule.

BEFORE-SCHOOL CARE SCHEDULE

7:00 AM Arrival
Television cartoons
Light arts and crafts
7:45 AM Outside
8:20 AM Dismissal to rooms

AFTER-SCHOOL CARE SCHEDULE

2:00 PM Attendance, snacks (Snacks are provided by the program)
2:20 PM Outside—supervised play
3:15 PM Quiet time—homework, games, and puzzles
4:30 PM Outside—supervised play, or inside—movies (half a movie is shown one day and the other half the next day).
5:15 PM Filmstrips
6:00 PM After-school care closes. Parents who pick their children up after 6:10 PM are charged a $5.00 late fee.

In order for parents to enroll their children in the program, they must purchase school insurance, agree to abide by the school discipline code, and sign their child in and out of child care each day. Also, any person other than the parent picking up the child must provide photographic identification, usually a driver's license.

All care-givers are licensed by the State of Florida. This licensing procedure includes a background check, fingerprinting, and completion of training programs including CPR and basic child development. Care-givers in the program are teachers, teachers' aides, college students, and parents.

The number of children who require after-school care is significant, as shown in Table 11–5.

Latchkey Children—Caring for Themselves

Eleven-year-old Lisa Martinez, an only child, takes the school bus home each day from school,

TABLE 11–5

AFTER-SCHOOL CARETAKER OF 5- TO 13-YEAR-OLD CHILDREN ENROLLED IN SCHOOL, BY LABOR FORCE STATUS OF MOTHER AND RACE, DECEMBER 1984 [NUMBERS IN THOUSANDS]

Status	Number	Caretaker (by percent)				
		Parent	Adult sibling	Other relative (percent)	Non-relative	No adult
All children:						
All races	28,852	75.5	2.7	6.6	7.8	7.2
White	23,350	75.4	2.6	5.7	8.3	7.8
Black	4,316	75.9	3.0	10.7	5.6	4.3
Mother in labor force:						
All races	17,027	63.2	4.1	9.5	11.8	10.9
White	13,715	62.5	3.9	8.6	12.7	12.0
Black	2,626	67.2	4.7	13.4	8.1	5.9
Mother employed full time:						
All races	10,559	54.3	5.2	11.7	14.8	13.5
White	8,307	52.8	5.0	10.8	15.9	15.0
Black	1,788	60.9	5.5	15.2	10.3	7.4

Source: Bruno, Rosalind R., 1987, After-School Care of School-Age Children, December 1984, Special Studies, Series P-23, No. 149, U.S. Department of Commerce, Bureau of the Census.

lets herself in with a key hung around her neck and cares for herself from 3:30 till 6:00 PM, when her parents arrive home. Some of the Martinez's neighbors think it is terrible that poor Lisa has to stay by herself. What is more, they think the Martinez's are "bad parents" for doing such a thing. After all, how could parents who love their children leave them alone while they are at work? The general perception by the public is that children who take care of themselves before and after school, *latchkey children*, are at risk and are somehow suffering irreparable consequences. But is this true? Does being a latchkey child *per se* mean that something bad is happening to the child's cognitive and social development? Let's find out.

First, the research regarding the effects of self-care by latchkey children is conflicting and confusing (Robinson, Coleman, & Rowland, 1986; Vandell & Corasaniti, 1988). Some studies (Long & Long, 1983) indicate that latchkey children are lonely, fearful, and stressed. Other studies (Rod-

man, Prato, & Nelson, 1985; Steinberg, 1986) show no differences between latchkey and other children.

Second, where a latchkey child lives makes a difference regarding the effects of her self-care. Urban latchkey children are at higher risk for psychological harm than rural or suburban children. Children who live in cities are more confined and face greater threats of personal intrusion and accidents (Robinson, Coleman, & Rowland, 1986). In rural and suburban areas, on the other hand, latchkey children, when compared to their adult-supervised counterparts, adjust equally well socially and academically (Robinson, Coleman, & Rowland, 1986). In a study of suburban, middle-class children, researchers found no evidence that third grade latchkey children did more poorly than children who returned home to their mothers. Their standardized test scores were comparable, and parents and teachers rated them similarly on emotional well-being, how they get along with their

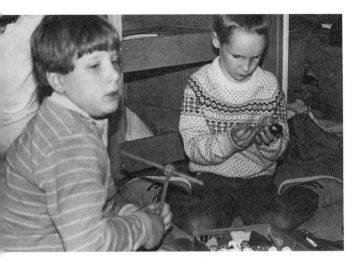
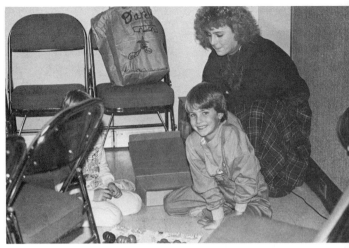

FIGURE 11-9 For many children with working parents the school day is an extended one beginning with before-school care and ending with after-school care. For some children this means a school day of ten or more hours. Consequently, these programs must be more than just baby-sitting services.

peers, and work/study skills (Vandell & Corasanati, 1988). So when talking about latchkey children in general, it pays to know the population we are talking about in order to make general statements about the effects of self-care on child development.

Third, the age at which children are providing themselves with self-care certainly is a factor that must be considered in any discussion of whether or not self-care has or has not any influences on children's development. Certainly a first grade child providing self-care for herself is different from a third grade child providing care for herself.

Fourth, there are different kinds of self-care. For example, when Lisa arrives home, she immediately calls her mother at work and "checks in." Also, she has a list of dos and don'ts she follows, and she has the telephone numbers of other people she can call if she needs help. In these ways, Lisa is really cared for "in absentia." This supervision of a latchkey child is entirely different from the situation in which a child gets little if any help from parents or others.

So, before we can say that the effects of self-care on latchkey children are positive or negative,

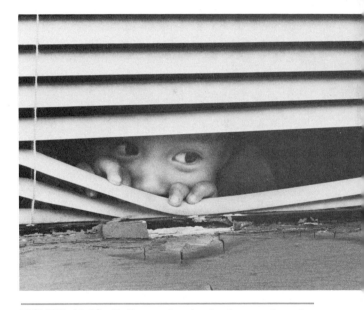

FIGURE 11-10 Self care is standard procedure for some children whio do not have the benefits of extended day care. For some children this is a satisfactory arrangement. Many agencies have support services such as emergency and homework telephone hot-lines to provide latch-key children with security and assistance.

we need to know the context and circumstances of their care. Keep in mind, too, that there are many individual circumstances surrounding children's care. Just because a child lives in an urban setting and is a latchkey child does not necessarily mean that the experience is harmful to her.

TRANSITIONS

A child faces a transition whenever there is a change in environment, in how schooling is conducted, and in the children and adults with whom they will interact. The preschool and kindergarten years are full of transitions. Major transitions involve leaving preschool to enter kindergarten, and leaving kindergarten to enter first grade. This transition may not be too difficult for children housed in the same school as the primary grades. For others, for whom the preschool or kindergarten is separate from the primary program, or who have not attended preschool or kindergarten, the experience can be unsettling and traumatic, or joyful and rewarding. Transitions can influence, positively or negatively, children's attitudes toward schooling. Children with special needs who are making a transition from a special program to a mainstreamed classroom need extra transitional attention and support.

The reputations children establish may follow them for a long time and may enhance or inhibit their learning and development. Therefore, when forecasting the outcomes of the transition period, particular attention needs to be paid to children's emerging peer status and to teachers' perceptions of their interpersonal and task-related behaviors (Ladd & Price, 1987). For this reason, the interpersonal characteristics of children in former settings and the peer composition of the transition setting are important predictors of peers' and teachers' perceptions. Consequently, there are a number of factors about children's characteristics and the pre- and post-transitional settings that are important for teachers and parents to know and take into consideration. These are (Ladd and Price, 1987):

- Children with higher levels of cooperative play in preschool and a pattern of extensive positive contacts among classmates tend to become better liked by peers in kindergarten and are perceived by teachers as more involved with their classmates.
- Children who spend more time engaging in aggressive behavior and who have a broader range of antisocial peer contacts in preschool tend to become disliked by their kindergarten classmates and are perceived as hostile toward others by their kindergarten teachers.
- For males in particular, the tendency to engage in antisocial interactions transcends school environments and predicts negative peer and teacher perceptions in present and future settings.
- Both the quality and the range of children's peer relationships are instrumental in the development of their social reputations in the larger peer group.
- Children's aggressive behavior and their negative peer contacts may influence teachers' perceptions of social maladjustment.
- The transition context is a predictor of children's peer status in kindergarten.
  1. The presence of familiar peers in children's classrooms has a facilitative influence on their peer acceptance.
  2. Familiar classmates provide children with a "secure base" from which to develop new relationships and extend their social ties.
  3. Children tend to perceive and rate familiar classmates as more likable.
- Children who like school less are absent more often and make more requests to see the school nurse. Also, children who are absent from school more often tend to display higher levels of anxiety in the classroom and also make more requests to see the school nurse.
- Time spent by a child with younger companions in preschool is negatively related to liking school, both at the beginning and at the end of kindergarten. Thus, overinvolvement with younger companions may impede later school adjustment.

- Prior school experiences prepare children for the stress and demands of the kindergarten setting.
- Perhaps preschoolers who have regular contact with peers in several community settings are less stressed by environmental alterations or have developed more adaptive coping styles for new or novel situations.
- Stable peer relationships facilitate school adjustment. Children who retain a larger proportion of their nonschool peer relationships have more favorable school attitudes at the beginning of kindergarten.
- Children who have a large number of familiar peers in their classroom tend to view kindergarten more positively.

Helping Children Make Transitions

Given these findings, what can teachers and parents do to facilitate their children's transitions to and adjustment in kindergarten? There are a number of things (Ladd and Price, 1987):

1. Educators can recognize that transition processes provide both opportunities and risks for children's development and school success.
2. Transitions that represent alteration in the peer system can provide opportunities for children to develop new reputations.
3. Preventative efforts involving preparing preschoolers for the challenges of the new setting should occur prior to and after the transition.
4. Teachers and parents can help children refrain from aggressive acts and pursue more positive peer contacts prior to kindergarten entrance.
5. Parents and teachers can arrange for children to attend preschool and spend more time with their agemates prior to kindergarten.
6. Parents can help children maintain ties among friends and associates outside the school environment as a means of assuring continuity in one social domain while the other domain, the transition from preschool to kindergarten, is changing.

7. School administrators can plan the peer composition of kindergarten classrooms, taking into consideration prior friendships and acquaintances, in order to facilitate early school adjustment.
8. Parents can help their children become acquainted with peers who are likely to attend the same school as their children.

In addition, there are other guidelines teachers, care-givers, parents, and others may wish to employ to lessen the stress of any transition (Morrison, 1988, pp. 283, 286):

- Alert and educate children ahead of time to the new situation. For example, children can visit, for a short time or for a day or two, the kindergarten they will be entering, and they can practice doing things in preschool the way they are done in the kindergarten and primary grades.
- Work with parents to educate them to the new setting and the expectations regarding dress, behavior, achievement, and parent-teacher relationships. A parent handbook is useful for this purpose.
- Educate parents to the curriculum their children will use by showing them books and conducting sample lessons with them; this helps parents understand what their children will learn.
- Work with parents of children with special needs to help them become familiar with and understand the new program. In particular, bilingual parents and parents with handicapped children will need extra transitional support.
- Teachers can work with, train, and orient each other as to what they do in each program. Visiting each other's classrooms for a day gives teachers insight into the programs from which they receive children and those to whom they send children.
- Teachers and coordinators can coordinate curriculum between programs so that what children do in preschool relates to what they will do in kindergarten and first grade.

■ Establish a "transition committee" of teachers and parents to help identify activities and processes for facilitating transitions.

The nature, extent, creativity, and effectiveness of transitional experiences for children, parents, and staff will be limited only by the commitment of all involved. If educators and parents are interested in providing good preschools, kindergartens, and primary schools, then they must include transitional experiences in the curricula of all the programs.

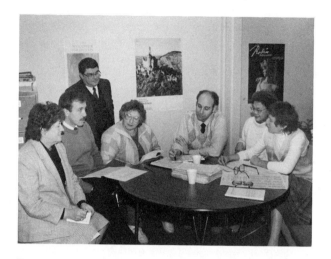

FIGURE 11-11 Transitions from one setting or program to another can be a stressful time in children's lives. More parents, teachers and school administrators are involved in processes and programs designed to help children and their parents prepare for and have good transitions.

*I*N THE SPOTLIGHT

THE DIETING CRAZE

In addition to all the other pressures society places on children, another that can be added to the list is the fear of fat. As a result, preadolescent dieting has increased greatly in recent years (Seligmann, Joseph, Donovan, & Gosnell, 1987). The weight and body image obsession begins early. In one survey 494 school girls described themselves as overweight, although only 15 percent actually were. Eighteen of the ten-year-old girls in the study were dieters.

There are several reasons for the early concern regarding weight and body image. First, girls are reaching puberty earlier (see Chapter Twelve). The early development of their breasts and hips may signal to them that they are getting fat. They see dieting as one way to deal with their changing body. Second, with the changing sexual mores of society, females are becoming sexually assertive at earlier ages. And, they think that boys don't make passes at fat girls. Third, attitudes about weight and diet filter down from parents to children. A mother who is constantly concerned about her weight and who is constantly dieting may encourage her daughter to do the same, even though the daughter isn't overweight. Also, some parents may go overboard in impressing on their children the importance of physical fitness and eating "healthy foods."

SUMMARY

- As society changes, so, too, does the curriculum of the nation's schools. Not only does the curriculum of the schools reflect efforts to help society solve its problems, it also indicates professionals' efforts to teach children in new and different—and hopefully better—ways.
- Cooperative learning is a new method for teaching and is viewed as a way of boosting student achievement and enhancing self-esteem. In cooperative learning, students are encouraged or required to work together on academic tasks.
- Many advocates of basic education maintain that thinking is the ultimate basic. In classrooms that emphasize thinking, students are encouraged to use their "power of analysis" and teachers are asking higher level questions. Teachers are encouraged to challenge their children to think critically and creatively rather than just giving back memorized responses.
- In the information processing approach to learning, the human mind is conceived of as a complex cognitive system, analogous in some ways to a digital computer. Like a computer, the system manipulates or processes information coming in from the environment or already stored within the system.
- Perception, attention, motivation and memory all play important functions in how children learn and in the information processing theory about how children learn. Memory is either long or short term. Metamemory is an individual's knowledge or cognition about anything pertaining to memory.
- Educators and psychologists are very much interested in the process of metacognition, an individual's knowledge of the factors that affect cognitive and learning activity and the control of these factors. How to apply the ideas of metacognition to the curriculum is an important educational consideration.
- Just as there is much interest in metacognition, there is also much interest in the two hemispheres of the brain, the right and the left. Educators are developing curriculum and programs to help students learn with both hemispheres.
- The kindergarten movement is growing in the United States, and now most children have a kindergarten program available to them. Most of the issues in kindergarten education today focus on the appropriateness of half- versus whole-day programs, the best age for beginning attendance, and what constitutes developmentally appropriate practice.
- Emerging literacy is based on the idea that reading and writing are cognitive and social abilities that involve many meaning-gaining strategies. It recognizes that most children begin to read and write long before they arrive at school, and that literacy emerges not in a systematic, sequential manner, but as a response to the printed language and the social environment.
- Some children come to school speaking nonstandard English. The Bilingual Education Act authorizes providing transitional programs for teaching children English. This and other bilingual programs are controversial in nature.
- With the increase in the number of working mothers, there has also been an increase in the need for before- and after-school child care. Many children care for themselves both before and after school. They are known as latchkey children. Where latchkey

children live—urban or suburban areas—makes a difference in the nature and the quality of their care. Also, the age of the children providing self-care and the nature of their support services also determine the quality of their care.

■ Transitions are important in children's lives. Teachers and parents can help with transitions from preschool to kindergarten, kindergarten to first grade, and from elementary to middle or junior high school. Particular attention should be paid to children's emerging peer status and to teachers' perceptions of their interpersonal and task-related behaviors. The nature, extent, creativity, and effectiveness of transitional experiences for children, parents, and staff will be limited only by the commitment of all involved.

QUESTIONS TO GUIDE YOUR REVIEW

1. How has the middle years curriculum changed over the past several decades? Why has it changed?
2. What is cooperative learning and why is it being used in the elementary grades?
3. How does cooperative learning benefit children?
4. What are the pros and cons of cooperative learning?
5. Why is thinking being taught in the elementary grades?
6. How are teachers teaching thinking?
7. What are the differences between ordinary thinking and critical thinking?
8. What is information processing and why is it receiving so much attention?
9. What are the similarities between information processing and the way computers function? Are these comparisons valid?
10. What roles do attention, perception, and motivation play in human learning?
11. What are the differences between long- and short-term memory? How does each work?
12. What are some ways you can enhance your ability to remember?
13. What functions do mnemonics play in the ability to remember?
14. What is metacognition and what role does it play in learning?
15. How do the two brains differ in their functional processes?
16. Is it true that humans only think with one side of their brain?
17. What can teachers do to encourage children to use both sides of their brains?
18. How did Froebel influence kindergarten education?
19. What is meant by "school readiness" and what are the controversies involved in getting children "ready" for school?
20. How have kindergartens changed over the last twenty years?
21. What are some examples of developmentally appropriate practices in the kindergarten?
22. What is meant by "emerging literacy"? What are the beliefs that form the foundation of emerging literacy?
23. What can teachers do to help speakers of black English learn to read and write standard English?
24. Why are programs of bilingual education necessary?
25. What is a program of transitional bilingual education?

26. Why is before- and after-school care of school-age children necessary?
27. Are all latchkey children equally at risk?
28. What are the factors that determine the quality of care latchkey children provide themselves?
29. How do transitions from preschool to kindergarten and first grade affect children?
30. What can teachers and parents do to promote effective transitions for young children?
31. How do teachers' perceptions of children influence and affect children's transitions from preschool to kindergarten and first grade?
32. In what ways has new knowledge of child development changed how you think about children in grades K–6?
33. What has been the most interesting topic for you in this chapter? Why?

CTIVITIES FOR FURTHER INVOLVEMENT

1. Although in many areas such as reading, writing, and arithmetic the school curriculum changes slowly, in many other ways it changes quickly and significantly.
   a. In what ways does the school curriculum mirror or reflect the problems, conditions, and concerns of society?
   b. Visit schools in your area and identify new curricular topics and ways of teaching. Why were these new topics introduced into the school curriculum? Are the topics and the methods for teaching them developmentally appropriate?
2. Educators and others seem to be infatuated with the brain and seek to know how to base methods for teaching and learning on what we know about the brain and how it functions.
   a. Visit schools and identify activities and curricula that are based on right and left brain research. Do you think they are effective?
   b. Do you think that students have benefited from participating in curricula based on brain research? Provide evidence for your opinions.
3. Kindergarten education is now almost universally available to most of the nation's five-year-old children.
   a. Why has kindergarten education become so popular?
   b. Visit private and public kindergartens and assess the developmental appropriateness of their curricula.
   c. Outline what you think would be appropriate goals for a kindergarten program.
4. Before- and after-school care for the nation's children is an issue that many parents would like to see have top priority.
   a. How can quality before- and after-school care contribute to children's normal growth and development?
   b. How can the absence of quality before- and after-school child care negatively influence children's social and emotional development?
5. Visit a public school that conducts a program of bilingual education.
   a. Interview parents, children, and teachers to determine the pros and cons of conducting a bilingual program.
   b. Is a program of bilingual education necessary for the normal growth and development of multicultural children?

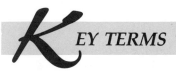

KEY TERMS

Attention The selective focusing of concentration.

Cooperative learning A set of instructional methods in which students are encouraged or required to work together on academic tasks.

Creative thinking Divergent thinking, in which a child generates many different answers, solutions, and approaches to a particular problem.

Critical thinking Reasonable, reflective thinking that is focused on deciding what to believe or do.

Developmental age The age of a child developmentally as opposed to his chronological age. If a child of chronological age five is demonstrating the behaviors of a four-year-old, then he has a developmental age of four.

Information processing The study of human cognition in which the human mind is conceived of as a complex cognitive system, analogous in some ways to a digital computer.

Latchkey children School-age children who provide self-care before and/or after school.

Metacognition An individual's knowledge of the factors that affect cognitive and learning activity and the control of these factors.

Metamemory An individual's knowledge or cognition about anything pertaining to memory.

Mnemonic Any system, strategy, or plan to develop or improve the memory.

Perception The ability of children to recognize, organize, and interpret sensory data and experiences.

Readiness The sum total of a child's physical, cognitive, social, and emotional development at a particular time in relation to particular tasks, especially those associated with schooling.

Transitional bilingual education programs Programs that incorporate a native language instructional component into their curriculum and instructional programs.

ENRICHMENT THROUGH FURTHER READING

Benderly, B. L. (1987). *The myth of two minds: What gender means and doesn't mean.* New York: Doubleday.

> The author presents a compelling case that gender stereotypes, rather than originating in physiological differences originate in culture. She argues that three longheld "truths" about differences between genders are false: That men and women think, feel and act differently; that gender differences are physiologically based; and that physiology explains the different male and female roles observed in many cultures.

Franklin, J. (1987). *Molecules of the mind.* New York: Athenaeum.

> Franklin maintains that every human thought, hope, fear, passion, yearning, and insight results from chemical interactions between transmitters and receptors. He also suggests that the main difference between the mind and an Apple computer is complexity.

Minsky, M. (1987). *The Society of mind.* New York: Simon & Schuster.

> Marvin Minsky, an artificial intelligence expert, writes about how the mind works

by writing self-contained essays about mental processes, such as how long- and near-term memory work and how an infant learns the concept of "more." Minsky is convinced that the mind works like a machine with an enormous number of parts.

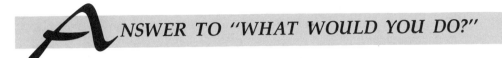

ANSWER TO "WHAT WOULD YOU DO?"

What You Expect Is What You Get

If you want a child to do poorly or fail at a task, communicating that expectation will help you achieve your goal. You are probably thinking, "Nobody wants a child to do poorly in anything! Teachers and parents should want their children to do well in all things." I'm glad you feel the way you do. However, not all parents or teachers do, as you can determine from Mrs. Baylish's comments. They may say they want their children to do well, but you and I have heard people say such things as this to children, "You're so dumb, you can't do anything!" Then, too, while some parents and teachers may not *tell* children they are dumb, how they *treat* children nevertheless communicates the same message.

Throughout school, the negative expectations children encounter from teachers constrains their opportunities to learn according to their abilities (Brophy, 1983). What is more, younger school children—ages six and seven—are as aware as older children—ages ten and eleven—of differences in teacher treatment of high- and low-achieving students (Weinstein, Marshall, Sharp, & Botkin, 1987). Furthermore, as you would expect, children's patterns of self-expectation mirror teachers' expectations (Weinstein et al., 1987).

So, your advice to Mrs. McCallum can be guided by the following:

1. The McCallums can ask for a conference with the principal and the teacher to discuss Mercedes' achievement. Suggest to them that they tell Mrs. Baylish and the principal that they will not accept the evaluation that Mercedes is a poorer student now than she was before and that they expect to see an improvement in Mercedes' achievement.
2. If Mrs. Baylish is telling Mrs. McCallum that her child is a poorer student, then she probably is doing this with other parents as well. If this is so, perhaps a group of parents can ask for a conference. The parents should stress that the reason for the meeting is in order to have the best education possible for their children.
3. It may well be that Mercedes is not as good a student as her previous grades would indicate. Nevertheless, she still has a right to be challenged to work to the best of her ability in a humane setting, free from negative expectations.
4. As a last resort, Mr. and Mrs. McCallum could ask that Mercedes be transferred to another teacher or another school. Generally, though, principals are reluctant to do this.
5. Whatever the school outcome, the McCallums should provide opportunities in the home and elsewhere (Girl Scouts, for example) for Mercedes to accomplish things and feel good about herself. Parents can help offset the negative messages children get throughout their school careers.

BIBLIOGRAPHY

Berger, J. (1988, June 1). Fourth graders writing biography and opening a door to history. *The New York Times*, p. 24.

Brandt, R. (1987). On cooperation in schools: A conversation with David and Roger Johnson. *Educational Leadership, 45,* 14–19.

Brophy, J. E. (1983). Research on the self-fulfilling prophecy and teacher expectations. *Journal Educational Psychology, 75,* 631–661.

Brown, A. L. (1978). Knowing when, where, and how to remember: A problem of metacognition. In R. Glaser (Ed.), *Advances in Instructional Psychology* (pp. 77–165). Hillsdale, NJ: Lawrence Erlbaum.

Bruno, R. R. (1987). *After-school care of school-aged children, December 1984,* (Special Studies, Series P-23, No. 149). U.S. Bureau of the Census. Washington, DC: U.S. Government Printing Office.

Chance, P. (1986). *Thinking in the classroom: A survey of programs.* New York: Teachers College Press.

Dewey, J. (1975). *Interest and effort in education.* Carbondale, ILL: Southern Illinois University Press.

Donovan, J. R. (1989, March 28). Letters to the editor. *The New York Times*, p. 21.

Doutre, C. B. (1988). Put on their creative thinking caps and add sparkle and verve to the whole curriculum. *Learning 88, 17,* 28–32.

Ennis, R. H. (1987). A taxonomy of critical thinking, dispositions, and abilities. In J. B. Baron, & R. J. Sternberg, (Eds.), *Teaching thinking skills: Theory and practice* (pp. 9–26). New York: W. H. Freeman.

Fiske, E. (1988, May 24). In Indiana, public school makes "frills" standard. *The New York Times*, p. A16.

Flavell, J. H. (1985). *Cognitive development* (2nd ed.). Englewood Cliffs, NJ: Prentice-Hall.

Gallup, A. M. (1986). The eighteenth annual Gallup poll of the public's attitude towards the public schools. *Phi Delta Kappan, 68,* 55–56.

Goodman, Y. (1980). "The roots of literacy." In M. P. Douglas (Ed.), *Reading: A humanistic experience.* Claremont, CA: Claremont Graduate School.

Hall, N. (1987). *The emergence of literacy.* Portsmouth, NH: Heinemann.

Johnson, J. (1989, March 8). Curriculum seeks to lift blacks' self-image. *The New York Times*, p. 1.

Kass, S. A. (1989, January 8). Recess, an endangered playtime. *The New York Times*, Section 4A, pp. 7–8.

Ladd, G. W., & Price, J. M. (1987). Predicting children's social and school adjustment following the transition from preschool to kindergarten. *Child Development, 58,* 1168–1189.

Lipman, M. (1988). Critical thinking—what can it be? *Educational Leadership, 46,* 40.

Long, T. J., & Long, L. (1983). *The handbook for latchkey children and their parents.* New York: Arbor House.

McTighe, Jay. (n.d.). *Improving the quality of student thinking.* Baltimore, MD: Maryland State Department of Education.

Markham, L. R. (1984). Assisting speakers of black English as they begin to write. *Young Children, 39,* 15–24.

Miller, G. A. (1956). The magical number seven, plus or minus two: Some limits on our capacity to process information. *Psychological Review, 63,* 81–97.

Morrison, G. S. (1988). *Early childhood education today* (4th ed.). Columbus, OH: Charles E. Merrill.

Murphy, D. F. (1988). The just community at Birch Meadow Elementary School. *Phi Delta Kappan, 69,* 427–428.

O'Neil, J. (1989). "Whole language": New view of literacy gains in influence. *ASCD Update, 31,* 1, 6–7.

Palincsar, A. S., & Ransom, K. (1988). From the mystery spot to the thoughtful spot: The instruction of metacognitive strategies. *The Reading Teacher, 41,* 784–789.

Picton, T. W., Stuss, D. T., & Marshall, K. C. (1986). Attention and the brain. In S. L. Friedman, K. A. Klivington, & R. W. Peterson, (Eds.). *The brain, cognition and education* (pp. 19–79). Orlando: Academic Press.

Restak, R. (1986). *The infant mind.* Garden City, NY: Doubleday.

Rhodes, R. (1986). *The making of the atomic bomb.* New York: Simon & Schuster. p. 28.

Robinson, B. E., Coleman, M., & Rowland, B. H. (1986). The after-school ecologies of latchkey children. *Children's Environments Quarterly, 3,* 4–8.

Rodman, H., Prato, D., & Nelson, R. (1985). Child care arrangements and children's functioning: A comparison of self-care and adult-care children. *Developmental Psychology, 21,* 413–418.

Seligmann, J., Joseph, N., Donovan, J., & Gosnell, M. (1987, Fall). Dieting, just like mommy. *Newsweek on Health,* p. 18.

Siegler, R. S. (1988). Individual differences in strategy choices: Good students, not-so-good-students, and perfectionists. *Child Development, 59,* 833–851.

Simon, H. A. (1986). The role of attention in learning. In S. L. Friedman, K. A. Klivington, & R. W. Peterson (Eds.). *The brain, cognition and education* (pp. 105–115). Orlando: Academic Press.

Slavin, R. E. (1987a). Cooperative learning and the cooperative school. *Educational Leadership, 45,* 7–13.

Slavin, R. E. (1987b). Developmental and motivational perspectives on cooperative learning: A reconciliation. *Child Development, 58,* 1161.

Smith, F. (1982). *Writing and the writer.* London: Heinemann.

Snow, C. (1987). Relevance of the notion of a critical period to language acquisition. In M. Bornstein (Ed.), *Sensitive periods in development: Interdisciplinary perspectives.* Hillsdale, NJ: Lawrence Erlbaum.

Springer, S. P., & Deutsch, G. *Left brain, right brain.* New York: W. H. Freeman.

Stark, E. (1984). Thanks for the memories. *Psychology Today, 18,* 80–81.

The statistical trends. (1985, May). *The Principal, 16,* 16.

Steinberg, L. (1986). Latchkey children and susceptibility to peer pressure: An ecological analysis. *Developmental Psychology, 22,* 433–439.

Stewner-Manzanares, G. (1988, Fall). *The bilingual education act: Twenty years later* (New Focus No. 6). Silver Spring, MD: National Clearing House for Bilingual Education.

Vandell, D. L., & Corasaniti, M. A. (1988). The relation between third graders' after-school care and social, academic, and emotional functioning. *Child Development, 59,* 868–875.

Weinstein, R. S., Marshall, H. H., Sharp, L., & Botkin, M. (1987). Pygmalion and the student: Age and classroom differences in children's awareness of teacher expectations. *Child Development, 58,* 1079–1093.

CHAPTER TWELVE

Development during the adolescent years

◆

VIGNETTES
INTRODUCTION: THE
  ADOLESCENT YEARS—
  WAITING FOR MATURITY
WHY AN ADOLESCENT PERIOD
  OF DEVELOPMENT?
PHYSICAL DEVELOPMENT
Important Terms
Pubescence
The Growth Spurt
Primary and Secondary Sexual
  Characteristics
Physical Growth
In the Spotlight: Preventing Bone
  Loss
In the Spotlight: Cracking Voices
The Role of Hormones in
  Adolescent Development
In the Spotlight: Winning and
  Losing an Olympic Gold Medal
Reproductive Functions
PUBERTY AND SELF-IMAGE

ADOLESCENTS AND SUICIDE
Personal Story: Carmen Espinosa
  and Project TRUST
In the Spotlight: Mirror, Mirror,
  On the Wall
MADONNA "WANNABEES"
PARENTING AND ADOLESCENT
  CONFLICTS
RECKLESSNESS AND FOOLISH
  RISKS
ANOREXIA NERVOSA
In the Spotlight: Understanding
  Anorexia Nervosa
BULIMIA
PEER GROUPS
THE WORLD OF WORK
Facilitating Teenagers' Work
Is Working Good for Teenagers?
ADOLESCENT RUNAWAYS
JUVENILE DELINQUENCY
TEENAGE ALCOHOLISM
WHY DO ADOLESCENTS

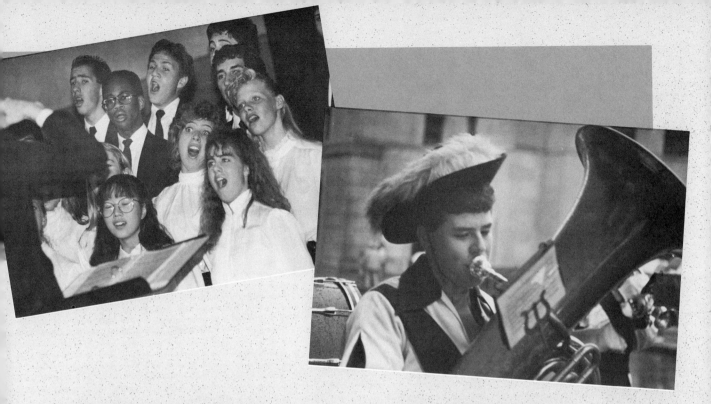

ENGAGE IN SUBSTANCE
  ABUSE?
Implications
TEENAGE SEX
Early Sex
Survival Sex
TEENAGE PREGNANCY—
  PREMATURE PARENTHOOD
Introduction
Teenage Pregnancy as a Social
  Problem
In the Spotlight: A Freudian View
  of Teenage Pregnancy
Reasons for Teenage Pregnancy
Consequences of Teenage Pregnancy
Consequences for Children of
  Teenage Mothers
Programs for Preventing Teenage
  Pregnancy
In the Spotlight: A Dollar a Day
  Keeps the Stork Away
What Would You Do?
Programs for Pregnant Teenagers

and Adolescent Parents
The Parent-child Education Center
Project PARENTING
In the Spotlight: TAPP (Teenage
  Parenting Program)
Teenage Pregnancy and Public
  Policy
HOMOSEXUALITY
Sexual Identity
Childhood Sexual Behaviors and
  Homosexuality
Homosexuality and AIDS
SUMMARY
QUESTIONS TO GUIDE YOUR
  REVIEW
ACTIVITIES FOR FURTHER
  INVOLVEMENT
KEY TERMS
ENRICHMENT THROUGH
  FURTHER READING
ANSWER TO "WHAT WOULD
  YOU DO?"
BIBLIOGRAPHY

481

⌣IGNETTES

As she was growing up, sixteen-year-old Shalonda Moore loved to babysit for her young nephew, Lavester. She treated him like a baby doll and came to think of him as her own. "I loved to dress Lavester up and take him all over town," bragged Shalonda. "People really made a fuss about us. When someone asked who his mother was, I told them, 'I am!'"

Shalonda doesn't have to pretend anymore. She now has a baby of her own, four-month-old Cantrell. Shalonda and Cantrell live with her mother, a niece, and a nephew in a two-room apartment of an inner city housing project. Shalonda returned to school after Cantrell's birth and is enrolled in a special program designed for teenage mothers. Shalonda wanted to go to college, but now she hopes to be a beautician. "If that don't work out I can clerk at the corner store," says Shalonda. "The owner already offered me a job." But this dream of work may not become a reality. Buster Bailey, Shalonda's eighteen-year-old boyfriend, wants her to have another baby. "Buster likes babies and he keeps after me to have another one. It's hard to say 'no' to Buster. He's real determined," she admits. As for Buster, he doesn't worry if Shalonda gets pregnant, "All I'm interested in, man, is getting it on and off." However on the topic of marriage, both Shalonda and Buster share the same feeling. "When you get married, you lose all your freedom," says Shalonda, while Buster grinningly nods in agreement.

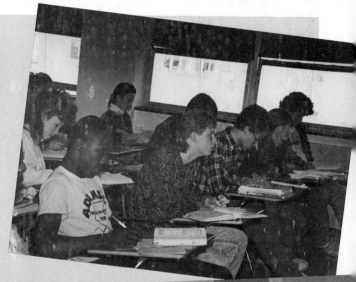

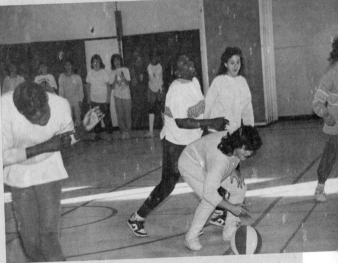

Juan and Maria are in love—at least for the time being. Both are fourteen and in the eighth grade at Hancock Junior High School. For Juan, it was love at first glance. "I saw her in the hall and knew she was for me," brags Juan. "I met her and I liked her personality and her looks." Maria thinks Juan is "beautiful." The newly-in-love couple spend all their time between classes holding hands and cuddling. A week ago, Juan was in love with thirteen-year-old Marta, a seventh grader. But as he explains it, "We don't get along anymore. Once I got to know her real well, I didn't like her personality and actions. Besides, there were too many other guys interested in her." Maria and Juan don't do much actual dating. They usually go to the local mall (they are dropped off separately by their parents) and then go to a movie where, with many other young teenage couples, they "make out," often oblivious to what is happening on the silver screen.

Mary Beth Streeter, seventeen and a junior at Northridge High School, is already a two-career woman. From 7:30 AM to 2:00 PM she takes a full schedule of classes, including advanced algebra and Latin, and is president of her class. By 2:30 PM each day, Mary Beth is in a different world, the world of work at Bascomb Hospital, where she files medical records for $6.25 per hour. Mary Beth works from 2:30 PM to 7:00 PM on weekdays, and from 7:00 AM to 3:00 PM on Sundays—a total of 32 hours for an income of $800 per month. On Saturdays Mary Beth catches up on her homework, conducts school and class-related business, cleans her room, and sleeps. She and her boyfriend always eat out on Saturday nights, generally at one of the better restaurants in town. "It is a hectic schedule, but I'm saving my money for college and I do like to travel," says Mary Beth. "I went to Europe last summer and I want to go to Australia this coming year." Mary Beth's mother, who is divorced, likes to see Mary Beth work, because, she says, "When Mary Beth's working, I don't worry about her being home alone."

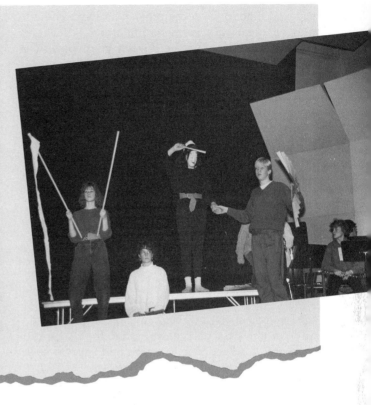

WHY AN ADOLESCENT PERIOD OF DEVELOPMENT?

The Adolescent Years—Waiting for Maturity. Did you ever wonder where the word *adolescence* comes from? It comes from the Latin word *adolescere,* "to grow up." The years from twelve to twenty are those in which youth mature into adulthood. Adolescence is a developmental period in which youth mature physically, socially, and emotionally in order to enter adulthood and assume adult-like responsibilities. *Adolescence* is the *transitional* period from youth to adulthood and represents a major transition period in the course of human development.

Adolescence is a period of profound and significant physical growth and changes. With the possible exception of the neonatal and infant periods, more biological and physical changes occur in adolescence than at any other time in human development. Adolescence is the period during which the much discussed and often publicized "growth spurt" occurs.

There is more to maturation than physical growth. Adolescents also develop in all the other areas, too—intellectual, emotional, and social. In fact, the biological developments of the adolescent are accompanied by some extremely powerful social and emotional developments as well. The adolescent years are years of important social and cultural significance in the lives of youth and their families.

The adolescent years, with the transition to adulthood, provide us with a window through which we may look in on adult development. While we cannot do that in this book, insights we gain about adolescents and the adolescent years enable us to more fully understand adult behavior. In this sense, the adolescent is the mother and the father of the adult he or she will become.

It was not always so. In colonial America, adolescence was only for the rich, and children, viewed as sources of cheap labor, were working at an early age (Greenberger & Steinberg, 1986). In fact, it has been only in the past decades that a period of time has been set aside as a time called adolescence. There are a number of reasons for this, mainly social and economic. First, it has been only in the last half-century that the American economy has been able to afford and support such a large number of people. There are 34,798,00 adolescents in the United States between the ages of twelve and nineteeen (U.S. Bureau of the Census, 1988). This represents about 16 percent of the population. Put another way, it is only for a relatively brief and recent period of history in the United States that people in this age bracket have not had to work full-time, either to support themselves or others. Thus, teenagers in general are dependent on and supported by their parents for longer periods of time than was customary in past decades.

Industrialization has brought with it longer periods of schooling, which, in turn, have extended the time youth are economically dependent on their parents. This then has lengthened the period of adolescence. Additionally, the industrialization of America has increased the concentration of population into large urban centers, which has encouraged consolidated schools and large school districts. These "mega" school districts, such as the Dade County Florida School District with 267,000 students and Miami Sunset High School (the largest high school in the State of Florida) with 3,200 students in grades ten, eleven, and twelve, enable large numbers of teenagers to come together, creating large and identifiable groups of peers. Without such congregation in a group distinct from adults, it is doubtful if there would be such opportunities for the development and expression of teenage culture.

But having to wait for maturity is one of the frustrating problems associated with adolescence and the source of much parental and societal frustration as well. Physically, mentally, and sexually, teenagers are at or near the pinnacle of their powers. Yet, they find themselves literally put on hold while completing their educations and arriving at that time when adults will view them responsible enough to take on adult responsibilities.

PHYSICAL DEVELOPMENT
Important Terms

In our discussion of adolescence, as in our study of children in previous chapters, specialized terminology helps us understand this developmental stage. *Puberty* is the time when an individual reaches sexual maturity and fertility. Both sexes are capable of procreation. (The word puberty comes from the Latin *puber*, meaning "adult".) *Pubescence* is the two-year period that precedes puberty and is the time during which profound physical changes of height, weight, and physiological functioning occur. Also, during pubescence, individuals develop the primary and secondary sexual characteristics that will characterize them as adults and capable of reproduction. (Pubescent also means covered with fine hair, from the Latin *pubescere*, meaning "to become hairy.") *Postpubescence* is the two-year period following puberty when growth is completed and reproductive functions are fully established.

Adolescence, which is the transitional period from youth to adulthood, begins with the physical changes of the pubertal period and ends when these physical changes are completed at around ages eighteen to twenty. Sometimes experts place the end of adolescence as occurring with marriage or economic independence. However, with the deliberate postponement of marriage common in today's world, and with many working and college youth economically dependent on their parents, tying the end of adolescence to marriage or economic independence does not do justice to all the youth who reach adulthood long before these two events occur. Keep in mind that adolescence is both a period of time *and* a process of psychological, social, and physical development initiated by pubertal changes. Then, too, some youth (see Chapter Thirteen, "Dropping Out") do not have the luxury of extending their dependency much beyond the early teens.

Pubescence

The beginning of pubescence varies for both males and females. For individuals in both groups the age of onset also varies, with some girls beginning as early as seven or eight years while others may not begin until age eleven or twelve. The same is true for boys, except that the beginning of pubescence is about two years later than in females. Consequently, some boys begin pubescence at ten while others may not begin until they are well into their teens. But the point about pubescence is this: during this time, dramatic physical changes occur in a short period of time and have profound influences on individuals for the rest of their lives.

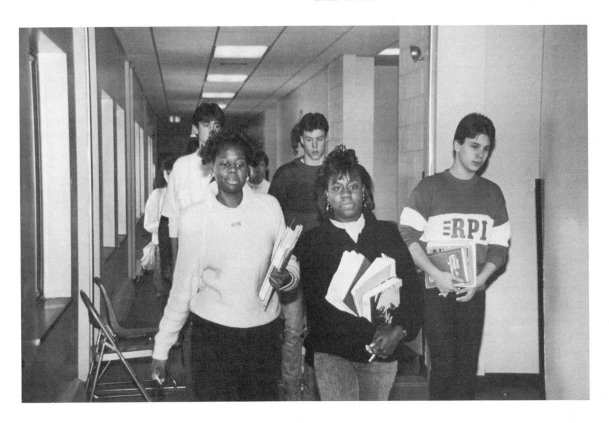

FIGURE 12-1 Adolescence is a time for growing up and for the many transitions that accompany the adolescent years. While there are many differences in how adolescents develop in and respond to this important time of life, adolescence is not now considered the turbulent time it once was.

BREAST DEVELOPMENT IN THE FEMALE

Stage 1
  Prepubescent appearance
  Elevated nipple

Stage 2
  Appearance of breast buds (may be unequal)
  Increased diameter of areola (area surrounding the nipple)

Stage 3
  Continued enlargement of breast buds and areola
  No separation of contours between breast and
    nipple

Stage 4
  Secondary mound formed by areola and nipple
  Increased breast size

Stage 5
  Mature appearance
  Recession of areola; projection of the nipple only
    from the contour

FIGURE 12-2 One result of estrogen production in female adolescents is breast development. Breasts are composed primarily of adipose tissue (tissue that contains stored cellular fat). Breasts also have mammary glands which produce milk during pregnancy and when the mother nurses. (From Lesner/PEDIATRIC NURSING, copyright 1983 by Delmar Publishers Inc.)

PUBIC HAIR DEVELOPMENT IN THE FEMALE

Stage 1
  No evidence of pubic hair

Stage 2
  Presence of small amount of pubic hair, which is
    usually straight, sparsely pigmented, and
    downy

Stage 3
  Darker in color, more coarsely textured, and
    curlier

Stage 4
  Thicker, curlier, and coarsely textured
  Covers entire mons veneris

Stage 5
  Abundant; adult in quantity and type
  Present on medial aspect of thighs

FIGURE 12-3 Pubic hair development in females is a secondary sex characteristic. Pubic hair is first straight and then turns kinky. After breast development, more public hair develops. (From Lesner/PEDIATRIC NURSING, copyright 1983 by Delmar Publishers Inc.)

The Growth Spurt

Throughout this text we have studied and discussed the predictable and orderly development of children through the prenatal, neonatal, infant, preschool, and elementary school years. Clearly, much of what occurs during the course of normal growth and development is determined by biological influences. The same is true for the adolescent period, so we must examine biological events to help us explain the adolescent growth spurt as well as the development of primary and secondary sexual characteristics.

The onset of the events that occur during pubescence and result in puberty begins with a hormonal signal. Hormones (chemical substances) that influence growth are secreted into the blood by endocrine glands. It is as though the growing individual has been preparing for the time when her biological alarm clock will ring and adolescence development will begin.

Primary and Secondary Sexual Characteristics

Physical changes of puberty involve both primary and secondary sexual characteristics. Primary sexual characteristics are the external and internal organs associated with reproductive functions. In the female, these are the ovaries, fallopian tubes, uterus, and vagina. In males, they are penis, tes-

---

GENITAL DEVELOPMENT IN THE MALE

Stage 1
Prepubescent testes, scrotum, and penis
Similar size and proportion to that present in
early childhood

Stage 2
Enlargement of the scrotum and testes
Reddened scrotal skin with rougher texture
Unchanged penile size or only slightly enlarged

Stage 3
Increase in penile length
Increased maturation of testes and scrotum

Stage 4
Increase in penile size and thickness, glans penis
more developed
Enlarged, darker scrotum

Stage 5
Adult development in both size and shape

FIGURE 12-4 Reproductive maturation in males is signaled by the growth of the penis and testicles. (From Lesner/PEDIATRIC NURSING, copyright 1983 by Delmar Publishers Inc.)

PUBIC HAIR DEVELOPMENT IN THE MALE

Stage 1
No evidence of pubic hair

Stage 2
Presence of small amount of pubic hair, which is
usually long and straight, and downy in
texture
Predominant at the base of the penis

Stage 3
Darker in color, curlier, and more coarsely
textured
Sparsely spread over mons veneris

Stage 4
Thicker, curlier, and coarsely textured
More evident over mons veneris

Stage 5
Abundant in amount
Adult in type, texture, and appearance

FIGURE 12-5 Pubic hair is also a secondary sex characteristic for males. Through the adolescent years, the pubic hair becomes thicker and coarser. (From Lesner/PEDIATRIC NURSING, copyright 1983 by Delmar Publishers Inc.)

---

ticles, seminal vesicles, and prostate gland. Secondary characteristics are the characteristics that distinguish males from females but play no direct role in reproduction. In females, these secondary characteristics include breasts, pubic and underarm hair, increased width and depth of pelvis, and changes in voice and skin. In males, these include pubic, underarm, and facial hair, broadening of the shoulders, and changes in voice and skin.

The stages of secondary sexual development have been closely studied and documented in both females and males. For example, five stages of female and male development are recognized and are referred to as *Tanner Stages* (Tanner, 1962). Figure 12-2 depicts stages of breast development in adolescent girls, and Figure 12-3 shows pubic hair development in adolescent girls. Stages of

male genital development are demonstrated in Figure 12-4, and Figure 12-5 shows stages of pubic hair development in adolescent boys.

Physical Growth

Physical growth during the adolescent years is rather pronounced and dramatic. This is the time of the much-discussed "growth spurt," during which the final 25 percent of height gain occurs in a two- to three-year period. Girls will gain two to eight inches in height and fifteen to fifty-five pounds in weight. Males, on the other hand, will gain four to twelve inches in height and fifteen to sixty-five pounds in weight. The weight and height norms for ages 2 to 18 are shown in Figures 12-6 and 12-7.

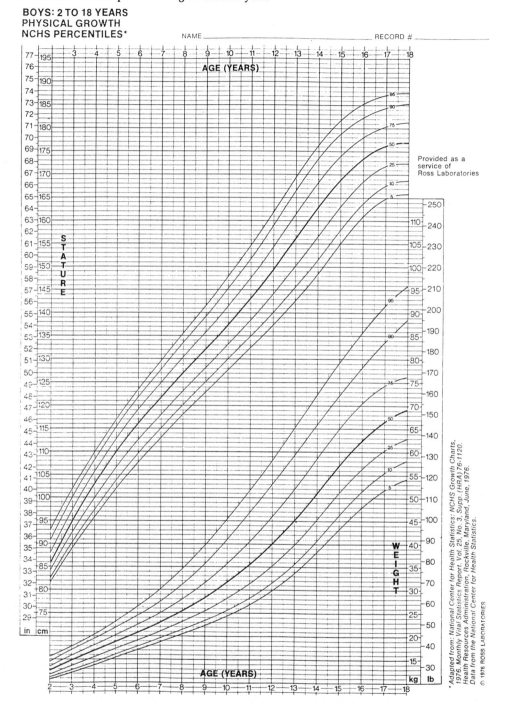

BOYS: 2 TO 18 YEARS
PHYSICAL GROWTH
NCHS PERCENTILES*

FIGURE 12-6 Weight and height norms for males. By the end of the adolescent years, boys weigh more than girls basically because of the higher proportion of muscle tissue (Used with permission of Ross Laboratories, © 1982)

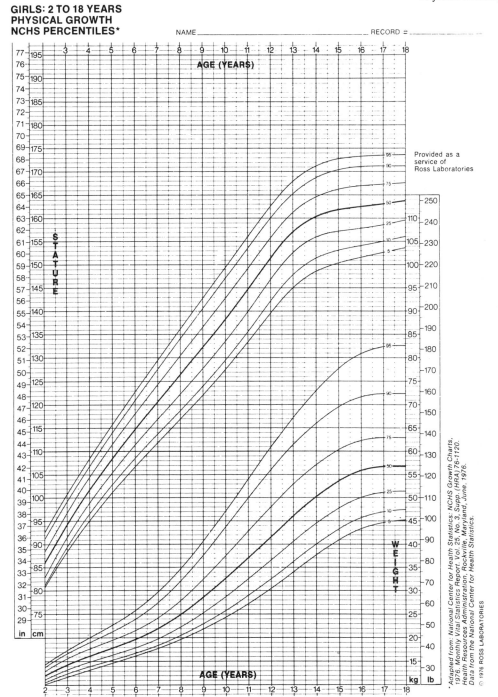

**GIRLS: 2 TO 18 YEARS
PHYSICAL GROWTH
NCHS PERCENTILES***

NAME _____ RECORD # _____

AGE (YEARS)

STATURE

WEIGHT

Provided as a
service of
Ross Laboratories

*Adapted from: National Center for Health Statistics: NCHS Growth Charts, 1976. Monthly Vital Statistics Report. Vol. 25, No. 3, Supp. (HRA) 76-1120. Health Resources Administration, Rockville, Maryland, June, 1976. Data from the National Center for Health Statistics.

© 1976 ROSS LABORATORIES

FIGURE 12-7 Weight and height norms for females. At the end of adolescence, girls are shorter than boys by about five inches. (Used with permission of Ross Laboratories, © 1982)

*I*N THE SPOTLIGHT

PREVENTING BONE LOSS

You have probably been reading and hearing a great deal lately about calcium supplements and osteoporosis, or bone loss, among the elderly. Part of the controversy revolves around whether or not calcium supplements later in life counteract bone loss. Included in the latest thinking, however, is the hypothesis that teenagers may be the ones to benefit most from calcium supplements. According to B. Lawrence Riggs of the Mayo Clinic in Rochester, Minnesota, increased calcium intake during the adolescent growth spurt and the following ten years may result in heavier and denser skeletons that are more resistant to fractures later in life. (Brody, 1987).

A social, health, and demographic phenomena of the last two decades is that young women are getting fatter. Over the last several decades, women between the ages of eighteen and thirty-four are increasing body mass and are overweight. This same trend is not true for men. The greatest increases in weight were for women with low levels of education and income (Leary, 1989). This trend has serious implications not only for women in the designated age bracket, but also for teachers and parents of teenagers. The time to address causes of being overweight are in the elementary, junior/middle and high school years. Practicing good nutrition, learning the importance of physical exercise, and developing a life-style conducive to good health should be part of public school curriculums.

Other differences between males and females are apparent in their growth patterns, such as skeletal development. Males are not only taller than females, but their arms and legs are longer, and their shoulders are broader.

Enlargement of the larynx and vocal cords occurs in males and females and both experience voice changes. Females' voices become slightly deeper and fuller. Males undergo a dramatic "voice change" with the characteristic deeping of the voice.

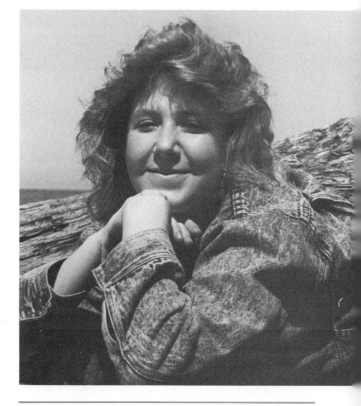

FIGURE 12-8 A fact of teenage life is that adolescents, especially girls, are getting heavier. Preventive measures include nutrition education and emphasis on the need for exercise throughout life.

IN THE SPOTLIGHT

CRACKING VOICES

It has probably happened to most boys during adolescence. They start to say something and their voice cracks, or suddenly in the middle of a word or sentence their voice goes from bass to soprano. This is one of the most embarrassing things that can happen to an adolescent boy. Why does it happen? The larynx is one of the organs targeted for change during adolescence. As the larynx enlarges in response to increased sex hormones, the Adam's apple develops and the vocal cords grow. With this sudden increase in size, there is a temporary loss of muscle control. The voice-change period lasts about four to six months, but it is several years before the full change—about an octave lower—takes place.

Increased muscle development occurs in both sexes. However, in males, there is more muscle development and consequently, males are more muscular than females.

Hormone activity is also responsible for growth in skin and hair. The sebaceous glands are very active during adolescence and this accounts for acne, one of the more publicized and advertised problems of adolescence (see "What Causes Acne?"). Generally, too, hair darkens in color, becomes coarser and grows longer. Pubic hair is more extensive in males, and they develop hair on the face and chest, and sometimes on the back and shoulders.

The characterization of teenagers as long-limbed and gawky is not accidental. They are just that! But there is a good reason for such appearance. Their physical growth occurs in characteristic ways, with arms, legs, and neck reaching adult length before other parts of their bodies reach adult proportions.

The Role of Hormones in Adolescent Development

Hormonal influences cause many of the events involved in puberty. *Somatotropin*, produced by the anterior pituitary gland, is the primary "growth hormone" and the one that generally stimulates growth and influences overall body size prior to puberty. However, at puberty, it relinquishes its primacy as a growth regulator to the gonadal hormones (Katchadourian, 1977, pp. 88–89). During adolescence, the primary hormones affecting growth are *testosterone* and *estrogen*. These hormones are called the "sex hormones" because they are produced by the gonads and because of their influence on sexual development and the growth spurt. In males, the masculining hormones are called *androgens*, the principal one being testosterone. Produced by the testes, testosterone promotes growth of the reproductive system and muscles, and is responsible for the voice change and development of secondary sexual characteristics.

In females, the primary sex hormones are *estrogen* and *progesterone*, which are produced by the ovaries and function in females much the same way testerone functions in males. They account for the maturation of the reproductive system and the development of secondary sexual characteristics. As such, they account for the growth of body hair and generally contribute to the growth spurt. In Chapter Three we discussed the reproductive function of the testes and ovaries. Now we see that they have a dual function as well, producing hormones.

Sex hormones in males and females are also produced by the outer layer (cortex) of the adrenal glands, located on the upper surface of the kidneys. However, the gonads are primarily responsible for the production of sex hormones. Sex hormones, both male and female, are present in all of us, but in different amounts (Katchadourian, 1977). Figure 12–9 shows the effects of hormones on development at puberty.

THE EFFECTS OF HORMONES ON PUBERTAL DEVELOPMENT

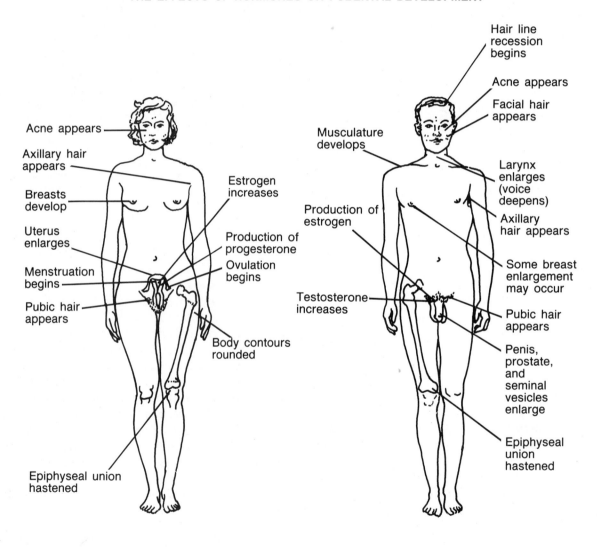

FIGURE 12-9 The majority of changes that occur during adolescence are due to the hormonal influences. The effects of these hormones are seen here.

*I*N THE SPOTLIGHT

WINNING AND LOSING AN OLYMPIC GOLD MEDAL

There is much publicity about the use of steroids by athletes. The most celebrated case of all involved Ben Johnson and the 100-meter dash at the 1988 World Olympics. Johnson won the gold medal in the 100-meter contest, but was subsequently disqualified and stripped of his gold medal because a urine test following the race revealed that he had used steroids prior to the race as a means of enhancing his athletic performance. *Steroids*, taken as a collective whole, are all of the hormones produced by the gonads and adrenal cortex of both sexes. So, the hormones that play such an influential role in adolescent growth and development are those taken by some athletes to give them that winning edge.

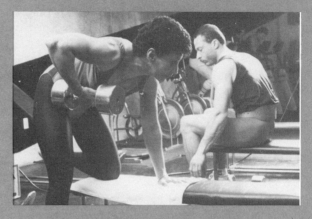

FIGURE 12-10 The media has given considerable attention to athletes who use steroids to enhance their physical development and consequently their athletic performance. In much the same way, steroids play a role in adolescent growth and development.

Reproductive Functions

In females, the secretion of estrogen occurs in a cyclic pattern, about one to two years before the onset of menstruation. About two years after the beginning of pubescent changes, initial menstruation or *menarche* begins. The normal age range of menarche is ages ten to fifteen years, with the average age being twelve and one-half years. The menstrual periods are usually irregular for a period of one to two years, and may or may not be accompanied by ovulation. After this time, the menstrual cycle and ovulation become regular. However, the establishment of the ovulation cycle, like so much of what we say about adolescent development, is highly individualized.

The most frequently cited perceptions by female adolescents regarding menstruation are the inconvenience and normalcy of menstruation. Initial reactions to menstruation include surprise, fear, and embarrassment (Havens & Swenson, 1986).

There is no sudden change in males to mark the beginning of reproductive functions. By seventeen, most males are producing sperm. One sign of mature reproductive ability is the beginning of nocturnal emissions, the involuntary ejaculation of seminal fluids during sleep. These emissions are a result of the buildup of semen in the genital ducts and will occur about every two weeks into adulthood.

PUBERTY AND SELF-IMAGE

According to researcher Ann Petersen (1987), the timing of puberty does influence how one views oneself and others. Among seventh and eighth graders, girls who are more physically mature are generally less satisfied with their appearance and weight than are their less mature classmates. The opposite is true for males. The more physically mature are more satisfied with their weight and appearance. Also, boys who reached puberty report more positive moods than their prepubertal classmates. Petersen believes that pubertal change is a positive one for boys but a negative one for girls. Apparently one reason for the more negative pubertal experience for girls is that it places more restrictions on them.

The timing of puberty also affects academic achievement, with adolescents who mature early getting better grades than their late-maturing peers. Petersen attributes this to the tendency of teachers to give more positive ratings to larger pupils.

How the adolescent changes physically is not all that there is to changes in adolescence. The adolescent's subjective reactions to these changes are also important. As an early-maturing girl commented about early maturation, "I tried to hide it. I was embarrassed and ashamed." By eighth grade however, the same girl remarked, "By then everyone wore a bra and had their period. I was normal" (Petersen, 1987, p. 30).

A great deal has been written about the turbulent adolescent years. While everyone agrees they are times of change and stress, we are now coming to understand that stress and turmoil are not necessarily the norm for all teenagers. Many teenagers make it through their adolescent years with little or no turmoil. Indeed, adolescents are not more intrinsically disturbed than adults and the percentage of adolescents that are disturbed in some way is about 20 percent, the same as the adult population. This means that 80 percent are not in constant turmoil. (Offer, 1987). Furthermore, the stresses and strains associated with puberty are not all due to biology. Other social and environmental forces, such as changing schools, the death of a parent, and family turmoil also contribute to adolescents' moods, behaviors, and achievements. However, given that 20 percent of the teenage population is disturbed in some way,

then this means that 3.4 million need some kind of mental health intervention (Offer, 1987).

Although in many ways adolescence, as we study and perceive it, is a unique period of life and development, in many other ways it is no different from other stages of life in that there are certain "tasks" that must be mastered. For adolescents, these include: (Simmons & Blyth, 1987)

1. The need to establish a positive self-image
2. The necessity of forgoing closer peer relationships
3. The need to attain a higher degree of independence
4. The establishment of plans for adulthood
5. The need to deal with conformity/deviance issues in school (p. 345)

It is how these tasks are mastered that is usually the source of many adolescent problems.

ADOLESCENTS AND SUICIDE

The growing incidence of suicide among teenagers was even more dramatically brought to the nation's attention when the Fairview School District in Fairview, Pennsylvania canceled its graduation program in which 150 seniors were to receive their diplomas. The cancellation occurred because school authorities feared that some students might try to commit suicide on stage at the graduation ceremonies ("Rumors of Suicide," 1988).

However, the incidence of the suicide rate in the adolescent population is deceptive. While the suicide rate among adolescents tripled from 1956 to 1977, it has since leveled off, and suicide rates correspond to increases and decreases on the proportion of adolescents in the population. Table 12–1 shows the actual and predicted suicide rates and population changes in the fifteen to twenty-four year age group in the United States from 1977 to 1985.

In a study 7,828 black children ages eleven to eighteen who were admitted on a first-time basis to in- and out-patient psychiatric facilities, re-

TABLE 12–1

SUICIDE RATES PER 100,000 POPULATION, 15-24 YEAR OLDS, UNITED STATES[a]

Year	Rate
1977	13.6
1978	12.4
1979	12.4
1980	12.3
1981	12.3
1982	12.1
1983	11.9
1984	12.5
1985	12.0[b]

[a] Sources of data: National Center for Health Statistics, 1981–1986 (for 1977–1981 data); National Center for Health Statistics, 1984 (for 1982 data); and National Center for Health Statistics, unpublished data (for 1982–1985 data).
[b] Based on a 10% sample.

searchers Bettes and Walker (1986) found that for both male and female adolescents who have suicidal thoughts and who display suicidal acts, depression is the most common symptom. For nonsuicidal adolescents, anger is the most common symptom. Other common symptoms exhibited by suicidal male teenagers are: anxiety, anger, assaultiveness, paranoia, sleep problems, antisocial acts, isolation, hyperactivity, inappropriate affect, and hallucinations. Symptoms characteristic of suicidal female adolescents are: anger, sleep problems, antisocial acts, anxiety, isolation, hallucinations, paranoia, and inappropriate affect. General symptoms for both sexes are depression as signaled by isolation, sleeping or eating too much or too little, apathy, hostility, alcohol or drug abuse, and writing, thinking, and talking about suicide.

There is a definite gender difference in suicidal behavior, with more girls expressing suicidal thoughts than boys. The overwhelming majority of girls who engage in suicidal acts express their intention to do so (Bettes & Walker, p. 596). Furthermore, for both males and females, there is a significant increase in suicidal behaviors with age. For males, the increase is from 3.5 percent for eleven to twelve-year-olds to 14.5 percent at ages seventeen to eighteen. The increase for females across ages is 8.72 percent for eleven to twelve-year-olds and 30.6 percent for seventeen to eighteen-year-olds (Bettes & Walker, 1986, p. 596).

Frequently, too, you may hear about how fictional films significantly increase the number of teenage suicides. The data, however, do not support such a conclusion. After studying the effects of such televised films in California and Pennsylvania, Phillips and Paight (1987) reported, "We conclude that it is premature to be concerned about the possibly fatal effects of fictional televised films about suicide" (p. 809).

During the teenage years, adolescents have a tendency to act in self-destructive ways. School-based programs such as Project TRUST, operated by the Dade County, Florida Public Schools are designed to help students cope and deal with their problems during these formative years. One TRUST school counselor is assigned to each of the county's forty-nine junior high schools.

Personal Stories

CARMEN ESPINOSA AND PROJECT TRUST

Carmen Espinosa is a Project TRUST counselor in grades seven to nine at W. R. Thomas Middle School. Prior to her work in the middle school, Carmen was a counselor in an allied drug prevention program called Project HOPE. Now she works in a project called "To Reach Ultimate Success Together" (TRUST). As Carmen explains it, "Trust is when two people share something in confidence. It's personal and it's not to be repeated to anyone else. It could be words, feelings, or emotions that people have a hard time expressing, due to shame and fear."

A student gets into the TRUST program, either through teacher referral or because Carmen or another counselor identifies them through the computer printout of all "at-risk" students in the junior high school. In Dade County Public Schools, "at risk" includes the numbers of subjects a student has failed, the number of times a student has been referred to an administrator, number of tardies to class, truancies, defiance, disruption, apathy, and other self-destructive behavior.

Carmen provides the following example of how the program works: "I met Gloria, age fifteen, last year, and I was able to get her in the program due to the fact that she used to practically live in the office since she was often truant from school. Her parents divorced, and her father has remarried for the third time. Gloria saw her mother lose control of the family and duties as a parent, thus Gloria's parents had difficulty supervising their daughter. Also, Gloria would come home late at night with all sorts of stories as to why she was late. Her school behavior was terrible, especially with the truancy problem. Gloria, in my opinion, was never a drug abuser. She did experiment at some point but not to the extreme of labeling her as a drug "user." Gloria failed every single class one semester. Toward the end of the year, she was a basket case of problems. I referred her and the parents to family counseling, however, her parents refused to participate in any kind of counseling as a family unit. There was a lot of hostility existing between both parents regarding a mistress who later became the father's third wife. Gloria's mother was his second wife."

"Gloria has shown a lot of progress this year. At the beginning, she started doing better. She would still be truant, but not as often. Now, attendance has improved a great deal. Several people helped Gloria through this phase of her life. One person in particular was the 4-H Club sponsor together with her students. The 4-H Club has a dropout prevention program for at-risk students. The club sponsor helped Gloria stay in school by getting her involved in school activities. Whenever the club had a field trip such as to the county jail, Gloria went with the group. Another project was the planting of trees out in front of the school and we discovered Gloria had a green thumb. The idea was to keep Gloria interested and motivated in school. Other people who made a difference were the administrators and Gloria's teachers. Our school principal, Jeff Miller, also took the time to talk to Gloria and her family. Due to cooperative and caring staff members, our school has been nominated at a national level for our successful substance prevention programs. Gloria made it through junior high and is doing very well emotionally, as well as academically, thanks to everyone involved."

"Our support group at our school is a place where Gloria and other members like her can share their feelings regarding issues that are of concern to them. The support group was great! Gloria would ramble on and on about any arguments she had with her mom or dad; she'd cry, and sometimes she'd scream. Sometimes, the group didn't like what Gloria said and sometimes she said something that even she was aware wasn't called for. The point was for her to say what she had to say and let it bounce off her peers. For example, she would say, 'I hate my mother. She tries to get my father against me but that's O.K. because I've got another game planned!' Gloria would actually have something planned! The other kids in the peer group would criticize her and say that she was real selfish! By the end of the year, the support group to some degree is practically a family. It contains a variety of surrogate brothers and sisters, and very good friends. If worse comes to worse, members can go out with each other on weekends, and call each other if they like."

Carmen believes her knowledge of child development is very helpful in her day-to-day job! "I definitely need to know certain basic child development concepts, such as how things like peer pressure influence adolescents. Peer pressure is very important at this age and is one of the factors that causes kids to contemplate using drugs and getting others involved in substance abuse. Knowing about adolescents in general and the fact that there is a lot of stress involved is also important. Also knowing the importance of learning how to relate to teenagers. Adolescents need to learn and understand certain skills, such as how to communicate with others and make decisions in order to surpass their adolescent phase successfully."

"The adolescent years are tender years. Students are not yet adults, and we adults often treat them as youngsters. For instance, the other day I went to a group and I asked the president, 'Are you going to get your club sponsor a gift at the end of this year? If so, I've got something I know she likes.' This young lady got very defensive and then, through the grapevine, I heard she felt insulted. She probably felt as though I didn't think she was responsible enough to take care of this task by herself. In essence, teenagers may feel that we adults treat them as children and we do not mean any harm."

Carmen believes that peer pressure plays a strong role in the lives of teenagers, but this is not the only pressure on them. She explains, "It's not always another adolescent influencing another. In my first year as a Project HOPE facilitator, a parent said to me, 'I'll be truthful with you, if my kid wants to get high, I want him to get high with me.' It is very sad and frustrating to work with the kind of mentality that truly rationalizes this behavior."

"At our middle school, there are a lot of students who do not live with their parents; they live with their grandparents, aunts and uncles, or foster parents. This is primarily because of divorce, and also because of the political realities of this area. We have a lot of children who have come from South America because of the wars and unrest there. Consequently, students have a lot of stress. Divorce is a stressor, too, along with drugs. Students also worry about not being grown up, if they look good, where they want to go, or if they can get into nightclubs without getting carded. Sex is another stressor. Girls especially worry about losing their virginity, getting pregnant, and abortion. These issues are very important to them at this point in their lives."

Carmen is very clear about her motivation for becoming a counselor: "I've always wanted to be a counselor since I was very young. I experienced some difficult moments in my adolescent years, because I lost significant people in my life; one loss was through a breakup of a relationship, another was someone close to me who committed suicide. All this affected me tremendously. I lost too many significant people at once, all in about a year or so. I changed schools; I went from one Catholic school to another. All of my friends attended different high schools; I had very few at my new school. After one full year at a new school with new friends, I had to change schools again, this time to a public high school, which was a culture shock for me. All these transitions made adolescence a turbulent time for me. I was lucky I had a good counselor in high school who helped me through these difficult times. He is a very special man and a good role model for students."

"My overall philosophy regarding adolescents is to keep them busy, be a positive role model, make sure they have a sense of identity, teach them to be cautious in a world full of trickery and negative influences, and without smothering them, give them responsibilities, obligations, and above all, *give them your time and love.*"

*I*N THE SPOTLIGHT

MIRROR, MIRROR, ON THE WALL

You stand in front of the mirror and examine your face for any signs of an impending eruption. Your best friend is covered with it and regularly visits a dermatologist. You don't want it to happen to you! You do what you consider all the "right" things, because you don't want to get it! You wash your face regularly, watch what you eat, and only occasionally yield to a chocolate bar. Breathing a sigh of relief, you turn from the mirror, confident that for today, at least, you don't have that dreaded teenage curse—ACNE!

What Causes Acne? Teenagers are particularly vulnerable—although adults have acne, too—because of a hereditary predisposition to it and the spurt of androgen, produced by both males and females, which stimulates the sebaceous glands and thus the production of sebum (Brody, 1988). Acne is formed in the skin's pores. These pores are constantly shedding cells that are washed to the surface by an oily substance called *sebum,* produced by sebaceous glands at the base of the pore. In acne, these glands are overactive, producing more oil than necessary. Thus, when the linings of the pores do not flake easily, they narrow and eventually become plugged with the sebum. When a pore is trapped to the outside, a whitehead or pimple occurs. Sebum blackens when exposed to the outside air, resulting in a blackhead. Painful lesions and ruptures occur when bacteria feed on the trapped sebum and produce irritable byproducts. Figure 12–11 provides a graphic description of how acne occurs.

In most people, diet is not a factor in causing acne, although it can be for some. Causes of acne include any substance that tends to clog pores, such as cosmetics, sunscreens, and oil from the environment. (In this case, making the french fries may be worse than eating them!) Other causes can be birth control pills and medications that trigger hormone production. Treatments for acne include everything from washing the face with mild soap, good hygiene, and good nutrition to over-the-counter medications and the latest in prescription drugs, such as Retin-A and Acutane.

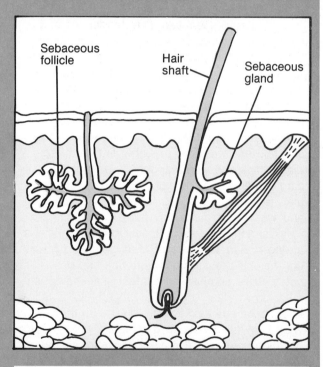

FIGURE 12-11   Acne is formed in the skin's pores.

MADONNA "WANNABEES"

Some teenagers want to be different from what they are—they "wannabee" like others—successful, beautiful, handsome, rich, popular, and at the center of attention. They "wannabee" what they are not and they "wannabee" someone other than who they are. They are known as the Madonna "Wannabees" of the twentieth century.

PARENTING AND ADOLESCENT CONFLICTS

Exists there a parent and a teenager who have not had their share of conflicts and confrontations? These contentious encounters cover the gamut of emotions involved in everyday family living. What family has not argued about whose turn it is to do what chores, the most appropriate time to be home at night, and the cost of clothing and records? Are these intergenerational infightings inherently inevitable? Apparently so. Laurence Steinberg (1987), who has spent much time studying adolescence, believes that parent-youth conflicts—nagging, squabbling, and bickering—begin with the biological event of puberty and suggests that such behavior is evolutionarily adaptive. Let's see how. Steinberg believes that in other animal species as well as in humans, there are biological and social mechanisms at work encouraging the young adolescent to leave the family group at the beginning of puberty. For example, if when young gibbon monkeys reach puberty they don't naturally emigrate, they are literally thrown out of the group. Reasons for emigration include that it enhances reproductive fitness, prevents inbreeding, and increases the gene pool, all of which are beneficial to the species.

In the United States and other industrialized countries, industrialization has provided its participants with many benefits, including improved nutrition, sanitation, and health. This in turn has *lowered* the beginning of puberty in the United States by about four years. Yet, at the same time, industrialization has increased the economic dependence of youth on their parents and compulsory schooling extends the time children are in the home. So, instead of leaving home to start a family of their own, today's youth, who are maturing earlier and who are more economically dependent on their parents for longer periods of time, find themselves in inevitable conflict with their parents, even in those families in which close ties already exist.

According to Steinberg, the good news is that conflict in the form of squabbling, nagging, and bickering is seldom fatal to close emotional bonds between parents and teenagers, and that such squabbling is usually temporary, lasting only until ages fifteen or sixteen. This is news that almost all parents are happy to hear.

Researcher Anne C. Petersen (1987) also agrees that puberty alone does not have the overwhelming psychological impact earlier clinicians and researchers assumed it did. In fact, today many of the myths of teenage life are being exploded. For example, instead of the view that teenagers are rambunctious, raging, and rebellious, and that the teenage years are a maddening time of life for all involved, the contemporary view supported by increasing numbers of psychologists and child developmentalists is that the vast majority of teenagers are well adjusted and get along well with their peers and parents (Flaste, 1988).

So while we can say that for teenagers *per se* tumult and negativism are not inevitable, we nonetheless, as consistently stressed in this text, focus on *individual* teenagers. While adolescent changes are not difficult for all youth, they are for some children, under some circumstances. Individual reactions to the changes of adolescence depend on the characteristics of the change, the characteristics of the individual, and the area in which change occurs (Simmons et al., 1987; p.346).

RECKLESSNESS AND FOOLISH RISKS

Why is it that teenagers take so many foolish risks? From acrobatic gyrations on skateboards to Russian roulette, the reckless abandon of teenagers is notorious and accounts for many accidents and deaths. Teenagers seem to live in a world unconstrained by the reasonable limits of the adult world. Teenagers have a natural desire to impress their peers and an urge to try on new roles, both of which would help explain their willingness to take risks. Then, too, risk-taking is a natural part of asserting independence and getting recognition from others.

Also, the tendency to take risks may result from a natural adolescent cognitive deficit in the ability to judge the personal danger involved in risk-taking.

ANOREXIA NERVOSA

Anorexia nervosa (anorexia is Greek and literally means "without a longing") is a severe loss of appetite. The name "Anorexia Nervosa" (AN) was first coined by Sir William Gill in 1874 to describe the syndrome of not eating and an aversion to food. Anorexics are often referred to as "starvers," because they fast to lose weight. Anorexia is manifested primarily in women and its incidence is relatively small, about 0.24 to 1.6 per 100,000 population (Murray, 1986). In this sense, then, the attention to and publicity about AN is large in proportion to its occurrence. This exaggerated attention can be attributed in part to public interest in rarities, the physical condition and mental state of persons with AN, and a number of famous people who have demonstrated AN symptoms. Primary anorexia is displayed through hypermotor activity, relentless pursuit of thinness, and delusional qualities in the perception of the dimensions of the body (Murray, 1986). Viewed in this way, anorexia nervosa is self-starvation, characterized by extreme prolonged dieting and weight loss and an intense preoccupation with food, weight, and exercise.

The following criteria characterize a person with AN (Murray, 1986):

1. Age of onset is prior to twenty-five. Most anorexics are teenagers.
2. Loss of at least 25 percent of original body weight.

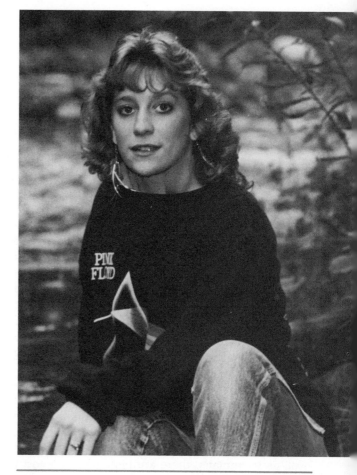

FIGURE 12-12   Anorexia nervosa usually strikes teenage girls. The deaths of public celebrities, especially singer and drummer Karen Carpenter, created much interest into the causes and consequence of anorexia nervosa.

3. Distorted implacable attitude toward eating or weight, which overrides hunger, thirst, admonitions, or assurances.
4. No known psychiatric disorder.
5. No known illness that could account for anorexia or weight loss.
6. At least two of the following: absence of menstruation; fine, soft hair; abnormally slow heartbeat; bouts of bulimia (insatiable appetite); periods of overactivity; and vomiting (may be self-induced). (p. 9)

In spite of a great deal of research, there is no universal agreement regarding why a person becomes anorexic. Some explanations for AN include (Caffary, 1987):

1. Psychoanalytic—Emphasis is placed on ego development interpretations, for example, food rejection is a symbol of disturbed relations with others, especially the mother. Also, the youth fails to develop an accurate set of internal cues needed to regulate hunger and satiation. Additionally, a youth makes a desperate attempt to gain control over her body as an attempt to regain her sense of self.
2. Ego weakness and interpersonal disturbances—These include lack of confirming responses by parents in early childhood, and individual overcontrolling, rigidity, and inadequacy in coping with stress and conflict.
3. Overestimation of body proportions, especially body width (Murray, 1986).

A full explanation of AN is very complex and the factors that cause a person to be an anorexic probably develop and operate in different people in different ways. Szmukler (1988) proposes the following causal factors for AN, some of which are listed according those that predispose, and those that precipitate.

Predisposing Factors

1. Sociocultural—for example, slimness as an ideal, and racial and social class view of the body. It is very possible that a young girl equates slimness with success.
2. Familial—Family history of affective disorder, alcoholism, AN, high aspirations, family dynamics, for example, the "psychosomatic family."
3. Psychological—Specific deficits, such as body image disturbance, sense of ineffectiveness, fear of maturation, personality, for example, perfectionism.
4. Biological—Genetic, such as Turner's syndrome, and illnesses such as diabetes.

Precipitating Factors

1. Some external precipitant, such as a family setting that does not value independence; dissatisfaction with life.
2. The need to be in control of some aspect of life and the positive reinforcement resulting from losing weight.

Treatment of AN includes hospitalization, behavior therapy, psychotherapy, family therapy, and drug therapy.

*I*N THE SPOTLIGHT

UNDERSTANDING ANOREXIA NERVOSA

We often wonder how someone comes to be an anorexic. Szmukler (1987) provides the following interesting portrait involving both cause and effect.

Many adolescents experience problems associated with establishing autonomy, separating from the family, coming to terms with sexual feelings, accepting peculiarities, developing satisfactory peer relationships, and achieving confidence in work and studies. A particular adolescent may attribute the cause of her problems to a particular source, for example, body shape. Unlike many other problems, body shape has the quality of being controllable. As a result:

The adolescent girl may decide that some weight loss would improve her figure and she may be influenced in this by the message from our culture that slimness is an important key to success. A perfectionist girl may embark on the enterprise of weight loss with method and determination and should she succeed, she will find some obvious rewards. Her appearance may improve and invite compliments from others. She may find the weight loss especially gratifying if she values the feeling of being in control. If her problems remain unaltered, she may intensify her efforts to diet in the hope that this will help more. With the investment of so much energy in losing weight this may become a special preoccupation. However, the more she starves, the more she will be troubled by her hunger and the more she will fear losing control. Once the diet is broken, her special achievement will be lost and so she may seek to establish a margin of safety so that, even if she should "break out," it will not represent a total disaster. Her starvation may thus become further intensified and as a consequence of this so will her preoccupation with weight and food. Other means may be introduced to keep her weight in check: exercise, purgatives, and vomiting. Since an ever increasing amount of energy is being expended on weight control she finds it difficult to maintain her other interests. Her social life begins to suffer, in part because eating with others is to be avoided. This can be embarrassing and the situation might prove irresistibly tempting. Alternative sources of satisfaction become fewer so that her special achievement assumes even greater importance. She has little energy to cope with the tasks of adolescent development and she falls progressively behind her peers. In face of the failures in these areas her weight control assumes even greater importance. (p. 30).

BULIMIA

In *bulimia*, (from the Greek *bous*, meaning "ox" and *limos*, meaning "hunger," literally "the appetite of a cow") the individual periodically fasts and binges on food, followed by self-induced vomiting. Bulimics are often referred to as "gorgers or vomiters," because of a binge-purge syndrome. Suffers have periods of high caloric consumption, followed by starvation, vomiting, excessive exercise, and the use of laxatives, diet pills, or diuretics. People with bulimia show the following behaviors: they are outgoing, have strong appetites, vomit more, show anxiety, exhibit depression and guilt, report more body-related complaints, are more sensitive in interpersonal relations, and do not sleep as well as fasting anorexics do (Caffary, 1987, p. 46). *Bulimarexia* is a combination of anorexia and bulimia, characterized by extreme dieting and purging.

PEER GROUPS

You have all heard about peer groups and more than likely you were and perhaps are a member of one. Why are such peer groups formed? Essentially to fulfill the needs of the adolescents who join them. Peer groups help adolescents develop an identity, adapt to their environment, and structure interpersonal relationships and activities.

In one study of peer group influences on decisions about schooling, (Delgado-Gaitan, 1986) four peer groups were identified: jocks, lowriders, eggheads, and freaks. The jocks were those who played sports, lowriders organized around their interest in cars, eggheads were in the college preparatory track, and freaks dressed atypically, including brightly colored hair.

However, when teenagers want freedom from parental authority and when parents free their children of parental authority, then what happens is that teenagers come under the control of another authority, even more demanding and rigorous than that of their parents. This is the authority of their peers. So most teenagers, rather than escaping from authority, become members of a very authoritarian peer group that dictates many and varied behavioral conformities.

We tend to think that peer groups are developed and maintained solely by the adolescents who are a part of them, but parents and teachers also play a role in peer group definition and maintenance. For example, parents and school personnel create clearly defined attributes for each group and tend to reinforce the expectations each group has for itself (Delgado-Gaitan, 1986, p. 456). Could it be that parents and teachers exercise their authority after all, but in a vicarious way?

THE WORLD OF WORK

Three-quarters of all high school seniors hold part-time jobs and work an average of sixteen to twenty hours per week (Bachman, 1987, p. 6). At first glance these figures may look good. Certainly a job helps develop all those qualities that are important—responsibility, autonomy, the ability to make decisions, and self-reliance. However, there is a flip side to this coin of work. Long hours of part-time work are also linked to weak school performance, low college aspirations, and higher drug use (Bachman, 1987, p. 7). In addition, as Table 12–2 shows, while there many positive benefits that can accrue to teenagers from working, over the last quarter century, the impact of youthwork has shifted from the positive and neutral to the negative (Greenberger & Steinberg, 1986, p. 51).

A major reason for the negative impact youthwork has on the lives of adolescents is the nature of the jobs that they have. Many of these jobs are considered by adults as "bad jobs" for a number of reasons. They pay low wages, offer less than full-time employment, have irregular shifts, are at night and on weekends, have low job security, provide few or minimal job benefits, and have poor prospects for promotion (Greenberger & Steinberg, 1986, p. 25).

TABLE 12–2

DIMENSIONS OF ADOLESCENT WORK EXPERIENCES

	Context		
	Educational	Economic	Social
Positive	Imparts skills, knowledge, habits, or attitudes that are valuable for successful assumption or performance of adult work roles	Serves some economic necessity to family and/or community (work is necessary for family's or community's well-being)	Brings youth into contact with adults and fosters meaningful intergenerational relationships
Neutral	Does not affect the acquisition of work-relevant skills, knowledge, habits, or attitudes	Work is not required by family or community but may benefit either financially	Neither facilitates nor impedes intergenerational ties
Negative	Fosters habits or attitudes or teaches skills that may be undesirable for future work roles	Work serves financial needs of individual youth exclusively and earnings are used chiefly for immediate consumption of nonessentials	Furthers separation of young people from adults; strengthens peer culture and accentuates intergenerational differences

Note. From *When Teenagers Work* (p. 52) by E. Greenberger and L. Steinberg, 1986, New York: Basic Books.

Facilitating Teenagers' Work

There are a number of reasons why youthwork is more available to teenagers today than it was in the past (Greenberger & Steinberg, 1986, pp. 75–77). First, is the match or fit between the hours of schooling and jobs available in the workplace. Today, the school day does not present a scheduling conflict for many part-time and service jobs.

TABLE 12–3

WHAT HIGH SCHOOL SENIORS RATE AS VERY IMPORTANT IN A JOB		
	1976	1986
Good chance for advancement and promotion	57%	67%
Chance to earn a good deal of money	47	58
Chance to participate in decision making	27	33
High status or prestige	20	32
Interesting to do	88	87
Uses skills and abilities	71	72
Predictable, secure future	62	64
Chance to make friends	54	53
Worthwhile to society	45	41

Note. From ''An Eye on the Future'' by J. Bachman, 1987, *Psychology Today, 21,* p. 8.

Second, many retail and service jobs are located where teenagers live, in the suburbs. Thus many jobs are readily accessible to teenagers. Third, the advertising industry's efforts to create teenage consumption have worked. Teens need more money to buy the products advertisers entice them to buy.

What is it that teenagers look for in their work? Table 12–3 provides the answer.

The sweat shops of the eighteenth century prompted many of the child labor laws prohibiting the exploitation of children, but today's labor shortage in the service industry and youth's insatiable appetite for consumer goods combine to make working after school and on weekends a way of life for many teenagers. The mall shops, department stores, and fast-food establishments provide youth opportunities to put designer clothes on their backs and help pay for their cars, most at the minimum wage. For many of America's teenagers, the transition from the world of childhood and basic dependency to the status of employee and consumer is coming earlier and earlier. Many teenagers are caught up in the work-spend ethic.

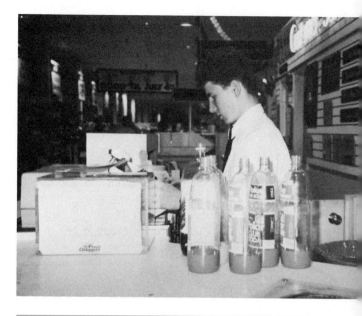

FIGURE 12-13 Many teenagers earn extra money and enhanced self-esteem through part-time work. Not everyone agrees, however, that part-time work is beneficial for teenagers. Undoubtedly however, more teenagers will continue to work as the demand for their services increases.

Is Working Good For Teenagers?

The conventional wisdom is that working is good for teenagers. Many parents probably encourage their teenagers to get involved in the world of work, as illustrated in the vignette at the beginning of the chapter. But is this a good idea? Some adolescents undoubtedly benefit, many others probably don't. In general, the effects of youthwork on adolescent development are bleak:

It is clear that in these three areas (educational, economic and social) the jobs available to young people in the new adolescent workplace do not generally provide environments conducive to psychological growth and development. Indeed, we would argue the counterintuitive findings. . . . that working is more likely to interfere with than enhance schooling; promotes pseudomaturity rather than maturity; is associated in certain circumstances with higher, not lower, rates of delinquency and drug use; and fosters cynical rather than respectful attitudes toward work—can be explained by deficiencies in the work experiences typically available to youngsters. It is precisely because the typical adolescent's experience in the new workplace is educationally irrelevant, economically unnecessary, and largely age segregated that adolescent employment has the impact it does. It promotes autonomy only in its most individualistic sense and social responsibility, little or not at all (Greenberger & Steinberg, 1986, p. 235)

Regardless of this dreary assessment of the impact of youthwork on adolescent development, the economic realities of our capitalist society will necessitate even more involvement by youth in the workplace. The need for hiring more teenagers is necessitated by (Joselow, 1989): (1) the nation's low unemployment rate; (2) a shrinking number of older teenagers in the labor pool; (3) more teenagers indulging in sophisticated consumer tastes; and (4) parents who approve of teenagers' work as a means of helping to offset stagnating real family incomes.

Our economic system is dependent on youth to fill many of the minimum-wage service jobs. The efforts of service industries to recruit senior citizens to fill jobs typically held by teenagers is vivid testimony to the number of service jobs that need to be filled. Then, too, the insatiable consumer appetites of teenagers will continue to motivate them to enter the workplace. After all, it is the American way.

ADOLESCENT RUNAWAYS

Have you ever thought about running away from home? Why did you want to run away from home? At one time or another, most children have contemplated running away from home. Dissatisfied with how they are treated and angry with their parents, they envision a life that is better, where people understand them and are sensitive to their needs. Indeed, much of adolescent literature is populated by runaway heroes such as Tom Sawyer and Huckleberry Finn. What was once

considered a romantic adventure and tolerated as a stage of growing up has now turned into a national crisis, and runaways are seen as being at risk for many different kinds of problems. Indeed it is difficult to go grocery shopping without seeing runaways' pictures on grocery bags. And, as you pour milk on your breakfast cereal, runaways' pictures stare at you from the milk carton.

The tragic death of Adam Walsh in 1981 heightened public awareness of the plight of missing children and precipitated passage of child protection laws, including the Missing Children's Assistance Act of 1984. As a result of this act, the National Center for Missing and Exploited Children was established. The Center, created through a cooperative arrangement with the United States Department of Justice, Office of Juvenile Justice and Delinquency Prevention, serves as a clearinghouse for information on missing and exploited children; provides training assistance to law enforcement and child protection agencies; assists individuals, agencies, and state and local governments in locating missing children; and administers a national toll-free hot line (800-843-5678) to receive information regarding missing children. The address is: National Center for Missing and Exploited Children, 1835 K Street, N.W., Suite 700, Washington, D.C. 20006. There is also a National Runaway Hot Line and Youth Assistance Program (800-448-4663). This hot line serves runaway children, children having problems, and parents of children having problems.

The Runaway and Homeless Youth Act (RHYA), which is Title III of the Juvenile Justice and Delinquency Prevention Act, is administered through the Department of Health and Human Services. This program provides funds to state and local governments and private agencies to meet the needs of runaway and homeless youth and their families with temporary shelter, counseling, and aftercare services. The 1987 reauthorization of this act also included funds to strengthen families through parent-adolescent mediation and the linking of social services, youth employment services, and private sector initiatives (Garrison, 1987).

JUVENILE DELINQUENCY

The national concern about juvenile crime and the need for an enhanced federal involvement in juvenile delinquency prevention and justice lead to the passage of the Juvenile Justice and Delinquency Prevention Act (JJDPA) of 1974. The latest reenactment was in 1987. The purpose of JJDPA is to provide necessary federal resources, leadership, and coordination for delinquency prevention, research, training, standards development, and aid to runaway and homeless youth (JJDPA, 1985). Two important agencies created by JJDPA are the Office of Juvenile Justice and Delinquency Prevention (OJJDP) and the National Institute for Juvenile Justice and Delinquency Prevention (NIJJDP). The OJJDP administers the JJDPA; collects and disseminates information regarding prevention, treatment, and control of juvenile delinquency; trains individuals; and conducts research with particular emphasis to prevention and treatment. Suggested topics for research include: family-based delinquency prevention and treatment; gang intervention; the treatment of juveniles in the juvenile justice system; the roles of family violence,

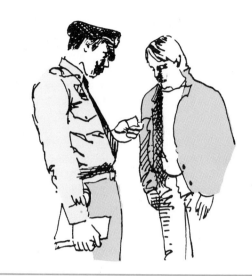

FIGURE 12-15 In trouble with the law! Many experts feel that the direction from which help comes must be from parents and school programs. (From Bailey/WORKING SKILLS, copyright 1990 by Delmar Publishers Inc.)

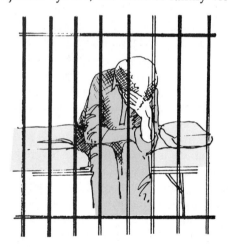

FIGURE 12-14 The atypical behaviors of teenagers are well documented in the daily press. Much of society's effort to effectively address these problems focuses on preventative efforts. (From Bailey/WORKING SKILLS, copyright 1990 by Delmar Publishers Inc.)

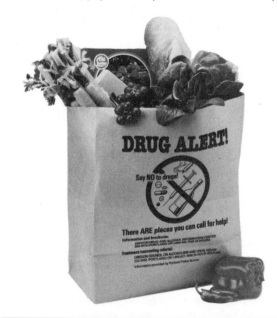

FIGURE 12-16 Many prevention programs for helping youth with problems of substance abuse and resulting consequences are school-based. After-care, better prevention and counseling are the new ABCs of many high school curricula. (From Bailey/WORKING SKILLS, copyright 1990 by Delmar Publishers Inc.)

sexual abuse, media violence and special remedial education in juvenile delinquency; and the differential treatment of youth by the juvenile justice system based on race, sex and family income (Garrison, 1987).

One of the determiners of future delinquent behavior is how early a youth starts his or her delinquent career. Youth who start their delinquent career early (ages eleven to twelve) exhibit more delinquent behavior *and* do so across the spectrum of types and seriousness of offenses. On the other hand, youth who begin delinquent behavior at later ages fifteen to eighteen may be doing so in order to "try on" social roles in relation to internalizing social values. When the delinquent behavior has fulfilled its developmental purpose, it diminishes (Tolan, 1987).

TEENAGE ALCOHOLISM

One of the problems facing teenagers is the use and abuse of alcohol. Consider the following (Ramsey, 1988, p.1):

- The average age children start drinking is twelve.
- Alcohol is the most commonly abused drug among adolescents.
- One out of twenty students will drink daily by their senior year in high school.
- More than 3,500 teens died in alcohol-related accidents in 1986.

That's the bad news. The good news is that alcohol and other drug use by high school seniors is decreasing ("Seniors Reported," 1989). For example, the number of seniors reporting they had a drink in the week prior to the survey dropped from 66 percent in 1987 to 64 percent in 1988. Thirty-three percent of the seniors reported using marijuana, down from 36.3 percent in 1987 and from 50 percent in 1980. The reason for the decline in drug use is attributed to teenagers heeding the messages about the risks associated with drugs.

WHY DO ADOLESCENTS ENGAGE IN SUBSTANCE ABUSE?

When you ask others why people use drugs, you get many answers. One reason frequently given is that personality plays a role. For example, Kitty Dukakis, wife of former Democratic presidential candidate Michael Dukakis, is characterized as having a "drug-dependent" personality. Other reasons often cited are role models, peer pressure, poor self-esteem, neighborhood environment, family dysfunctions, media and advertising, and a genetic predisposition.

There are a number of theories about the causes, reasons, and origins of drug use. A social learning theory explanation (Akers, Khron, Lanze-Kaduce & Rasosevich, 1979) maintains that operant conditioning and imitation are important factors. The social psychological explanation (Jessor and Jessor, 1978) is based on the belief that in teenagers' "problem behavior process"—which is the resultant interaction of individual values, expectations, beliefs, and attitudes with the surrounding environment, its supports, controls, models and expectations—can lead to drug use depending on the nature of the indicated variables and the nature of their interaction. Peer pressure and peer interaction are often given as a reason for drug use (Kandel, Kessler, & Margulies, 1978). Drug use as an effort to raise self-esteem is another leading theory for drug involvement (Kaplan, Martin, & Robbins, 1982).

One other reason for or cause of drug use in adolescence that is of particular interest is the connection between early personality characteristics and substance abuse. Researchers Block, Block, and Keyes (1988) explain their findings this way:

The nursery school personality precursors of adolescent drug usage are numerous, unique, and implicative. Among girls and boys, personality characteristics are identifiable at an early age (three to four years) that persist over time and are conducive to later involvement with drugs. No important differences were observed, at these earlier ages, between the path to later marijuana and the path to later hard drug use. For both sexes, the constellation of personality characteristics encompassed by the concept of ego under control (inability to delay gratification, rapid tempo, emotional expressiveness, mood liability [changes], overactivity, etc.) correlationally foretold later drug use: for girls, but not for boys, an absence of ego resiliency (i.e., adaptional insufficiencies leading to a personality vulnerability) also presaged drug usage in adolescence (p. 350).

The researchers' findings regarding the family antecedents of drug use in adolescence are equally informative and fascinating:

Boys who are uncontrolled at an early age are more likely to go on in adolescence to use drugs: their tendency to use drugs does not appear to be attenuated or amplified by parental and environmental characteristics (p. 351).

For girls, however, "various parental and environmental attributes, in interaction with personality qualities of the child, related to subsequent drug use" (p. 351). What are these antecedents of drug use? The researchers continue:

The early family variables foretelling later drug use in girls are a mixed bag of antecedents requiring an interpretive leap for their reconciliation. These precursors include a cluster of parenting and environmental qualities that, taken together, connote a permissiveness and relaxedness of parents with their daughters. Thus, traditional values were not inculcated and home situations were highly interactive, informal, and unconventional. Early independence of the daughters was fostered. Mothers encouraged their daughters to think and wonder about life. Sex-typing was not emphasized. Emotional expression in the form of crying, spontaneity of play, and the challenging of mother and teachers was acceptable.

A constellation of other variables, however, suggests to us that the seeming "progressiveness" of these parents may have stemmed from parental insufficiencies and parental distractions rather than principled, value-based parental choices. Thus, the unconventional home was also unmannerly, noisy, and carelessly organized. The daughters who were pressed toward early independence also were generally not pressed to achieve. The mothers who encouraged their daughters to contemplate the nature of life also expressed disappointment and anger with their daughters, for whom they felt they had given up some of their own interests.

Such parental inconsistencies would have to register, affectively, upon the developing daughters. We suggest that, to evolving, structure-seeking, and structure-building girls, such indifferent or disorganized parents would not appear to be suitable models for emulation or sufficient providers of the instruction and reassurance required for the identification process that leads to identity development. Given the self-uncertainty that this kind of family environment would engender, it would not be surprising if later vulnerability to peer influence was observed in these girls (pp. 351–352).

IMPLICATIONS FOR PARENTS

Several implications based on the cited research findings seem clear. Schools and other public agencies would do well in their programs of drug prevention to include components that enable parents to learn about and implement effective parenting skills. Second, such programs could model as well those behavioral and personal characteristics appropriate to effective parenting. We know that knowledge of what constitutes a good parent does not necessarily translate into being a good parent. Third, such parenting programs should be provided for parents of young children and for parents-to-be in order that they can be good parents from the beginning of their parenting careers rather than having to try to rectify their and their children's deficiencies after it is obviously too late.

TEENAGE SEX

Many of the developmental tasks of the teenage years are also bound to developing sexuality.

Early Sex

A simple fact of teenage life is that teenagers are having sex earlier in their lives than teenagers did a decade ago. Table 12–4 shows the ages and percentages at which teenagers are having sex.

Survival Sex

Some teenagers, especially those who are homeless and live on the street, barter sex for the necessities of life—food, clothing, and shelter. To identify this kind of sex and to distinguish it from prostitution, Gary Yates and his coworkers at Children's Hospital's High Risk Project in Hollywood, California have coined the term *survival sex*. Children of both sexes, many in their early teens, use sex to meet immediate needs by trading sex for food, shelter, and drugs.

TEENAGE PREGNANCY— PREMATURE PARENTHOOD

Introduction

Pregnancy at any age engenders developmental change; in the immature, it creates developmental crisis. Pregnancy during adolescence thus compounds the stress of two normative developmental stages and endangers the successful resolution to

TABLE 12–4

	TEEN SEX BY AGE AND PERCENT			
	Survey Year			
Race and Age	1971	1976	1979	1982
TOTAL	(N = 2,739)	(N = 1,452)	(N = 1,717)	(N = 1,157)
15–19	30.4	43.4	40.8	44.8
15	14.8	18.9	22.8	17.0
16	21.8	30.0	39.5	29.0
17	28.2	46.0	50.1	41.0
18	42.6	56.7	63.0	56.6
19	48.2	64.1	71.4	72.0
WHITE	(N = 1,758)	(N = 881)	(N = 1,034)	(N = 767)
15–19	26.4	38.3	46.8	43.3
15	11.8	14.2	18.5	15.4
16	17.8	25.2	37.4	27.3
17	23.2	40.0	45.8	39.4
18	38.8	52.1	60.3	56.3
19	43.8	59.2	68.0	70.4
BLACK	(N = 981)	(N = 571)	(N = 683)	(N = 390)
15–19	53.7	66.3	66.2	53.6
15	31.2	38.9	41.7	24.6
16	46.4	55.1	50.9	37.6
17	58.4	71.9	74.8	49.4
18	62.4	76.4	77.0	73.6
19	76.2	85.3	88.7	81.4

* Note. From "Premarital Sexual Activity Among US Teenage Women over the Past Three Decades" by S. Hoffarth, J. R. Kahn and W. Baldwin, 1987, *Family Planning Perspectives, 19*, pp. 46–53.

either one. Childbirth and parenthood add tasks, choices, and responsibilities. Developmental failures in parents place their children at biological, psychological, and social risk. Among crises during adolescence, pregnancy endangers not only the individual and society, but also the unborn child (Group for the Advancement of Psychiatry, 1986, p. xix).

Teenage Pregnancy as a Social Problem

When describing and/or addressing the topic of teenage pregnancy, people who work in the field as well as the public in general use such words as "crisis," epidemic," and "national disease," with the teenage parents and their children both characterized as "victims." Clearly, in today's world, teenage pregnancy is viewed as a social problem, necessitating the marshalling of economic and political forces to solve it. Why is this?

Teenage pregnancy and parenthood is not a new phenomena in the United States. At the height of the baby boom—about 1957—half of all women married while in their teens and over 25 percent of all women gave birth to their first child before age twenty (Frustenberg, Brooks-Gunn, & Morgan, 1987, p. 1). Why all the fuss then about teenage pregnancy? Three phenomenon have helped focus the public's attention on pregnant teenagers.

First, the number of *unmarried* teenagers who give birth has increased dramatically, to about 470,000 a year (Buie, 1987). Second, during the 70s and 80s, the age at which people marry increased, thus the delay of marriage focused attention on premarital pregnancy, especially where teenagers are concerned. While 14 percent of teenage births were out of wedlock in 1955, this percentage skyrocketed to 56 percent by 1984! (Frustenberg et al., 1987, p. 4) Third, as a result of the 1973 Supreme Court decision, *Roe* v. *Wade*, which legalized abortion, many pregnant teenagers opted for abortions over marriage. In fact, about 400,000 teenagers have abortions every year (Buie, 1987). The legalization of abortion made marriage after pregnancy unnecessary for some teenagers, thus severing the link between marriage and pregnancy.

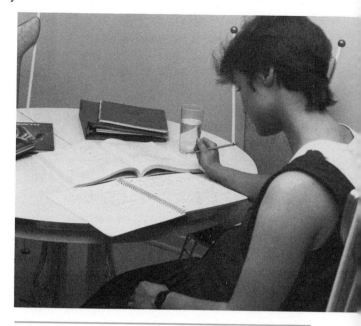

FIGURE 12-17 In spite of the wide-spread availability of contraception information and products, many teenagers continue to become pregnant during their high school years. The consequences of teen-age pregnancies are many and far reaching, affecting not only pregnant mothers but their children, families and society.

All of which tended to further focus attention on teenage pregnancy.

More teenagers, especially those under sixteen, are becoming sexually active at earlier ages (Hofferth, Kahn, & Baldwin, 1987). In the 1960s and 1970s there was not only a social revolution, but a sexual revolution as well, resulting in an increase in sexual activity among teenagers. While this increase occurred first in older teenagers, it also spread to younger teenagers as well. And younger teenagers are at higher risk for unintended pregnancy because they are slow to use contraceptive measures after their first intercourse. For example, only 23 percent of women under age fifteen at first intercourse started using a contraceptive method within the first month of becoming sexually active. This compares with 53 percent of the eighteen and nineteen-year-olds, who used a contraceptive within the first month after becoming sexually active (Hofferth et al., 1987).

*I*N THE SPOTLIGHT

A FREUDIAN VIEW OF TEENAGE PREGNANCY

Development of sexuality plays a powerful role in the lives of children and youth. The resolution of sexual desires and conflicts thus contributes to ego development as well as normal psychosexual development. The following is a Freudian interpretation of the psychic motivations for and causes of teenage pregnancy.

For a girl, having ideas of a fetus being part of herself, of her own nourishment, and inseparable as a distinct being may blur her own boundaries; having a baby to nourish and nurture may be like nourishing her still-infantile self or being nurtured again by her own mother. In this way she may express the need to remain mother's cared for and dependent child. At the same time, the baby may be considered as competing for nurture as a sibling, arousing jealousy and rage. A baby may be a precious gift for mother or a bodily product to be withheld in defiance. The baby as something mother cannot force her to give up, may be valued as proof of autonomy; the baby may be devalued and rejected if associated with disgusting products of elimination.

Such fantasies may occur in young healthy girls from emotionally healthy families. They diminish in intensity as girls separate from their childhood-dependent relationship with their parents, integrate their sexuality into a mature body image and sexual identity, and focus their drives on appropriate heterosexual objects and actions. If there is interference with the resolution of such concepts, they may be acted out through premature pregnancy and may lead to harmful interaction between the girl, her parents, and the father (Group for the Advancement of Psychiatry, 1986, p. 11).

Reasons For Teenage Pregnancy

In addition to the social and demographic patterns of teenage pregnancy discussed, we need to examine the reasons why teenagers become pregnant.

First, some teenagers, especially those from low-income families, may feel that they are trapped in a life that offers little in terms of their present condition. For them, the future outlook may be equally bleak, with little opportunity to share in the wealth of the middle class through higher education, better jobs, and higher incomes. Faced with such a bleak future, a child may be one way to achieve status and demonstrate self-expression. For these youth then, it makes little difference if they have a child at sixteen or twenty-six.

Second, for some teenagers, having a baby is a rite of passage from childhood to adulthood (Read, 1988). Thus those teenagers who have babies are viewed as "normal," while those who do not are viewed as "having something wrong with them." Certainly the reality that some teenagers become pregnant because they want to cannot be dismissed. Landry and her associates (1986) report that the majority of teens in their study knew about birth control and knew where to get it, yet only 12 percent of the child bearers and 23 percent of the pregnancy terminators claimed to be using a contraceptive method at the time they became pregnant (p. 273).

A third reason would seem to be the persistent resistance of the American public and the schools to making contraceptive information available to teenagers. Ninety-six percent of the school districts in the United States do not provide birth control information to their students (Buie, 1987).

A fourth reason relates to a developmental phenomena, the *secular* trend. One effect of the secular trend, the onset of puberty at earlier ages, is that it prolongs adolescence. Thus instead of a two-, three-, or four-year period, it now is for some teenagers who begin menarche at age twelve or earlier, a period as long as six to eight years. Thus, the window of opportunity for a teenager to become pregnant as a teenager is longer than it might have been in years gone by.

Consequences of Teenage Pregnancy

Teenage pregnancy can kill hopes and dreams. For some, hopelessness and helplessness result. One concrete and economic consequence is that "women who have had a child either before leaving high school or within a number of months of leaving school are far less likely to have eventually obtained a secondary credential than are women who have postponed childbearing until their 20s" (Mott & Marsiglio, 1985, p. 237).

The cognitive and emotional immaturity of a teenager makes the decision to abort or have the child even more difficult. For a young pregnant teenager, decisions for abortion or childbirth may reflect more of her parents' values than her own, especially when she has not been able, because of developmental age, to develop self-autonomy.

Many teenagers are becoming parents when they are children themselves. Frequently what happens is that they remain economically and emotionally dependent on their parents. They thus remain cared-for children while attempting to be parents who must care for their own children. In this sense, teenage pregnancy robs children of their own childhood, and has a number of negative consequences on the life choices and chances of adolescent parents.

Let's look at these:

1. Teenage mothers do not achieve as much education as mothers who delay childbearing.
2. Teenage mothers are less likely to find stable and remunerative employment than women who delay childbearing. Thus they are more likely to receive public assistance.
3. The children of early childbearers may be disadvantaged in comparison to the offspring of women who delay childbearing, because they are more likely to grow up in a single-parent home and are more likely to be poor (Furstenberg et al., 1987).
4. Much has been written about the cognitive and educational effects of teenage parenting on the children of teenagers. For example, one study (Coll, Hoffman, & Oh, 1986), found that infants of teenage parents had lower mental functioning at eight months of age than did the children of nonteenage parents.

However, in general, children of adolescent mothers are not at substantially increased risk for deficits in cognitive or academic functioning (Kinard & Reinherz, 1987). The critical variable, rather, is maternal education. Consequently, the extent to which children of adolescent mothers are at risk for poor educational achievement seems to be a function of low maternal educational attainment (Kinard & Reinherz, 1987). Thus, the child of a teenager who gave birth at fourteen and who did not complete her junior high school education is at greater educational risk than the child of a teenager who gave birth at nineteen after completing her high school education.

Consequences For Children of Teenage Mothers

Whereas two decades ago unwed teenage mothers tended not to raise their own children, today things are different. The overwhelming majority—93 percent—now raise their own children (Coll, Hoffman, Oh, & Vohr, 1987). This providing of primary maternal care for their children by teenage mothers has a number of consequences for children.

Teenage parents have unique parenting practices that have particular and important implications for their children. For example, Caucasian adolescent mothers rely more frequently on other teenagers for help in caring for their infants (Coll et al., 1987). The fact that infants of teenage mothers rely on their peers for help in care-giving may mean, depending on individual circumstances, that the children are receiving less than optimal care. This is particularly true when considered within the finding that adolescent mothers tend to be less verbal, less emotionally positive, and less didactic with their children (Coll et al., 1987).

Adolescent maternal behavior is a combined function of the mother's developmental history and her current social support (Crockenberg, 1987). This combination of how adolescents were raised and their supportive or nonsupportive relationships has implications for how an adolescent mother raises her child. For example, when teenage mothers experienced both rejection during pregnancy and low current support from their partners they were likely to exhibit a pattern of angry and punitive parenting (Crockenberg, 1987). This pattern of parenting style is reciprocal in that when mothers are angry and punitive, then children are angry and noncompliant, distance themselves from their mothers, and exhibit little confidence in their ability to cope with challenging tasks (Crockenberg, 1987). In effect, then, one challenge facing professionals and developers of social policy is to find ways to intervene in adolescent mothers' parenting patterns to provide them with the parenting skills and support systems that will enable them to be effective parents.

Furthermore, teenage parents are at greater risk for abusing their children. Teenage parenting is stressful and this situation lowers the ability of the parents to cope with further stress (Gelles, 1986). Also, as we have discussed, when an adolescent parent has a background of rejection and a current context of low support for their roles as parents, this leads to angry and punitive parenting. These two behavioral reactions—anger and punitiveness—are ingredients of child abuse.

One key to healthy sexual development in teenagers is a good family experience in which the teenager is loved and respected; where a value system is both implicitly and explicitly stated and followed; where opportunities are provided for involvement in a wide range of interests; and in which opportunities for autonomy, responsibility, and decision making are a normal part of living.

Programs For Preventing Teenage Pregnancy

While everyone talks about teenage pregnancy, preventing it is difficult. Program intervention efforts are mainly based on two approaches, sex education and contraceptive services. Quinn (1986) believes the following four themes, identified in the research literature, offer the best basis for designing teenage pregnancy prevention programs. These themes are:

1. Interventions aimed at fostering more effective parent-child (especially mother-daughter) communication around sexual issues have a good record in the important areas of delaying the onset of sexual activity among teenagers and of encouraging contraceptive use among sexually active teens.
2. Involvement in sexual activity is not the norm for younger teens and this group should be encouraged to postpone sexual involvement for several developmental reasons, including the fact that they are known to be careless contraceptive users.
3. Programs that provide experiences directly related to behavioral goals can change behaviors.
4. Across cultural groups, young women with higher educational and career aspirations are less likely to become teenage parents than their classmates with lower aspirations or less clear life goals (pp. 101–102).
5. Programs that teach adolescent sexual abstinence. (See the answer to "What Would You Do?" for more details.)

A unique and radical approach to the prevention of teenage pregnancy is the formation of "adolescent development zones . . . in which teenage girls actually receive periodic payments for remaining childless" (Belsky & Draper, 1987, p. 23). Here is what the researchers propose:

We can imagine young adolescents, receiving when they turn eleven (and six months later) a cash payment of, say, $50 if they report to the school nurse and can be certified, simply on the basis of external (visual) examinations, as not being pregnant. When these girls turn thirteen this twice-a-year award would increase to $75. At fifteen, payments would become both larger and more frequent, with teenagers receiving $100 every four months. Teenagers remaining childless until eighteen years of age would qualify for a cash bonus of $500. Graduation from high school would carry

with it an additional $500 cash bonus along with $2,000 in educational benefits to be used to secure additional training (academic or vocational) within the next two years (Belsky & Draper, 1987, p. 23).

They would reward the mothers of teenagers as well.

We propose that the mother or legal guardian of a teenage girl residing in our adolescent development zones receive cash payments of $250 if the teenager is childless at age twelve, $400 if still childless at fifteen, and $600 if she reaches the age of eighteen without having become pregnant or born a child (p. 24).

*I*N THE SPOTLIGHT

A DOLLAR A DAY KEEPS THE STORK AWAY

Paying teenagers not to become pregnant is exactly what happens at La Mariposa Health Station in Denver, Colorado (Zaslowsky, 1989). Teenagers are paid a dollar a day—seven dollars a week—for not becoming pregnant—again. In 1985, the Educational Endowment Committee of Planned Parenthood of the Rocky Mountains contracted with the Denver Children's Home to conduct the "Dollar-a-Day" Program to prevent repeat pregnancies in high-risk Hispanic adolescents at Mariposa (Mariposa means "butterfly" in Spanish) Health Station in Denver.

The program includes two phases: identifying a group of high-risk females with a history of at least one pregnancy by the age of sixteen, and recruiting each girl to voluntarily attend a meeting once each week at a neighborhood health station. The girls come to the meetings as long as they are not pregnant and it is made clear that membership ends if pregnancy occurs. The girls complete the program by attending 100 sessions or when they turn eighteen (Anderman, 1988).

When the girls check in each week and receive their money, they stay a while and discuss topics of interest to them. In many ways, the "Dollar-a-Day" group is a basic support group that provides informal socialization for the teenage girls. In this regard, the program is similar to Alcoholics Anonymous (AA) and other support groups, such as Narcotics Anonymous (NA), which rely on the group to help enforce and reinforce commitments to the group goal—in this case, not becoming pregnant.

The program is successful in preventing teenage pregnancy. Over a period of two years, only three of the original group of eighteen experienced pregnancy, and two of these three returned to the group in an attempt to avoid becoming pregnant again.

The reasons for the program's success are (Anderman, 1988):

- Group homogeneity—The teenagers know one another, attend the same school, and socialize together. The location of the

weekly meetings are in a neutral facility in a homogeneous, monoracial neighborhood.
- Financial incentive—The dollar-a-day serves as an incentive for group membership.
- Continuity and consistency—The program staff did not miss any group sessions. Through their attention and involvement, they communicate a feeling of commitment and camaraderie to the group.

- Refreshments—Food and beverage serve as a motivator and central organizing feature for these needy, low-income Hispanic teenagers.
- Staff training—The staff are well trained in counseling and group process skills.
- Expectations—The group is a nonthreatening one. As such, it does not attempt to overpower participants through an education or formal dissemination model.

Based on what we know, it is necessary to start teenage pregnancy prevention programs early, before teenagers become teenagers.

From time to time, you may hear people say that sex education is the responsibility of the parents and that parents need to talk more with their children about sex. But does parent-child communication about sex do any good in relation to children's sexual behavior? Apparently not. Newcomer and Udry (1985) collected data from teenagers and their mothers, and concluded that "the data reveal little effect of parental attitudes or parental-child communication on either the child's subsequent initiation of coitus or his or her contraceptive behavior. The reason may be that parental communication about sex is generally so vague or so limited as to have no impact" (p. 174). The implication for the first theme mentioned is that parents do need support that will enable them to develop effective communication with their children.

Another reason for the fact that parent-child communication about sex and sexual practices does little good is that teenagers feel that they alone should govern their sexual behavior (Williams, 1989). This attitude seems to be an outgrowth of social changes of the 60s and 70s and is reinforced by television advertising and clinics, and counselors and parents whom teenagers see as preaching one way and living yet another. Sexual behavior,

then, is viewed by teenagers as a matter of personal choice rather than a matter of parental or adult control, with sex being their right. (Williams, 1989).

What Would You Do?

As you know by now, there is a great deal of discussion about teenage pregnancy, and it seems as though there are more solutions for pregnancy prevention formulated every time you read the newspaper. The other day, your friend, Mary Lou, attended a local discussion group where the speaker talked about teenage pregnancy. Her main thesis was that "just saying 'No' " is an effective method for avoiding an unwanted pregnancy.

Mary Lou can hardly contain her laughter as she tells you about the meeting. "Just saying 'No' " is the dumbest thing I've ever heard of! How can you expect to combat such a national epidemic with such a simplistic approach?"

How are you going to respond to Mary Lou?

Programs for Pregnant Teenagers and Adolescent Parents

Title XX of the Public Health Service Act of 1981 authorized Adolescent Family Life Demonstration Projects. This legislation provided for services such as pregnancy testing; maternity counseling and referral; family planning; primary and preventative health services, including pre- and postnatal care, nutritional information, counseling, and referral; education in sexuality and family life; child care consumer education; and transportation and counseling for the extended family. Such comprehensive programs, however, face four serious obstacles to their implementation: inadequate financial support; an insufficient health and social welfare infrastructure; negative public and political attitudes; and unproven intervention technology, for example, programs make claims about services that they are not able to keep or provide (Weatherley, Perlman, Levine, & Klerman, 1986).

The Parent-child Education Center

It is currently a common practice for many high schools to have nurseries for the children of teenage parents. Whereas once teenage mothers quit school in shame and were banned to a world of isolation, now programs like these school nurseries are designed to keep teenage mothers from dropping out. They also serve several other functions as well. They provide opportunities for other students to learn parenting skills.

One such program is the Parent-child Education Center at Weaver High School, a large urban high school in Hartford, Connecticut (Cobb, 1985). Located in the home economics department, the multipurpose room provides space where infants sleep and play, and where they are fed and changed. It is also the site of the parenting classes.

How The Parent-child Center Works   The Parent-child Education Center provides parent training to Weaver High School students (Cobb,

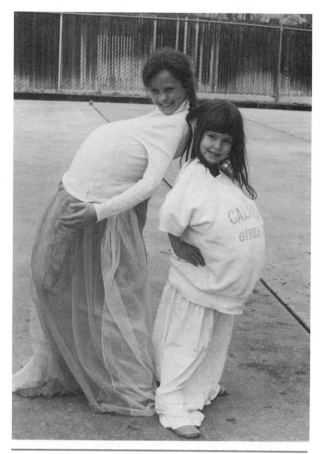

FIGURE 12-18   While these two are only kidding, teenage pregnancy is no joking matter! Many teenage parents are still children themselves and do not have the skills necessary to adequately parent their new children. Many high-school based programs provide both academic and parenting education for young teenage mothers.

1988). A course called "Parenting" is offered by the Home Economics Department and provides parenting education and hands-on experiences working with infants. The course is offered on both the academic and general levels, and includes units in self-awareness, reproductive health issues, pregnancy and delivery, developmental tasks and skills, infant and child health care and safety, and behavior and discipline. Students who enroll their infants at the Center must take the course. For all other students at Weaver High, the course is an elective.

Student parents who wish to continue their education are eligible to enroll their children on a space-available basis, with preference given to juniors and graduating seniors. Infants must be at least one month old and may stay until about one year of age. Parents must agree to follow the rules of the Center. There is no charge for infant care and the parents are aware that other students will be caring for their children during the day. The Center is staffed by the director, a paraprofessional, and a foster grandparent, who are responsible for the care of between six and ten infants during the course of a year. Transportation is provided in the winter months for the student/parents and their infants.

Salaries for the teacher/director and the paraprofessional are partially reimbursed by the Day Care Division of the State Department of Human Resources.

The Parent-child Education Center helps teen parents in the following ways:

- Gives support to the teen parent by acting as a mentor/tutor in her studies.
- Brings the teen back into the social setting where she can interact with her peers.
- Lowers the chances of child abuse by monitoring the teen and baby.
- Enhances the teen's self-image by giving her confidence as a care-giver.
- Encourages the teen parent to use positive efforts to discipline her child.

The parenting course helps all students, teenage parents and nonteenage parents, by:

- Teaching them to have reasonable expectations of a child's accomplishments through the study of developmental tasks and skills.
- Exposing them to the effects of sexually transmitted diseases on themselves, their partners and others, especially fetuses.
- Demonstrating recognition of a sick and a well child; learning protocol used in examining a child; and mastering the reading of a thermometer.
- Helping them discover the positive and negative sides of reproductive health issues and demonstrating knowledge of these issues through role playing.
- Teaching them to assess their homes to assure a safe environment for their children.

Teen parents are supportive and enthusiastic about the Parent-child Center. As one teen mother expresses her feelings, "I have no money to pay for a baby-sitter. Without this program, I would have to drop out of school."

Project PARENTING

Project PARENTING (*Proactive Assessment and Regulation of Environmental Nurturing and Teaching Interventions for Normal Growth*) in the Pitt County School System of North Carolina is based on the premise that, even under the best of conditions, parenting is a stressful job and that supportive interventions are necessary for teenage mothers and their children (Taylor, 1988).

The goals of Project PARENTING Center are to:

- Decrease the rate of abuse and neglect among adolescent mothers and their children.
- Help adolescent parents improve their child-rearing skills.
- Increase adolescent mothers' knowledge of child development.
- Assist adolescent mothers in meeting the health care needs of their children.
- Build the self-esteem of adolescent mothers.
- Help adolescent mothers plan for the future.

Project PARENTING activities for the teenage mothers include:

- Assessment of each teenage mother with the Nursing Child Assessment Satellite Training (NCAST) scales in order to assess the home environment and parent-child interaction.

- Visitation to each home by a project social worker.
- Use of a toy, book, and materials lending library.
- Participation in group and individual meetings to offer support, information, and encouragement.
- Interaction with mentors/role models through an Adopt-a-Mom program. Mentors are education students at East Carolina University.

In addition, Project PARENTING has initiated a teenage pregnancy prevention program designed to provide recognition and reinforcement to teenagers who are at risk for becoming pregnant. A major goal of this preventative program is to improve the self-esteem of at-risk teenagers. Emphasis is placed on the responsibilities of being a parent and how being a parent affects future plans. In addition, delaying pregnancy is stressed.

A common component of these and other programs is child development knowledge and information. While such programs attempt to increase teenagers' knowledge of child development,

there may not be any changes in maternal attitudes toward their children. Thus, teenagers may learn the importance of being warm and loving and providing a caring environment, but their attitudes toward their children may keep them from putting their new-found information into action. So programs that attempt to help teenagers be better parents should focus on helping them accept their responsibility for their children (Roosa, 1984).

Also, one of the goals of Project PARENTING is to enhance and build the teenage parents' self-esteem. This is an important area that needs to be targeted by all such programs, since adolescent unwed mothers as a group project poor self-esteem and feelings of inadequacy and unworthiness, and are more dissatisfied with their family relationships and feel that what happens to them can generally be attributed to fate. Given these attributes teenage unwed mothers exhibit, programs designed to help them should include parenting skills, job-entry skills, the enhancement of social competence, and the development of effective interpersonal relationships (Thompson, 1984).

*I*N THE SPOTLIGHT

TAPP (TEENAGE PARENTING PROGRAM)

Emerson Teenage Parent Program, Jefferson County Public Schools, Louisville, Kentucky This school-based program is comprehensive in nature and is designed to meet the needs of pregnant and parenting adolescents and their families. Its primary objective is to provide an academic program with in-house medical and social service supports to reduce pregnancy-related school dropouts and ensure uninterrupted academic progression during pregnancy. Students are referred to TAPP by school counselors, social service

agencies, medical clinics, doctors, churches, and individual inquiry.

Program components include:

- Academic component—The academic program consists of a regular middle and high school program of studies and services. Each student's academic program is individually scheduled and planned. The instructional program includes: English, mathematics, science, social studies, home economics, business education, art, foreign language, and special education.

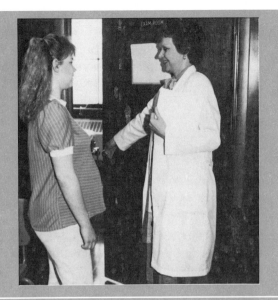

FIGURE 12-19 The Louisville, Kentucky Teenage Pregnancy Program is a nationally recognized agency which provides a wide range of services to teenage mothers, fathers and their children and families.

- Medical/Health component—This component provides complete prenatal and post-partum care and family planning services. The school-based clinic collaborates with the University of Louisville School of Medicine to provide year-round obstetrical services. Three registered nurses are available to assist and monitor students on a daily basis.
- A mid-morning breakfast and a lunch program is provided to meet the increased nutritional needs of the pregnant teen.
- A Women, Infants and Children (WIC) clinic is housed in the school building. WIC is a Federal program that provides food to pregnant women, nursing mothers, infants, and children.
- Social services component—This component provides individual and group counseling, instruction in parenting and baby care skills, and makes referrals to social services.

- Co-op infant care—The infant care program provides quality infant care services for infants between the ages of ten days and eighteen months. Open between 7:00 AM and 3:00 PM, the co-op training center provides experience in early childhood education and job training.
- Fatherhood component—This component provides young fathers with prenatal classes, instruction in parenting and family planning, and individual and group counseling. A simulated apartment, complete with a nursery, provides the instructional setting for couples to learn parenting skills.
- Grandparents component—This component provides evening group sessions for the parents/guardians of the teen mother and/or teen father.
- Extended family component—This component provides outreach workers to make home visits to help family members:

1. Develop open communication with and support one another;
2. Become part of a support network of other families facing similar issues;
3. Become knowledgeable about community resources and learn how to use them;
4. Increase family awareness of issues related to sexual responsibility so as to prevent unwanted pregnancies among female relatives;
5. Increase the family's potential economic self-sufficiency.

TAPP won the 1986 Meritorious Service Award presented by the National Organization on Adolescent Pregnancy and Parenting (NOAPP).

[*Special thanks to Georgia Chaffee, Principal, and the staff and students of TAPP for providing the author with information and material during an on-site visit.*]

Teenage Pregnancy and Public Policy

When all things are said and done, the fact remains that parents and professionals must develop programs for teenage parents that are designed to deal with the long-term policy implications involved. The following are some general public policy implications derived from research conducted by the Child Welfare League of America on childbearing and childrearing by young adolescent mothers twelve to fifteen years of age (Miller, 1983):

- Age-specific differences within adolescence must be understood and respected, and the different consequences of unplanned pregnancies or births for various age groups, such as the younger teenager's greater chance of bearing premature and low-birth-weight babies and greater likelihood of increased dependence on her family, must be considered on policy development and service delivery.
- To have a long-term impact on the lives of pregnant adolescents, young mothers, and their children, services must continue for a longer time after delivery, preferably at least until the children enter school.
- Programs for pregnant teenagers and young mothers should focus their limited resources on clearly defined, agreed-upon goals, such as high school completion, adequate medical care and nutrition, stable child care and living arrangements, and so forth. All programmatic objectives should be aimed at meeting these goals. Only by a systematic approach to service delivery will unproductive service efforts be eliminated and progress toward the identified goals be achieved most efficiently and effectively.
- The pregnant teenager's or young mother's extended family (often including the baby's father) is her first source of support and must be recognized and respected. Social service providers' efforts should be directed toward enhancing what the family already provides

or offering what the family cannot, instead of duplicating assistance that is already available. The positive behaviors and strengths of teenage parents have to be acknowledged and built upon. Few people are giving these young mothers positive reinforcement, encouragement, and praise for handling a variety of demands and responsibilities fairly well.

HOMOSEXUALITY
Sexual Identity

When you think of sexual identity, what comes to your mind? For some, clothing and hair styles may be the key. For others, body build and sexual preference may be the answer. For Richard Green (1987), there are three components of sexual identity:

1. Anatomic identity—a person's identity as either male or female.
2. Gender-role behavior—sex-typed behavior, or masculinity and femininity.
3. Sexual orientation—sexual partner preference, or sexual object choice (p. 6).

Sexual identity begins early. At one year, infants can discriminate between male and female age-mates; at one year, males look longer at male faces and females look longer at female faces. This "like-me/not-like-me" orientation may be innate and is the first component of sexual identity (Green, 1987, pp. 28–29).

Childhood Sexual Behaviors and Homosexuality

Sexual orientation early in life can influence later sexual identification and behavior. While true for both sexes, it is especially true for males. Boyhood cross-gender behaviors can be significantly associated with adolescent and adult homosexuality (Green, 1982). Cross-gender behaviors that for males indicate an opposite sex orientation include cross-dressing; engaging in mannerisms considered "feminine," such as playing with dolls; not engaging in rough-and-tumble activities; playing almost exclusively with girls; and assuming the female role in make-believe play.

But how do boys become homosexual? There are a number of plausible explanations. Two that make sense are those formulated by researcher Green (1987, pp. 379–381). The first is a developmental track that leads from "feminine" boy to homosexual adolescent and adult. It includes innate contributions of the child, psychological features of the parents, and sociological patterns of the environment. Let's look at each of these developmental influences. First, the level of prenatal androgen influences later postnatal behavior, such as timidity, aggression, participation in rough-and-tumble play and interest in newborns (and by extension, baby dolls). Second, parents are not neutral in their relationships with their children. For example, parents who wanted a girl instead of a boy may contribute to an impression that the boy may possess feminine traits. Another example. Fathers are usually the enforcers of sex-role behaviors. Father absence—either absolute or relative—during the initiation of a boy's cross-gender behavior may result in a lack of direction toward traditional sex-role behavior. Third, when the child enters a school setting, it may be difficult for him to move off the "feminine" developmental track because he lacks masculine skills. He is labeled a "sissy" and is further isolated from males.

What parents need to understand is that children are different. There is not one "cause" to explain why children grow up to be homosexual. Parents do exercise control over their children's development and, to this extent, they are contributory agents to their children's behavior. However, it is unlikely that parents can point to one thing they did and say that it "caused" their children to be homosexual. What is of most importance is that parents provide a loving, stable, and accepting environment in which their children can grow and develop in accordance within their biological and developmental contexts.

Homosexuality and AIDS

The current AIDS epidemic poses a particular threat to gay teenagers, whose incidence of homosexuality is about the same as in the general population, one in ten. Gay teenagers also share with their heterosexual contemporaries the same sense of immortality and invincibility. Furthermore, their teenage impulsiveness frequently involves them in life-threatening affairs. The teenagers' sense of immortality and tendency to have all the answers also make it difficult to provide AIDS information and counseling.

Nationally, about 8,000 teenagers, mostly males, have AIDS. This number is rising and even more alarmingly, the age of AIDS victims is dropping.

SUMMARY

■ Adolescence is a period of profound physical, emotional, and social development. The adolescent years have important social and cultural significance in the lives of youth and their families.

■ During puberty, individuals reach sexual maturity, and procreation is possible. The beginning of puberty varies for both males and females as a group and also for individuals within each group. Many physical changes occur during puberty, including the "growth spurt" and the development of secondary sexual characteristics. Many of these changes are due to hormonal influences. Puberty influences how adolescents see themselves and others. The adolescent period of development is not now thought to be the tempestuous period of development it was once thought to be.

■ Suicide is in the national spotlight and there is much public concern about the numbers of teenagers who commit suicide. Depression is a common symptom of teenagers who have suicidal thoughts and who commit suicide. There is a gender difference in suicide rate, with more girls than boys committing suicide. Many school-based programs such as Project Trust conducted by Carmen Espinosa are designed to help teenagers cope with the problems of adolescence.

■ Acne is something most teenagers dread. It is caused by overly active sebaceous glands that clog pores with sebum, an oily substance. Acne can be caused by substances that clog the pores or medications or drugs that trigger hormone production.

■ There are several reasons for the inevitable conflicts that occur between parents and youth in the adolescent years. First, the beginning of puberty is beginning earlier and second, youth are dependent on their parents for longer periods of time. Today, most researchers agree that puberty, by itself, does not have the overwhelmingly negative impact on parent-youth relationships once previously thought.

■ Anorexia nervosa (AN) is a syndrome in which an individual has an aversion to food and literally starves himself. There are many explanations of AN, and the origin and course of AN is different in different people.

■ Adolescent peer groups are formed by teenagers themselves to fulfill the needs of the members. However, parents and teachers reinforce group attributes and membership.

■ Three-quarters of all high school seniors work. However, not everyone agrees that such work is good for adolescent psychological development. Nonetheless, youthwork is a reality and will likely continue.

■ Runaway youth are a serious national concern and a number of national agencies are devoted to helping runaway children, children contemplating running away, and parents of runaways.

■ Juvenile delinquency is an important national concern. The Juvenile Justice and Delinquency Prevention Act is designed to provide federal resources to address issues related to juvenile delinquency and runaway and homeless youth.

■ Teenage pregnancy is viewed as a serious social problem and schools, and federal, state, and local agencies have developed many programs to address the problem. The focus on teenage pregnancy results from the increase in the number of unwed teenagers giving birth and the severing of the link between pregnancy and marriage.

Teenage pregnancy has many negative consequences for teenagers and their children.

■ Some teenagers may have a baby because they feel trapped; for others it is a rite of passage; and for others, ignorance of contraception results in pregnancy. Teenagers in general have a longer period of time in which to become pregnant.

■ Teenage pregnancy and parenting has a number of serious consequences for both mothers and children. A primary one is lack of maternal education attainment, which influences children's educational achievement.

■ Many programs exist to help teenagers prevent becoming pregnant and to provide them and their families with comprehensive services following the birth of a child.

■ Sexual identity consists of three parts: anatomical, gender, and sexual. Homosexuality in males may occur through a developmental track or through being subjected to a number of variables that are associated with homosexual development. AIDS is a particular health risk for homosexual teenagers.

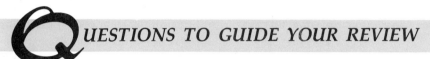

QUESTIONS TO GUIDE YOUR REVIEW

1. Why is it possible to have an adolescent period of development?
2. What important developmental changes occur during the adolescent period?
3. What role do hormones play in adolescent development?
4. What significant physical changes occur during the adolescent years?
5. What is the "growth spurt" and what causes it?
6. What are the secondary female and male sex characteristics that develop during the adolescent years?
7. What effects does puberty have on adolescent self-image?
8. What are the root causes of adolescent suicide?
9. How does acne occur and what can be done to prevent it?
10. How do the adolescent years influence and affect parent-youth relationships?
11. What is anorexia nervosa and what causes it?
12. Are there any cures for anorexia nervosa? What are they?
13. How would you describe someone with anorexia nervosa?
14. How does bulimia differ from anorexia nervosa?
15. In what ways do peers and peer groups influence adolescent behavior?
16. What are the major issues surrounding the question of whether or not working is good for teenagers?
17. What major agencies are involved in preventing and dealing with the problem of teenage runaways? What services do they provide?
18. What are the key features and services of programs that are designed to address problems, such as substance abuse, facing today's teenagers?
19. Why is there so much current interest in teenage pregnancy?
20. How does teenage pregnancy affect both mother and child?
21. What are the social and developmental causes of teenage pregnancy?
22. What are the basic features of programs designed to help prevent teenage pregnancy?
23. What are programs doing to help pregnant teenagers, young mothers, their children, and their families?
24. Can you explain how a child grows to be homosexual rather than heterosexual?

ACTIVITIES FOR FURTHER INVOLVEMENT

1. Experts in adolescent development generally agree that adolescent development today is different from what you, your parents and your grandparents experienced.
   a. Interview people regarding their experiences and remembrances of adolescence. How do these recollections differ from adolescent experiences and behavior today?
   b. How is the adolescent period of development in other cultures similar to and different from adolescent development in the United States?
   c. What are the major biological, social and cultural factors that account for changes in behavior during the adolescent years?
2. Transitions are very important in all children's lives, but they assume significant importance during the adolescent years.
   a. What transitions play a particularly important role in teenagers' lives? How and why are they important? In what ways do transitions influence adolescent development?
   b. Interview teenagers to determine what activities, information and understandings would be most helpful to them in making the transition from adolescence to adulthood.
3. Visit school-based and agency sponsored programs designed to provide counseling and other services to teenagers, their parents and families.
   a. How successful are these programs at meeting their stated purposes?
   b. What do teenagers like best about such programs? What suggestions do they have for improvement?
4. The opening lines of *Turning Points: Preparing American Youth for the 21st Century*, the report on the Carnegie Council's Task Force on Education Of Young Adolescents, state: "Young adolescents face significant turning points. For many youth 10 to 15 years old, early adolescence offers opportunities to choose a path toward a productive and fulfilling life. For many others, it represents their last best chance to avoid a diminished future." (P.8).
   a. What are the significant turning points in teenagers' lives? How do these turning points differ for different youth according to their culture and socio-economic status?
   b. How do turning points in adolescents' lives lead to diminished futures?
5. The consequences of teenage pregnancy are significant for mothers, fathers, families and children.
   a. In what ways are people's lives changes by teenage pregnancy?
   b. Developmentally, how are children of teenage parents at risk? What can be done to reduce developmental risk for these children?

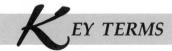

KEY TERMS

Adolescence The *transitional* period from youth to adulthood; represents a major transition period in the course of human development.

Androgens Hormones that stimulate male characteristics.

Anorexia nervosa Severe loss of appetite. Used to describe a constellation of symptoms associated with extreme fasting and weight loss, primarily in teenage women.

Bulimia A condition in which periodically an individual alternately fasts and binges on food.

Bulimarexia A combination of anorexia and bulimia, characterized by extreme dieting and purging.

Estrogen A female sex hormone.

Menarche The beginning of menstruation.

Postpubescence The two-year period following puberty when growth is completed and reproductive functions are fully established.

Progesterone A female sex hormone.

Pubescence The two-year period that pre-cedes puberty and is the time during which profound physical changes of height, weight, and physiological functioning occur.

Puberty The time when an individual reaches sexual maturity and fertility. Both sexes are capable of procreation.

Sebum An oily substance produced by sebaceous glands.

Steroids Taken as a collective whole, all of the hormones produced by the gonads and adrenal cortex of both sexes.

Tanner stages The stages of growth in secondary sex characteristics.

Testosterone A male sex hormone.

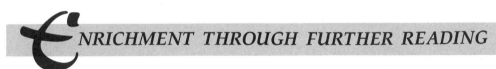

ENRICHMENT THROUGH FURTHER READING

Engel, Joel. (1989). *Addicted: Kids talking about drugs in their own words.* New York: A Tom Doherty Associates Book/Tor.

Engel chronicles the experiences of ten youths who started with alcohol and marijuana and ended up addicted to drugs. These interviews provide an interesting insight into early backgrounds and experiences of drug-using teenagers.

Foster, S. (1981). *The one girl in ten: A self portrait of the teen-age mother.* Claremont, CA: Arbor.

This is a book about being pregnant and being a teenage mother, as told by women who had a child while they were of school age. Covers material relating to first sexual experiences, the crisis produced by the pregnancy, and life after childbirth.

Humphreys, J. (1988). *Rich in love.* New York: Viking.

A bright and vigorous story of Lucille Odom, the adolescent heroine who demonstrates charm, intelligence, and a humorous insight into life and the process of growing up.

Kett, J. (1977). *Rites of passage.* New York: Basic Books.

This book is informative because of the historical insights it provides into adolescence in America from 1790 to 1977. The reader will find it interesting to contrast what we presently know about adolescence and our changing view of adolescence to previous notions about adolescence.

Powell, D. H. (1986). *Teenagers: When to worry and what to do.* Garden City, NY: Doubleday.

Deals with specific concerns of the teenage years, such as sexuality, alcohol, moodiness, eating habits, and identity. Provides parents with specific advice about how to help their teenagers and themselves.

Williams, Terry. (1989). *Cocaine kids: The inside story of a teenage drug ring*. Reading, MA: Addison-Wesley Publishing Company.

> Sociologist Terry Williams spent five years conducting ethnographic research with teenage drug dealers in Spanish Harlem. The result is a fascinating description of youth at work and play in the underground economy of drugs.

 NSWER TO "WHAT WOULD YOU DO?"

Well, as you know by now, not too many things in life are as simple as they first appear. Although at first glance, "just saying 'No!'" may seem too simplistic an approach to preventing teenage pregnancy, the commitment behind saying "No!" is what makes it possible for a teenager—or any other woman for that matter—to avoid becoming pregnant. When girls have the right support and encouragement, they can avoid teenage pregnancy regardless of their circumstances. The major factors that affect risk are (Blake, 1988):

- Parenting—Among blacks, close parental supervision reduces the number of unwed mothers. Among whites, a high-quality relationship with parents lowers girls' chances of pregnancy.
- Religious commitment—Religious commitment, especially among Hispanics, is an important factor in avoiding pregnancy.
- Willingness—Girls who think it is unacceptable to have a baby out of wedlock usually avoid it. This "mind over risk" is very important for black teenagers. For white teenagers, the attitudes of their classmates strongly affect their willingness to become pregnant.
- Problem behavior—Girls who have acted up in other ways are more likely to become pregnant.
- Opportunity costs—Girls who plan to continue their education are less likely to have babies before they marry. Black girls, especially those who plan on college, understand what they stand to lose with a pregnancy.

So, in response to your friend Mary Lou's laughter, you can share this information with her. Saying "No!" is an effective way of preventing pregnancy, especially when the response is based on and grows out of other life and behavioral factors.

Furthermore, there are programs that are specifically designed to promote teen abstinence, which is the ultimate "No!" Such programs usually emphasize six approaches to abstinence. They are (Peterson, 1989):

- Health concerns—Two of the most forceful arguments against having early sex are the danger of catching AIDS or a venereal disease and the danger of pregnancy "ruining one's life." So these and other health risks involved are often included in the curriculum emphasizing abstinence. (Keep in mind not only the health risk to the young teenager but also to her child.)
- Values education. Rather than be "value free" in their teaching, staff are encouraged to support such values as respect for oneself and others, honesty in relationships, and the destructiveness of sexual coercion.

- Decision making—Helping adolescents develop decision-making skills gives them the power to see situations in a new light. Also, teens need to learn that there is a link between current decisions and their future plans for family, jobs, and life goals.
- Refusal skills—Teaching girls *and* boys skills associated with saying "No!" as well as how to say "No!" is critical in any program of abstinence.
- Helping parents—Programs frequently include activities to increase parent involvement and promote parent-child communication. Such activities help win parent support for sexuality education and provide a means and opportunity for parents to share their values with their children.
- Comprehensive sexuality education—Teenagers need to have accurate and up-to-date information, and have opportunities to discuss their feelings and beliefs about sexuality. Such information also assists in good decision making.

ℬIBLIOGRAPHY

Akers, R. L., Khron, M. D., Lanze-Kaduce, L., & Rasosevich, M. (1979). Social learning and deviant behavior: A specific test of a general theory. *American Sociological Review*, 44, 636–655.

Anderman, E. (1988). Correspondence of Ellen Anderman to Mary Gittings, Program Director, The Piton Foundation; sent by Diane Medena of La Mariposa to the author.

Bachman, J. G. (1987). An eye on the future. *Psychology Today*, 21, 6–8.

Belsky, J. & Draper, P. (1987). Reproductive strategies and radical solutions. *Society*, 24, 23–24.

Bettes, B. A., & Walker, E. (1986). Symptoms associated with suicidal behavior in childhood and adolescence. *Journal of Abnormal Child Psychology*, 14 591–604.

Blake, L. M. (1988). Babies: Just say no. *Psychology Today*, 22, 16.

Block, J. Block, J. H., & Keyes, S. (1988). Longitudinally foretelling drug usage in adolescence: Early childhood personality and environmental precursors. *Child Development*, 59, 336–355.

Brody, J. E. (1988, May 26). The reality of adult acne, and the arsenel of weapons available for its treatment. *The New York Times*, p. 20.

Brody, J. E. (1987, February 17). Dozens of factors critical in bone loss among elderly. *The New York Times*, p. 17.

Buie, J. (1987). Teen pregnancy: It's time for the schools to tackle the problem. *Phi Delta Kappan*, 68, 738.

Caffary, R. A. (1987). Anorexia and bulimia—the maladjusting coping strategies of the 80s. *Psychology of the Schools*, 24, 45–48.

Cobb, P. C. (1988) Personal correspondence with the author. Patricia Cobb provided the information and description of the Parent-child Education Center.

Cobb, P. C. (1985, November-December). How infants in high school keep their parents in school. *Illinois Teacher*, pp. 50–53.

Coll, C. G., Hoffman, J., & Oh, W. (1986). Maternal and environmental factors affecting developmental outcomes of infants of adolescent mothers. *Developmental and Behavioral Pediatrics*, 7, 230–236.

Coll, C. G., Hoffman, J., Oh, W., and Vohr, B. R. (1987). The social ecology and early parenting of Caucasian adolescent mothers. *Child Development*, 58, 955–963.

Crockenberg, S. (1987). Predictions and correlates of anger toward and punitive control of toddlers by adolescent mothers. *Child Development, 58,* 964–975.

Delgado-Gaitan, C. (1986). Adolescent peer influence and differential school performance. *Journal of Adolescent Research, 1,* 449–462.

Flaste, R. (1988, October 9). The myth about teen-agers. *The New York Times Magazine,* p. 76.

Frustenberg, F., Brooks-Gunn, J., & Morgan, S. P. (1987). *Adolescent mothers in later life.* Cambridge, England: Cambridge University Press.

Garrison, E. G. (1987). The juvenile justice and delinquency prevention act. *Social Policy Report, 11,* 4.

Gelles, R. J. School-age parents and child abuse. In J. B. Lancaster, & B. A. Hamburg (Eds.), *School-age pregnancy and parenthood: Biosocial dimensions* (pp. 347–359) New York: Aldine De Gruyter.

Green, R. (1987). *The sissy boy sydrome and the development of homosexuality.* New Haven: Yale University Press.

Green, R. (1982). Relationship between "feminine" and "masculine" behavior during boyhood and sexual orientation during manhood. In *Sexology—Sexual Biology, Behavior and Therapy: Selected Papers of the 5th World Congress of Sexology.* Jerusalem, Israel, June 21–26, 1981.

Greenberger, E. & Steinberg, L. (1986). *When teenagers work.* New York: Basic Books.

Group for the Advancement of Psychiatry. (1986). *Crisis of adolescence: Teenage pregnancy, impact on adolescent development.* New York: Brunner/Mazel.

Havens, B., & Swenson, I. (1986). Menstrual perceptions and preparation among female adolescents. *Journal of Obstetric, Gynecologic and Neonatal Nursing, 15,* 406–411.

Hofferth, S., Kahn, J. R., & Baldwin, W. (1987). Premarital sexual activity among U.S. teenage women over the past three decades. *Family Planning Perspectives, 19,* 46–53.

Hollinger, P. C., Offer, D., & Zola, M. A. (1988). A prediction model of suicide among youth. *The Journal of Nervous and Mental Disease, 170,* 277.

Jessor, R., & Jessor, S. L. (1978). *Problem behavior and psychological development: A longitudinal study of youth.* New York: Academic Press.

Joselow, F. (1989, March 26). Why business turns to teen-agers. *The New York Times,* Section 3, pp. 3, 6.

Juvenile Justice and Delinquency Prevention Act of 1974 (Public Law 93-415 as amended through September 30, 1985) 42 U.S.C. §5601 (1985).

Kandal, D. B., Kessler, R. C., & Margulies, R. Z. (1978). Antecedents of adolescent initiation in stages of drug use: A developmental analysis. In D. B. Kandel (Ed.), *Longitudinal research in drug use* (pp. 73–99). New York: John Wiley.

Kaplan, H. B., Martin, S. S., & Robbins, C. (1982). Application of a general theory of deviant behavior: Self-derogation and adolescent drug use. *Journal of Health and Social Behavior, 23,* 274–294.

Katchadourian, H. (1977). *The biology of adolescence.* San Francisco: W. H. Freeman.

Kinard, E. M., & Reinherz, H. (1987). School aptitude and achievement in children of adolescent mothers. *Journal of Youth and Adolescence, 16,* 69–87.

Landry, E., Bertrand, J. T., Cherry, F., & Rice, J. (1986). Teen pregnancy in New Orleans: Factors that differentiate teens who deliver, abort and successfully contracept. *Journal of Youth and Adolescence, 15,* 259–274.

Leary, W. E. (1989, February 23). Young women are getting fatter, study finds. *The New York Times*, p. 20.

Miller, S. H. (1983). *Children as parents: Final report on a study of childbearing and child rearing among 12-to-15-year-olds*. New York: Child Welfare League of America, p. 111.

Mott, F., & Marsiglio, W. (1985). Early childbearing and completion of high school. *Family Planning Perspectives, 17*, 234–237.

Murray, J. B. (1986). Psychological aspects of anorexia nervosa. *Genetic, Social, and General Psychology Monographs, 112*, 5–40.

Newcomer, S. F., & Udry, R. J. (1985). Parent-child communication and adolescent sexual behavior. *Family Planning Perspectives, 17*, 169–174.

Offer, D. (1987). In defense of adolescents. *Journal of the American Medical Association, 257*, 3047–3408.

Petersen, A. C. (1987). Those gangly years. *Psychology Today, 21*, 28–34.

Phillips, D. P., & Paight, D. J. (1987). The impact of televised movies about suicide. *The New England Journal of Medicine, 317*, 809–11.

Quinn, J. (1986). Rooted in research: Effective Adolescent pregnancy prevention programs. *Adolescent Sexualities*. Falls Church, VA: Haworth.

Ramsey, B. (1988) Kids who drink: Nursing the bottle? *Family Album*. Miami: Charter Hospital.

Read, E. W. (1988, February 2). Birth cycle. *The Wall Street Journal*, p. 1.

Roosa, M. W. (1984) Short-term effects of teenage parenting programs on knowledge and attitudes. *Adolescence, XIX*, 659–666.

Rumors of suicides cancel graduation. (1988, June 6). *The Miami Herald*, p. 2A.

Seniors' reported drug use lowest in years, poll finds. (1989, March 8.). *Education Week*. p. 17.

Simmons, R. G., Blyth, D. A. (1987). *Moving into adolescence: The impact of pubertal change and school context*. New York: Aldine De Gruyter.

Steinberg, L. (1987). Bound to bicker. *Psychology Today, 21*, (9) 36–39.

Szmukler, G. I. (1987). Anorexia nervosa: A clinical view. In R. A. Boakes, D. A. Popplewell, & M. J. Burton (Eds.), *Eating habits: Food, psychology and learned behavior* (pp. 25–44). Chichester, England: John Wiley.

Taylor, B. H. (1988). Project PARENTING: An education program for adolescent mothers and their children. *Elementary School Guidance and Counseling, 22*, 320–324.

Thompson, R. A. (1984, May). The critical needs of the adolescent unwed mother. *The School Counselor*, pp. 460–466.

Tolan, P. H. (1987). Implications of age of onset for delinquency risk. *Journal of Abnormal Child Psychology, 15*, 47–65.

U.S. Bureau of the Census. (1988, March). *Current population report, July 1, 1987. (Series P-25, No. 1022, Table 1). Washington, D.C.: U.S. Government Printing Office.*

Weatherly, R. A., Perlman, S. B., Levine, M. H., & Klerman, L. V. (1986). Comprehensive programs for pregnant teenagers and teenage parents: How successful have they been? *Family Planning Perspectives, 18*, 73–78.

Williams, L. (1989, February 27). Teen-age sex: New codes amid the old anxiety. *The New York Times*, pp. 1, 12.

Zaslowsky, D. (1989, January 19). Denver program curbs teen-agers' pregnancy. *The New York Times*, p. 8.

CHAPTER THIRTEEN

Learning and education in the adolescent years

◆

VIGNETTES
INTRODUCTION: ADOLESCENT
  DEVELOPMENT IN
  PERSPECTIVE
SCHOOLING AND
  TRANSITIONS
Arenas of Comfort
EDUCATIONAL AND SOCIAL
  POLICY IMPLICATIONS
ESSENTIAL FEATURES OF
  MIDDLE SCHOOLS
In the Spotlight: Loggers' Run
  Middle School
HIGH SCHOOLS
High School Counseling Services
In the Spotlight: Students Helping
  Students
DROPPING OUT
REMEMBERING YOU
In the Spotlight: Reconsidering
  Adolescent Development

What Would You Do?
CHARACTER EDUCATION IN
  THE HIGH SCHOOLS
PARENTING THE TEENAGER
Too Independent Too Soon
"I Didn't Do It!"—Teenagers and
  Lying
In the Spotlight: The Shopping
  Mall as Surrogate Family
PREVENTION PROGRAMS
Implications
SUMMARY
QUESTIONS TO GUIDE YOUR
  REVIEW
ACTIVITIES FOR FURTHER
  INVOLVEMENT
KEY TERMS
ENRICHMENT THROUGH
  FURTHER READING
Answer to "What Would You Do?"
Bibliography

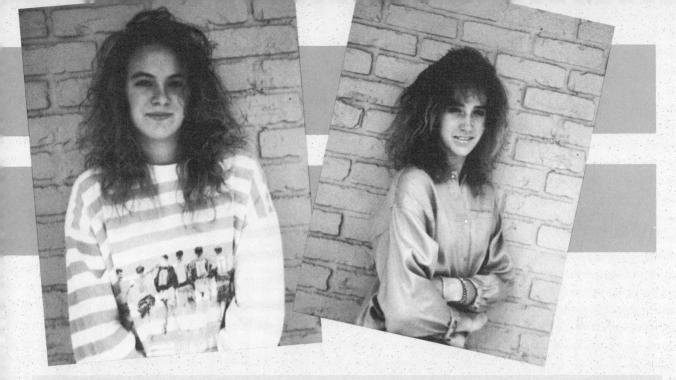

Vignettes

My Typical Day, by Brandy June "Every morning, I get up at 6:30 sharp to get in the shower. Now, I don't have to be at the bus stop until 8:15, but I need a lot of time to get ready. As a newly initiated teenager, I have to look perfect before I walk out of the door. If I'm not satisfied, I miss the bus and keep working to look good, and then my parents drive me to school. If I do catch the bus, as I usually do, I have an adventure riding it. Five miles to school, kids are screaming, the bus driver is yelling—real fun! The bus is a social definer, the cool kids sit in the back, and the nerds sit in the front. Everyone starts out in the front, and gradually they move back. As an eighth grader, I have the back seat of the bus— the coolest possible. It all seems stupid to adults, but to us, it's very important! I've worked for three years to be in the back!"

"We finally get to school, and the miniature 'soap opera' begins. There's always a new crisis, every morning. A boyfriend and a girlfriend have broken up, a dog has died, a detention . . . there's so many things that we consider horrible. Occasionally, a good thing happens. Then everybody is happy, and smiling. I am very close to all of my friends, and they are what the school day orbits around, except when I am learning. We all go to our classes together, write notes to each other, and go to lunch together. After six classes, I am usually pretty tired. I take the wonderful bus home, and get started on my homework."

"At least three of the five days of the week I have meetings to attend after school. I am on newspaper and Honor Society. I am also the Student Council President; all of these things keep me busy, plus I usually do homework until 10:30 or 11:00 at night. I do other activities, like acting, singing lessons, and guitar lessons, which also take up my free time. By 11:30 I've turned in for the night. I always lay awake for an hour or so— thinking about school, my social life, guys, life in general, and of course, what I am going to wear to school the next day.

"I love my life, and wouldn't want to be somebody else right now, as a lot of people are trying to. I am happy to be me, because I am an interesting person. I've made myself that way. I have a lot of high goals for myself, and I know

I'll achieve them. I've promised myself that I will be famous one day. But for now, I am having a hard enough time dealing with the pressure. I don't want to grow up, just yet!"

A Typical Day for José Avillo One year ago, fourteen-year-old Jose Avillo lived with his grandmother and sister in a small village outside the Nicaraguan town of Boaco. Jose was constantly in fear of being drafted into the military. One day he was wounded in the leg during a skirmish for his village between the Sandanista and Contra forces. Jose and his family decided it was time for him to come to the United States. Alone, he traveled through Nicaragua, Honduras, Guatemala and then Mexico. Jose carried bricks for a construction company in Mexico to get enough money to pay the border smugglers. Once in the United States at Brownsville, Texas, Jose boarded a bus and headed for Miami to join the thousands of other Nicaraguan refugees.

Today, Jose is in the ninth grade at Seaside Middle School. He is enrolled with twenty other children in a bilingual class designed to help them speak English. Jose is not having too much success with his English, however. It takes about two years for a student to become proficient in English and Jose is very impatient. Jose's classmates sometimes make fun of his attempts at English, so he avoids it as much as possible and prefers to talk in Spanish to his friends.

Jose's teacher is not optimistic for his success in school, saying that, "Jose may mean well, but he doesn't pay attention in class or to schoolwork. He needs more attention than I can give him. He really needs individual attention and I can't do that with all the kids I have to teach."

Jose wants to quit school and work at a fast-food restaurant in order to help bring his grandmother and sister to the United States. Many refugee adolescents from Central America prefer to work at places where they don't have to speak English or where their peers are from the same background. In addition, Jose, like most of the other adolescent refugees, is used to manual labor, not schoolwork.

Jose will almost certainly drop out of school and join the other immigrants who see America as a land of opportunity. Through hard work and connections in the Nicaraguan community, Jose plans to live the American dream. As Jose puts it, "If I work hard, I know I can make it."

My Typical Day, By Terri Finnigan "Waking up at 6:50 in the morning is awful! However, waking up to the radio isn't so awful! After my radio sounds I usually lay in bed for a few minutes stretching, moaning, groaning, and just thinking about going back to sleep and what I could actually do for the day if I accidentally missed the bus and stayed home instead of going to "Alcatraz"! Really, school isn't as bad as kids say it is! Where else could you see all your friends in one place and get to converse with them while passing notes? But, before I go to school, the long haul of getting prepared for it is needed. First, there's a shower, then getting dressed, then doing my hair. . . . Oh, no! That's another thing, hair! My hair is especially unpleasant to deal with because it is in that lovely stage of trying to grow it long and not being able to do anything with it because no matter how many cans of hair spray you use, it just doesn't feel like working with you! Then I eat while watching the most infamous 'Smurfs!' Brush the teeth, check the hair once more, then I'm good as gone!

"School is great, especially since I'm in 8th grade, and I rule the school! By now I've gotten pretty friendly with my teachers and my school, so my classes are pretty fun. This year I got awful classes, though, because all my friends signed up for a class that I didn't! I consider myself in 'nerd heaven.' Anyway, after school, I usually have basketball, or student council, or tutoring, or something to keep me busy.

"When I get home, which is usually around 6:00, I have dinner and then there's homework. I simply must finish before 8:00 because on Monday, there's 'Alf'; Tuesday, there's 'Who's the Boss'; Wednesday, there's 'Head of the Class'; Thursday, there's 'Cosby'; and Friday, there's 'Full House' (and on weekends, I can see a movie with my friends!). Now it's 10:30 or 11:00, and I am blowing a kiss to my Madonna poster, and I am falling off into dreamland. . . .

Adolescent Development in Perspective. Much of adolescent development has been and is attributed to hormonal development, as we discussed in Chapter Twelve. However, as we have also disccussed, there is less of a tendency today to rely solely on biology for explanations regarding adolescent behavior. Rather, there is more emphasis on the contextual and ecological influences on development. For example, we now are more interested in how others (parents and peers, for example) react to teenage behavior and how this reaction in turn determines how teenagers respond and behave. Likewise, a teenager's perception of her body image by others helps reinforce or alter her self-perception about how she looks. This cyclical pattern of interactions now receives as much attention as a pure biological explanation of adolescent development.

Early adolescence, in particular, is a time when dramatic changes occur within a teenager and within the context in which that teenager lives, in other words, entrance into high school and the dynamic interaction between the two. Consequently, adolescent development is influenced and shaped by biological factors; the interactions of the adolescent with others and environmental settings; and adaptive changes the adolescent makes to her interactions with others and the environment.

SCHOOLING AND TRANSITIONS

Many adolescents change school during their pubertal years, moving from the comforting confines of a neighborhood elementary school to a large middle/junior high school or high school. Such moves disrupt familiar peer group structures, introduce youth to different standards and achievement expectations, and provide opportunities for new extracurricular activities, both licit and illicit (Petersen, 1987b). Petersen also found in her study of adolescents that youngsters who change school within six months of peak pubertal change report more depression and anxiety than those whose school and biological transitions are more separated by time (Petersen, 1987). Consequently, social changes and transitions may play as important a role in adolescent behavior as the biological event of puberty. Also, from the standpoint of the influences of school on development, grade in school is at least as powerful an influence on adolescents as chronological age (Petersen, 1987a).

In Chapter Twelve we said that in any consideration of the effects of adolescent transitions, we must consider individuals. Some youth, as individuals belonging to a particular group, are at greater risk than others during the adolescent years. These "at-risk" individuals are girls; students experiencing many simultaneous life changes; children who are allowed early independence from their parents; children who have been or are being victimized by their peers; and children with disadvantages, such as low self-esteem, lack of popularity, dissatisfaction with their looks, and a history of problem behavior in the elementary grades (Simmons & Blyth, 1987).

In addition, there are *normative transitions*, or transitions that all adolescents must face. These include changing schools, the onset of puberty, and dating. Then there are *nonnormative transitions*, such as geographical relocation and parental marital change, that affect only some adolescents (Simmons, Burgeson, Carlton-Ford, & Blyth, 1987). Generally, adolescents can cope with individual transitions, but the problems occur when they must cope with several transitions at once. The effects of having to engage in multiple coping are several: girls suffer losses in self-esteem; both boys and girls exhibit declines in GPA (Grade Point Average) and extracurricular participation; and for girls, with each successive transition, the coping process becomes more difficult (Simmons et al., 1987).

Arenas of Comfort

One way of coping with the discomfort and stress of transitions is through the establishment or maintenance of *'arenas of comfort.'*

If the child is comfortable in some environments, life arenas, and role relationships, then discomfort in another arena should be able to be tolerated and mastered. Children appear less able to cope if at the same time they are uncomfortable with their bodies because of physical changes, with family because of changes in family constellation, with home because of a move, with school because of a great discontinuity in the nature of the school environment, and with peers because of the emergence of opposite-sex relationships and the disruption of prior peer networks. There needs to be some arena of life or set of role relationships with which the individual can feel relaxed and comfortable, to which he or she can withdraw and become reinvigorated (Simmons, Burgeson, Carlton-Ford, 1987).

EDUCATIONAL AND SOCIAL POLICY IMPLICATIONS

Since schools play such an important part in the life of teenagers, there are a number of policy implications for teachers and school officials. One of these is that the *middle school,* serving children in grades six to eight (ages ten to fourteen), provide an earlier, first transition from the elementary school. (There are many grade configurations for middle schools, including five to seven and seven to nine. Some junior high schools have changed their names to middle schools.) Ideally, this transition enables children involved to accustom themselves to their new school environment *prior to* having to cope with the changes of puberty. What is developmentally wrong with the graded structure of most junior high schools consisting of grades seven to nine is that children must make the transition to a large, impersonal atmosphere with many unknown peers at the same time they are making one of life's most significant developmental transitions.

Furthermore, "Middle school advocates have always stressed the need of every early adolescent to experience success on a regular basis" (George, 1988, p. 15). As such, the middle school, probably more than any other school configuration and organization, has been and is perceived as a school that focuses on the characteristics and needs of its students. In this regard, middle schools are perceived as a major way to provide an arena of comfort to young teenagers at a time when it is needed in their lives.

For this reason, middle schools are increasing in popularity and number, and are viewed as places in which youth can make more gradual, peaceful, and less discontinuous transitions. In fact, the term *middle level of schooling* is used to denote this level of education and to refer to educators' attempts to provide unique experiences for young adolescents in response to their developmental needs. Middle schools are now the most predominant form of school organization for early adolescents. Currently, there are about 12,000 middle-level schools, enrolling well over eight million boys and girls ("Recognition of the Middle Level" 1988).

ESSENTIAL FEATURES OF MIDDLE SCHOOLS

There are a number of essential features that characterize quality middle schools, enabling them to provide essential services to meet the special needs of children in grades six to eight or five to seven. These essential features are guidance, transition programs, organizing for instruction, team teaching, teaching strategies, exploration and athletics (Cawelti, (1988).

Guidance   An effective guidance system provides youth with an adult who has the time and responsibility for providing advice on academic, personal, and social matters. Guidance counselors have traditionally provided such services. However, the counselor-student ratio is often too high to provide the quality of services necessary. Accordingly, a number of viable alternatives are currently used.

One is the *'home base'* plan, in which each teacher in the middle school is assigned a group of advisees. Using the teachers' classrooms as a "home base," these students receive daily counseling on academic, social, and career matters. Not surprisingly, the most relevant guidance activity is in the area of personal and social, advice, and career matters. Generally, students are assigned to the same home base over the three-year period of their middle school experience. Such programs help reduce anonymity and isolation while at the same time assuring continuity and consistency.

Transition Programs   *Transitions*, or the process of helping children (and often their parents, too) make the passage from one setting to another is a very big topic in the entire field of preschool to high school education. It is not surprising, then, that middle schools are more concerned than ever before with helping children and youth make the transition from the elementary grades to the middle school and from the middle school to the senior high school. Transition programs are designed to help minimize distress. Transition activities include the orientation of students prior to their arrival in a new school; the orientation of parents to the philosophy of the school and providing parents with the opportunity to visit classes; having students already enrolled at a school provide newly arriving students with information; and having teachers visit the homes of their students.

Organizing for Instruction   One problem students face once they go to middle, junior or senior high school is that their daily schedules become fragmented, with much time spent in changing classes and other nonessential activities. Increasingly, more middle schools are arranging student schedules in *blocks* of time, so that several or more traditional class periods are combined in a block of time. The idea is that a teacher or group of teachers can provide more meaningful programs,

instructions, and activities in the larger time blocks.

Team Teaching   Or *interdisciplinary teaching* as it is more frequently known, enables groups of teachers to cooperatively plan and teach as a team a group of students assigned to the larger time periods or blocks of time. Thus, interdisciplinary teaching/teaming and block scheduling are viewed as two ideal ways to organize for instruction in order to meet the unique needs of early adolescents.

Teaching Strategies   Middle schools provide unique opportunities for faculty to address the individual needs and learning styles of their students. Indeed, over the last decade, there has been a significant increase in efforts by teachers to match their instructional methods to the unique learning styles of their students. Frequently reported teaching strategies include inquiry teaching, cooperative learning, independent study, and teaching to learning styles.

Exploration and Athletics   Middle school students need opportunities to make informed choices. These opportunities in turn help students become more independent and self-reliant. *Exploration* plays a large role in the lives of adolescents. Exploration of careers and opportunities through courses and curricula enables youth to explore and satisfy their needs for exploration through socially approved activities and in "safe" ways. Some courses that provide exploratory opportunities are art, computer education, industrial arts, music, home economics, technology education, typing, fine arts, career education, and community service.

Interscholastic athletic activities can provide significant opportunities for middle school students. However, there should be provisions for all students to have such opportunities through intramural programs as well.

*I*N THE SPOTLIGHT

LOGGERS' RUN MIDDLE SCHOOL

A visitor to Loggers' Run Middle School in Boca Raton, Florida can't help but be impressed by the visible signs of excellence. In the school office, plaques line the wall attesting to student and faculty involvement and achievement—The United Way Gold Award, 100 percent Faculty PTA Membership, the Palm Beach County School District "Reach for Excellence" Award, the Florida Department of Education "Outstanding Secondary School Program" Award and a framed letter from the State Commissioner of Education awarding a $20,000 grant to pilot an advisor-advisee program.

The middle school exudes a home-like atmosphere, which is exactly what it is supposed to do. In Principal Juanita Lampi's office, impressionist prints line the wall and a couch with soft pillows and end tables with lamps create the feeling that this is a place to relax and feel secure and comfortable. The earthtone colors and the exterior and interior designs promote a calm and relaxed atmosphere. This school is home away from home. This is a place where the principal reassures students that, "At Loggers' Run, you have somebody who loves you."

The home-like image, atmosphere, and security at Loggers' Run is not an accidental happenstance. Everything from the decor to the class schedules to the teachers are planned and designed that way. As Principal Lampi says, "When I interview teachers, I look for the Loggers' Run image, which is one of caring, energy and creativity. If they don't have it, I don't hire them. I tell them I think they would be happier teaching someplace else."

The faculty at Loggers' Run uses a "home base" approach to further give students a feeling of home. Students spend the first hour and fifteen minutes of the day with their home base teacher. The first fifteen minutes is devoted to "home base" activities, such as helping students get organized for the day, taking turns doing announcements, and making decisions about home base projects, for example, how they will do the school's opening activities when it is their turn, and individual guidance activities. Teachers work on forming attachments with their students and, as eighth grade teacher Carolyn Horkey says, "There are many times during the home base period and throughout the day that I play a mother's role. Just last Monday, fourteen-year-old Cindy was sobbing when she came to school. I put my arms around her, gave her a reassuring hug, and asked her what was wrong. She said that on Saturday, her dad slapped her mom and stormed out of the house. They haven't heard from him since then. Cindy was all torn up." Teachers and students in the home base program become attached to each other, which promotes a climate in which youth will share and seek help.

Forty percent of the children in this middle- to upper-middle-class community come from single-parent homes, so there is a lot of mothering to do. According to seventh grade teacher Janice Faustin, "Children who come from single-parent homes look for more attention. They also generally lack discipline and therefore are harder to handle in school. This is one reason we work so much on self-discipline and responsibility."

Loggers' Run provides thirteen clubs, such as the Computer Club, the Drama Club and the Junior Astronaut Club, in which children can also have access to strong role models. Extracurricular sports, such as soccer and track, also provide an opportunity for further involvements and interpersonal interactions. The swimming team, which has fifty members, practices at Mission Bay, an Olympic training facility located a mile away. Also, as sixth grade teacher Claudia English points out, "Sports help kids learn how to abide by rules and this carries over into the classroom and home."

At Loggers' Run, teachers and administrators have certain goals for the 1,425 sixth, seventh and eighth grade students. These goals are designed to:

- Help students make transitions from the elementary to the middle school and from the middle school to the high school. At the first of the year especially, teachers work with parents and students to inculturate them into the policies, rules, and procedures of the school. A transition activity for eighth graders is a study skills course in which they are taught how to study, how to plan for and do homework, and what homework to do first, the hard or the easy.
- Develop good habits of organization. Teachers help children learn organization skills, for instance, having a notebook for each class, how to organize their notes, planning for the things they will need to take to their classes, and budgeting time for homework.
- Help students be responsible for what they do. The teachers help students develop attitudes and skills by which they can learn to be responsible for themselves, rather than being dependent on others to help them be responsible.
- Help students set goals for their personal and academic lives.

Expectations are high at Loggers' Run for teachers and for students. The school motto is "We have CLASS." CLASS stands for *C*aring, *L*earning, *A*chieving, *S*haring, and *S*uccess. "We try to give each student an opportunity to be involved in each of these areas," emphasizes Juanita. "We put our motto into practice and the students and others benefit." The emphasis on academic achievement is apparent by the number of students in the school's Honors Program—about one-quarter of each of the three grade levels.

The daily schedule for a typical student at Loggers' Run is similar to the following:

8:00–8:55 AM—Clubs, activities, and sports on an elective basis.

8:55 AM (Opening bell)—Students enter the school.

9:00–10:04 AM—Home base and first period class—science. If the home base teacher needs more time to engage in guidance activities, she has the opportunity and freedom to do so.

10:08–11:03 AM—Math

11:07 AM–12:02 PM—Physical education or another elective. In Florida, physical education is an elective. Other electives are language (Spanish), chorus, band, shop or vocational "wheel" (If this elective is selected, then every nine weeks the student takes different classes from the vocational core, or "wheel," for example, computers, art, home economics, and business).

12:06–12:35 PM—Lunch. Students can bring their own lunch or have their choice of a hot lunch or salad bar in the cafeteria. Also, students may purchase ice cream, milk shakes, french fries, and similar foods.

12:39–1:31 PM—English

1:35–2:30 PM—Social Studies

In an eighth grade, gifted social studies class, teacher Donna Baker literally lets the students run the classroom. As Donna says, "I'm a facilitator. I let the students do most of the planning and decision making. I find they are much more challenging to themselves and to their peers when they have the responsibility for making decisions about how things should be run. Also, I believe in hands-on learning, so we do a lot of projects."

2:34–3:30 PM—Elective

At Loggers' Run there are the usual cliques that exist at all middle and junior high schools. Youth this age don't want to stand out, they want to fit in, so their need to identify is strong. Just as in adult life, so, too, in teenage life, like attracts like and kids join groups according to the clothes they wear, the music they listen to, and hair styles. There are the "Surfers" and the "Bassers" and other groups in which youth experiment with who they are and join with youth every-

where in seeking an ego identity. This is when Erickson's Stage of Role Identity vs. Role Diffusion is visually played out before one's eyes. Teenagers intuitively realize that childhood is almost past and that adulthood looms on the horizon. Questions about "Who am I?" and "What am I going to do with my life?" indicate ego confusion in daily attempts to resolve the identity conflict. One universal way to deal with the conflict is to select role models—the "Surfers," the "Punks," "Heavy Metal Freaks"—with which to identify. Membership is tight and restrictions about who can get in and out are rigid. In this way, the group and the role defends the searching ego from role confusion. The teenager is somebody because of the group.

Nurturing and academics play major roles at Loggers' Run Middle School. Both are essential ingredients that make the transition from youth to adult more manageable and productive for youth, parents, and teachers.

HIGH SCHOOLS

The American high school is also receiving its share of attention. In particular, there is a national interest in the curriculum of the high school, with a decided emphasis on the academics necessary for a sound education. Some people see contemporary high school curricula as fragmented and filled with too many courses in such areas as physical education and work experiences. One of these critics was William Bennett, U.S. Secretary of Education during the Reagan Administration. Bennett developed a curriculum for all American students called *James Madison High School* (Bennett, 1988). The curriculum Bennett proposes (Figure 13–1) is designed to maintain high academic standards and is to be taught to all students.

As you might expect, not everyone finds the *James Madison* curriculum acceptable. First, critics

maintain that it is educationally unsound to expect one curriculum to fit everyone; that all students are not college bound and consequently it fails to provide for the practical needs of students entering the world of work; and that it is elitist in concept and content (Parnell, 1988).

However, in the Duval County Public Schools, Jacksonville, Florida, 40,000 students in sixteen high schools are involved in the James Madison curriculum. In addition to the curriculum, however, other standards of expectation, such as attendance and discipline, are equally important. According to Mike Walker, Director of Programs of Academic Instruction, "The program works because everyone is devoted to it. It has positive public support from the top down. If everyone in the community promotes and supports high expectations, then they are possible. Our superintendent has a favorite saying—'Students rise to the level expected.'"

The Program In Brief: A Four-Year Plan				
SUBJECT	**1st YEAR**	**2nd YEAR**	**3rd YEAR**	**4th YEAR**
ENGLISH	Introduction to Literature	American literature	British Literature	Introduction to World Literature
SOCIAL STUDIES	Westerm Civilization	American History	Principles of American Democracy (1 sem) and American Democracy & the World (1 sem)	
MATHEMATICS	Three Years Required From Among the Following Courses: Algebra I, Plane & Solid Geometry, Algebra II & Trigonometry, Statistics & Probability (1 sem), Pre-Calculus (1 sem), and Calculus AB or BC			
SCIENCES	Three Years Required From Among the Following Courses: Astronomy/Geology, Biology, Chemistry, and Physics or Principles of Technology			
FOREIGN LANGUAGE	Two Years Required a Single Language From Among Offerings Determined by Local Jursidictions		*ELECTIVE*	
PHYSICAL EDUCATION/ HEALTH	Physical Education/ Health 9	Physical Education/ Health 10		
FINE ARTS	Art History (1 sem) Music History (1 sem)			

FIGURE 13-1 The James Madison curriculum is an example of efforts of educational reformers to re-emphasize the basics in the high school curricula.

High School Counseling Services

Just as counseling services are important in the middle and junior high school, they are also a necessary part of high school programs. However, just as in middle schools where there are too few guidance counselors to go around, high schools turn to alternative programs to provide students the counseling services they need. One of these is *peer counseling,* in which specially trained classmates, also called *peer helpers,* talk to and listen to their peers, help them explore their attitudes, and when necessary, make referrals to school personnel. Some schools provide extensive training for their peer counselors, including credit and noncredit courses and seminars.

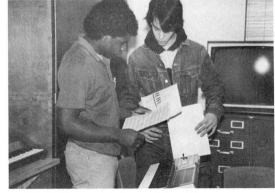

FIGURE 13-2 Peer counseling is growing in popularity in high schools across the United States. Peers have the ability to relate to and provide their classmates the support and reinforcement they need in times of crisis.

*I*N THE SPOTLIGHT

STUDENTS HELPING STUDENTS

Seventeen year old Rebecca Richmond is pregnant, lonely, and frightened. She is swept by feelings of guilt and despair. She needs to talk to someone, but who? She knows her parents will be upset and her mother will be hysterical when she finds out about the pregnancy. But she needs to tell someone. After days of inner turmoil, Rebecca finally decides to confide in her best friend, Melissa.

Melissa is happy Rebecca has confided in her, but she realizes too that Rebecca needs help. She suggests that Rebecca needs to talk to one of the school's peer counselors. Melissa approaches counselor Mary Ellen Strawser, "I have a friend who needs to talk to a peer counselor. I want her to talk to Vivian; she's in my Spanish class, and I know we can trust her."

Vivian is happy to meet with Rebecca and after listening to her story, encourages her to talk about all the solutions she has for her problem of being pregnant. Eventually—after three sessions—Rebecca trusts Vivian enough that Vivian can say, "I think we ought to talk this over with Mrs. Strawser. If you trust me you can trust her." Rebecca meets with Mrs. Strawser, who counsels her to tell her mother about being pregnant and to bring her in on the decision about what course of action is best: "I'll be glad to be with you when you tell your mother and I'm sure Vivian would be present, too, if you want her. Your mother will be upset, but after she settles down, we will all decide what's best."

At Coral Park Senior High School in Miami, Florida, school counselor Mary Ellen Strawser is a specialist in a unique, innovative, and successful program called, PRIDE (Profes-sional *R*esources in *D*evelopmental *E*ducation). PRIDE is a peer counseling program designed to provide the high school with peer counselors who are trained and able to intervene with their peers, who are referred by teachers, parents, and other students.

At the end of each school year, students try out to be peer counselors, just like actors try out for a play. PRIDE counselors interview anyone who wants to be a counselor. In the 1987–1988 school year, over 200 juniors applied for eighteen slots. Such competition is no accident. Students know what counselors can do and they are anxious to help others. Also, as Mary Ellen explains, "We try to get as much variety in our Counselor Corps as possible. We balance the counselors ethnically. For example we have an American Indian, Nic-araguans, African Americans, Hispanics, and Anglos. We also try to get counselors who have personal experience with a particular problem or area. For example, we have a former drug user, a girl whose father died in her arms, and a former anorectic. They all have scars, but they managed to deal with and get over their problems, and then got on about the business of living their lives."

Mary Ellen trains the peer counselors in a wide range of topics: "I train the eighteen peer counselors in communication, both oral and body language, psychological theories (Freud, Skinner, Maslow), positive feedback, group techniques, and interpersonal relation-ships."

During the school year, the peer coun-selors are required to have a case load of three students in each of the eight marking periods, or a total of twenty-four clients with whom they are working throughout the year. Counselors keep accurate records and write a synopsis of each session on a peer counseling form, and Mary Ellen keeps a case card for her records. Mary Ellen gives counselors free reign to counsel their clients as they feel appropriate, except in cases of abuse and suicide. "Counselors tell their clients up front that their conversations are confidential except in cases of abuse or suicide. If they encounter either of these two areas, they have to tell me. I have to go through the proper channels with this."

The peer counselors get a lot of satisfaction and rewards. For example, a former counselor, who is now a college freshman, came back to school during one of her breaks and asked to see one of her former clients. When the client came into the room, she hugged her former counselor and said, "Look at me—would you recognize me now? I'm a different person because of you!"

Each peer counselor also has a group of twenty-five to thirty peers with whom they work in weekly sessions. Students sign up for the sessions on club day. The peer counselor picks the topic, writes a lesson plan, and is in complete charge of the group. Topics include such concerns as family violence, death, alcoholism, suicide, and AIDS.

Peer counselors also visit an elementary school four times a year and make morning presentations to the elementary students on such topics as good self-concept, peer pressure, and developing a positive attitude. Then in the afternoon, they see students who are referred by the teachers and school guidance counselor. These referrals include children of divorce, students who have recently experienced a death in the family, drug users, and students with discipline problems.

Counselors get one academic credit for their year's work in PRIDE. They also receive "letter sweaters," just like athletes. Mary Ellen explains, "There is real esprit de corps—a sense of family. The counselors have a deep sense of pride knowing that they are really making a difference. This kind of program reaffirms my belief that schools underutilize students. Schools should turn students on to using their hearts as well as their heads. Peer counseling does just that!"

In the accompanying "In the Spotlight" section, you will notice that the first person Rebecca confided in was her best friend, Melissa. Is this unusual? Why did Rebecca confide first in her best friend and not her mother? The reason is that pubertal maturation is associated with increased emotional distance between adolescents and their parents (Steinberg, 1987). Additionally, while adolescents of both sexes tend to disclose embarrassing events more to their mothers, girls' first preference for self-disclosure is to female friends. On the other hand, mothers are boys' first preference for disclosure (Denholm & Chabassol, 1987). So, it was normal rather than unusual for Rebecca to disclose to Melissa, her best friend.

DROPPING OUT

The school dropout problem is a serious issue facing schools and society. Dropping out also poses a serious threat to those who do drop out, and places them at risk for poor jobs, lower wages, and an improvised life-style. When we talk about dropouts, we have to understand what a dropout is. Most states have a definition such as the one in Florida, which defines *dropout* this way: "A dropout is a student who during a particular school year is enrolled in school and leaves such school for any reason, except death, before graduation or completion of a program of studies and without transfer to another public or private school or other educational institution'' (Florida State Statute 228.041). The interesting thing about this definition is that the data on dropouts based on such a definition is delimited to a ''particular year,'' so we are unable to determine the dropout rate for a cohort group.

In the Dade County, Florida Public School District, the nation's fourth largest school system, the eighth grade cohort group for June 1980 to January 1985, consisting of 18,829 students, had a cumulative dropout rate of 29.5 percent (Stephenson & Wilbur, 1985, p. 43). This represents 5,555 students in the cohort who dropped out of school. The dropout rate for whites was 29.5 percent, for blacks, 33.9 percent, for Hispanics, 29.3 percent and for Asians, 19 percent. For males, the dropout rate was 32.1 percent, and for females, 26.8 percent.

While you may think these dropout rates are high, in one New York high school, of the 1,221 students in one ninth grade cohort, only 20 percent graduated from that high school and only 33 percent of the group graduated from any high school. This means the dropout rate in this ninth grade cohort group was 66% (Fine, 1986)!

Fine (1986) identifies four types of circumstances under which students drop out of high school prior to graduation:

1. Those who leave with an articulated critique of the schools and/or a negative appraisal of the relation of schooling to labor market success. Fine provides two excellent examples:

Leo, who left in his senior year after scoring 1200 on the SAT, speaks about his social studies teacher, ''Every time she would write something on the board, even if students contradicted it and made a good point, if it was in her notes we had to write it down. Like there was no discussion. . . . Then why did she ask us our opinions? I couldn't go to that class.'' Broderick left because he saw no relation between schooling and future income. He dropped out at age 16 to sell drugs. ''Where else am I going to earn this kind of money even with a diploma?''

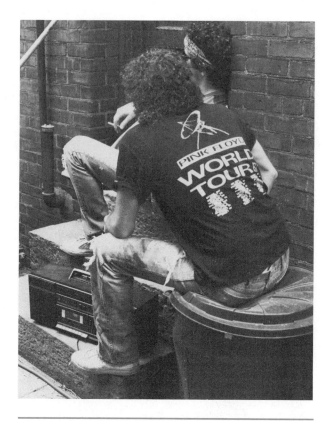

FIGURE 13-3 The number of students who drop out of school is increasing at an alarming rate. Many programs are designed to prevent students from dropping out. Some states such as West Virginia and Florida have passed laws which take away from students their driver's license if they drop out of school.

2. Those who leave to attend to their families' social and health needs, making schooling irrelevant. Diana, seventeen, is typical.

''My mother has lupus [a skin disease]. She's dying and those doctors are killing her. Nobody speaks English good in my family and she wants me there. My brothers and sisters are little and they need me.''

3. Those who leave because they are surrounded by unemployment and poverty, have expe-

rienced failure, have been held back at least once, feel terrible about themselves, and see little hope.

4. Those who are literally thrown out or discharged from school for some reason.

While the number of high school dropouts is high, the number of Hispanic youth that dropout is even higher, averaging two or three times the rate for other students. Some of the reasons for this higher rate of Hispanic (Mexican-American, Puerto Rican, Dominican, and Cuban) dropout are attributed to language problems, poverty, teenage pregnancy, and cultural differences, such as the Hispanic family's traditional nonrelationship with the public schools (Carmody, 1988). What is even more puzzling to school authorities is that the Hispanic dropout rate is high even among those who are not at risk for dropping out, the children from middle class homes who are doing academically well in school. It is estimated that 45 percent of eighteen- and nineteen-year-old Hispanic students have not completed high school and that the Hispanic dropout rate for New York State in 1986 was 62 percent (Carmody, 1988).

A number of strategies are designed to address the Hispanic school dropout rate. They include:

- Special programs designed to specifically target Hispanic students at risk for dropout.
- Improving the teaching and Learning of English.
- Parent communication, contact, and involvement programs.

Many of the dropout prevention programs are justified on an economic model. First, students who drop out of school as a group are not able to have as well-paying jobs as those who don't drop out, therefore dropouts have a lower income over their lifetime. The second justification is related to the first. With a large number of currently employed workers ready to retire—the so-called graying of the work force—many economists are fearful that youth who are dropping out today will not earn enough money to pay the Social Security taxes necessary to support those who contributed most of their work lives to the Social Security fund. Economists also cite the increased costs of providing welfare benefits for those who cannot find a job due to a lack of skills.

Although the peer group frequently is blamed for adolescents dropping out of school, this is not necessarily so. Peer groups are only part of the dynamic involvement in decisions regarding schooling. Home and school also play important roles. Adolescents need to be supported in their efforts to interact positively in both home and school. This support will enable them to change their self-concepts of powerlessness and failure to ones whereby they see themselves as having options that will create results for themselves (Delgado-Gaitan, 1986).

Yet, at the same time, the testing and excellence movements have combined to create school programs and climates in which it is harder for youth to stay in school and easier than ever to leave.

REMEMBERING YOU

How are you remembered by your high school classmates? Are you remembered by them the way you hoped you would be? Everyone wants to be remembered. Memories of one's high school years recur periodically throughout life. How one is remembered is important. But what are the important elements of being remembered? Well, it depends. Males' criteria for popularity for themselves and for females differ from females' criteria for males and for themselves (see Table 13–1).

There are several interesting things about teenager popularity. First, being an athlete is a high status symbol for males as rated by male and female adolescents. Second, in spite of the trend toward participation in sports by females, "being an athlete" does not carry high social status. Third, group membership—"being in the right crowd"—is important for both males and females, and is consistent with what we would expect, given the importance of groups in the lives of teenagers.

TABLE 13–1

CRITERIA FOR ADOLESCENT POPULARITY

Males for Males	Females for Males
Be an athlete—2.20	Be an athlete—2.19
Be in the leading crowd—2.21	Be in the leading crowd—2.28
Leader in activities—3.01	Come from the right family—3.30
High grades, honor roll—3.38	Have a nice car—3.42
Come from the right family—4.05	High grades, honor role—3.50
Females for Females	**Males for Females**
Be in the leading crowd-2.11	Be in the leading crowd—2.08
Leader in activities—2.95	High grades, honor role—2.88
Be a cheerleader—3.67	Come from the right family—3.07
High grades, honor role—3.76	Athletic star—3.34
Be an athlete—4.01	Have a nice car—3.36

Note. The rating scale was from 1–5. The lower scores indicate more importance. From "Sport and Social Status for Adolescent Males and Females" by L. Thirer and S. Wright, 1985, *Sociology of Sport Journal, 2,* pp. 167–169.

*I*N THE SPOTLIGHT

RECONSIDERING ADOLESCENT DEVELOPMENT

During our discussion of moral development in Chapter Ten, we were challenged by Carol Gilligan to reconsider traditional views of moral development to include moral views held by girls and women. Now, Gilligan (1987) challenges us to reconsider adolescent development in relation to changes in modern society and a reconceptualized view of moral development. Gilligan's ideas have particular implications for secondary school education.

Gilligan believes it is appropriate to reconsider contemporary psychology of adolescent development for four reasons. First, contemporary views of childhood have remarkably changed over the last several decades. This is particularly true in terms of how infants and children relate to others. The child is now viewed as a person who can initiate and sustain connections with others and who shows empathy and concern for others. Gilligan argues,

If social responsiveness and moral concern are normally present in early childhood, their absence in adolescence becomes surprising. Rather than asking why such capacities have failed to emerge by adolescence, implying that the child is stuck at some earlier or lower stage, one would ask instead what has happened to the responsiveness of infancy, how have the child's capacities for relationship been diminished or lost? (p. 65)

Second, Gilligan maintains that there is a particular emptiness in adolescent literature as it relates to girls and women. Gilligan contends,

Thus to say what is true—that girls and women have not been much studied—is only to begin to appreciate what such study might entail. To reconsider adolescent development in light of the inattention to girls and women is to hold in abeyance the meaning of such key terms of psychological analysis as *self* and *development* and perhaps above all *relationship* (p. 66).

Third, Gilligan believes that the definition of cognition in a narrow, Piagetian perspective, in other words, mathematical and scientific thinking, has virtually ruled out other views of cognition as well as narrowing the school curricula. Gilligan asserts,

This [Piagetian] conception of cognitive development conveys a view of the individual as living in a timeless world of abstract rules. Within this framework, there is no rationale for teaching history or languages or writing or for paying attention to art and music. In fact, the flourishing of Piagetian theory within psychology over the past two decades has coincided with the decline of all these subjects in the school curriculum (p. 67).

Fourth, Gilligan maintains that much of our current thinking about adolescent development is based on the processes of separation, individuation, and independence. Given this perspective, the outcome of adolescent development is self-sufficiency. Gilligan argues that such a view is insufficient.

To see self-sufficiency as the hallmark of maturity conveys a view of adult life that is at odds with the human condition—a view that cannot sustain the kinds of long-term commitments and involvements with others that are necessary for raising and educating a child

or for citizenship in a democratic society. The equation of development with separation and maturity with independence presumes a radical discontinuity of generations and encourages a vision of human experience that is essentially divorced from history and time (pp. 67–68).

What implications do Gilligan's ideas have for educational practice? Several. First, Gilligan maintains that mothers and teachers play significant roles in adolescent development.

Yet mothers of adolescents are increasingly single parents living in poverty, and teachers at present are generally unsupported and devalued. Psychological development in adolescence may well hinge on the adolescent's belief that her or his psyche is worth developing, and this belief in turn may hinge on the presence in a teenager's life of an adult who knows and cares about the teenager's psyche. Economic and psychological support for the mothers and the teachers who at present are the primary adults engaged with teenagers may be essential to the success of efforts to promote adolescent development (p. 82).

Second, society and educators must provide opportunities to talk about and integrate into activities and curricula issues of care and concern. Gilligan suggests that,

If at present a care perspective offers a critical lens on a society that seems increasingly justice focused, it is also one that clarifies and makes sense of the activities of care that teenagers describe [in their discussions]—not only helping others but also creating connections with others, activities they link with times when they feel good about themselves (p. 87).

Third, Gilligan thinks that research involving teenagers and their particular moral dilemmas, for example, abortion, may serve both an intervention and educational function. Gilligan states,

It may be that asking teenagers to talk about their own experiences of moral conflict and choice in itself constitutes an effective intervention, as some preliminary evidence suggests. Such questioning may reveal to teenagers that they have a moral perspective, something of value at stake, and thus that they have grounds for action in situations where they may have felt stuck or confused or unable to choose between alternative paths. . . . For the adolescent, the realization that he, and perhaps especially she, has a moral perspective that an adult finds interesting, or a moral voice that someone will respond to, shifts the framework for action away from a choice between submission and rebellion (action defined in others' terms) and provides a context for discovering what are one's own terms. In adolescence, this discovery galvanizes energy and stimulates initiative and leadership (pp. 88–89).

What Would You Do?

Janice and Jim Capaletti are concerned about their daughter, Julie, an only child who has just finished her sophomore year at Thomas Jefferson Senior High School. The school is overcrowded. Many classes are held in hallways and storage areas and the student teacher ratio is about 35:1. Julie was an excellent student throughout elementary and junior high school, but she has just managed to get all B's at Thomas Jefferson. "Julie used to be interested in her studies and really was involved academically," laments Janice. "Now she seems so distracted by a lot of other activities." What concerns the Capaletti's the most is that Julie is developing a negative attitude toward school and for her junior year wants to register in general education courses rather than the college-bound track.

The Capaletti's are at their wits' end and are willing to try anything. They already have had Julie to a counselor, but without demonstrable results. Last week, in exasperation, Janice and Jim contacted a local Catholic girls' school and inquired about their program.

The Capaletti's have learned that you are home for summer vacation from the state university. Since you are their next-door neighbor, they feel they can ask you for your opinion about enrolling Julie in an all-girl high school. What can you say to the Capaletti's that will help them make their decision?

CHARACTER EDUCATION IN THE HIGH SCHOOLS

An increasing number of problems are facing society and intimately involve our children. Many of these are characterized as "psychosocial epidemics" and include family disruption, sexual behavior, births to unwed mothers, child neglect and abuse, alcohol and drug use by children, children's suicide, and the high school dropouts rate (London, 1987). For these reasons, character education is now advocated as one of the basics many schools should include in their curricula.

Character education consists of two facets: "(1) Education in *civic virtue* and in the qualities that teach children the forms and rules of citizenship in a just society; and (2) education in *personal adjustment*, chiefly in the qualities that enable children to become productive and dependable citizens" (London, 1987).

PARENTING THE TEENAGER
Too Independent Too Soon

We have stressed in this text the importance of independence in the lives of children. However, during the years prior to and during adolescence, the abandonment of too much parental supervision too soon is not in the best interests of individual children. The problem is that precisely at the time children need supervision—during the transition to junior or senior high school—is the time when

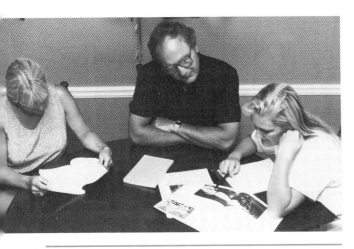

FIGURE 13-4 Interaction between family members is crucial for true communication.

many parents have abandoned or are abandoning their supervisory role. Part of this stems from the fact that many parents are afraid to say "no" to their children. As a consequence, parents do not assume their responsibility to provide their children with the guidance they need during the time they need it most.

"I Didn't Do It!"—Teenagers and Lying

Many parents believe their children are always right. Perhaps this is only natural, given the trusting relationships that parents strive for with their children. However, lying on the part of teenagers is very common.

*I*N THE SPOTLIGHT

THE SHOPPING MALL AS SURROGATE FAMILY

For many of today's teenagers, the shopping mall has replaced the family as a place for values and entertainment. Social values are being defined by advertisements and product promotions. Materialism becomes a value focus, with malls promoting the feeling that you can have all you want of anything you want. Be all you want to be at your local mall. The good life is yours and always will be. Amid the opulence, abundance, and variety, it is difficult to think beyond oneself to others. How could others be in need of food or clothing when there is so much here? Mall stores reinforce the image of consumerism with teenage advisory boards helping to promote the idea that if your peers approve, it is okay to do or buy.

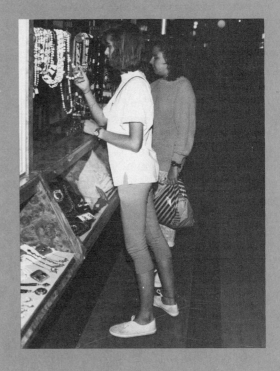

FIGURE 13-5 For many teenagers the shopping mall is the home away from home as well as the place to go when they want to get away from home. Many mall merchants specifically cater to teen wants and needs with the latest fashions and products. Teens, for their part, are more than happy to have places to spend their time and money.

PREVENTION PROGRAMS

Given all the problems facing today's youth—suicide, substance abuse, delinquency, running away, dropping out of school, and general alienation—it is little wonder that communities, schools, and state, local, and private agencies have developed programs to help youth and society deal with these problems.

One program that has achieved success and national attention is the "KNOW THE SCORE" program of the McKeesport Area School District in McKeesport, Pennsylvania. This program is a combined substance and suicide prevention program and has the following components (Sofo & Champagne, 1989):

■ Drug prevention curriculum—This curriculum, "Here's Looking at You, Two" spans grade levels K–12 and includes topics on the harmful effects of drugs, the importance of using refusal skills, and developing a healthy self-concept.
■ Elementary Absenteeism Program (EAP)—This program is designed to reduce unexcused school absenteeism, which is a common indicator of future academic, emotional, and social problems.
■ Middle/High School Student Assistance Program (SAP)—SAP consists of a core team of school personnel who are trained to serve as a data collection and referral source for youth who display significant behavioral patterns indicating substance abuse or depression. Core teams work with community drug/alcohol and mental health professionals to help provide community-based helping services. SAP also operates bi-weekly aftercare programs for youth returning to school from residential treatment centers.
■ Peer Awareness and Support System (PAWSS)—This is a "kids helping kids" peer program that emphasizes positive peer influence as a means of prevention.
■ Parent education program—Parents, along with peer pressure, are two of the most powerful sources of drug abuse prevention. The program increases parental awareness concerning youth substance abuse and suicide, and provides information regarding access to professional helping services.

At the Upper Moreland Middle School in Hatboro, Pennsylvania, school officials focus on parents by providing education, training, and discussion opportunities as a means of helping the parents improve their parenting skills so they can effectively cope with the needs of their early adolescents and nurture a cooperative partnership between the home and school (Lessa & Smith, 1989).

The first level of parenting education includes topics on preadolescent development, strengthening a child's self-concept, approaches to discipline, and parents and schools—a cooperative effort.

The second level of the parent education program includes topics on drug and alcohol use, crisis intervention, sexuality and dating, and stress management. The topics on sexuality and dating are taught by an obstetrician/gynecologist, Morgan T. Smith, M.D., a member of the Adolescent Sexuality Task Force for the American College of Obstetrics and Gynecology.

The middle school also conducts an Early Family Intervention Program. In this program, a core of professional staff, including administrators, counselors, a psychologist, and a social worker work with families of students who were previously identified as having learning or social problems at the elementary level. In this way, students and families are provided services *prior* to the youth's entry into middle school. In addition, the school also conducts an ongoing support group for parents with children in special education.

In the Richardson Independent School District, Richardson, Texas, administrators, teachers, and students have established a Student Assistance Program designed to prevent substance abuse and assist students and their families (Onley, Weckerly, & Puckett, 1989). Teachers refer students to an intervention team of teachers, administrators and counselors. Teachers use a Referral Concern Form to identify students who exhibit "signs of concern."

These signs include lower grades, lower achievement, absenteeism, tardiness, increased visits to the school nurse, erratic behavior, and sleeping in class. When the intervention team receives a Referral Concern Form, they meet and assess the student's behavior and develop an intervention plan. This plan can include meeting with the parents and student, and referral to public and private community agencies where students are treated on an outpatient, inpatient, and/or aftercare basis. The school district also has on the school site support groups such as AA and NA, enabling students to have a safe place to meet with adult facilitators.

IMPLICATIONS FOR PARENTS

It is interesting to note that in combating and preventing problems facing today's adolescents, the schools and the public are shifting their focus to what happens to children early in their schooling experiences. For example, high school dropout problems are seen as having part of their root causes in early life problems, such as preschool, kindergarten, and primary grade absenteeism, grade failure; and impaired family relationships. Thus it is not unusual to see comprehensive programs designed to prevent substance abuse, delinquency, and school dropout targeting young preschool and elementary children and their families.

More school districts and school personnel are realizing that they alone cannot solve or resolve all the social problems facing today's youth. Increasingly, they are developing comprehensive programs that involve the parents, the community, and existing community agencies. Realizing the wastefulness of duplicating services and mindful that many community agencies have well-trained and dedicated personnel, schools are reaching out and linking. They have adopted a motto of our founding forefathers—"United we stand, divided we fall,"—especially when it comes to the war on drugs, dropouts, and delinquency.

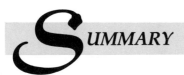

SUMMARY

- Whereas in the past, the majority of the causes of adolescent behavior and development were attributed to hormones, today there is more emphasis on the interactions of biological, parental, and social forces as determiners of behavior and development. In particular, the school is seen as exerting significant influence on teenagers.
- Transitions from elementary school to middle and high schools disrupt familiar peer group structures, introduce youth to different standards and achievement expectations, and provide opportunities for positive and negative extracurricular activities.

- Two types of transitions teenagers face are normative—those faced by all teenagers—and nonnormative transitions, such as geographical relocation, faced only by some teenagers.
- Middle schools and middle-level schooling are designed to be socially and educationally responsive to the developmental needs of young adolescents. Essential characteristics of middle schools include an emphasis on guidance and transition activities, block scheduling, team teaching, tailoring teaching to students' learning styles, and exploration of careers and opportunities.
- High schools also are undergoing changes. There is more of an emphasis on academics and providing all students with essential knowledge, and learning and thinking skills.
- Student counseling services are emphasized in both middle and senior high schools. Peer counseling in particular is increasing in popularity and effectiveness.
- Dropping out of school is a serious problem facing both youth and society. Students drop out because they see little relation of schooling to work and life, they are needed to help their families, they are dealing with life events and environmental circumstances that provide them with little hope for the future, and they are literally thrown out of school.
- Being an athlete is one of the primary criteria for male popularity in high school. Being in the right crowd is an important determiner of popularity for both males and females.
- Carol Gilligan advocates a reconsideration of adolescent development because views of childhood have changed, girls and women have been left out of adolescent literature, cognitive development has been too narrowly defined, and self-sufficiency is not necessarily the only or desired outcome of adolescent development. The educational implications of such views are that adolescents need teachers who care about them, issues of care and concern must be integrated into curricula, and teenagers can be helped to develop moral perspectives that are respected by adults.
- Prevention programs have assumed a prominent role in helping parents and youth deal with many of the problems facing today's adolescent, such as substance abuse, suicide, and delinquency.

QUESTIONS TO GUIDE YOUR REVIEW

1. How has our conception of adolescent development changed through the years?
2. What influences does schooling have on adolescent development?
3. What roles do transitions play in adolescent life?
4. Why are transition activities important in helping adolescents adjust? How do such transitional activities help?
5. What are the educational and developmental justifications for middle schools?
6. What are important characteristics of middle schools?
7. What are considered important activities and services in middle schools?
8. How is Loggers' Run Middle School different from the middle/junior high schools with which you are familiar?

9. How are high schools changing academically?
10. How is the James Madison Curriculum similar to or different from the curriculum you studied in high school?
11. What are the major reasons youth drop out of school?
12. What are some measures that are recommended for preventing school dropouts?
13. What are major theories for explaining why youth engage in substance abuse?
14. What are some essential features of programs designed to prevent substance abuse?
15. Why does Carol Gilligan want to reconsider adolescent development? Are these valid reasons?
16. What implications do Gilligan's ideas have for educational practice?

 ACTIVITIES FOR FURTHER INVOLVEMENT

1. In both Chapters Twelve and Thirteen, considerable attention is paid to the discussion of *transitions.*
   a. Interview teenagers at local middle and high schools to determine what transitions were most stressful for them, and solicit their suggestions for how to reduce the stress associated with these transitions.
   b. Recall your own teenage years, for positive and or negative stressful transitions. How were you affected by these?
2. Middle schools are viewed as one way of helping adolescents cope with the stress of the pre- and adolescent years.
   a. Visit middle schools in your area and interview both teachers and students to determine what they believe are the benefits of middle schools.
   b. What do you think are topics that should be included in middle school curricula that would most likely help students adjust to the teenage years?
3. Society and the business community view the high school dropout problem as a serious threat to the nation's well-being and economy.
   a. Interview high school students to determine the reasons that students give for dropping out.
   b. What do you think would be positive solutions to the dropout problem?
4. Prevention programs designed to help prevent many of the problems facing today's youth are very popular in the nation's high schools.
   a. Visit local high schools and make a survey of the prevention programs available.
   b. What prevention programs should be available, and are not? What are the reasons for their lack of availability? What are the most successful programs?
5. Teenagers engage in faddish behavior in order to fit in with the group and maintain a self-identity.
   a. What are some of the latest teenage fads, and how do they help teenagers fit in?
   b. What fads or teenage practices tend to endure from one generation to the next? Why?

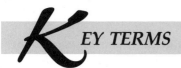

KEY TERMS

Arenas of comfort Relationships or environments in which youth can feel emotionally and physically comfortable.

Home base The educational practice in which a teacher acts as a counselor to a group of students. The home-base meeting generally occurs at the beginning and end of the day.

Middle level of schooling Denotes level of education in grades six to eight and educators' attempts to provide unique experiences for young adolescents in response to their developmental needs.

Middle school A school specifically designed to meet the developmental needs of youth in grades six to eight.

Nonnormative transitions Transitions that affect only some adolescents, such as geographical relocation.

Normative transitions Transitions that all adolescents must face. These include changing schools, onset of puberty, and dating.

Peer counseling Specially trained student classmates, also called *peer helpers,* who talk to and listen to their peers and help them explore their attitudes and when necessary, make referrals to school personnel.

Team teaching An educational practice of having to cooperatively plan and teach a group of students. Also known as *interdisciplinary teaching.*

Transition The process of helping children (and often their parents, too) make the passage from one setting—usually a school—to another.

ENRICHMENT THROUGH FURTHER READING

Brumberg, J. J. (1988). *Fasting girls: The emergence of anorexia nervosa as a modern disease.* Cambridge, MA: Harvard University Press.

A fascinating study of this much-discussed but little understood disease.

Oakes, J. (1985). *Keeping track: How schools structure inequality.* New Haven, CT: Yale University Press.

The author maintains that tracking practices (homogeneous grouping) of America's junior and senior high schools create and perpetuate inequality. Oakes believes that cooperative learning can provide more equity in schooling and society.

ANSWER TO "WHAT WOULD YOU DO?"

Where the Boys Aren't

The idea of coeducation is almost universally accepted in the United States. Almost everyone assumes that in this day of equality and equal access that coeducation should be the normal course of events for America's boys and girls. Faced with declining

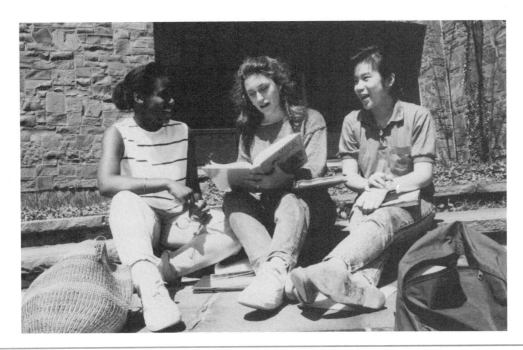

FIGURE 13-6 For some girls, single-sex schools offer opportunities for success and achievement they might not find in co-educational schools.

enrollments, single-sex schools are like an endangered species and are threatened with extinction. So, perhaps your first reaction was that the Capalettis' idea of sending Julie to an all-girl school wasn't a very good idea. (You resisted the thought of calling it a stupid idea!)

But, is single-sex education necessarily all bad? Not if you believe the research of Valerie Lee and Anthony Bryk (1986). According to them, single-sex Catholic high schools have many positive benefits, especially for girls. All-girl schools evidenced consistant and positive effects on student attitudes towards academics and the girls were more likely to associate with academically oriented peers and to express specific interest in mathematics and English. Additionally, girls in all-girl schools took more mathematics, vocational offerings, and social sciences than did their coeducational counterparts.

The news is even better when we look at the achievement of girls in single-sex schools. Beginning in the sophomore year, students in the all-girl schools outperformed their coed counterparts in reading and science. In addition, "These girls' schools showed some positive effects on students' locus of control, and the girls were less likely to see themselves in sex-stereotyped adult roles" (p. 394).

Commenting on the beneficial effects of single-sex schools' sensitizing influence on young women to their occupational and societal potentials, Lee and Bryk comment, "Adolescence is a critical period for the formation of attitudes about oneself. It may be that some separation of students' academic and social environments removes the distractions that can interfere with the academic development of some students" (p. 394).

How do you explain the effects of the single-sex schools? What makes the difference? Lee and Bryk attribute the effects to the schools themselves—the schools are smaller, the student-teacher ratio is smaller and the schools have a less "diverse array of courses. As a result, students are more likely to take a similar course of study, and this homogeneity of experiences could conceivably produce beneficial effects" (p. 392).

So, while you can't say that the school the Capalettis are thinking about will have the same positive impact on Julie that the research reports, you can share the Lee and Bryk study with them. This information can form the basis for some good questions they can ask when they visit the girls' school and meet with the principal.

*B*IBLIOGRAPHY

Bennett, W. J. (1988, June-July). A curriculum for American students: James Madison High School. *AACJC Journal*, 10.

Carmody, D. (1988, August 17). Hispanic dropout rates puzzling. *The New York Times*, p. 26.

Cawelti, G. (1988, November). Middle schools a better match with early adolescent needs, ASCD survey finds. *ASCD curriculum update*, pp. 1–12.

Delgado-Gaitan, C. (1986). Adolescent peer influence and differential school performance. *Journal of Adolescent Research*, 1, 461.

Denholm, C. J., & Chabassol, D. J. (1987). Adolescents' self disclosure of potentially embarrassing events. *The Journal of Psychological Reports*, 60, 45–46.

Fine, M. (1986). Why urban adolescents drop into and out of public high school. *Teachers College Record*, 87, 393–409.

George, P. (1988). Education 2000: Which way the middle school? *The Clearing House*, 62, 15.

Gilligan, C. (1987, Fall). Adolescent development reconsidered. In C. E. Irwin, Jr. (Ed.), *Adolescent Social Behavior and Health* (New Directions for Child Development, No. 37). San Francisco: Josey-Bass.

Lee, V. E., & Bryk, A. S. (1986). Effects of single sex secondary school on student achievement and attitudes. *Journal of Educational Psychology*, 78, 381–395.

Lessa, W. A., & Smith, M. T. (1989, March). *Coping with the adolescent years: An interdisciplinary approach to parent education*. A paper presented at the 44th Annual Conference of the Association for Supervision and Curriculum Development, Orlando, FL.

London, Perry. (1987). Character education and clinical intervention: A paradigm shift for U.S. schools. *Phi Delta Kappan*, 68, 667–673.

Onley, P., Weckerly, E., & Puckett, K. (1989, March). *Loving intervention for teens*. A paper presented at the 44th Annual Conference of the Association for Supervision and Curriculum Development, Orlando, FL.

Parnell, D. (1988, June-July) Does one curriculum really fit all? *AACJC Journal*, 11.

Petersen, A. C. (1987a). The nature of biological-psychological interactions: The sample case of early adolescence. In R. M. Lerner & T. T. Foch (Eds.), *Biological-psychological interactions in early adolescence*. Hillsdale, NJ: Lawrence Erlbaum.

Petersen, A. C. (1987b). Those gangly years. *Psychology Today*, 21, 28–34.

Recognition of the middle level of schooling. (1988). *Middle School Journal, 19,* 27.

Simmons, R. G., & Blyth, D. A. (1987). *Moving into adolescence: The impact of pubertal change and school context.* Hawthorne, NY: Aldine.

Simmons, R. G., Burgeson, R., Carlton-Ford, S. & Blyth, D. A. (1987). The impact of cumulative change in early adolescence. *Child Development, 58,* 1220–1234.

Sofo, R., & Champagne, D. W. (1989, March) *Students-drugs, suicide, stress, life, growth, health-choices.* Paper presented at the 44th Annual Conference of the Association for Supervision and Curriculum Development, Orlando, FL.

Steinberg, L. (1987). Impact of puberty on family relations: Effects of pubertal status and pubertal timing. *Developmental Psychology, 23,* 451–460.

Stephenson, R., & Wilbur, K. (1985). *A study of the longitudinal dropout rate: 1980 eighth grade cohort followed from June, 1980 through February, 1985.* Miami, FL: Dade County Public Schools.

Thirer, L., & Wright, S. D. (1985). Sport and social status for adolescent males and females. *Sociology of Sport Journal, 2,* 167–169.

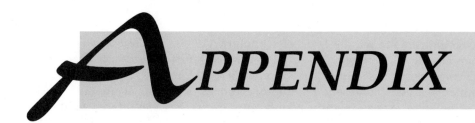

APPENDIX

Journals & publications relating to child development

Advances in Child Development and Behavior
Academic Press, Inc.
1250 Sixth Ave.
San Diego, CA 92101

Advances in Learning and Behavioral Disabilities
J A I Press, Inc.
55 Old Post Rd., No. 2, Box 1678
Greenwich, CT 06836–1678

American Journal of Orthopsychiatry
American Orthopsychiatric Association, Inc.
19 W. 44th St.
New York, NY 10036

BC Journal of Special Education
Special Education Association
Dept. of Special Education, University of British Columbia
2075 Wesbrook Mall
Vancouver, B.C. V6T 1W5, Canada

Child Development
University of Chicago Press, Journals Division
5720 S. Woodlawn Ave.
Chicago, IL 60637

Child Education
Scholastic Publications
Marlborough House
Hollywalk, Leamington Spa
Warks CV32 4LS, England

Child Psychiatry and Human Development
Human Sciences Press, Inc.
72 Fifth Ave.
New York, NY 10011

Child Study Journal
State University of New York, College at Buffalo
Bacon Hall 312 J, 1300 Elmwood Ave.
Buffalo, NY 14222–1095

Childhood Education
Association for Childhood Education International
11141 Georgia Ave., Ste. 200
Wheaton, MD 20902

Children's Environments Quarterly
City University of New York, Graduate Center
Environmental Psychology Program
33 N. 42nd St.
New York, NY 10036

Developmental Psychobiology
John Wiley & Sons, Inc. Periodical Division
605 Third Ave.
New York, NY 10158

Early Childhood Research Quarterly
Ablex Publishing Corporation
355 Chestnut St.
Norwood, NJ 07648

Early Human Development
Elsevier Scientific Publishers Ireland Ltd.
PO Box 85
Limerick, Ireland

Educational Research
Carfax Publishing Co.
85 Ash St.
Hopkinton, MA 01748

Educational Studies
American Educational Studies Association
c/o John E. Carter, Ed.
School of Education, Indiana State University
Terre Haute, IN 47809

Gifted Child Quarterly
National Association for Gifted Children
4175 Lovell Rd., Ste. 140
Circle Pines, MN 55014–3501

Gifted Children Monthly
Gifted and Talented Publications, Inc.
213 Hollydell Dr.
Sewell, NJ 08080

Gifted Education International
AB Academic Publishers
Box 97, Berkhamsted
Herts HP4 2PX, England

Gifted International
Trillium Press, Inc.
Box 209
Monroe, NY 10950

Journal for the Education of the Gifted
University of North Carolina Press
Box 2288
Chapel Hill, NC 27515–2288

Journal of Abnormal Child Psychology
Plenum Press

233 Spring St.
New York, NY 10013

Journal of Adolescence
Academic Press, Ltd.
24-28 Oval Rd.
London NW1 7DX, England

Journal of Adolescent Research
H.E.L.P. Books, Inc.
1201 E. Calle Elena
Tucson, AZ 85718

Journal of Child Language
Cambridge University Press
Edinburgh Bldg., Shaftesbury Rd.
Cambridge CB2 2RU, England

Journal of Child Psychology & Psychiatry
Pergamon Press, Inc., Journals Division
Maxwell House, Fairview Park
Elmsford, NY 10523

Journal of Development and Behavioral Pediatrics
Williams & Wilkins
428 E. Preston St.
Baltimore, MD 21202

Journal of Early Adolescence
H.E.L.P. Books, Inc.
1201 E. Calle Elena
Tucson, AZ 85718

Journal of Educational Psychology
American Psychological Association
1200 17th St., N.W.
Washington, DC 20036

Journal of Genetic Psychology
Heldref Publications
4000 Albermale St., N.W.
Washington, DC 20016

Journal of Learning Disabilities
5341 Industrial Oaks Blvd.
Austin, TX 78735

Journal of Pediatric Nursing
Grune & Stratton, Inc., Journals Department
Orlando, FL 32887–0018

Journal of Pediatric Psychology
Plenum Press
233 Spring St.
New York, NY 10013

Journal of Pediatrics
C.V. Mosby Co.
11830 Westline Industrial Dr.
St. Louis, MO 63146

Journal of Perinatal and Neonatal Nursing
Aspen Publishers, Inc.
1600 Research Blvd.
Rockville, MD 20850

Journal of Practical Approaches to Developmental Handicap
University of Calgary, Rehabilitation Studies
Education Tower
Alta T2N 1N4, Canada

Journal of Reading Behavior
National Reading Conference, Inc.
11 E. Hubbard St., Ste. 200
Chicago, IL 60611

Journal of Reading, Writing & Learning Disabilities International
Hemisphere Publishing Corporation
79 Madison Ave., Ste. 1110
New York, NY 10016–7892

Journal of Special Education Technology
Association of Special Education Technology
Developmental Center for Handicapped Persons,
Utah State University
UMC 68
Logan, UT 84322

Journal of Youth and Adolescence
Plenum Press
233 Spring St.
New York, NY 10013

Maternal-Child Nursing Journal
University of Pittsburgh
Maternity Nursing and Nursing Care of Children
Departments
437 Victoria Bldg.
3500 Victoria St.
Pittsburgh, PA 15261

MCN American Journal of Maternal Child Nursing
American Journal of Nursing Co.
555 W 57th St.
New York, NY 10019

Merrill-Palmer Quarterly
Wayne State University Press
Leonard N. Simons Bldg.
5959 Woodward Ave.
Detroit, MI 48202

New Directions for Child Development
Jossey-Bass, Inc., Publishers
350 Sansome St.
San Francisco, CA 94104

Perceptual and Motor Skills
Dr. C.H. Ammons & Dr. R. B. Ammons
Box 9229
Missoula, MT 59807

Pre and Peri Natal Psychology Journal
Human Sciences Press, Inc.
72 Fifth Ave.
New York, NY 10011

Psychological Reports
Dr. C. H. Ammons & Dr. R. B. Ammons
Box 9229
Missoula, MT 59807

Psychology in the Schools
Clinical Psychology Publishing Co., Inc.
4 Conant Square
Brandon, VT 05733

Psychology of Women Quarterly
Cambridge University Press
Edinburgh Bldg.
Shaftesbury Rd.
Cambridge CB2 2RU, England

Reading Research Quarterly
International Reading Association, Inc.
800 Barksdale Rd., Box 8139
Newark, DE 19714–8139

Sex Roles
Plenum Press
233 Spring St.
New York, NY 10013

Special Services in the Schools
Haworth Press, Inc.
12 W 32nd St.
New York, NY 10001

Young Children
National Association for the Education of Young
Children
1834 Connecticut Ave., N.W.
Washington, DC 20009

BIBLIOGRAPHY

Accreditation criteria and procedures of the National Academy of Early Childhood Programs. (1984). Washington, DC: National Association for the Education of Young Children.

Adachi, T. & Okada, H. (1985). Acoustic properties of infant cries and maternal perception. *Tohoku Psychologica Folia, 44,* 51–58.

Adams, R.J., Maurer, D., & Davis, M. (1986). Newborns' discrimination of chromatic from achromatic stimuli. *Journal of Experimental Child Psychology, 41,* 267–281.

Agency for Toxic Substances and Disease Registry (July, 1988). *Nature and extent of lead poisoning in children in the United States: A report to congress July, 1988.* Atlanta, GA: Agency for Toxic Substances and Disease Registry. p. 4.

AIDS infant malformed. (1986, August 12). *The New York Times.*

Ainsworth, M., Blehar, M., Waters, E., & Walls, S. (1978). *Patterns of Attachment.* Lawrence Erlbaum.

Akers, R.L., Khron, M.D., Lanze-Kaduce, L., & Rasosevich, M. (1979). Social learning and deviant behavior: A specific test of a general theory. *American Sociological Review, 44,* 636–655.

All fall down. (1986, July-August). *American Health,* p. 29.

Am, E. (1986). Play in the preschool: Some aspects of the role of the adult. *The International Journal of Early Childhood, 18* (2), 90–97.

Amdur, J.M., Mainland, M.C., & Parker, K.C.H. (1984). *Diagnostic inventory for screening children.* San Antonio, TX: The Psychological Corporation.

American Academy of Pediatrics. (1982). Promotion of breast feeding. *Pediatrics, 69,* 654–660.

American Academy of Pediatrics and The American College of Obstetricians and Gynecologists. (1983). *Guidelines for prenatal care.*

American College of Obstetricians and Gynecologists, The. (1987, October). Patient choice: maternal-fetal conflict. *ACOG Committee Opinion,* No. 55, Washington, DC: The American College of Obstetricians and Gynecologists.

American Heritage Dictionary, The. (1982). Boston, MA: Houghton-Mifflin.

Ames, L.B. (1987). Respect for readiness. In E. Shiff (Ed.), *Experts advise parents.* New York: Delacorte, pp. 123–145.

Ames, L.B. & Chase, J.A. (1980). *Don't push your preschooler.* New York: Harper & Row.

Anderman, E. (1988). Correspondence of Ellen Anderman to Mary Gittings, Program Director, The Piton Foundation; sent by Diane Medena of LaMariposa to the author.

Annest, J.L. et al. (1982, May 12). *Blood lead level for persons 6 months to 74 years of age: U.S. 1976–1980. (Vital and health statistics).* National Center for Health Statistics (Advance Data, No. 79). pp. 1–24.

Anspaugh, D., Ezell, G., & Goodman, K.N. (1987). *Teaching today's health.* Columbus, OH: Merrill.

Ansul, S.E., DiBase, R., & Weintraub, M. (1987, April). *The effects of maternal employment and child sex.* Paper presented at the biennial meeting of the Society for Research in Child Development, Baltimore, MD.

Apgar, V. (1966). The newborn (Apgar) scoring system, reflections and advice. *Pediatric Clinic of North America, 13m* 645.

Archambault, R.D. (Ed.). (1964). *John Dewey on education-selected writings.* New York: Random House.

Aronson, S.S. & Osterholm, M.T. (1986). Infectious diseases in child day care: Management and prevention summary of the symposium recommendations. *Reviews of Infectious Diseases, 8,* 672–679.

Azmitia, M. (1988). Peer interaction and problem solving: When are two heads better than one? *Child Development, 59,* 87–96.

Bachman, J.G. (1987, July). An eye on the future. *Psychology Today, 21,* 6–8.

Baily, W.T. (1987, Spring). On avoiding subject attrition in longitudinal research. *SRCD Newsletter,* p. 2.

Bandura, A. (1977). *Social learning theory.* Englewood Cliffs, N.J.: Prentice-Hall.

Banks, M.S. & Dannemiller, J.L. (1987). Infant visual psychophysics. In P. Salapatek & L. Cohen (Eds.), *Handbook of infant perception* (Vol. 1. From sensation to perception, pp. 115–184). Orlando: Harcourt Brace Jovanovich.

Baranowski, T., Rassin, D., Richardson, C.J., Brown, J. & Bee, D. (1986). Attitudes toward breast feeding. *Developmental and Behavioral Pediatrics, 7,* 367–372.

Barclay, L. (1985). *Infant development.* New York: CBS College.

Barrett, D. (1987). Undernutrition and child behavior: What behaviors should we measure and how should we measure them? In J. Dobbing (Ed.). *Early nutrition and later development.* London: Academic Press.

Bassuk, B. & Rubin, L. (1987). Homeless children: A neglected population. *American Journal of Orthopsychiatry, 57,* 279–285.

Bates, B., et al. (1988). *From first words to grammar,* Cambridge, England: Cambridge University Press.

Baumrind, D. (1971). Current patterns of parental authority. *Developmental psychology monograph, 4,* p. 2.

Baumrind, D. (1967). Child care practices anteceding 3 patterns of preschool behavior. *Genetic psychology monographs,* 43–88.

Bax, M. (1985). Crying: A clinical overview. In B. Lester & C.F.Z. Boukydis (Eds.). *Infant Crying* (pp. 341–348). New York: Plenum Press.

Bayless, M.D. (1984). *Reproductive Ethics.* Englewood Cliffs, N.J.: Prentice-Hall.

Belsky, J. & Draper, P. (1987). Reproductive strategies and radical solutions. *Society, 24,* 23–24.

Belsky, J. & Rovine, M.J. (1988). Non-maternal care in the first year of life and the security of infant-parent attachment. *Child Development, 59,* 157–167.

Bennett, W.J. (1988, June-July). A curriculum for American students: James Madison High School. *AACJC Journal,* 10.

Berch, D.B. & Bender, B.G. (1987, December). Margins of sexuality. *Psychology Today,* pp. 54–57.

Berger, J. (1988, June 1). Fourth graders writing biography and opening a door to history. *The New York Times*, p. 24.

Berk, L.E. (1986). Private speech: learning out loud. *Psychology Today, 20,* 35–42.

Berk, L.E. (1985). Why children talk to themselves. *Young Children, 40,* 46–52.

Berk, L.E. & Garvin, R.A. (1984). Development of private speech among low-income Appalachian children. *Developmental Psychology, 20,* 271–286.

Berrueta-Clement, J.R., Schweinhart, L.J., Barnett, W.S., Epstein, A.S., & Weikart, D.P. *Changed lives: The effects of the Perry preschool program on youths through age 19.* Ypsilanti, MI: The High/Scope Press.

Bettes, B.A. & Walker, E. (1986). Symptoms associated with suicidal behavior in childhood and adolescence. *Journal of Abnormal Child Psychology, 14,* 591–604.

Bettleheim, B. (1987). *A good enough parent.* New York: Alfred A. Knopf.

Biber, B. (1984). *Early education and psychological development.* New Haven: Yale University Press.

Bithoney, W.G. & Newberger, E.H. (1987). Child and family attributes of failure to thrive. *Developmental and Behavioral Pediatrics, 8,* 32–36.

Blake, L.M. (1988). Babies: Just say no. *Psychology Today, 22,* 16.

Blakeslee, S. (1987, December 14). New attention focused on infant organ donors. *The New York Times*, p. 18.

Block, J., Block, J.H., & Keyes, S. (1988). Longitudinally foretelling drug usage in adolescence: Early childhood personality and environmental precursors. *Child Development, 59,* 336–355.

Bloom, L. (1970). *Language development: form and function in emerging grammars.* Cambridge, MA: MIT Press.

Bobak, I.M. & Jensen, M.D. (1987). *Essentials of maternity nursing: the nurse and the childbearing family* (2nd ed.). St. Louis: C.V. Mosby.

Boston Children's Hospital. (1986). *Parents' guide to nutrition.* Reading, MA: Addison-Wesley.

Boston Woman's Health Book Collective, (1976). From infancy to old age: Development across the lifespan. *Our Bodies, Ourselves.* New York: Simon and Schuster.

Bowlby, J. (1969). *Attachment.* New York: Basic Books.

Bradley, R. (1981). *Husband-coached childbirth* (3rd ed.). New York: Harper & Row.

Brandt, R. (1987). On cooperation in schools: A conversation with David and Roger Johnson. *Educational Leadership, 45,* 14–19.

Brazelton, T.B. (1973). *The neonatal behavioral assessment scale.* Philadelphia: J.B. Lippincott.

Breese, K.M., Director of Employee Relations, Oster/Sunbeam. (1988, July 13). Telephone conversation with the author.

Brody, J.E. (1988, May 26). Reality of adult acne, and the arsenal of weapons available for its treatment, The. *The New York Times*, p. 20.

Brody, J.E. (1987, February 17). Dozens of factors critical in bone loss among elderly. *The New York Times*, p. 20.

Bronfenbrenner, U. (1979). *The ecology of human development: Experiments by nature and design.* Cambridge, MA: Harvard University Press.

Brophy, J.E. (1983). Research on the self-fulfilling prophecy and teacher expectations. *Journal Educational Psychology, 75,* 631–661.

Brown A.L. (1978). Knowing when, where, and how to remember: A problem of meta-cognition. In R. Glaser (Ed.), *Advances in Instructional Psychology*. Hillsdale, NJ: Lawrence Erlbaum, (pp. 77–165).

Brown, R. (1973). *A first language*. Cambridge, MA: Harvard University Press.

Bruner, J.S. (1983). *Child's talk: Learning to use language*. New York: W.W. Norton.

Bruno, R.R. (1987). *After-school care of school-aged children, December 1984*. (Special Studies, Series P-23, No. 149), U.S. Bureau of the Census. Washington, DC: U.S. Government Printing Office.

Buckner, L.M. (1988). On the fast track to. . . ? Is it early childhood education or early adult education? *Young Children, 43*, 5.

Buie, J. (1987). Teen pregnancy: It's time for the schools to tackle the problem. *Phi Delta Kappan, 68*, 738.

Bureau of Labor Statistics, U.S. Department of Labor. (1988). Telephone interview with Howard Hayght, June 2, 1988.

Bus, A.G. & van Ijzendoorn, M.H. (1988). Mother-child interactions, attachment, and emergent literacy: A cross-sectional study, *Child Development, 59*, 1262–1272.

Bybee, R.W. & Sund, R.B. (1982). *Piaget for educators* (2nd ed.). Columbus, OH: Merrill.

Caffary, R.A. (1987). Anorexia and bulimia—the maladjusting coping strategies of the 80s. *Psychology of the Schools, 24*, 45–48.

Capute, A.J. & Accardo, P.J. (1978, November). Linguistic and auditory milestones during the first two years of life: A language inventory for the practicioner. *Clinical Pediatrics, 17*, 847–853.

Capute, A.J., Shapiro, B.K., Wachtel, R.C., Gunther, V.A., & Palmer, F.B. (1986). The clinical linguistic and auditory milestone scale (CLAMS): Identification of cognitive defects in motor delayed children. *American Journal of Diseases of Children, 140*, 694–698.

Carey, S. (1978). The child as word learner. In M. Halle, J. Bresnan, & G.A. Miller (Eds.), *Linguistic theory and psychological reality*, (pp. 263–293). Cambridge, MA: MIT Press.

Carmody, D. (1988, August 17). Hispanic dropout rates puzzling. *The New York Times*, p. 26.

Cawelti, G. (1988, November). Middle schools a better match with early adolescent needs, ASCD survey finds. *ASCD Curriculum Update*, pp. 1–12.

Centers for Disease Control. (1989, July). *HIV-AIDS surveillance report*.

Centers for Disease Control. (1987). Rubella vaccination during pregnancy. *Morbidity and Mortality Weekly Report, 36*, 460–461.

Chaiklin, H., Mosher, B.S., & O'Hara, D.M. (March, 1985). The social and the emotional etiology of childhood lead poisoning. *Journal of sociology and social welfare, XII*, 62–78.

Chambers, M. (1987, February 27). Case against woman in baby death thrown out. *The New York Times*. p. 5.

Chance, P. (1986). *Thinking in the classroom: A survey of programs*. New York: Teachers College Press.

Charlesworth, W.R., (March, 1987). *Revision submitted to Council for the Committee for Ethical Conduct in Child Development Research*. Society for Research in Child Development. Chicago: Approved by the Governing Council of SRCD at the Biennial Meeting of the SRCD. Kansas City, April 1989.

Charlesworth, W.R. & Dzur, C. (1987). Gender comparisons of preschool behavior and resource utilization in group problem solving. *Child Development, 58*, 192.

Chess, S. & Thomas, A. (1987). *Know your child.* New York: Basic Books.

Child development: Language takes on new significance. (May 5, 1987). *The New York Times,* p. 23.

Childbearing occupies short period of woman's life in developed world. (1987, March-April). *Family Planning Perspectives, 19,* 85.

Chomsky, N. (1965). *Aspects of the theory of syntax.* Cambridge, MA: MIT Press.

Clark, E.V. (1983). Meanings and concepts. (in J.H. Flavell & E.M. Markman (Eds.). *Cognitive Development.* Vol. 3 of *Handbook of child psychology,* (4th ed.), P.H. Mussen. New York: John Wiley.

Cobb, P.C. (1988) Personal correspondence with the author. Patricia Cobb provided the information and description of the Parent-child Education Center.

Cohen, D. (1983). *Piaget: critique and assessment.* New York: St. Martin's Press.

Coles, R. (1970). *Erik H. Erikson: the growth of his work.* Boston: Little, Brown.

Coll, C., Garcia, T., Hoffman, J., Oh, W., & Vohr, B.R. (1987). The social ecology and early parenting of Caucasian adolescent mothers. *Child Development, 58,* 955–963.

Coll, C.G., Hoffman, J., & Oh, W. (1986). Maternal and environmental factors affecting developmental outcomes of infants of adolescent mothers. *Developmental and Behavioral Pediatrics, 7,* 230–236.

Colombo, J. (1982). The Critical period concept: Research methodology and research issues. *Psychological Bulletin, 81,* 260–275.

Conners, K.C. & Blouin, A.G. (1983). Nutritional effects on behavior of children. *Journal of Psychiatric Research, 17,* 193–201.

Cornell, B. (1988, February 18). Drug speeds development of fetuses in ailing women. *The Miami Herald,* pp. 1, 16A.

Corsini, R.J. (Ed.). (1984). *Encyclopedia of Psychology* (Vol. 2). New York: John Wiley & Sons.

Craig, G. (1986). *Human Development* (4th ed.). Englewood Cliffs, N.J.: Prentice-Hall.

Crnic, K. & Greenberg, M. (1987, April). *Early family predictors of developmental and social competence of risk and normal children at age five.* Paper presented at the biennial meeting of the Society for Research in Child Development, Baltimore, MD.

Crockenberg, S. (1987). Predictions and correlates of anger toward and punitive control of toddlers by adolescent mothers. *Child Development, 58,* 964–975.

Crockenberg, S. & McCluskey, K. (1986). Change in maternal behavior during the baby's first year of life. *Child Development, 57,* 746–753.

Crook, C. (1987). Taste and olfaction. In P. Salipatek & L. Cohen (Eds.). *Handbook of infant perception: Vol 1. From perception to sensation,* (pp. 237–264). Orlando: Harcourt Brace Jovanovich.

Crook, C. (1979). The organization and control of infant sucking. In H. Reese & L.P. Lipsitt (Eds.). *Advances in child development and behavior* (Vol. 14 pp. 209–251). New York: Academic Press.

Current Population Survey, October, 1986. Telephone interview with Paul Siegel, June 2, 1988, regarding the U.S. Bureau of the census.

Curtiss, S. (1977). *Genie: A psycholinguistic study of a modern day wild child.* New York: Academic Press.

Cutrona, C.E. & Troutman, B.R. (1986). *Child Development, 57,* 1507–1518.

Dale, P.S. (1976). *Language Development* (2nd ed.). New York: Holt, Rinehart & Winston.

DeCasper, A.J. & Fifer, W.P. (1980). Of human bonding: newborns prefer their mothers' voices. *Science, 208,* 1174–1176.

DeFries, J.C., Plomin, R., & LaBuda, M.C. Genetic stability of cognitive development from childhood to adulthood. *Developmental Psychology, 23* (1), 4–12.

Delgado-Gaitan, C. (1986). Adolescent peer influence and differential school performance. *Journal of Adolescent Research, 1,* 449–462.

DeLuccie, M. (1989). Mothers as gatekeepers: A model of maternal mediators of father involvement. Paper presented at the biennial meeting of the Society for Research in Child Development, Kansas City, MO.

Denholm, C.J. & Chabassol, D.J. (1987). Adolescents' self disclosure of potentially embarrassing events. *The Journal of Psychological Reports, 60,* 45–46.

DeStefano, J. (1978). *Language, the learner and the school.* New York: John Wiley.

deVilliers, P.A. & deVilliers, J.G. (1979). *Early language.* Cambridge, MA: Harvard University Press and William Collins.

DeVries, R. (1987). *Programs of early education: The constructivist view.* New York: Longman.

Dewey, J. (1975). *Interest and effort in education.* Carbondale, IL: Southern Illinois University Press.

Dickie, N.H., & Bender, A.E. (1982). Breakfast and performance in schoolchildren. *British Journal of Nutrition, 48,* 482–496.

Dick-Read, G. (1959). *Childbirth without fear.* New York: Harper & Row.

Dimidjian, V.J. (1986). Helping children in times of trouble and crisis. *Journal of children in contemporary society, 17,* 113–128.

Discount Store News. (1988, May 9). p. 85.

Donovan, J.R. (1989, March 28). Letters to the editor. *The New York Times,* p. 21.

Doutre, C.B. (1988). Put on their creative thinking caps and add sparkle and verve to the whole curriculum. *Learning 88, 17,* 28–32.

Eagan, A.B. (1985, December). Two hundred years of childbirth. *Parents, 60,* p. 188.

Egeland, J.A., Gerhard, D.S., Pauls, D.L., Sussex, J.N., Kidd, K.K., Allen, C.R., Hostetter, A.M., & Housman, D.E. (1987). Bipolar affective disorders linked to DNA markers on chromosome 11. *Nature, 325,* 783–787.

Elkind, D. (1987). *Mid-education: Preschoolers at risk.* New York: Alfred A. Knopf.

Elkind, D. (1987, May). Superkids and super problems. *Psychology Today,* p. 60.

Elkind, D. (1986). Formal education and early education: An essential difference. *Phi Delta Kappan, 67,* 634.

Elkind, D. (1984). *All grown up and no place to go.* Reading, MA: Addison-Wesley.

Elliman, A.M., Bryan, E.M., & Elliman, A.D. (1986). Low birth weight babies at 3 years of age. *Child Care, Health and Development, 12,* 287–311.

Emihovich, C., Gaier, E.L., & Cronin, M.C. (1984). Sex role expectation changes by fathers for their sons. *Sex roles, 11,* 861–868.

Ennis, R.H. (1987). A taxonomy of critical thinking, dispositions, and abilities. In J.B. Baron and R.J. Sternberg (Eds.). *Teaching thinking skills: Theory and practice* (pp. 9–26). New York: W.H. Freeman.

Erikson, E. (1963). *Childhood and society.* New York: Norton.

Espenschade, A.S. & Eckert, H.M. (1980). *Motor development* (2nd ed.). Columbus, OH: Merrill.

Ethical considerations of the new reproductive technologies. *Fertility and Sterility Supplement 1, 46.* 57S.

Evans, R.I. (1973). *Jean Piaget: The man and his ideas.* New York: E.P. Dutton.

Evans, R.I. (1968). *B.F. Skinner: The man and his ideas.* New York: E.P. Dutton.

Fabrizi, M.S. & Pollo, H.R. (1987). A naturalistic study of humorous activity in a third, seventh, and eleventh grade classroom. *Merrill-Palmer Quarterly, 33,* 107–128.

Falbo, T. (Ed.). (1984). *The single-child family.* New York: The Guilford Press.

Fantz, R. (1961). The origin of form perception. *Scientific American, 204,* 66–72.

Farber, E.A. & Egeland, B. Developmental consequences of out-of-home care for infants in a low-income population. In E.F. Zigler & E.W. Gordon (Eds.). *Day Care: Scientific and social policy issues,* (pp. 102–125). Boston: Auburn House.

Feinbloom, R.I., and The Boston Children's Medical Center. (1979). *Pregnancy, birth and the newborn baby.* New York: Delacorte Press.

Field, D.E. (1987, April). *Television coviewing related to family characteristics and cognitive performance.* Paper presented at the bienneal meetings of the Society for Research in Child Development, Baltimore, MD.

Field, T. (1987). Baby research comes of age. *Psychology Today, 21,* 46.

Field, T., Woodsen, R., Greenberg, R., & Cohen, D. (1982). Discrimination and imitation of facial expressions by neonates. *Science, 218,* 179–181.

Fine, G.A. (1987). *With the boys Little League baseball and preadolescent culture.* Chicago: The University of Chicago Press.

Fine, M. (1986). Why urban adolescents drop into and out of public high school. *Teachers College Record, 87,* 393–409.

Fiske, E. (1988, May 24). In Indiana, public school makes "frills" standard. *The New York Times,* p. A16.

Flaste, R. (1988, October 9). The myth about teen-agers. *The New York Times Magazine,* p. 76.

Flavell, J.H. (1985). *Cognitive development* (2nd ed.). Englewood Cliffs, NJ: Prentice Hall.

Fong, B.C. & Resnick, M.R. (1986). *The Child: Development through adolescence* (2nd ed.). Palo Alto, CA: Mayfield.

Forman, M.R., Meirik, O., & Bracken, M.B. (1987). Delayed childbearing: No evidence for the increased risk of low birth weight and preterm delivery. *American Journal of Epidemiology, 125,* 101–109.

Forrester, J.D. (1987, May-June). Has she or hasn't she? U.S. Women's Experiences with contraception. *Family Planning Perspectives, 19.* 113.

Fowler, M.G. & Cross, A.W. (1986). Preschool risk factors as predictors of early school performance. *Developmental and Behavioral Pediatrics, 7,* 237–241.

Francher, R.E. (1979). *Pioneers of psychology.* New York: W.W. Norton.

Frankenburg, W.K., Fanctal, A.W., Sciarillo, W., & Burgess, D. (1981). The newly abbreviated and revised Denver Developmental Screening Test. *The Journal of Pediatrics, 99,* 995–999.

Freud, S. (1973). *An outline of psychoanalysis.* London: Hogarth.

Fruedenheim, M. (1988, December 28). In pursuit of the punctual baby. *The New York Times,* p. 25.

Frustenberg, F., Brooks-Gunn, J., & Morgan, S.P. (1987). *Adolescent mothers in later life.* Cambridge, England: Cambridge University Press.

Futrell, M.H. (1987). Public schools and four-year olds. *American Psychologist, 42,* 251–253.

Gallup A.M. (1986). The eighteenth annual Gallup poll of the public's attitude toward the public schools. *Phi Delta Kappan, 68,* 55–56.

Garrard, K.R. (1986). Helping young children develop mature speech patterns. *Young Children, 42,* 16–21.

Garrison, E.G. (1987). The juvenile justice and delinquency prevention act. *Social Policy Report, 11,* 4.

Gay, L.R., (1987), *Educational research: Competencies for analysis and application* (3rd Ed.). Columbus, OH: Merrill.

Gelles, R.J. School-age parents and child abuse. In J.B. Lancaster & B.A. Hamburg (Eds.). *School-age pregnancy and parenthood: Biosocial dimensions.* (pp. 347–359). New York: Aldine DeGruyter.

George, P. (1988). Education 2000: Which way the middle school? *The Clearing House, 62,* 15.

Gesell, A. (1928). *Infancy and human growth.* New Haven, CT: Gesell Institute of Human Development.

Gesell Institute of Human Development. (1978). *Preschool readiness test.* New Haven, CT: Author.

Gibson, E.J. & Walk, R.D. (1960). The visual cliff. *Scientific American, 202,* 64–71.

Gilligan, C. (1987, Fall). Adolescent development reconsidered. In C.E. Irwin, Jr. (Ed.). *Adolescent social behavior and health.* (New Directions for Child Development, No. 37). San Francisco: Josey-Bass.

Ginsburg, H. & Opper, S. (1979). *Piaget's theory of intellectual development.* Englewood Cliffs, NJ: Prentice-Hall.

Gold, S. (1983). Parent-infant bonding: Another look. *Child Development, 54,* 1355–1382.

Goldstein, B.E. (1984). *Sensation and perception* (2nd ed.). Belmont, CA: Wadsworth.

Goleman, D. (1988, October 6). Aggression in children can mean problems later. *The New York Times,* p. 22.

Goleman, D. (1988, February 2). The experience of touch: Research points to a critical role. *The New York Times,* pp. 17 and 20.

Goleman, D. (1987, August 25). Embattled giant of psychology speaks his mind. *The New York Times,* p. 17.

Goodman, Y. (1980). The roots of literacy. In M.P. Douglas (Ed.). *Reading: A humanistic experience.* Claremont, CA: Claremont Graduate School.

Gould, S.J. (1982). Human babies as embryos. In J. Belsky (Ed.). *In the Beginning: Readings in infancy.* New York: Columbia University Press.

Green, R. (1987). *The sissy boy syndrome and the development of homosexuality.* New Haven: Yale University Press.

Green, R. (1982). Relationship between "feminine" and "masculine" behavior during boyhood and sexual orientation during manhood. In *Sexology—sexual biology, behavior and therapy: Selected papers of the 5th World Congress of Sexology,* Jerusalem, Israel, June 21–26, 1981.

Greenberger, E. & Steinberg, L. (1986). *When teenagers work.* New York: Basic Books.

Greenhouse, Linda. (1989). A right is challenged—Justices accept more cases on the issue. *The New York Times,* July 4, 1989.

Groller, I. (1987, October), Is surrogate motherhood okay? *Parents,* p. 28.

Gromley, A.V., Gromley, J.B., & Weiss, H. (1987). Motivations for parenthood among young adult college students. *Sex roles, 16,* 34–36.

Group for the Advancement of Psychiatry. (1987). *Crisis of adolescence: Teenage pregnancy, impact on adolescent development.* New York: Brunner/Mazel.

Guillen, M.A. (1984, December). The first cause. *Psychology Today,* pp. 72–73.

Haith, M. (1986). Sensory and perceptual processes in early infancy. *The Journal of Pediatrics, 109,* 158–171.

Hall, N. (1987). *The emergence of literacy.* Portsmouth, NH: Heinemann.

Hamill, P.V.V., Drizd, T.A., Reed, R.B., Johnson, C.L., Roche, A.F., & Moore, W.M. (1979). Physical growth: National Center for Health Statistics Percentiles. *The American Journal of Clinical Nutrition, 32,* 607–629.

Hanafin, H. *Surrogate parenting: Reassessing human bonding.* Paper presented at the convention of the American Psychological Association. New York. (1987, August 28).

Harlap, S. (1979, June 28). Gender of infants conceived on different days of the menstrual cycle. *New England Journal of Medicine, 300,* 1447.

Harlow, H.F. & Harlow, M.K. (1962). Social deprivation in monkeys. *Scientific American, 207,* 136–144.

Hartup, W.W., Laursen, B., Stewart, M.I., & Eastenson, A. (1988). Conflict and the friendship relations of young children. *Child Development, 59,* 1590–1600.

Havens, B. & Swenson, I. (1986). Menstrual perceptions and preparation among female adolescents. *Journal of Obstetric, Gynecologic and Neonatal Nursing, 15,* 406–411.

Haviland, C.E. & Lelwica, M. (1987). The induced affect response: Ten-week-old infants' responses to three emotional expressions. *Developmental Psychology, 23,* 97–104.

Henig, R.M. (1988, May 22). Should baby read? *The New York Times Magazine,* pp. 37–38.

Hetherington, E.M. & Parke, R.D. (1986). *Child psychology: A contemporary viewpoint.* New York: McGraw-Hill.

Hicky, T.L. & Peduzzi, J.D. (1987). Structure and development of the visual system. In P. Salapatek & L. Cohen (Eds.). *Handbook of infant perception* (Vol. 1. From sensation to perception, pp. 1–42). Orlando: Harcourt Brace Jovanovich.

Ho, Hsiu-Zu, Glahn, T.J., & Ho, Ju-Chang. (1986). The fragile-x syndrome. *Developmental medicine and child neurology, 30,* 252–265.

Hofferth, S., Kahn, J.R., & Baldwin, W. (1987). Premarital sexual activity among U.S. teenage women over the past three decades. *Family Planning Perspectives, 19,* 46–53.

Hogue, C. (1981). Coffee consumption in pregnancy. *Lancet, 1,* 554.

Holden, C. (1987, September). Genes and behavior: A twin legacy. *Psychology Today,* p. 18.

Hollinger, P.C., Offer, D., & Zola, M.A. (1988). A prediction model of suicide among youth. *The Journal of Nervous and Mental Disease, 170,* 277.

Homann, M., Banet, B.F. & Weikart, D.P. (1979). *Young children in action.* Ypsilanti, MI: The High/Scope Press.

Hoskisson, K. & Tompkins, G.E. *Language arts: Content and teaching strategies.* Columbus, OH: Merrill.

Howes, C. (1988). Peer interaction of young children. *Monographs of the Society for Research in Child Development, 53* (Serial No. 217).

Huston, A.C. (1983). Sex-typing. In P.H. Mussen, & E.M. Hetherington (Eds.). *Socialization, personality and social development* Vol. 4. New York: John Wiley.

Invention eases colic symptoms. (1988, January-February). *Children Today, 17,* 2.

Jambor, T. (1986). Risk-taking needs in children: An accommodating play environment. *Children's Environment Quarterly, 3,* 22–25.

Jankowski, C.B. (1986, March). Radiation and pregnancy: Putting the risks in proportion. *The American Journal of Nursing, 86,* 260–265.

Jessor, R. & Jessor, S.L. (1978). *Problem behavior and psychological development: A longitudinal study of youth.* New York: Academic Press.

Johnson, J. (1989, March 8). Curriculum seeks to lift blacks' self-image. *The New York Times,* p. 1.

Johnson, J.E., Christie, J.F., & Yawkey, T.B. (1987). *Play and early childhood development.* Glenview, IL: Scott, Foresman.

Johnson, W.G. & Corrigan, S.A. (1987). The behavioral treatment of child and adolescent obesity. *Journal of Child and Adolescent Psychotherapy, 4,* 91–100.

Jones, E. (1961). *The life and work of Sigmund Freud.* (J. Trilling & S. Marcus, eds). New York: Basic Books.

Jones, T. (1988, June 1). Quebec tries to buck trend, kindle baby boom with cash. *The Miami Herald,* p. 2A.

Joselow, F. (1989, March 26). Why business turns to teen-agers. *The New York Times,* Section 3, pp. 3, 6.

Judd, D.M., Siders, J.A., Siders, J.Z., & Atkins, K.R. (1986). Sex-related differences on fine-motor tasks at grade one. *Perceptual and Motor Skills, 62,* 307–312.

Juvenile Justice and Delinquency Prevention Act of 1974 (Public Law 93–415) as amended through September 30, 1985). 42 U.S. Code Section 5601). (1985).

Kagan, J.J., Reznick, S., & Snidman, N. (1988). Biological bases of childhood shyness. *Science, 240,* 167–171.

Kahn, F. (1943, 1971). *Man in structure and function.* New York: Alfred A. Knopf.

Kamii, C. (1981). Application of Piaget's theory to education: The preoperational level. In I.E. Sigel, D.M. Brodzinsky, R.M. Golinkoff, (Eds.). *New directions in Piagetian theory and practice.* Hillsdale, N.J.: Lawrence Erlbaum Associates.

Kandal, D.B., Kessler, R.C., & Margulies, R.Z. (1978). Antecedents of adolescent initiation in stages of drug use: A developmental analysis. In D.B. Kandel (Ed.). *Longitudinal research in drug use.* (pp. 73–99). New York: John Wiley.

Kaplan, H.B., Martin, S.S., & Robbins, C. (1982). Application of a general theory of deviant behavior: Self-derogation and adolescent drug use. *Journal of Health and Social Behavior, 23,* 274–294.

Kass, S.A. (1989, January 8). Recess, an endangered playtime. *The New York Times,* Section 4A, pp. 7–8.

Katchadourian, H. (1977). *The biology of adolescence.* San Francisco: W.H. Freeman.

Keller, B. (1987, December 26). Mother Russia makes a comeback on births. *The New York Times.* pps. 1, 4.

Kellog, R. (1970). Understanding children's art. In P. Cramer (Ed.). *Readings in developmental psychology today.* Delmar, CA: CRM Books. (pp. 31–39).

Kinard, E.M. & Reinherz, H. (1987). School aptitude and achievement in children of adolescent mothers. *Journal of Youth and Adolescence, 16,* 69–87.

Klaus, M.H. & Kennell, J.H. (1982). *Parent-infant bonding* (2nd ed.). St. Louis: C.V. Mosby.

Klebanoff, M.A., Koslowe, P.A., Kaslow, R., & Rhoades, G.G. (1985). Epidemiology of vomiting in early pregnancy. *Obstetrics and Gynecology, 66,* 612–616.

Kline, M. (1989, April). *Work and family life during the transition to parenthood.* Paper presented at the "Becoming a Family" Project Symposium at the biennial meeting of the Society for Research in Child Development, Kansas City, MO.

Kogan, S.C., Doherty, M., & Gitschier, J. (1987, October 15). An improved method for prenatal diagnosis of genetic diseases by analysis of amplified DNA sequences. *New England Journal of Medicine, 317,* 985–990.

Kohlberg, L. (1973, October 25). The claim to moral adequacy of a highest state of moral judgement. *The Journal of Philosophy, 70,* 630–646.

Kolata, G. (1988, October 4). New egg-implanting technique avoids surgery. *The New York Times,* p. 27.

Kolata, G. (1988, May 24). Children and AIDS: Drug tests raise hope and ethical concerns. *The New York Times,* p. 23.

Kolata, G. (1988, April 22). Anti-acne drug faulted in birth defects. *The New York Times,* p. 1.

Kolata, G. (1988, February 15). New obesity studies indicate metabolism is often to blame. *The New York Times,* pp. 15, 19.

Kolata, G. (1984). Studying learning in the womb. *Science, 225,* 302–303.

Konner, M. (1989, January 8). Where should baby sleep? *The New York Times Magazine,* pp. 39–40.

Konstantareas, M.M., Hauser, P., Lennox, C., & Homatidis, S. (1986). Season of birth in infantile autism. *Child Psychiatry and Human Development, 17,* 53–65.

Korner, A.F. & Thoman, E.B. (1977). The relative efficacy of contact and vestibular-proprioceptive stimulation in soothing neonates. *Child Development, 43,* 443–453.

Kostelink, M.J., Stein, L.C., Whiren, A.P., & Soderman, A.K. (1988) *Guiding children's social development.* Cincinnati, OH: South-Western Publishing Co. pp. 359–362.

Kryukova, N. (1987, June). Child of the sea. *Soviet Life,* pp. 22–25.

Kuhn, D. (1984). Cognitive development. In M.H. Bernstein & M.E. Lamb (Eds.). *Developmental psychology: An advanced textbook.* pp. 133–180. Hillsdale, N.J.: Lawrence Erlbaum Associates.

Kuhn, D. (1981). The role of self-directed activity in cognitive development. In I. Sigel, D.M. Brodzinsky, & R.M. Golinkoff (Eds.). *New directions in Piagetian theory and practice.* (pp. 353–363). Hillsdale, NJ: Lawrence Erlbaum.

Ladd, G.W. & Price, J.M. (1987). Predicting children's social and school adjustment following the transition from preschool to kindergarten. *Child Development, 58,* 1168–1189.

Lamaze, F. (1970). *Painless childbirth,* Chicago: Henry Regnery.

Lamb, M.E. (1981). *The role of the father in child development* (2nd Ed.). New York: John Wiley.

Lambert, B. (1988, January 13). One in 61 babies in New York has AIDS antibodies, study says. *The New York Times,* p. 1.

Landry, E., Bertrand, J.T., Cherry, F., & Rice, J. (1986). Teen pregnancy in New Orleans: Factors that differentiate teens who deliver, abort and successfully contracept. *Journal of Youth and Adolescence, 15,* 259–274.

Lang, S.S. (1986). Tots on wheels. (1986, July-August). *American Health,* p. 86.

Langlois, J.H., Roggman, L.A., Cassey, R.J., Ritter, J.M., Rieser-Danner, L.A., & Jenkins, V.Y. (1987). Infant preferences for attractive faces: Rudiments of a stereotype? *Developmental Psychology, 23,* 363–369.

Lapierre, D. (1985). *The city of joy.* Garden City, NY: Doubleday.

LeBoyer, F. (1975). *Birth without violence.* New York: Alfred Knopf.

Lee, V.E. & Bryk, A.S. (1986). Effects of single sex secondary school on student achievement and attitudes. *Journal of Educational Psychology, 78,* 381–395.

Lessa, W.A. & Smith, M.T. (1989, March). *Coping with the adolescent years: An interdisciplinary approach to parent education.* A paper presented at the 44th Annual Conference of the Association for Supervision and Curriculum Development, Orlando, FL.

Lester, B.M. (1985). There's more to crying than meets the ear. In B.M. Lester and C.F. Boukydis (Eds.). *Infant crying.* (pp. 1–27). New York: Plenum Press.

Lewin, T. (1987, August 16). Medical uses of fetal tissue spurs new abortion debate. *The New York Times,* p. 16.

Lewis, M. (1988). Infant concern. *Working Parents, 5,* 14–15.

Lewis, M. & Michalson, L. (1985). The gifted infant. In J. Freeman (Ed.). *The psychology of gifted children.* New York: John Wiley.

Lieberman, P. (1984). *Biology and the evolution of language.* Cambridge, MA: Harvard University Press.

Lipman, M. (1988). Critical thinking—what can it be? *Educational Leadership, 46,* 40.

Lipsitt, L.P. (1986). Learning in infancy: Cognitive development in babies. *The Journal of Pediatrics, 109,* 173.

Lipsitt, L.P. (1977). Taste in human neonates: Its effects on sucking and heart rate. In J.M. Weiffenbach (Ed.). *Taste and development: The genesis of sweet preference.* (pp. 125–140).

Lipsitt, L.P. & Kaye, H. (1964). Conditioned sucking in the human newborn. *Psychometric Science, 1,* 29–30.

London, Perry. (1987). Character education and clinical intervention: A paradigm shift for U.S. schools. *Phi Delta Kappan, 68,* 667–673.

Long, T.J. & Long, L. (1983). *The handbook for latchkey children and their parents.* New York: Arbor House.

Longstreth, L.G. (1980). Human handedness: More evidence for genetic involvement. *The Journal of Genetic Psychology, 137,* 275–283.

Lowery, G.H. (1986). *Growth and development of children* (8th Ed.). Chicago: Year Book Medical.

Lowery, R.J. (1973). *A.H. Maslow: An intellectual portrait.* Belmont, CA: Wadsworth.

Lynn, K.S. (1987). *Hemingway.* New York: Simon and Schuster.

Maccoby, E.E. & Jacklin, C. (1974). *The psychology of sex differences.* Stanford, CA: Stanford University Press.

Maccoby, E.E. & Martin, J.A. (1983). Socialization in the context of the family: parent-child interaction. In *Socialization, personality and social development.* E. Hetherington (ed). Vol. 4 of Mussen (ed). *Handbook of child psychology.* New York: John Wiley.

MacFarlane, A. (1977). *The psychology of childbirth.* Cambridge, MA: Harvard University Press.

Macnamara, J. (1982). *Names for things.* Cambridge, MA: MIT Press.

Madrazo, I. et al. (1988), Transplantation of fetal substantia nigra and adrenal medulla to the caudate nucleus in two patients with Parkinson's disease. (Correspondence). *New England Journal of Medicine, 318,* 51.

Mama, talk to your baby. (1987, November 2). *Newsweek,* p. 75.

Maranto, G. (1984, October). Choosing your baby's sex. *Discover,* pp. 25–27.

Mardell-Czudnowski, C. & Goldenberg, D. (1983). *DIAL-R: Developmental indicators for the assessment of learning—revised.* Edison, NJ: Childcraft.

Markham, L.R. (1984). Assisting speakers of black English as they begin to write. *Young Children, 39,* 15–24.

Maslow, A.H. (1970). *Motivation and personality.* New York: Harper & Row.

Maslow, A.H. (1968). *Toward a psychology of being.* Princeton, N.J.: Van Nostrand.

McCarthy, P.A. (1983, January). Fetal alcohol syndrome and other alcohol-related birth defects. *Nurse-practicioner, 8,* 34.

McCarthy, P.A. (1983). *American Journal of Primary Health Care, 8,* 34.

McFarlane, A. (1978). What a baby knows. *Human Nature, 1,* 74–81.

McKay, H., Sinisterra, L., McKay, A., Gomes, H., & Lloreda, P. (1978). Improving cognitive ability in chronically deprived children. *Science, 200,* 270–278.

McMillan, J.H. & Schumacher, S. (1984). *Research in education: A conceptual approach.* Boston: Little, Brown.

McTighe, J. (nd). *Improving the quality of student thinking.* Baltimore, MD: Maryland State Department of Education.

Meltzoff, A. & Moore, K.M. (1983). Newborn infants imitate adult facial gestures. *Child Development, 54,* 703–709.

Merahn, S., Shelov, S., & McCracken, G. (1988, March). AIDS: What teachers, directors and parents want to know. *Scholastic Pre-K Today,* pp. 3–6.

Michel, G.F., Ovrut, M.A., & Harkins, D.A. (1985). Hand-use preference for reaching object manipulation in 6- through 13-month-old infants. *Genetic, Social, and General Psychology Monographs, 111,* 422.

Miller, A. & Gilda, P.M. (1987, September). How children learn words. *Scientific American, 257,* 94–99.

Miller, E., Cradock-Watson, J.E., & Pollock, M. (1982). Consequences of confirmed maternal rubella at successive stages of pregnancy. *The Lancet,* 781–784.

Miller, S.H. (1983). *Children as parents: Final report on a study of childbearing and child rearing among 12- to 15-year-olds.* New York: Child Welfare League of America, p. 111.

Miller, W. (1983), Chance, choice and the future of reproduction. *American Psychologist, 38,* 1198–1205.

Montessori, M. (1967). *The discovery of the child.* Notre Dame, IN: Fides.

Moore, K.L. (1974). *Before we are born.* Philadelphia: Saunders. p. 96.

Morrison, G.S. (1988). *Early childhood education today* (4th Ed.). Columbus, OH: Charles E. Merrill.

Morrison, G.S. (1988) *Education and development of infants, toddlers and preschoolers.* Glenview, IL: Scott, Foresman.

Moss, R.C.S. (1986). Frank Lake's maternal-fetal distress syndrome and primal integration workshops—part II. *Pre- and Perinatal Psychology, 1,* 52–53.

Mott, F. & Marsiglio, W. (1985). Early childbearing and completion of high school. *Family Planning Perspectives, 17,* 234–237.

Muhlen, L., Pryke, M., & Wade, K. (1986). Effects of type of birth and anesthetic on neonatal behavioral assessment scale scores. *Australian Psychologist, 21,* 253–270.

Mulinare, J., Cerdero, J., Erickson, D.J., & Berry, R.J. (1988). Periconceptional use of multivitamins and the occurrence of neural tube defects. *JAMA, 260,* 3141–3145.

Murphy, D.F. (1988). The just community at Birch Meadow Elementary School. *Phi Delta Kappan, 69,* 427–428.

Murray, A.D., Dolby, R.M., Nation, R.L., & Thomas, D.B. (1981). Effects of epidural anesthesia on newborns and their mothers. *Child development, 52,* 71–82.

Murray, J.B. (1986). Psychological aspects of anorexia nervosa. *Genetic, Social, and General Psychology Monographs, 112,* 5–40.

Murray, P., (1987, April). *Infants' responsiveness to modeling vs. instruction.* Paper presented at the biennial meeting of the Society for Research in Child Development, Baltimore, MD.

Myers, B.J. (1987). Mother-infant bonding as a critical period. In M.H. Bornstein (Ed.), *Sensitive periods in development: Interdisciplinary perspectives.* Hillsdale, N.J.: Lawrence Erlbaum Associates.

National Association for the Education of Young Children. (1986, September). Position statement on developmentally appropriate practice in early childhood programs serving children from birth through age four. *Young Children, 41,* 4–29.

National Center for Health Statistics. (1988). *Advanced report of final divorce statistics, 1985.* (Monthly Vital Statistics Report, Vol. 36, No. 8 Supplement, DHHS Publication No. (PHS) 88–1120). Hyattesville, MD: Author.

National Center for Health Statistics. (1986, June). *Maternal weight gain and the outcome of pregnancy, United States, 1980.* (Vital and Health Statistics. Series 21, No. 44, DHHS Publication No. PHS 86–122.) Washington, DC: Public Health Service.

National Council on Radiation Protection and Measurement. (1977). *Review of NCRP radiation dose limit for embryo and fetus in occupationally exposed women.* (NCRP Publication No. 53). Washington, DC: U.S. Government Printing Office.

National Institutes of Health. (1984). Consensus Development Conference. *Diagnostic ultrasound imaging in pregnancy.* National Institute of Health.

National Institutes of Health (1980). *Cesarean Childbirth.* National Institutes of Health Consensus Development Conference Summary.

Neeson, J.D. & May, K.A. (1986). *Comprehensive maternity nursing.* Philadelphia: J.B. Lippincott.

Nelson, M. et al. (1980). Randomized clinical trial of the LeBoyer approach to childbirth. *The New England Journal of Medicine, 302,* 655–659.

New York Times, The. (July 4, 1989). Excerpts from the court decision on the regulation of abortion. p. 10.

Newcomer, S.F. & Udry, R.J. (1985). Parent-child communication and adolescent sexual behavior. *Family Planning Perspectives, 17,* 169–174.

Newman, J.M. (1985). *Whole language: Theory in use.* Portsmouth, NH: Heinemann.

Newport, E.L., Gleitman, H., & Gleitman, L. (1977). Mother, I'd rather do it myself: Some effects and non-effects of maternal speech style. In C.E. Snow & C.A. Ferguson (Eds.). *Talking to children: Language input and acquisition.* Cambridge, England: Cambridge University Press, (pp. 112–129).

Nickel, R.E., Forrest, B.C., & Lamson, F.N. (1982). School performance of children with birth weights of 1,000 g or less. *American Journal of Disabled Children, 136,* 105–110.

Nilsson, L. (1977), *A child is born.* New York: Delacorte Press/Seymour Lawrence, p. 22.

1988 world population data sheet. (1988, April). Washington, DC: Population Reference Bureau.

Norton, A.J. (1987, July-August). Families and Children in the year 2000. *Children Today,* 16.

Nowlis, G.H. & Kessen, W. (1976). Human newborns differentiate differing concentrations of sucrose and glucose. *Science, 191,* 865.

Offer, D. (1987). In defense of adolescents. *Journal of the American Medical Association, 257,* 3047–3408.

O'Neil, J. (1989). Whole language: New view of literacy gains in influence. *ASCD Update, 31,* 1, 6–7.

Onley, P., Weckerly, E., & Puckett, K. (1989, March). *Loving intervention for teens.* A paper presented at the 44th Annual Conference of the Association for Supervision and Curriculum Development, Orlando, FL.

Otten, A.L. (1988, May 18). Study cites lack of success with in vitro fertilization. *The Wall Street Journal,* p. 33.

Owen, A.L. (1980). *Feeding guide: A nutritional guide for the maturing infant.* Bloomfield, N.J.: Health Learning Systems.

Palinscar, A.S. & Ransom, K. (1988). From the mystery spot to the thoughtful spot: The instruction of metacognitive strategies. *The Reading Teacher, 41,* 784–789.

Papousek, H.A. (1967). Conditioning during early postnatal development. In Brackbill & G.B. Thompson (Eds.). *Behavior in infancy and early childhood.* New York: Free Press.

Parent's Guide to Infant Nutrition. (1986). Evansville, IN: Mead, Johnson.

Parnell, D. (1988, June-July). Does one curriculum really fit all? *AACJC Journal,* 11.

Parten, M. (1932). Social play among preschool children, *Journal of Abnormal and Social Psychology, 27,* 243–269.

Patterson, D. (1987, August). The causes of Down Syndrome. *Scientific American, 257,* 52.

Pederson, D. & TerVrught, D. (1973). The influence of amplitude and frequency of vestibular stimulation on the activity of two-month-old infants. *Child Development, 44,* 122–128.

Petersen, A.C. (1987). Those gangly years. *Psychology Today, 21,* 28–34.

Petersen, A.C. (1987). The nature of biological-psychological interactions: The sample case of early adolescence. In R.M. Lerner & T.T. Foch (Eds.). *Biological-psychological inter-actions in early adolescence.* Hillsdale, NJ: Lawrence Erlbaum.

Phillips, D.P. & Paight, D.J. (1987). The impact of televised movies about suicide. *The New England Journal of Medicine, 317,* 809–811.

Phipps-Yonas, S. (1980, October). Teenage pregnancy and parenthood: A review of the literature. *American Journal of Orthopsychiatry, 50,* 403–431.

Piaget, J. (1970). *Genetic epistemology.* (E. Duckworth, Trans.). New York: Columbia University Press.

Piaget, J. (1965). *The child's conception of number.* New York: W.W. Norton.

Piaget, J. (1962). *Play, dreams and imitation in childhood.* New York: W.W. Norton.

Piaget, J. (1952). The origins of intelligence in children. (Cook, Trans.). New York: International Universities Press.

Piaget, J. (1932). *The moral judgement of the child.* (M. Gabin, Trans.). New York: The Free Press.

Piaget, J. & Inhelder, B., (1958). *The growth of logical thinking from childhood to adolescence.* Trans. (A. Parsons & S. Seagrin). New York: Basic Books.

Picton, T.W., Stuss, D.T., & Marshall, K.C. (1986). Attention and the brain. In S.L. Friedman, K.A. Klivington, & R.W. Peterson (Eds.). *The brain, cognition and education,* (pp. 19–79).

Pollitt, E. (1988, Winter). A child survival and developmental revolution: GOBI-FFF. *SRCD Newsletter,* p. 4.

Post-graduate pharmacist/continuing education drugs and the human fetus. (1981, March). *U.S. Pharmacist, 6,* 44–61.

Potts, L. (1980, October). Considering parenthood: Group support for a critical life decision. *American Journal of Orthopsychiatry, 50,* 629–638.

Predicting diseases. *U.S. News and World Report,* (1987, May 25), p. 65.

Public Citizen Health Research Group. (1989, January/February). C-section rates remain high, but postcesarean vaginal births are rising. *Family planning perspectives, 21,* 36–37.

Pulaski, M.A.S. (1980). *Understanding Piaget.* (rev. ed.). New York: Harper & Row.

Quinn, J. (1986). Rooted in research: Effective adolescent pregnancy prevention programs. *Adolescent sexualities.* Falls Church, VA: Haworth.

Ramsey, B. (1988). Kids who drink: Nursing the bottle? *Family Album.* Miami, FL: Charter Hospital.

Raper, J. & Aldridge, J. (1988, February). What every teacher should know about AIDS. *Childhood Education,* pp. 146–149.

Read, E.W. (1988, February 2). Birth cycle. *The Wall Street Journal,* p. 1.

Recognition of the middle level of schooling. (1988). *Middle School Journal, 19,* 27.

Reinhold, R. (1988, February 22). New law will warn Californians of chemical risks of modern life. *The New York Times,* pp. 1, 10.

Reisman, J.E. (1987). Touch, motion and proprioception. In P. Salapatek & L. Cohen (Eds.). *Handbook of infant perception: Vol. 1. From sensation to perception.* (p. 265). Orlando: Harcourt Brace Jovanovich.

Restak, R. (1986). *The infant mind.* Garden City, NY: Doubleday.

Rhodes, R. (1986). *The making of the atomic bomb.* New York: Simon & Schuster, p. 28.

Richmond, P. (1970). *An introduction to Piaget.* New York: Basic Books.

Richmond-Abbott, M. (1984). Sex role attitudes and children in divorced, single parent families. *Journal of divorce, 8,* 61–81.

Ricklefs, R. (1987, November 24), What a darling baby! Let's push, rewind and see her again. *The Wall Street Journal.* p. 1.

Robinson, B.E., Coleman, M., & Rowland, B.H. (1986). The after-school ecologies of latchkey children. *Children's Environments Quarterly, 3,* 4–8.

Robinson, C.C. & Morris, J.T. (1986). The gender-stereotyped nature of Christmas toys received by 36-, 48-, and 60-month-old children: A comparison between requested and nonrequested toys. *Journal of Sex Roles, 15,* 21–32.

Rodman, H., Prato, D., & Nelson, R. (1985). Child care arrangements and children's functioning: A comparison of self-care and adult-care children. *Developmental Psychology, 21,* 413–418.

Roosa, M.W. (1984). Short-term effects of teenage parenting programs on knowledge and attitudes. *Adolescence, XIX,* 659–666.

Rose, S., Schmidt, K., Riese, M., & Bridger, W. (1980). Effects of prematurity and early intervention on responsivity to tactile stimuli: A comparison of preterm and full-term infants. *Child Development, 51,* 416–425.

Rosenblith, J.F. & Sims-Knight, J.E. (1985). *In the Beginning: Development in the first two years.* Monterey, CA: Brooks/Cole.

Rosenstein, D. & Oster, H. (1988). Differential facial responses to four basic tastes in newborns. *Child Development, 59,* 1562.

Ross, H.S. & Lollis, S.P. (1987). Communication within infant social games. *Developmental Psychology, 23,* 241–248.

Rubin, N. (1988, February). Baby fat or just plain fat. *Parents,* p. 103.

Rumors of suicides cancel graduation. (1988, June 6). *The Miami Herald,* p. 2A.

Sadker, M. & Sadker, D. (1985, March). Sexism in the school room of the '80s. *Psychology Today,* 54–57.

Salkind, N.J. (1985). *Theories of human development.* New York: John Wiley & Sons, p. 6.

Sameroff, A.J., Seifer, R., Baldwin, C., & Baldwin, A. (1989, April). *Continuity of risk from early childhood to adolescence.* Paper presented at the biennial meeting of the Society for Research in Child Development, Kansas City, MO.

Save the Children Federation. (1985). *Hard choices: Portraits of poverty and hunger in America.* Westport, CT: Author.

Scarborough, H. & Wyckoff, J. (1986). Mother, I'd still rather do it myself: Some further non-effects of motherese. *Journal of Child Language, 13,* 431–437.

Scarr, S. (1984, May). Interview. *Psychology Today,* pp. 59–63.

Schaffer, R. (1977). *Mothering.* Cambridge, MA: Harvard University Press.

Schmeck, H.M.J. (1989, May 9). New methods fuel efforts to decode human genes. *The New York Times.* p. 23.

Schmeck, H.M.J. (1987, December 12). Single gene may determine the sex of a fetus. *The New York Times* p. 1.

Schneider, P., (1987, November). What it's like to adopt. *Parents,* p. 178.

Schweinhart, L.J. & Weikart, D.P. (1985). Evidence that good early childhood programs work. *Phi Delta Kappan, 66,* 545–548.

Sclarz, A.L. (1988, Winter). Homelessness: Implications for children and youth. *Social Policy Report: Society for Research in Child Development, 3,* 1–18.

Self, P.A., Horowitz, F.D., & Paden, L.Y. (1972). Olfaction in newborn infants. *Developmental Psychology, 7,* 349–363.

Seligmann, J., Joseph, N., Donovan, J., & Gosnell, M. (1987, Fall). Dieting, just like mommy. *Newsweek on Health,* p. 18.

Selman, R.L. & Selman, A.P. (1979, October). Children's ideas about friendship: A new theory. *Psychology Today, 13,* 71–114.

Seniors' reported drug use lowest in years, poll finds. (1989, March 8). *Education Week,* p. 17.

Serunian, S.A. & Broman, S.H. (1975). Relationship of Apgar scores and Bayley mental and motor scores. *Child Development, 46,* 699.

Shanberg, S.M. & Field, T.M. (1987). Sensory deprivation stress and supplemental stimulation in the rat pup and preterm human neonate. *Child Development, 58,* 1431–1447.

Shatz, M. (1983). Communication. In P.H. Mussen, J.H. Flavell, & E.M. Markman (Eds.). *Handbook of child psychology: Cognitive Development:* Vol. 3. New York: John Wiley.

Shyr, M.A., Klein, M.D., & Goodfriend, M. (1956). The effects of maternal narcotic addiction on the newborn. *American Journal of Obstetrics and Gynecology, 71,* 29–36.

Siegler, R.S. (1988). Individual differences in strategy choices: Good students, not-so-good-students, and perfectionists. *Child Development, 59,* 833–851.

Simmons, R.G. & Blyth, D.A. (1987). *Moving into adolescence: The impact of pubertal change and school context.* Hawthorne, NY: Aldine de Gruyter.

Simmons, R.G., Burgeson, R., Carlton-Ford, S., & Blyth, D.A. (1987). The impact of cumulative change in early adolescence. *Child Development, 58,* 1220–1234.

Simon, H.A. (1986). The role of attention in learning. In S.L. Friedman, K.A. Klivington, & R.W. Peterson (Eds.). *The brain, cognition and education.* (pp. 105–115). Orlando: Academic Press.

Simon, N. (1983). Preventing prematurity. *Parents,* pp. 74–79.

Singer, J.L. & Singer, D.G. (1986). Television-viewing and family communication style as predictors of children's emotional behavior. *Journal of Children in Contemporary Society, 17,* 75–91.

Singer, P. & Wells, D. (1985). *Making babies: The new science and ethics of conception.* New York: Charles Scribner's Sons.

Sinisterra, L. (1987). Studies on poverty, human growth and development: The Cali experience. In J. Dobbing (Ed.). *Early nutrition and later achievement.* London: Academic Press.

Skinner, B.F. (1979). *The shaping of a behaviorist.* New York: Alfred A. Knopf.

Skinner, B.F. (1967). Autobiography. In E.G. Boring & Gardner Lindzey, (Eds.). *A history of psychology in autobiography: Vol. 5.* New York: Appleton-Century-Crofts.

Slaughter, D., Oyemade, U.J., Washington, V., & Lindsey, R.W. (1988, Summer). Head Start: A backward and forward look. *Social Policy Report: Society for Research in Child Development,* 1–19.

Slavin, R.E. (1987). Cooperative learning and the cooperative school. *Educational Leadership, 45,* 7–13.

Slavin, R.E. (1987). Developmental and motivational perspectives on cooperative learning: A reconciliation. *Child Development, 58,* 1161.

Slobin, D.I. (1982). Universal and particular in the acquisition of language. In E. Wanner & L.R. Gleitman (Eds.). *Language acquisition: The state of the art* (pp. 128–170). Cambridge, England: Cambridge University Press.

Smith, F. (1982). *Writing and the writer.* London: Heinemann.

Snow, C. (1987). Relevance of the notion of a critical period to language acquisition. In M. Bornstein (Ed.). *Sensitive periods in development: Interdisciplinary perspectives.* Hillsdale, NJ: Lawrence Erlbaum.

Snow, C. (1979). Talking and playing with babies: The role of ideologies in child rearing. In M. Bullowa (Ed.). *Before speech: The beginning of interpersonal communication.* (pp. 269–288). Cambridge, England: Cambridge University Press.

Sofo, R. & Champagne, D.W. (1989, March). *Students—drugs, suicide, stress, life, growth health—choices.* Paper presented at the 44th Annual Conference of the Association for Supervision and Curriculum Development, Orlando, FL.

Sommerville, J. (1982). *The rise and fall of childhood.* Beverly Hills: Sage Publications.

Sontag, D. (1989, May 25). What's a name? *The Miami Herald,* p. 1F.

Spencer, H. (1878). *The principles of psychology.* London: Appleton.

Spitz, R.A. (1965). *The first year of life.* New York: International Universities Press.

Spock, B. & Rothenberg, M.B. (1985). *Baby and child care.* New York: E.P. Dutton.

Springer, S.P. & Deutsch, G. *Left brain, right brain.* New York: W.H. Freeman.

Sroufe, L.A. (1978, October). Attachment and the roots of competence. *Human Nature, 1,* 52.

Stark, E. (1984). Thanks for the memories. *Psychology Today, 18,* 80–81.

Statistical trends, The. (1985, May). *The Principal, 64,* 16.

Stein, A. (1987, January 17). New York's poor children: A tinderbox. *The New York Times,* p. 27.

Steinberg, L. (1987). Bound to bicker. *Psychology Today,* 36–39.

Steinberg, L. (1987). Impact of puberty on family relations: Effects of pubertal status and pubertal timing. *Developmental Psychology, 23,* 451–460.

Steinberg, L. (1986). Latchkey children and susceptibility to peer pressure: An ecological analysis. *Developmental Psychology, 22,* 433–439.

Stephenson, R. & Wilbur, K. (1985). *A study of the longitudinal dropout rate: 1980 eighth grade cohort followed from June 1980 through February, 1985.* Miami, FL: Dade County Public Schools.

Stewner-Manzanares, G. (1988, Fall). *The bilingual education act: Twenty years later.* (New Focus No. 6.). Silver Spring, MD: National Clearing House for Bilingual Education.

Surrogate grandma has triplets. (1987, October 1). *The Miami Herald* p. 23A.

Sutton, C. (1986, November 11). Why do boys score higher? *The Washington Post,* p. 85.

Szmukler, G.I. (1987). Anorexia nervosa: A clinical view. In R.A. Boakes, D.A. Popplewell, & M.J. Burton (Eds.). *Eating habits: Food, psychology and learned behavior.* (pp. 25–44). Chichester, England: John Wiley.

Tangney, J.P. (1988). Aspects of the family and children's television viewing content preferences. *Child Development, 59,* 1070–1079.

Taylor, B.H. (1988). Project PARENTING: An education program for adolescent mothers and their children. *Elementary School Guidance and Counseling, 22,* 320–324.

Tellegan, A. (1987, July). The recruitment bias in twin research: Rule of two-thirds reconsidered. *Behavior Genetics, 17* (4), 343–362.

Teller, D.Y. & Bornstein, M.H. Infant color vision and color perception. In P. Salapatek and L. Cohen (Eds.). *Handbook of infant perception: Vol. 1. From sensation to perception.* (pp. 185–263). Orlando: Harcourt Brace Jovanovich.

Thirer, L. & Wright, S.D. (1985). Sport and social status for adolescent males and females. *Sociology of Sport Journal, 2,* 167–169.

Thomas, A., Chess, S., & Birch, H. (1970, August), The origin of personality. *Scientific American, 223,* 102–109.

Thomas, R.M. (1979). *Comparing theories of child development.* Belmont, CA: Wadsworth.

Thompson, R.A. (1984, May). The critical needs of the adolescent unwed mother. *The School Counselor.* pp. 460–466.

Tolan, P.H. (1987). Implications of age of onset for delinquency risk. *Journal of Abnormal Child Psychology, 15,* 47–65.

Traub, J. (1986). Goodbye, Dr. Spock: Vignettes from the brave new world of the better baby. *Harper's Magazine, 272,* 57–64.

Turner, C.W., Simons, L.S., Berkowitz, L., & Frodi, A. (1977). The stimulating and inhibiting effects of weapons on aggressive behavior. *Aggressive Behavior, 3,* 355–378.

Tyack, D.L. (1981). Teaching complex sentences. *Language, Speech and Hearing Services in Schools, 17,* 160–174.

Unresolvable question, The. (1981, April 6), *Time,* p. 23.

U.S. Bureau of the Census. (1988, March). *Current population report.* July 1, 1987. (Series P25, No. 1022, Table 1). Washington D.C.: U.S. Government Printing Office.

U.S. Bureau of the Census (1987). (Current Population Reports, Series P-25, No. 1006). *United States population estimates and components of change: 1970 to 1986.* Washington, DC: U.S. Government Printing Office.

U.S. Bureau of the Census (1987). (Current Population Reports, Series P-23, No. 15). *Population profile of the United States: 1984–1985* Washington, DC: U.S. Government Printing Office.

U.S. Bureau of the Census (1986). (Current Population Reports, Series P-20, No. 441). *Household and family characteristics: March 1985.* Washington, DC: U.S. Government Printing Office.

U.S. Department of Health and Human Services. (1984, November). *Head start performance standards.* (45-CFR 1304) Washington, DC: U.S. Government Printing Office.

U.S. Nuclear Regulatory Commission. (1975). *Instruction concerning prenatal radiation exposure, (Regulatory guide* 8.13, Rev. 1), pp. 3–4.

Updated estimates of the costs of raising a child. (1986, April). *Family Economics Review,* 2, 34.

Valentine, D.P. (1982). The experience of pregnancy: a developmental process. *Family Relations, 31,* 243–248.

Van Petten, G. (1976). Principles of fetal pharmacology. In J.W. Gooden, J.O. Gooden, & G.W. Chance (Eds.)., *Perinatal medicine: the basic science underlying clinical practice* (pp. 286–302). Baltimore: Williams & Wilkins.

Vandell, D.L. & Corasaniti, M.A. (1988). The relation between third graders' after-school care and social, academic, and emotional functioning. *Child Development, 59,* 868–875.

Vaux, D. manager of the Repository for Germinal Choice. (1987, October 8). Information provided in a conversation with the author.

Watson, J.B. (1930). *Behaviorism* (rev. ed.). Chicago: University of Chicago Press.

Watson, J.B. (1913). Psychology as the behaviorist views it, *The Psychological Review, 20,* 158.

Weatherly, R.A., Perlman, S.B., Levine, M.H., & Klerman, L.V. (1986). Comprehensive programs for pregnant teenagers and teenage parents: How successful have they been? *Family Planning Perspectives, 18,* 73–78.

Weikart, D. & Tompkins, M. (1988, February). Introduction to the High/Scope curriculum. A paper distributed at the Florida Leadership Conference, Tampa, Florida.

Weinstein, R.S., Marshall, H.H., Sharp, L., & Botkin, M. (1987). Pygmalion and the student: Age and classroom differences in children's awareness of teacher expectations. *Child Development, 58,* 1079–1093.

Weintraub, K.S. & Furman, L.N. (1987, December). Child care: Quality, regulation, and research. *Social Policy Report, Society for Research in Child Development, 2,* (4), 1.

Welborn, S.N. Extroverts Are Born: Not Made. *U.S. News and World Report. 102,* 62.

Wells, M. (1988). The roots of literacy. *Psychology Today, 22,* 20–22.

Whaley, L.F. & Wong, D.L. (1985). *Essentials of Pediatric Nursing* (2nd ed.). St. Louis: C.V. Mosby.

Whaley, L.F. & Wong, D.L. (1983). *Nursing care of infants and children* (2nd ed.). St. Louis: C.V. Mosby.

Whaley, L.F. & Wong, D.L. (1982). *Nursing care of infants and children*. St. Louis: C.V. Mosby.

Wheeler, D. (1986, September 3). Researchers weigh a stepped-up effort to map the terrain of the human gene. *Chronicle of Higher Education*.

Wheeler-Liston, C. (1986). *Parents and premises: Nurturing the preemie*. Dallas: Touchpoints.

When life begins at two pounds. (1986, Fall). *Portraits* (Health and Wellness publication). Miami FL: North Shore Hospital and Medical Center.

White, B. (1985). *The first three years of life*. Englewood Cliffs, NJ: Prentice-Hall.

Whitehurst, G.J. & Valdez-Menchaca, M.C. (1988). What is the role of reinforcement in early language acquisition? *Child Development, 59*, 430–440.

Wieder, S. & Greenspan, S.I. (1987). Staffing, process, and structure of the clinical infant development program. In S.I. Greenspan et al. (Eds.), *Infants in multirisk families*. Madison, CT: International Universities Press. p. 11.

Williams, L. (1989, February 17). Teen-age sex: New codes amid the old anxiety. *The New York Times*, pp. 1, 12.

Willis, J. (1980, September). Genetic counseling: Learning what to expect. *FDA Consumer, 14*, 11–13.

Wintemute, G.J., Teret, S.P., Kraus, J., Wright, M.A., & Bradfield, G. When children shoot children. *Journal of the American Medical Association, 257*, 3107–3109.

Wolff, P. (1971). Mother-infant relations at birth. In J.G. Howels (Ed.), *Modern perspectives in international child psychiatry*. New York: Brunner/Mazel. pp. 20–97.

Wolff, P. (1973). The classification of states. In J.L. Smith, T. Henrietta, & L.B. Murphy (Eds.). *The competent infant*. New York: Basic Books. pp. 269–272.

Woman pregnant with twins from frozen embryos. (1987, July 15). *The Tampa Tribune*, p. 4A.

Woolston, J.L. (1987). Obesity in infancy and early childhood. *J. amer. acad. child adol. psychiat., 26*, 123–126.

Zaslowsky, D. (1989, January 19). Denver program curbs teen-agers' pregnancy. *The New York Times*, p. 8.

Zucker, K. (1987). Commentary of Kohlberg, Ricks, and Snarey's (1984): Childhood development as a predictor of adaption in adulthood. *Genetic, Social and General Psychology Monographs, 11*, 127–130.

$\mathcal{I}$NDEX

A

Abortion, 101
Accidents, preschoolers and, 340
Accommodation, Piaget and, 60
Accutane, pregnancy and, 168
Acne, adolescence and, *498*
Acquired immune deficiency syndrome. *See* AIDS
Act for Better Child Care, 312
ADA deficiency, 113
Adachi, T., 227
Adams, T., 202
Adamsons, Karlis, 156
Adaptation, Piaget and, 59
Additional consent, 23
Adolescence, 482–529
  acne and, *498*
  alcoholism and, 507
  anorexia nervosa and, 500–501
    understanding, *501–502*
  bulimia during, 502
  defined, 12–13, 483, 484
  female, weight and height norms, *489*
  high school and, 538–543
    counseling services in, 539, 541
    dropping out, 541–543
      prevention programs, 548–549
  homosexuality and, 520–521
  juvenile delinquency and, 506–507
  lying and, 547
  males, weight and height norms, *488*
  middle schools and, 534–535
  parenting the, 499, 546–547
  peer groups and, 502–503
  physical development during, 484–493
    bone loss prevention, *490*
    female breasts, *486*
    female pubic hair, *486*
    growth spurt, 486
    hormones, 491–492
    male genitals, *487*
    male pubic hair, *487*
    physical growth, 487, 489–491
    pubescence and, 485
    reproductive functions, 493
    sexual characteristics, 486–487
    voice changes, *491*
  popularity criteria, 543, *544*
  pregnancy during, 509–520
    consequences of, 512–513
    Freudian view of, *511*
    Parent-child Education Center and, 516–517
    prevention programs, 513–515
    programs for, 516
    Project PARENTING and, 517–518
    public policy and, 520
    reasons for, 511–512
    as a social problem, 510–511
    TAPP (Teenage Parenting Program) and, *518–519*
  Project TRUST and, *495–497*
  recklessness during, 499–500
  runaways and, 505
    toll free telephone number, 505
  schooling

social policy and, 534
transitions, 533–534
self-image and, 493–494
sexual activity and, 509
  age and percent, *509*
substance abuse and, 507–508
suicide, 494–495
work and, 503–505
  dimensions of, *503*
Adoption, 97–98
Adoption Factbook, 98
Adulthood, *51*, 55
Affective development, middle childhood and, family influences on, 421–422
AFP (alpha-fetoprotein test), 155–156
After-School Care of School-Age Children, 468
Agency for Toxic Substances and Disease Registry, lead poisoning and, 6
Age-stage approach to child study, 12–13
Aggression
  preschoolers and, 335–336
    biological factors, 335
    environmental/social factors, 335–336
    implications for parents, *336*
    sex differences in, 336
AIDS
  homosexuality and, 520–521
  preschoolers and, 347–349
    implications for parents, 348–349
    implications for public policy, 349
  pregnancy and, *189*
  sperm banks and, 99
Ainsworth, M., 264
Akers, R. L., 507
Alcohol, pregnancy and, *168*
Alcoholism, adolescence and, 507
All Fall Down, 340
Alliance for Better Child Care, 311–312
Alpha-fetoprotein test (AFP), 155–156
Alzheimer's disease, fetal tissue and, 157
Am, E., 337
Amdur, J. M., 378
American Academy of Pediatrics
  breast feeding and, 226
  circumcision and, *195*
  maternal weight gain and, 171
American Adoption Congress, 98
American College of Obstetricians and Gynecologists, *158*, 171
  maternal weight gain and, 171
American Fertility Society, 100
American Society for Psychoprophylaxis in Obstetrics, 161
Ames, L. B., 393
Amniocentesis, 114, 152–154
Amnion, 142
Amniotic fluid, 142–143
  purpose of, 143
Amphetamines, pregnancy and, *168*
Anal stage of development, 44, 45
Anderman, E., *514*
Androgens, 491
Anencephaly, 142
Angle's kiss, 187
Anonymity, research ethics and, 24
Anorexia nervosa

adolescence and, 500–501
  understanding, *501–502*
Anspaugh, D., 409
Ansul, S. E., 16, 19
Anthony, Pat, 96
Apgar, Virginia, 193
Apgar scoring system, 193
Aplastic anemia, fetal tissue and, 157
Aristotle, 113
Aronson, S., 310
Art of Sensual Massage, 43
Artificial insemination, *96*
As You Like It, 244
Aspirin, pregnancy and, *168*
Asynchrony, defined, 408
Atkins, K. R., 417
Attachment
  fathers and, 222
  infants and, 262–266
    fathers and, 265–266
    importance of, 263
    maternal responsiveness and, 264–265
    multiple, 263–264
    quality of, 264
    stages of, 262
  neonate and, 221–223
    sensitive periods for, 222–223
Attention, middle childhood and, 452
Auditory milestones, first year, *21*
Authoritarian parenting, preschoolers and, 345
Authoritative parenting, preschoolers and, 343

B

Babbling, infants and, 261
Babinski reflex, 197
Babkin reflex, 197
Baby. *See* Neonate
"Baby M", 96
Baby Tender, *68*
Bachman, J. G., 503, *504*
Bailey, W. T., 265–266
Baily, William, 21
Baldwin, W., 510
Bandura, Albert, 71, 336
Banet, B., 377
Bank Street College of Education, 368
Bank Street Program, 372–375
Banks, M. S., 253
Baranowski, T., 227
Barkan, S. E., 208
Bates, E., 330
Baumrind, D., 342, 345
Bax, M., 341
Bayley, Nancy, 21
Bayley Infant Mental and Motor Scales, 193
BEA (bilingual education act), 463
Beck, L. E., 331–332
Bee, D., 227
Behavior modification, behaviorists' definition of, 70
Behavioral adaptations, neonate and, 192–193
Behaviorism, 65–72
  advantages and disadvantages of, 71–72
  glossary of terms for, 70–71

operant conditioning and, 68
principles of, 70
social learning theory and, 71
teaching machines and, 69–70
Behaviorists, 41
Behram, R. E., *409*
Belsky, J., 514
Bender, A. E., 411
Bender, B. G., 116
Berch, D. B., 116
Berendes, H. W., 208
Berkley Growth Study, 21
Better Baby Institute, *307*
Bettes, B. A., 495
Bettleheim, B., 342
Biber, B., 374
Bilingual Education Act (BEA), 463
Bilingualism, middle childhood and, 463–465
Bilirubin, neonate and, 191
Binet, Alfred, 58
Biological father, 97
Biological processes, developmental
    processes and, 4
Birch, T., 111, 223
Birth, *186*
age, defined, 189
labor and, 159–160
premature, 208–217
    causes of, 208
    defined, 209–211
    ecological influences on, 220
    neonatal intensive care and, 211
    parenting and, 214–216
    preventing, *217*
timing of, 158
Birth Without Violence, 161
Birthing mother, defined, 97
Birthing practices, 160–164
cesarean births, 163, *164*
natural childbirth, 161–162
water babies, 162, *163*
Birthmarks, 187
Blakeslee, S., *221*
Blastocyst, *136*, 137
Blended family, 92
Block, J. and J. H., 507
Bloom, L., 301
Blos, Peter, 49
Blyth, D. A., 533
Boarder babies, 363
Bobak, I. M., 137, 140, 143
Bonding, neonate and, 221–223
Bone loss, preventing in adolescence, *490*
Bornstein, M. H., 254
Boston Woman's Health Book Collection, 95
Bottle feeding, 226–227
Bowlby, John, stages of attachment, 262
Bracken, M. B., 208
Bradley, R., 161
Brain
curriculum organization for, 457
dichotomies of left-right, *456*
organization of, 455–457
Brandt, R., 447–448
Braxton-Hicks contractions, 159
Brazelton, T. Berry, 194
Brazelton Neonatal Behavioral Assessment
    Scale, 194
Breast
development in female, *486*
feeding, 226–227
Breese, Kevin M., *217*
Bridger, W., 218
Broman, S. H., 193
Bronfenbrenner, U., 14
Brown, A. L., 455
Brown, J., 227
Brown, R., *301*

Brown fat, 192
Bruner, J. S., 258, 302
Bruno, R., 468
Budin, Pierre-Constantin, 211
Buie, J., 510, 511
Bulimia, adolescence and, 502
Burgeson, R., 533
Burgess, D., 378
Bybee, R. W., 417

C
C-section births, 163, *164*
Caffary, R. A., 501, 502
Caffeine, pregnancy and, *168*, 171
Cancer, cervical, diethylstilbestrol (DES)
    and, 167
Capute, A. J., 20
Cardiovascular system
embryo and, 140
neonate and, 190–191
Carey, S., 421
Carlton-Ford, S., 533
Carmody, D., 543
Carrying mother, defined, 97
Casa dei Bambini, 370
The Cat in the Hat, 150–151
Catheter fertilization, 99
Cawelti, G., 534
CCFP (School Breakfast and Child Care
    Food Program), 28
Center, childproofing, toddlers and, 307
Centers for Disease Control
lead poisoning and, 6
preschoolers with AIDS and, 347, 348
rubella vaccine and, 169
Cephalocaudal development, 250
Cervical cancer, diethylstilbestrol (DES) and,
    167
Cesarean births, 163, *164*
CF (cystic fibrosis), 118
Chaffee, Georgia, *519*
Chaiklin, H., 6
Chambers, M., 157
Champagne, D. W., 548
Chance, P., 450
Character education, 546
Charkovsky, Igor, 162
Charlesworth, W. R., 16, 19, 20, 22, 23
Chemicals, pregnancy and, 167
Chess, S., 111, 223, 342
Child Bearing Occupies, 95
Child care
before and after school, 467, *468*
center, childproofing, 307
infants and, 273–275
middle childhood and, 467–470
toddlers and
    care-givers and, 311
    curriculum and, 310–311
    environment and, 309–310
    social policy and, 311–312
Child Development, 22
Child development
career choices and, 9
defined, 3–4
ethics of, 22–25
    standards for, *23–25*
influences in, 25–28
    current areas of interest, 26–27
    early learning, 27
    ecological considerations and, 27–28
    life-span development and, 26
    "plasticity," 27
    social policy, 28
    sociobiology, 27
reasons for studying, 8–9
theory, 4
See also Development

Child study
life-span approach, 13
    ecological approach, 14
    multidisciplinary approach, 13
methods of, 12–14
    age-stage approach, 12–13
    topical approach, 13
Childbirth Without Fear, 161
Childproofing environment
neonates and, 271–272
toddlers and, 306–307
Children
cost of raising, *94*
reasons for having, 95
See also Middle childhood; Preschoolers
Children's Defense Fund, 28
Chomsky, N., 258
Chorionic villus sampling (CVS), 154
Christie, J. F., 337
Chromosome
abnormalities, 115–116
    Down syndrome, 115–116
    sex, 116–117
Circulatory system, fetal, 148–150
Circumcision, *195*
City College of New York, 72
Clark, E. V., 299
Classical conditioning, behaviorists'
    definition of, 70
Classification, middle childhood
    understanding of, 418–419
Cleavage, *136*, 13*7*
Cleft spine, 142
Cleveland Clinic, 99
Climbing
middle childhood and, 415
preschoolers and, *326*, 327
Cobb, P. C., 516
Codominance, 107
Cognitive development
middle childhood and, 417–422, 451–455
    family influences on, 421–422
    operational skills and, 417–420
neonate, 204–206
pendulum problem and, 64–65
Cognitive development theory, 58–64,
    204–206
constructivism and activity and, 60–61
equilibrium and, 60
stages of, 61–65
    concrete operations stage, 62, 63–64
    formal operations stage, 64
    preoperational stage, 62, 63
    sensorimotor stage, 62, 62–63
Cognitive equilibrium, 60
Cohen, D., 40, 57, 202
Cohort, defined, 21
Coleman, M., 468
Coles, R., 49
Colic, 229–230
Coll, C. G., 512, 512–513
Colombo, J., 6
Color
infants and, 254
neonates and, 202
Colostrum, antibodies received from, 192
Committee on Child Development and
    Social Policy, 28
Common Sense Book of Baby and Child Care,
    269
Comprehensive Early Childhood
    Development Program, 28
Concrete operations stage, *62*, 63–64
cognitive development and, 63
Confidentiality, research ethics and, 24–25
Congenital rubella syndrome (CRS), 169
Consanguineous relationships, 108
Constant Positive-Pressure Ventilation

Machine (CPPV), 211
Contingency management, behaviorists'
  definition of, 70
Contraceptives, use of by women, 94, 95
Control group, described, 17
Conversation, middle childhood and, 417–418
Cooing, infants and, 261
Cooperative education, middle childhood
  and, 446–448
Corasanati, M. A., 468, 469
Correlational research, 17
Corrigan, S. A., 409
Corsini, R. J., 21
Counseling services, high school, 539, 541
CPPV (Constant Positive-Pressure
  Ventilation Machine), 211
Crawling
  infants and, 251
  reflex, 197
Creative thinking, teaching, middle
  childhood and, 450
Creeping, infants and, 251
Crick, Francis, 104
Critical period, defined, 6
Critical thinking, 449–450
  ordinary thinking compared, 450
Crnic, K., 220
Crockenberg, S., 264, 513
Cronin, M. C., 427
Crook, C., 150, 203, 204, 226, 254
Cross, A. W., 378
Cross-sectional data gathering method,
  21–22
CRS (Congenital rubella syndrome), 169
Curtiss, S., 258
Cutrona, C. E., 265
CVS (chorionic villus sampling), 154
Cyropreservation of embryos, 99
Cystic fibrosis (CF), 118

D
Dale, P. S., 303
Dannemiller, J. L., 253
Davis, M., 202
DDST (Denver Developmental Screening
  Test), 378
de Villiers, J. G. and P. A., 261, 299–300
Deception, research ethics and, 24
Defense mechanisms in psychoanalytic
  theory, 46–47
DeFries, J. C., 111
Dehaan, Anne, child care program director,
  12
Dehydration, premature neonate and, 211
Delgado-Gaitan, C., 502–503, 543
DeLuccie, M., 266
Dental development
  infancy and, 248–249
  preschoolers and, 325
  toddlers, 288
Denver Developmental Screening Test
  (DDST), 378
Deoxyribonucleic acid (DNA), 104
  structure of, 105
Depth perception
  infants and, 252
  neonates and, 200
Descriptive research, 16–17
DeStefano, J., 421
Development
  behaviorists' definition of, 70
  defined, 4
  stage and nonstage explanations, 40–42
  theories of, 39–76
    defined, 39–40
    importance of, 40–42
    major developmental, 40

psychoanalytic theory, 42–49
  psychosocial theory, 49–57
  See also Child development
Developmental age, defined, 459
Developmental Indicators for the
  Assessment of Learning-Revised
  (DIAL-R), 378
Developmental processes, 4–8
  biological, 4
  critical periods of, 6–7
  environment and, 7
  environmental, 4–6
  heredity and, 7
  interaction of, 7–8
  learning, 7
Developmental stages of play, 338
DeVries, R., 373, 375
Dewey, John, 372, 452
Diabetes, fetal tissue and, 157
Diagnostic Inventory for Screening Children
  (DISC), 378
DIAL-R (Developmental Indicators for the
  Assessment of Learning-Revised), 378
Diazepam, pregnancy and, 168
DiBase, R., 16
Dick-Read, Grantly, 161
Dickie, N. H., 411
Diethylstilbestrol (DES), cervical cancer and,
  167
Dieting, preadolescent, 472
Disadvantaged children, preschools and,
  362–363
DISC (Diagnostic Inventory for Screening
  Children), 378
Divergent thinking, 450–451
Divorce, rate of, 363
Dizygotic twins, 114
DNA, 104
  structure of, 105
Dolby, R. M., 162
Doman, Glenn, 307
Dominant genes, 107
Donovan, J. R., 454, 472
Doutre, C. B., 450
Down, John, 115
Down syndrome, 115–116
  alpha-fetoprotein test (AFT) and, 155
  chorionic villus sampling and, 154
  mother's age and, 115, 116
Dr. Spock, parenting and, 269–270
Draper, P., 514
Drizd, T. A., 324, 325
Dropout
  defined, 541
  high school, 541–543
Drugs, pregnancy and, 167–168
Ductus arteriosus, 148, 190
Ductus venosus, 148, 190
Dukakis, Kitty and Michael, 507
Dzur, C., 19, 20, 22

E
Eagan, A. B., 160
Early Childhood Education, 371
Early Childhood Program at Sullivan
  County, 389
Echography, fetal biology and, 154–155
Eckert, H. M., 290, 325, 326, 415
Ecological approach to child study, 14
Ecological research, 19
Economic Opportunity Act, 368
Ectoderm, embryo and, 140
Ectopic pregnancies, 137
Education and Development of Infants, Toddlers,
  and Preschoolers, 367
Education for All Handicapped Children Act
  of 1975, 387
Education of the Handicapped Act

Amendments, 387–388
Education, sex, middle childhood and, 446
Egeland, B., 263
Egeland, J. A., 108
Ego, 43
  integrity, 55
  mediation by the, 45
Egocentric, 63
  formal operations stage and, 65
Egocentrism, preschoolers and, 329
Electra complex, 45
Elkind, D., 27, 65, 364
Embryo
  amniotic fluid and, 142–143
  cyropreservation of, 99
  developmental milestones, 140, 146–148
  germ layer development, 140, 141
  implantation, 96, 98–99
  neural tube defects and, 140, 142
  placenta and, 142
Emerging literacy, defined, 381
Emihovich, C., 427
Endoderm, embryo and, 140
English as a Second Language (ESOL), 463
Ennis, R. H., 450
Environment, developmental processes and, 7
Environmental infancy model, 246
Environmental processes, developmental
  processes and, 4–6
Ericsson, Ronald, 114
Erikson, Erik, 50, 52, 53, 55, 60, 224
  psychosocial theory and, 49–57
    implications of, 55
    stages of, 50–55
    strengths and weaknesses of, 56–57
Erogenous zones, 42
ESOL (English as a Second Language), 463
Espenschade, A. S., 290, 325, 326, 415
Estrogen, 491
  breast development and, 486
Ethics, 22–25
  dilemmas in, 25, 28
  fetuses' vs women's rights, 157
  issues of, 23, 25
  reproductiveness and, 100
  sex selection and, 114
  standards of, 23–25
  surrogate parenting and, 97
  in vitro fertilization and, 98–99
Ethics Committee of the American Fertility
  Society, 100
Eugenics, 99
Evans, Richard, 70
Experimental group, described, 17
Experimental research, 17–18
Extended family, 92
Extinction, behaviorists' definition of, 70
An Eye on the Future, 504
Ezell, G., 409

F
Fabrizi, M. S., 19
Failure to thrive (FTT), 224
Falbo, T., 94
Families
  American shrinking, 93–94
  changes in, 92–93
  changing, implications of, 95–96
  contemporary, 90–92
Fancher, R. E., 65
Fantz, R., 200
Farber, E. A., 263
FAS (fetal alcohol syndrome), pregnancy
  and, 170
Fathers
  attachment and, 222
  defined, 97
Federal Drug Administration

caffeine and, 171
  thalidomide and, 167
Feliciano, Sandra Garcia de, 156
Fertility rate, 93, *94*
Fertilization, 100–103
  age in weeks, *144*
  catheter, 99
  in vitro, 98–99
Fetal
  alcohol syndrome (FAS), pregnancy and, 170
  biology, 152–156
    alpha-fetoprotein test (AFP), 155–156
    amniocentesis and, 152–154
    chorionic villus sampling (CVS) and, 154
    fetoscopy and, 155
    percutaneous umbilical blood sampling (PUBS), 156
    ultrasound and, 154–155
  circulatory systems, 148–150
  development by trimester, *145*
  developmental stage, 143–145
  medicine, 156
  rights, 157
  therapy, 156–157
  tissues, medical use of, 157
Fetoscopy, 155
  fetal biology and, 155
Field, Diane E., 17
Field, T., 202, 243
Fine, G. A., *416*
Fine, M., 542–543
Fine motor skills
  middle childhood and, 417
  preschoolers and, 327
  toddlers and, 290–291
Fitness, preschoolers and, *340*
Fixation, 46
Flaste, R., 499
Flavell, J. H., 451, 454
Focal length, neonates and, 200
Follow Through program, 368
Fontanelles, *188*
Food and Drug Administration (FDA), caffeine and, 171
Foramen ovale, 148, 190
Form perception, neonates and, 200
Formal operations stage, *62*, 64
Forman, M. R., 208
Fowler, M. G., 378
Fragile-X syndrome, 117
Frandenburg, W. K., 378
Fraternal twins, 114
Freud, Anna, 50
Freud, Sigmund, 41, 45, 60
  children's play and, 337
  psychoanalytic theory and, 42–49
    anal stage, *44*, 45
    controversies about, 47
    criticisms of, 47
    defense mechanisms and, 46–47
    implications of, 47, 49
    latency stage, *44*, 46
    mature genital stage, *44*, 46
    oral stage and, *44*, 45
    personality traits development and, 46
    phallic stage, *44*, 45–46
Freudenheim, M., *217*
Froebel, Friedrick, 364, 457
Frustenberg, F., 510
FTT (failure to thrive), 224
Functional invariants, 41
Functional play, 337–338
Furman, L. N., 312
Futrell, M. H., 393

G

Gaier, E. L., *427*
Gale, Robert, 157

Gamete intra-fallopian transfer (GIFT), 99
Garrard, K. R., 330
Garrison, E. G., 505, 507
Garvin, R. A., 331
Gastrointestinal functions, neonate and, 191
Gavage feeding, 195
Gay, L. R., 15, 17
Gelles, R. J., 513
Gender development, preschoolers and, 334–335
Gene(s), 107
  mapping, 112–113
  therapy, 113
Genetic
  codes, 4
  counseling, 111, *112*
  diseases, 117–118
    number of people affected, *119*
    types of, *118*
  mother, defined, 97
  primer, *105*
  screening, 111–113
Genitals, male, development of, *487*
Genome, 113
Genotype, 104
George, P., 534
German measles, pregnancy and, 169
Gesell, Arnold, 393, 459
Gesell Institute of Child Development, 393
Gesell Institute of Human Development, 459
Gestation
  period, 134
  last menstrual period and, *134*
GIFT (gamete intra-fallopian transfer), 99
Gifted, preschoolers, 392
Gilda, P. M., *421*
Gill, Sir William, 500
Ginsburg, H., 65, 300
Give Your Child a Superior Mind, 245
Glahn, T. J., 117
Gleitman, H. and L., 301
Glossary, of behaviorist terms, 70–71
Gold, S., 223
Goldenberg, D., 378
Goleman, D., 423
Gomez, H., 267
Goodfriend, M., 170
Goodman, K. N., 409
Goodman, Yetta, 461
Gosnell, M., *472*
Gould, S. J., 246
Graham, Robert, 99
Grasping, infants and, 251
Grasping reflex, *251*
Green, R., 520–521
Greenberg, M., 220
Greenberg, R., 202
Greenberger, E., 484, 503, 504–505
Greenspan, S. I., 269
Grolitzer, Paul, teacher, emotionally disturbed adolescents, *11*
Gromley, A. V. and J. B., 95
Group for the Advancement of Psychiatry, 509–510, *511*
Growth, defined, 4
Guidance programs, middle schools and, 534–535
Guillen, M. A., 109
Gunther, V. A., 20

H

Habituation, behaviorists' definition of, 70
Hall, N., 461–462
Hammill, P. V. V., *324*, *325*
Hanafin, H., 97
Handedness, toddlers and, 291
Handicapped Infants and Toddlers Program, 387
Harkins, D. A., 291

Harlap, S., 114
Harlow, Harry, 218
Hauser, M. M., 158
Havens, B., 493
Haviland, J. M., 265
Hawkins-Stafford Elementary and Secondary School Improvement Act of 1988, 463
Head Start, 28, 363, 364, 368–370
  objectives of, 369–370
Hemingway, Ernest, 49
Hepatic functions, neonate and, 191
Heredity, 104–108
  developmental processes and, 7
  DNA, 104, *105*
  genetic primer, *105*
  laws of, 107–108
  personality and, *110*
  sex linked, 108
Heroin, pregnancy and, 170–171
Heterozygous gene pairs, 107
Hicky, T. L., 253
Hierarchy of needs, *73*, 74
High schools, 538–543
  adolescence popularity criteria, 543, *544*
  character education in, 546
  counseling services in, 539, 541
  teenagers dropping out of, 541–543
High/Scope Curriculum, 375–377
Ho, Hsiu-Zu and Ju-Chang, 117
Hofferth, S., 510
Hoffman, J., 512, 512–513
Holden, C., 111
Homann, M., 377
Homatidis, S., 158
Home
  childproofing
    neonates and, 271–272
    toddlers and, 306
Homeless, preschoolers, *346*
Homeostasis, 192
Homo sapiens, 104
Homosexuality
  adolescence and, 520–521
  AIDS and, 520–521
Homozygous gene pairs, *105*, 107
Hormones
  adolescent development and, 491–492
  pubertal development and, *492*
Horowitz, F. D., 203
Hoskisson, K., 422
How to Multiply Your Baby's Intelligence, 307
Human development, 3
Human life, beginning of, 103–104
Humanistic theory, 72–76
  hierarchy of needs, *73*, 74
  implications of, 74–75
  strengths and weaknesses of, 75–76
Huntington's chorea, fetal tissue and, 157
Huston, A. C., 334
Hydrocephaly, 142
Hypothesis, stating a, 15–16

I

Id, 42
Identical twins, 114
Imitation, neonates and, 202, *203*
Immunizations, infancy and, 272
Immunologic adaptations, neonate and, 192
Implantation, 137
In vitro fertilization (IVF), 98–99
  number per year, 100
Incentives, research ethics and, 24
Independent variable, defined, 18
Indifferent-uninvolved parenting, preschoolers and, 345–346
Individualized Family Services Plan (IFSP), 388
Infancy

attachment during, 262–266
  fathers and, 265–266
  importance of, 263
  maternal responsiveness and, 264–265
  multiple, 263–264
  quality of, 264
  stages of, 262–263
care of during, 271–272
changing views of, 243–245
child care during, 273–275
colors and, 254
defined, 12
immunizations during, 272
importance of, 246
intellectual development and, 254–257
language development and, 257–262
  behaviorism and, 257–258
  biology and, 259
  cognitive development and, 258
  emergence of, 261–262
  environmental influences and, 259
  heredity and, 256
  motherese and, 260
  social interactions and, 259–260
learning capability during, 14, 26
models of development, 246
mortality rates, 244, 245
nutrition and, 266–269
  bottle mouth and, 269
  caloric intake, 267–268
  needs, 267
  solid foods scheduling, 267, 268
  supplements and, 268
parenting during, 269
  Dr. Spock and, 269–270
physical development during, 246–252
  dental development, 248–249
  height and weight, 247–248
  motor development, 249–251
  visual development, 253–254
sexuality, 42
sleeping location, 270–271
stranger anxiety during, 272–273
taste and smell in, 254
touch and motion and, 254
Infant Colic Research Project, 230
Infant Success-Future Success, 245
Infantile
  apnea, 227
  genital period, 45–46
  sexuality, 42
Infants. See Infancy
Information processing, middle childhood
  and, 451–455
Informed consent, 23
Informing participants, research ethics and,
  24–25
Inheritance
  laws of, 107–108
  sex-linked, 108
Institute Jean-Jacques Rousseau, 58
Instruction, organizing for, middle schools
  and, 535
Intellectual development
  infancy and, 254–257
  neonate, stages of, 207
  preoperational, preschoolers and, 328–329
  preschoolers and, 328–330
    egocentrism and, 329
    implications for parents, 329–330
    motor skills implications and, 328
  toddlers and, 295–298
Intelligence, 111
Interactional infancy model, 246
Interactionism, preschooler language
  development and, 330
Interviews, research and, 18–19
Intrusive learning, 52–53
ISFP (Individualized Family Services Plan),

388
IVF (in vitro fertilization), 98–99
  number per year, 100

J
Jacklin, C., 425
Jacobs, Melody, 68
Jambor, T., 339
James Madison High School, 538
  curriculum, 539
Jankowski, C. B., 168, 169
Jensen, M. D., 137, 140, 143
Jeopardy, research ethics and, 24
Jessor, R. and S. L., 507
JIDPA (Juvenile Justice and Delinquency
  Prevention Act), 505, 506
Johnson, C. L., 324, 325
Johnson, Harriet, 368, 372
Johnson, J. E., 337
Johnson, W. G., 409
Jones, E., 42
Jones, T., 92
Joselow, F., 505
Joseph, N., 472
Joy of Sex, 43
Judd, D. M., 417
Juvenile delinquency, 506–507
Juvenile Justice and Delinquency Prevention
  Act (JIDPA) of 1974, 505, 506

K
Kagan, J. J., 425
Kahn, J. R., 510
Kamii, Constance, 60, 375
Kandal, D. B., 507
Kaplan, H. B., 507
Kaposi's Sarcoma, preschoolers with AIDS
  and, 347
Kass, S. A., 445
Katchadourian, H., 491
Kaye, H., 206
Keller, B., 92
Kellog, R., 290
Kennell, J. H., 222, 223
Kessen, W., 203
Kessler, R. C., 507
Keyes, S., 507
Khron, M. D., 507
Kidneys, neonate and, 191
Kinard, E. M., 512
Kindergarten
  defined, 12
  middle childhood and, 457–461
    basic skills orientation, 460
    reading in, 461
    purpose of, 458
    universal, 458
Kinesthetic awareness, neonates and, 202
The King, the Mice, and the Cheese, 151
Klaus, M. H., 222, 223
Klerman, L. V., 516
Kline, Marsha, 90
Klinefelter's syndrome, 116
Kogan, Scott, 113
Kohlberg, L., 428
Kolata, G., 99, 150, 348, 410, 411
Konstantareas, M. M., 158
Korner, A. F., 228
Kotselink, M. J., 425
Kryukova, N., 162
Kuhn, D., 65, 375

L
La Leche League International, 227
La Raza Medical Center, 157
Labor, 159–160
LaBuda, M. C., 111
LAD (language acquisition device), toddlers
  and, 301–302

Ladd, G. W., 470, 471
Lamaze, Fernand, 161
Lamaze method of childbirth, 161
Landry, E., 511
Language acquisition device (LAD), toddlers
  and, 301–302
Language development
  infancy and, 257–262
    behaviorism and, 257–258
    biology and, 259
    cognitive development and, 258
    emergence of, 261–262
    emotional influences and, 259
    heredity and, 256
    motherese and, 260
    social interactions and, 259–260
  middle childhood and, 421–422
    implications of, 422
    phonological development, 421
    sentence use, 421–422
    vocabulary development, 421
  neonates and, 224
  preschoolers and, 330–332
    complex sentences and, 331
    facilitating, 380
  toddlers and, 298–301
    first words, 299
    games and, 302
    holophrasic speech, 299–300
    implications for parents, 303
    LAD and LASS, 301–302
    motherese, 301
    negatives, 301
    relations expressed in, 301
    school and, 303–304
    symbolic representation, 300
    telegraphic speech, 300–301
    vocabulary development, 300
Language Experimental Approach (LEA), 330
Language support system (LASS), toddlers
  and, 301–302
Lanius, Andrew, 248
Lanius, Patricia, 165–166
Lanugo, 143
  neonate and, 185
Lanze-Kaduce, L., 507
LASS (language support system), toddlers
  and, 301–302
Latchkey children, middle childhood and,
  467–470
Latency stage of development, 44, 46, 51, 53
LEA (Language Experimental Approach), 330
Lead poisoning, children and, 6
Learning, neonate, 206–209
Learning processes, developmental
  processes and, 7
Leary, W. E., 490
LeBoyer, Frederick, 161
Lee, Anne, 90
Left Brain, Right Brain, 456
Legal problems, surrogate parenting and, 97
Lelwica, M., 265
Lennox, C., 158
Lester, B. M., 227, 228
Leukemia, fetal tissue and, 157
Levine, M. H., 516
Lewin, T., 157
Lewis, M., 392
Libido, 42, 45
Lieberman, P., 258
Life in the 30s, 154
Life-span
  approach to child study, 13
  development, 3, 13, 26
Liley, Sir William, 156
Limited English Proficient (LEP) students,
  463–464
Lindsey, R. W., 28
Linguistic milestones, first year, 21

Lipsitt, L. P., 199, 203, 206
Literacy
  defined, 381
  development, preschoolers and, facilitating,
    381–383
  middle childhood and, 461–463
Little League Baseball, middle childhood
  and, 416
Liver, neonate and, 191
Lloreda, P., 267
Locomotor-genital stage, 51, 52–53
Loggers' Run Middle School, 536–538
London, P., 546
Long, L. and T. J., 468
Long term memory (LTM), 453
Longitudinal data gathering method, 21
Longstreth, L. G., 291
Lowery, R. J., 72
LTM (long term memory), 453
Lynn, Kenneth, 49

M
McCartney, Kathleen, 109
McClelland, D., 376
McCluskey, K., 264
Maccoby, E., 342, 343, 345, 425, 427
McCracken, G., 348–349
McFarlane, A., 203
MacFarlane, A., 254
McKay, A. and H., 267
McMillan, J. H., 18
McTighe, J., 449
Madrazo, Ignacio, 157
Mainland, M. C., 378
Mainstreaming, preschoolers, 388
Manic depression, 108
Maranto, G., 114
Mardell-Czudnowski, C., 378
Margulies, R. Z., 507
Markham, Lynda, 463
Marshall, K. C., 452
Marsiglio, W., 512
Martin, J., 342, 343, 345
Martin, S. S., 507
Maslow, Abraham, 75
  humanistic theory and, 72–76
    hierarchy of needs, 73, 74
    implications of, 74–75
    strengths and weaknesses of, 75–76
Massage, benefits of, 218, 220
Match-up matrix, preschoolers, 388–391
Maternal nutrition, pregnancy and, 171
Mature genital stage of development, 44, 46
Maturity stage, 51, 55
Maurer, D., 202
May, K. A., 114, 142, 169, 190
Measurement terms, 427–428
Meconium, 191
Meiosis, 104
Meirik, O., 208
Meltzoff, A., 202
Memory
  middle childhood and, 453–454
    mnemonic devices and, 454
Merahn, S., 348–349
Mesoderm, embryo and, 140
Metabolic adaptations, neonate and, 192
Metabolism, defined, 410
Metacognition
  defined, 455
  middle childhood and, 454–455
Metamemory, 454
Michael Reese Hospital, first incubator
  used, 211
Michalson, L., 392
Michel, G. F., 291
Middle childhood
  affective development and, family
    influences on, 421–422

attention and, 452
  bilingualism and, 463–465
  child care and, 467–470
  cognitive development and, 417–422,
    451–455
    family influences on, 421–422
    operational skills and, 417–420
  cooperative education and, 446–448
  critical thinking and, 449–450
  defined, 12
  dieting and, 472
  information processing and, 451–455
  kindergarten and, 457–461
    basic skills orientation, 460
    reading in, 461
  language development and, 421–422
    implications of, 422
    phonological development, 421
    sentence use, 421–422
    vocabulary development, 421
  latchkey children and, 467–470
  literacy and, 461–463
  Little League Baseball and, 416
  memory and, 453–454
    mnemonic devices and, 454
  metacognition and, 454–455
  metamemory and, 454
  motor development during, 415, 417
  new curriculum for, 445
  nutrition during, 411–415
    food guide for, 413–415
  perception and, 452
  physical development and, 408–411
    average height of, 408
    physical appearance and, 409–411
    weight reduction and, 410, 411
    weights percentile chart, 409
  recess and, 445
  sensory processes and, 452
  sex education and, 446
  teaching thinking and, 448
  transitions, 470–472
    helping children make, 471–471
Middle schools
  features of, 534–535
  Loggers' Run Middle School, 536–538
Milia, 187
Milk spots, 187
Miller, E., 169
Miller, G. A., 421, 453
Miller, S. H., 520
Miller, W., 95
Minnesota Center for Twin and Adoption
  Research, 111
Missing Children's Assistance Act of 1984,
  505
Mitosis, 104
Mnemonic devices, memory and, 454
Mongolian spots, 187
Monozygotic twins, 114
Monson, Pamela, 157
Montessori, Maria, 333, 370
Montessori program, 370–372
  sensory development, toddlers and, 291–292
  sensory materials, 370, 371
Moore, K. M., 202
Moore, W. M., 324, 325
Moro reflex, 196
Morrison, G. S., 337, 367, 371, 471
Mortality
  gestational age, weight and, 210
  infant rates, 244, 245
Mosher, B. S., 6
Mother, defined, 97
Motherese, 260
  toddlers and, 301
A Mother's Story, 96
Mothers of Twins Clubs, Inc., 115
Motion

infants and, 254
  neonates and, 202
Motor development
  infancy and, 249–251
    milestones, 249, 250
  middle childhood, 415, 417
  preschoolers and, 325–328, 326
    climbing, 326, 327
    intellectual development implications and,
      328
    running, 325, 326
    walking, 325, 326
  toddlers, 289–291
Mott, F., 512
Mouth, neonates, 191
Muhlen, L., 162
Mulinare, J., 142
Multidisciplinary approach to child study, 13
Multiple births, 114–115
Murray, A. D., 162
Murray, J. B., 500
Murray, Patricia, 18
Muscular-anal stage, 51, 52
Mutual responsibility, research ethics and, 24
Myers, B. J., 222

N
Nation, R. L., 162
National Association for the Education of
  Young Children, 275
National Association for the Education of
  Young People, 310
National Center for Health Statistics, 363
National Center for Health Studies,
  maternal weight gain and, 171
National Center for Missing and Exploited
  Children, 505
National Committee on Adoption, 98
National Council on Radiation Protection
  and Measurements, 168
National Genetics Foundation, 112
National Institute of Child Health and
  Human Development, 230
National Institutes of Health, cesarean
  births and, 163
National Institutes of Health for the Human
  Genome Studies, 113
Natural childbirth, 161–162
Natural Childbirth, 161
Naturalistic observation, 19
Naturalistic Study of Humorous Activity in a
  Third, Seventh, and Eleventh Grade
  Classroom, 19
Neeson, J. D., 114, 169, 190
Negative reinforcer, behaviorists definition
  of, 70
Nelson, M., 161
Nelson, Meredith, neonatal nurse, 212–214
Nelson, R., 468
Nelson Textbook of Pediatrics, 409
Neonate
  abilities of, 199–204
    imitation, 202, 203
    kinesthetic awareness, 202
    olfaction, 202–203
    taste, 202–204
    touch and motion, 202
    vision, 200–202
  Apgar scoring system and, 193
  appearance of, 185–189
  at risk, 208–211, 214–216, 218, 220
  average vital statistics of, 193
  Bayley Infant Mental and Motor Scales, 193
  behavioral adaptations and, 192–193
  bonding and attachment, 221–223
  Brazelton Neonatal Behavioral Assessment
    Scale, 194
  breast or bottle question, 226–227
  cardiovascular system and, 190–191

care-giver styles and, 229
caring for, 224–227
circumcision, *195*
cognitive development, 204–206
colicky, 229–230
cries of, 227–230
defined, 12, 189
gastrointestinal functions and, 191
head of, *188*
hepatic functions and, 191
immunologic adaptations and, 192
individuality of, 223–224
intensive care and, 211
kidneys and, 191
language development, 224
learning, 206–209
massage and, 218–220
metabolic adaptations and, 192
naming the, *225*
neurological function of, 192
organ donations, *221*
period, 189
phenylketonuria (PKU) and, 194
physical tests and procedures, 194
premature, 208–217
  defined, 209–211
  ecological influences on, 220
  intensive care and, 211
  parenting the, 214–216
  psychosocial development, 224
reflexes of, 195–198
  babinski, 197
  babkin, 197
  crawling, 197
  grasping, 196–197
  implications, 197–198
  moro, 196
  plantar, 197
  rooting, 197
  stepping, 197
  sucking, 195–196
  swimming, 197
  tonic neck, 196
  walking, 197
respiration and, 190
social development of, 221–223
soothing the, 228–229
states of, 198–199
vitamin K injection to, 194
Nesson, J. D., 142
Neural tube
  defects of, 140, 142
  alpha-fetoprotein test (AFT) and, 155
Neurological function, neonate and, 192
Neuroses, 45
New York Times, 15, 154
Newcomer, S. F., 515
Newman, J. M., 381
Newport, E. L., 301
Newsweek, 151
Nicotine, pregnancy and, *168*
Nilsson, L., 101
Nobel Laureate Sperm Banks, 99
Non-harmful procedures, 23
Nonstage theory of development, 40
  common features of stage theory and, 41
Norton, A. J., 93
Nowlis, G. H., 203
NRC (Nuclear Regulatory Commission), 168
Nuclear family, 92
Nuclear Regulatory Commission (NRC), 168
Number, middle childhood understanding
  of, 419
Nurse practitioners, *9–10*
Nursery School of the Bureau of
  Educational Experiments, 368, 372
Nursery schools, 366, 368
  activities in, 368
Nutrition

children and, 4–5
infants and, 266–269
  bottle mouth and, 269
  caloric intake and, 267–268
  needs, 267
  solid food scheduling, *267*, 268
  supplements and, 268
middle childhood, 411–415
  food guide for, *413–415*
pregnancy and, 171
toddlers and, 293

O

Obesity
  defined, 409
  middle childhood and, 409–411
  weight reduction and, *410*, 411
Observation, data gathering through, 19–20
Oedipus complex, 45
Offer, D., 494
Office of Juvenile Justice and Delinquency
  Prevention (OJJDP), 506
Office of Technology Assessment, in vitro
  fertilization and, 100
Oh, W., 512, 512–513
O'Hara, D. M., 6
OJJDP (Office of Juvenile Justice and
  Delinquency Prevention), 506
Okada, H., 227
Old Order Amish, manic depression and,
  108
Olfaction, neonates and, 202–203
On Studying the Explanations of Children, 58
Operant conditioning, 68–69
  behaviorists' definition of, 70
Opper, S., 65, 300
Oral-sensory stage, 50, *51*, 52
Oral stage of development, *44*, 45
Organ donations, infant, *221*
Orgasm, 101
Oster, H., 204
Osterholm, M. T., 310
Otten, A. L., 100
Our Bodies, Ourselves, 95
Ovaries, 100–101
Ovrut, M. A., 291
Ovulation, fertilization and, 100
Ovum, 100, *101*
Owen, A. L., 226
Oxytocin, 162
Oyemade, U. J., 28

P

Paden, L. Y., 203
Pain, childbirth and, 162
Palincsar, A. S., 455
Palmer, F. B., 20
Papousek, H. A., 206
Parent Care, 220
Parental consent, 23
Parent-child Education Center, 516–517
Parenting
  adolescence and, 499
  contemporary, 90–92
  infants and, 269
    Dr. Spock and, *269–270*
  premature neonate, 214–216
  preschoolers, 341–346
    authoritarian, 345
    authoritative, 343
    indifferent-uninvolved, 345–346
    styles matrix, 342–343
  preschools and, working, 363
  psychoanalytic theory and, 47, 49
  psychosocial theory and, 55
  styles, children and, 5
  surrogate, 96–97
  toddlers, 305–306
Parents magazine, surrogate parenting and, 97

Parke, R. D., 335, 336
Parker, K. C. H., 378
Parkinson's disease, fetal tissue and, 157
Parten, Mildred, developmental stages of
  play, *338*
Participant observation, 19
Patent ductus arteriosus, 191
Pathologic jaundice, neonate and, 191
Patterson, D., 115
Pavlov, Ivan, 66
Pederson, D., 228
Pediatric nurse practitioner, *9–10*
Peduzzi, J. D., 253
Peer groups, adolescence and, 502–503
Pehrsson, B. H., 389
Pendulum problem, cognitive development
  and, 64
Penis envy, 46
Perception, middle childhood and, 452
Perceptual development, toddlers and,
  291–292
Perinatal, defined, 189
Perlman, S. B., 516
Permissive parenting, preschoolers, 345
Perry Preschool Program, 379
Personality, 108–110
  heredity and, *110*
  prenatal development of, 150
Petersen, A. C., 493–494, 499, 533
Phallic stage of development, *44*, 45–46
Phenotype, 104
Phenylketonuria (PKU), 118
  neonates and, 194
Phipps-Yonas, S., 95
Phonological development, middle
  childhood and, 421
Physical development
  adolescence and, 484–493
    bone loss prevention, *490*
    female breasts, *486*
    female pubic hair, *486*
    growth spurt, 486
    hormones, 491–492
    male genitals, *487*
    male pubic hair, *487*
    physical growth, 487, 489–491
    pubescence and, 485
    reproductive functions, 493
    sexual characteristics, 486–487
    voice changes, *491*
  infants and, 246–252
  middle childhood and, 408–411
    average height of, *408*
    physical appearance and, 409–411
    weight reduction and, *410*, 411
    weights percentile chart, *409*
  preschoolers and, 324–325
  toddlers and, 287–288
Physical growth, adolescence and, 487,
  490–491
*Physical Growth: National Center for Health
  Statistics Percentiles*, 324, *325*
Physiological jaundice, neonate and, 191
Piaget, Jacqueline, Laurent and Lucienne, 58
Piaget, Jean, 41, 58, 63, 64, 255
  clinical method of, 57–59
  cognitive development theory and, 57–65,
    204–206
    pendulum problem and, 64–65
    stages in, 58–64
    strengths and weaknesses of, 65
  language development and, 331
  middle childhood cognitive development
    and, 417
  symbolic play and, 337–338
  toddler experimentation and, 295
Picton, T. W., 452
Pitocin, 162
PKU (phenylketonuria), 118

neonates and, 194
Placenta, 137, 142
Plantar reflex, 197
Play
  defined, 337
    classifications of, 337–338
    competencies of, 338–339
    environments for, 339
    reasons for, 336–337
  social, 337
  toddlers and, *308*
Pleasure principle, 42
Plomin, R., 111
Pollitt, E., 244
Port wine stains, 187
Positive reinforcer, behaviorists' definition
  of, 70
Postnatal, defined, 189
Potts, L., 95
Prato, D., 468
Pratt, Caroline, 368
Preadolescent dieting, *472*
Pregnancy
  adolescence and, 509–520
    consequences of, 512–513
    Freudian view of, *511*
    Parent-child Education Center and, 516–517
    prevention programs, 513–515
    programs for, 516
    Project PARENTING and, 517–518
    public policy and, 520
    reasons for, 511–512
    as a social problem, 510–511
    TAPP (Teenage Parenting Program) and,
      518–519
  AIDS and, *189*
  developmental process of, 158–159
  influences on, 166–171
    caffeine and, 171
    chemicals and, 167
    drugs and, 167–168
    fetal alcohol syndrome (FAS) and, 170
    heroin and, 170–171
    nutrition and, 171
    radiation and, 168–169
    Rh blood factor and, 169
    rubella and, 169
    teratogenic substances, 167
    tobacco and, 169
  signs of, *137–138*
Premature births, 208–217
  causes of, 208
  defined, 209–211
  ecological influences on, 220
  neonatal intensive care and, 211
  parenting, 214–216
  preventing, *217*
Prenatal
  defined, 12
  development test, 133–134
  developmental stages, 134–145
    critical periods in, *139*
    embryo stage, 139–143
    fetal stage, 143–145
    primer of, 146–148
    zygote stage, 137, 139
  genetic screening, 113
  personality development, 150
  sensory development and, 150–151
Prenatal University, 151
Preoperational intelligence, preschoolers
  and, 328–329
Preoperational stage, *62*, 63
Preschool
  curriculum, 392–393
  defined, 12
  enrollment in, 362
  importance of, 363
  issues concerning, 392–393

popularity of, 362–363
programs, 365–366
  academic orientation of, 365–366
  preventative programs of, 366
  types of, *366–367*
screening, implications of, 379
trends in, *458*
value of, 379–380
Preschoolers
  accidents and, 340
  aggression of, 335–336
    biological factors, 335
    environmental/social factors, 335–336
    implications for parents, *336*
    sex differences in, 336
  AIDS and, 347–349
    implications for parents, 348–349
    implications for public policy, 349
  average heights for, *324*
  average weight of, *324*
  communication and, 383–384
    implications for parents and teachers, 384
  crisis and stress and, *394–395*
  dental development of, 325
  fitness of, *340*
  gender development of, 334–335
  gifted, 392
  homeless, *346*
  intellectual development of, 328–330
    egocentrism and, 329
    implications for parents, 329–330
    motor skills implications and, 328
    preoperational, 328–329
  language development of, 330–332
    complex sentences and, *331*
    facilitating, 380
  literacy development of, facilitating, 381–383
  mainstreaming, 388
  match-up matrix, 388–391
  motor development of, 325–328
    climbing, *326*, 327
    intellectual development implications and,
      328
    running, 325, *326*
    throwing, *326*, 327
    walking, 325, *326*
  parenting, 341–346
    authoritarian, 345
    authoritative, 343
    indifferent-uninvolved, 345–346
    styles matrix, 342–343
  peer interaction, *385–387*
  people's view of, 363–365
    as competent child, 364
    as future investments, 364–365
    as growing plants, 364
    as miniature adults, 364
  permissive parenting of, 345
  physical development of, 324–325
  play of
    classifications of, 337–338
    competencies of, 338–339
    environments for, 339
    reasons for, 336–337
  predicting success of, 377–379
  psychosocial development of, 332–334
  special needs of, 387
  tantrums and, 340–341
  transitions of, 377
  writing and, 381–383
Prevention programs, adolescents and,
  548–549
Price, J. M., 470, 471
Primary grades, defined, 12
Progesterone, 491
Project PARENTING, 517–518
Project TRUST, *495–497*
Projection, psychoanalytic theory and, 47
Pryke, M., 162

Psychoanalytic theory, 42–49
  anal stage, *44*, 45
  criticisms of, 47
  defense mechanisms and, 46–47
  implications for parents, 47, 49
  latency stage, *44*, 46
  mature genital stage, *44*, 46
  oral stage, *44*, 45
  personality traits development and, 46
  phallic stage, *44*, 45–46
Psychoprophylaxis, 161
Psychosocial development
  neonates, 224
  preschoolers and, 332–334
  toddlers and, 304
Psychosocial theory, 49–57
  implications of, 55
  stages of, 50–55
    adulthood, 55
    latency, 53
    locomotor-genital, *51*, 52–53
    maturity, 55
    muscular-anal, *51*, 52
    oral-sensory, 50, *51*, 52
    puberty and adolescence, 53–54
    young adulthood, 54–55
  strengths and weaknesses of, 56–57
Puberty
  adolescence stage and, *51*, 53–54
  defined, 484
  self-image and, 493–494
Pubescence, described, 485
Pubic hair
  female, development of, *486*
  male, development of, *487*
Public Citizen Health Research Group, 163
Public Health Services Act of 1981, 516
Public Law 94–142, 387
Public Law 99–457, 387–388
Public Law 100–403, 28
Public Law 100–435, 28
PUBS (percutaneous umbilical blood
  sampling), 156
Punishment, behaviorists' definition of, 70

Q
Qhuildlen, Anna, 154
Questionnaires, research and, 18–19
Quickening, 143
Quinn, J., 513

R
Radiation sickness, fetal tissue and, 157
Ramsey, B., 507
Ransom, K., 455
Rasosevich, M., 507
Rassin, D., 227
Rationalization, psychoanalytic theory and,
  46–47
Read, E. W., 511
Readiness
  school, *459*
  promoting, 459–460
Reading, kindergarten and, 461
Reality principle, 43
Recessive genes, 107
Recklessness, adolescence and, 499–500
Recognition of the Middle Level, 534
Reed, R. B., *324*, *325*
Reflexes
  neonate and, 195–198
    babinski, 197
    babkin, 197
    crawling, 197
    grasping, 196–197, *251*
    implications, 197–198
    moro, 196
    plantar, 197
    rooting, 197

stepping, 197
sucking, 195–196
swimming, 197
tonic neck, 196
walking, 197
Regression, psychoanalytic theory and, 46
Reilly, Maureen, pediatric nurse practitioner, 9–10
Reinforcement
 behaviorists' definition of, 70
 theory, 67
Reinforcer, behaviorists' definition of, 70
Reinherz, H., 512
Reinhold, R., 167
Reisman, J. E., 202, 228, 254
Reporting results, research ethics and, 24–25
Repository for Germinal Choice, 99
Repression, psychoanalytic theory and, 46
Reproduction, adolescence and, 493
Reproductive, technology, 96–97
Reproductiveness, ethical issues of, 100
Research, 14–15
 analyzing, 22
 data gathering, 18–20
 defined, 15
 determining development through, 20–22
  cross-sectional method, 22–23
  longitudinal method, 21
 dissemination, 22
 ethical standards of, 23–25
 hypothesis, 15–16
 methods, 16–18
  correlational, 17
  descriptive, 16–17
  experimental, 17–18
 scientific method, 15
  applying, 16
Respiration, neonates and, 190
Response
 behaviorism and, 67
 behaviorists' definition of, 70
Restak, R., 453
Reznick, S., 425
Rh blood factor, pregnancy and, 169
RHYA (Runaway and Homeless Youth Act), 505
Ribonucleic acid (RNA), 104
Richardson, C. J., 227
Richmond-Abbott, M., 427
Richmond, P., 59–60
Ricklefs, R., 94
Riese, M., 218
RISC (Risk Index of School Capability), 378–379
Risk, defined, 6
Risk Index of School Capability (RISC), 378–379
RNA, 104
Robbins, C., 507
Robinson, B. E., 468
Roche, A. F., 324, 325
Rodman, H., 468
Roe vs. Wade, 101, 510
Roosa, M. W., 518
Rooting reflex, 197
Rose, S., 218
Rosenblith, J. F., 139
Rosenstein, D., 204
Rousseau, Jean-Jacques, Institute of, 58
Rowland, B. H., 468
Rubella, pregnancy and, 169
Rubin, N., 411
Rumors on Suicide, 494
Runaway and Homeless Youth Act (RHYA), 505
Runaways
 adolescence and, 505
  toll free telephone number, 505
Running, middle childhood and, 415

S
Sadker, D. and M., 426
Safety
 infants and, 271
 toddlers and, 292
Salkind, N. J., 12
Samatotropin, 491
Sameroff, A. J., 7
Save the Children Federation, 362
SCA (Sex chromosome abnormalities), 116–117
Scarr, Sandra, 109, 111
Schaffer, R., 244
Schatz, M., 383
Schmeck, H. M., 113
Schmidt, K., 218
Schneider, P., 97
School-age children. See Middle childhood
School Breakfast and Child Care Food Program (CCFP), 28
School Readiness Test, 393
Schumacher, S., 18
Sciarillo, W., 378
Scientific method, 15
 applying, 16
Second language, learning a, 464–465
Self-image, adolescence, 493–494
Self, P. A., 203
Seligmann, J., 472
Selman, A. P. and R. L., 424
Semen, 101
Seniors Reported, 507
Sensorimotor stage, 62, 62–63, 205
Sensory development
 prenatal development of, 150–151
 toddlers, 291–292
Sensory processes, middle childhood and, 452
Seriation, middle childhood, understanding of, 418
Serunian, S. A., 193
Sex chromosome abnormalities (SCA), 116–117
Sex education, middle childhood and, 446
Sex selection, 113–114
Sex-typing, defined, 334
Sexual activity
 adolescence and, 509
 age and percent, 509
Sexual characteristics, adolescence and, 486–487
Shakers, 90
Shakespeare, 244
Shapiro, B. K., 20
Shelov, S., 348–349
Short term memory (STM), 453
Siamese twins, 114
Sickle-cell anemia, 117–118
Siders, J. A. and J. Z., 417
SIDS (Sudden Infant Death Syndrome), 227
Siegler, R. S., 455
Simmons, R. G., 499, 533
Simon, H. A., 452, 453
Simon, N., 208
Simon, Theodore, 58
Sims-Knight, J. E., 139
Simulated observation, 19
Singer, D. G. and J. L., 420
Single-parent family, 92
Sinisterra, L., 267
Skinner box, 69
Skinner, Burrhus Frederick
 behaviorism and, 65–72
  advantages and disadvantages of, 71–72
  glossary of terms for, 70–71
  operant conditioning and, 68
  principles of, 70
  social learning theory and, 71
  teaching machines and, 69–70

Slaby, R. G., 335, 336
Slaughter, D., 28
Slavin, R. E., 447
Sleep Tight, 229–230
Slobin, D. I., 258
Smiling, infants and, 261
Smith, F., 461
Snidman, N., 425
Snow, C., 258, 465
Snyder, L., 330
Social learning theory, 71
Social play, 337
Social policy, 28
Socialization in the Context of the Family; Parent-Child Interaction, 343
Society for Research in Child Development, 23, 28
Sociobiology, 27
Soderman, A. K., 425
Sofo, R., 548
Solarz, A. L., 346
Solid food, introduction of, 267, 268
Sommerville, J., 270
Sonography, fetal biology and, 154–155
Space, middle childhood understanding of, 419–420
Spencer, H., 337
Sperm, 101, 102
 banks, 99
 filtering, 114
Spermatozoa, 101, 102
Spina bifida, 142
 alpha-fetoprotein test (AFT) and, 155
Spock, Benjamin, parenting and, 269–270
Spontaneous abortion
 amniocentesis and, 154
 chorionic villus sampling and, 154
Sport and Social Status for Adolescent Males and Females, 544
Springer, S. P., 456
Sroufe, Alan, 229
Sroufe, L. A., 263
Stage theory of development, 40–42
Standard deviation, 432
Standard error of measurement, 428
Stark, E., 453
Status quo infancy model, 246
Stein, A., 363
Stein, L. C., 425
Steinberg, L., 468, 484, 499, 503, 504–505
Stepfamilies, 92
Stephenson, R., 542
Stepping reflex, 197
Sterilization, 94
Stern, Elizabeth and William, 96
Stewner-Manzanares, G., 463
Stimulus
 behaviorism and, 67
 definition of, 70
STM (short term memory), 453
Stork bite, 187
Strange Situation, 264
Stranger anxiety, infants and, 272–273
Strawberry marks, 187
Stuss, D. T., 452
Sublimation, psychoanalytic theory and, 47
Substance abuse, adolescence and, 507–508
Sucking reflex, neonate, 195–196
Sudden Infant Death Syndrome (SIDS), 227
Suicide, adolescence and, 494–495
Sund, R. B., 417
Superbabies, 307–308
Superego, 44–45
 defense mechanisms and, 46
 phallic stage and, 45
Surfactant, 143–144
Surrogate Grandma, 97
Surrogate parenting, 96–97
Surveys, research and, 18–19

Sutton, C., *427*
Sweinhart, L. J., 5
Swenson, I., 493
Swimming reflex, 197
Symbolic play, 338
Szmukler, G. I., 501

T

Tangney, J. P., 420
Tanner stages, 487
Tantrums, preschoolers and, 340–341
TAPP (Teenage Parenting Program), *518–519*
Taste
  infants and, 254
  neonates and, 202–204
Tay-Sachs disease, 118
Teaching Complex Sentences, 331
Teaching English to speakers of other
    languages (TESOL), 464
Teaching machines, behaviorists and, 69–70
Team teaching, middle schools and, 535
Teenage Parenting Program (TAPP), *518–519*
Teenager. *See* Adolescence
Telegraphic speech, toddlers and, 300–301
Television, environmental processes and, 6
Tellegen, A., 110
Teller, D. Y., 254
Temperament, *110*, 111
  neonate and, 223–224
Teratogenic substances, pregnancy and, 167
TerVrught, D., 228
TESOL (teaching English to speakers of
    other languages), 464
Testosterone, 491
Thalidomide, pregnancy and, 167–168
Theories. *See* Development, theories of
Theory, defined, 39
Thinking, teaching, middle childhood and,
    448–451
Thoman, E. B., 228
Thomas, A., 111, 223, 342
Thomas, D. B., 162
Thomas, Murray, 55
Thomas, R. M., 63
Thompson, R. A., 518
Thorndike, Edward, 66, 67
Throwing
  middle childhood and, 415
  preschoolers and, *326*, *327*
Time, middle childhood understanding of,
    420
To Reach Ultimate Success Together, *495–497*
Tobacco, pregnancy and, 169
Toddlerhood, defined, 12
Toddlers
  child care and, 309–310
    care-givers and, 311
    curriculum and, 310–311
    environment and, 309–310
    social policy and, 311–312
  childproofing environment of, 306–307
  dental development of, 288
  developmental milestones of, 304–305
  handedness of, 291
  independence of, 292
    implications for parents, *293–294*
  intellectual development of, 295–298
  language development of, 298–301
    first words, 299
    games and, 302
    holophrasic speech, 299–300
    implications for parents, 303
    LAD and LASS, 301–302
    motherese, 301
    negatives, 301
    relations expressed in, *301*
  school and, 303–304

symbolic representation, 300
  telegraphic speech, 300–301
  vocabulary development, 300
motor development of, 289–291
nutrition of, 293
objective permanence development and, *297*
parenting the, 305–306
perceptual development of, 291–292
physical development of, 287–288
playtime and, *308*
psychosocial development of, 304
safety of, 292
scribble stage, *291*
toilet training of, 294–295, 305
weight and height of, *287*
Toilet training, toddlers and, 294–295, 305
Tolan, P. H., 507
Tompkins, G. E., 422
Tompkins, M., 376
Tonic neck reflex, 196
Topical approach to child study, 13
Touch
  infants and, 254
  neonates and, 202
Touching, neonates, importance of, 218
Toys, influence on children, 5–6
Transactional infancy model, 246
Transition programs, middle schools and, 535
Transitional stools, 191
Triple-X syndrome, 116
Trophoblast, 137
Troutman, B. R., 264
Tubal ligations, 94
Turner's syndrome, 116
Twins, 114
Tyack, D. L., 331

U

U. S. Bureau of the Census, preschools and,
    362
U. S. Department of Health and Human
    Services
  cesarean births and, 163
  Head Start objectives and, 369–370
Udry, R. J., 515
Ultrasound, fetal biology and, 154
Umbilical cord, 142
Unconditioned response, 66
Unconditioned stimulus, 66
Unforeseen consequences, research ethics
    and, 24–25
UNICEF (United Nations Children's Fund),
    244
United Nations Children's Fund (UNICEF),
    244
United States Society of Believers in Christ's
    Second Coming, 90
University of California at San Francisco, 113
University of Minnesota, study of twins, 110
University of Puerto Rico School of
    Medicine, 156–157
Urine, neonates and, 191

V

Valdez-Menchaca, M. C., 299
Valentine, D. P., 158–159
Valium, pregnancy and, *168*
Van de Carr, Rene, 151
Van Petten, G., 167
Vandell, D. L., 468, 469
Vasectomies, 94
Vaughn, V. C., *409*
Vaux, D., 99
Vernix caseosa, 143, 148
Video Baby, 94
Vienna Psychoanalytic Society, 50
de Villiers, J. G. and P. A., 261, 299–300

Vision, neonates and, 200–202
Visual acuity, neonates and, 200, *201*
Visual development, infants, 253–254
Vocabulary development, middle childhood
    and, 421
Vohr, B. R., 512–513
Vygotsky, Lev, language development and,
    331

W

Wachtel, R. D., 20
Wade, K., 162
Walker, E., 495
Walking
  preschoolers and, 325, *326*
  toddlers and, 304–305
Walking reflex, 197
Walsh, Adam, 505
Washington, V., 28
Water babies, 162, *163*
Watson, J. B., 66, 67
Watson, James, 104
Watson, James D., 113
Weatherley, R. A., 516
Weider, S., 269
Weight gain, pregnancy and, 171
Weikart, D. P., 5, 376, 377
Weintraub, K. S., 312
Weintraub, M., 16
Weiss, H., 95
Wellborn, S. N., 110
What's a Name?, 225
Wheeler, D., 105
Wheeler-Liston, C., 216
When Life Begins, 184
When Teenagers Work, 503
Whiren, A. P., 425
Whitehead, Mary Beth, 96, 97
Whitehurst, G. J., 299
WHO (World Health Organization), 244
Whole language, defined, 381
Wilbur, K., 542
Williams, L., 515
Wilson, M. A., 389
Witches milk, 187
Wolff, P., 198, 224
Woman Pregnant, 99
Women
  contraceptive use by, 94, *95*
  in labor force, *363*
Women's rights, 157
Woodsen, R., 202
Woolston, J. L., 410
Work
  adolescence and, 503–505
  dimensions of, *503*
Working parents, preschools and, 363
World Health Organization (WHO), 244
Writing
  beginning of, 381–383
  cultural background and, 462–463

X

XYY syndrome, 116

Y

Yawkey, T. B., 337
Young adulthood, *51*, 54–55
*Young Children in Action: A Manual for
    Preschool Educators*, 65
*Young Children Reinvent Arithmetic:
    Implications of Piaget's Theory*, 65

Z

Zajonc, R. B., 94
Zucker, K., 425
Zygote, 103, 137, 139, 146